KGMU Textbook of
General Surgery for Dental Students
Theory and Practical

KGMU Textbook of

General Surgery for Dental Students

Theory and Practical

TC Goel

MS (Surgery), FLCS, DSc (Hons)
Emeritus Professor of Surgery
King George's Medical University
Emeritus Professor of Surgery and Postgraduate Teacher
Dr Ram Manohar Lohia Combined Hospital
Lucknow, Uttar Pradesh

Apul Goel

MS (Surgery), MCh (Urology), DNB, MNAMS
Professor of Urology
King George's Medical University
Lucknow, Uttar Pradesh

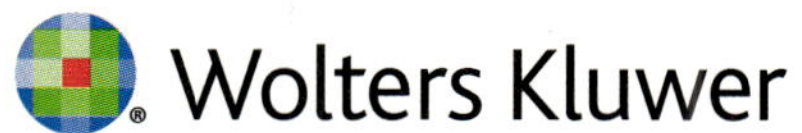

Publishing Manager: P Sangeetha
Development Editor: Dr Vallika Devi Katragadda
Production Editor: K Annie Devi
Assistant Manager-Manufacturing: Sumit Johry

10th Floor, Tower C, Building No. 10
Phase – II, DLF Cyber City, Gurgaon, Haryana – 122002

ISBN-13: 978-93-87963-39-9

Published by Wolters Kluwer (India) Pvt. Ltd., Gurgaon
Compositor: maniworks.com
Printed and bound at Sanat Printers, Haryana

For product enquiry, please contact – Marketing Department (marketing@wolterskluwerindia.co.in) or log on to our website www.wolterskluwerindia.co.in.

Dedication

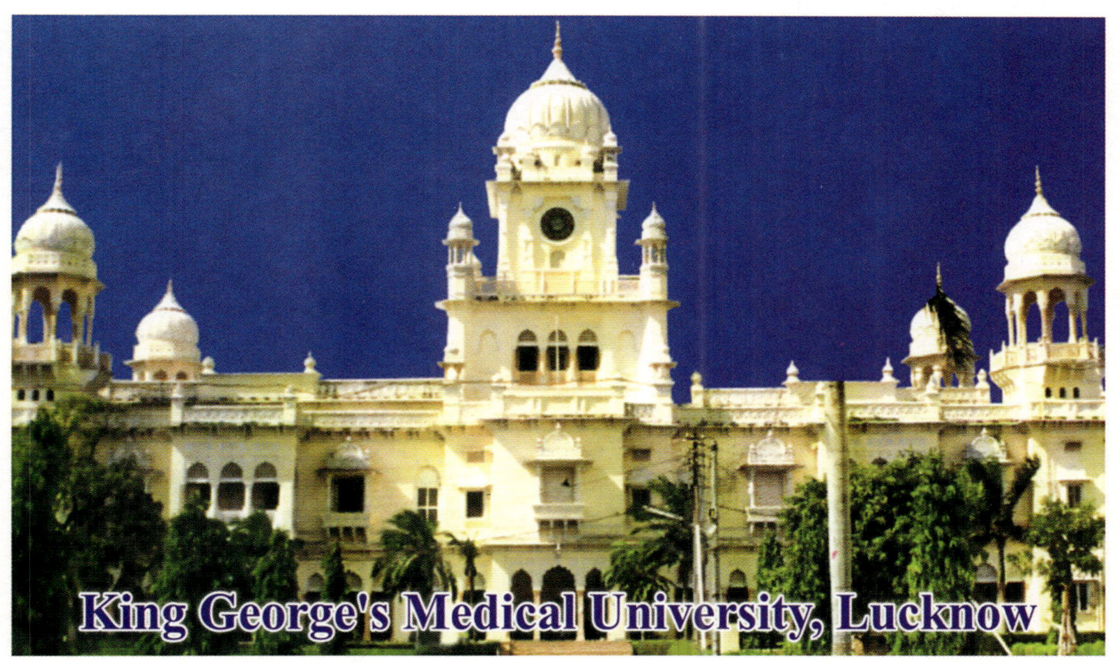

मातृदेवैः श्रीचरणे

Dedicated to the Holy Feet of our Mother Institution – KGMU

TC Goel
Apul Goel

Foreword

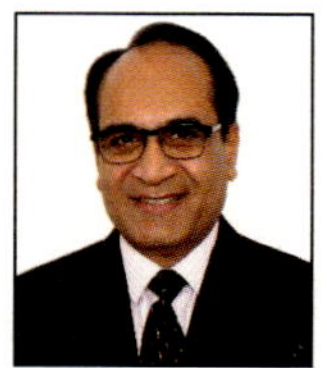

I congratulate the authors of *KGMU Textbook of General Surgery for Dental Students: Theory and Practical* for presenting the subject of General Surgery for Dental Students in a systematic manner for easy understanding and remembrance.

Emeritus Professor TC Goel, former Professor, Department of Surgery, King George's Medical University (erstwhile KGMC) and Dr Apul Goel, Professor, Department of Urology, King George's Medical University have authored many books. I had the opportunity to see them all and I can write confidently that this book is one of their best written works.

Dr TC Goel, the senior author taught (and examined) General Surgery to Dental students of this college (now University) from 1974–1999, then after retirement from 1999 to 2010 in Career Institute of Dental Sciences, Lucknow. He was one of the best teacher of his time and was given Best Teacher Award by Shri Atal Bihari Vajpayee, the then Prime Minister of India in the College Day Function in January 1999.

This book is written after long experience and tremendous effort. Language is very lucid and easily understandable with sketch diagrams and photographs which explain the topics very vividly. The chapters are supplemented with multiple choice questions at the end for the self-evaluation of the students. I am sure it will be of immense help to the dental students in understanding the subject of General Surgery.

With Best Wishes

Madanlal Bhatt.

Professor M.L.B. Bhatt
Vice Chancellor
King George's Medical University
Lucknow, Uttar Pradesh

Foreword

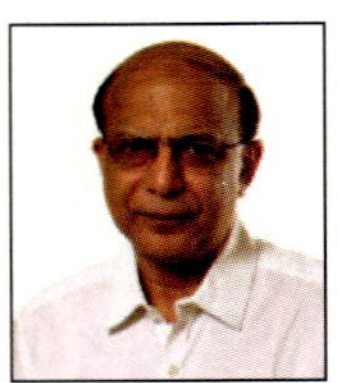

I first came in close contact with Professor TC Goel, one of the authors of this book, in 1984, when I joined as Lecturer in Surgery at King George's Medical College, Lucknow. An ardent teacher, excellent surgeon, and a frank human being, Prof. Goel was always seen reading and writing during his nonclinical time. He has written several textbooks in surgery, few of which I have read and reviewed. However, I consider the present book *KGMU Textbook of General Surgery for Dental Students: Theory and Practical* as one of the best books written by the author. King George's Medical College started a dental college under its premises much early in time. The standard of curriculum for teaching of surgery to the dental students was set here and most likely by the author of this text—Dr TC Goel who was associated with the responsibility of teaching surgery to dental students from very early days. Besides general surgery that includes wounds, ulcers, sinuses, fistulae, shock, hemorrhage, electrolyte imbalances, inflammation, systemic and regional surgery of the head and neck region form the part of the surgical curriculum of the dental students. The same has been extremely well covered in this book. Traditionally, surgeons have been entrusted with introducing the basics of anesthesiology and radiation treatment to the undergraduate students. These two subjects have also been covered in necessary detail in this textbook. Chapters on biopsy and electrocautery followed by surgical instruments, suture materials, pathology specimens, clinical cases and diagnostic images make it a complete book and a ready reckoner for a BDS student for his exams and reference. A single, yet concise, resource presenting a comprehensive selection of topics written in simple language is what this book is about. Of the currently available textbooks available to BDS students, I have no doubt that the present book stands out and is worthy of recommendation.

Dr Sandeep Kumar
MS, FRCS (Edinburgh), PhD (Wales), MMSc (Newcastle)
Professor and Head
Saraswati Medical College
Unnao, Uttar Pradesh

Foreword

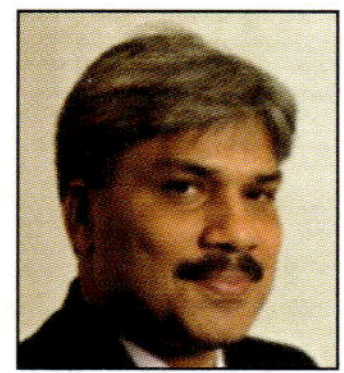

The present book covers the curriculum, theory as well as practical, of general surgery for undergraduate dentals students completely and comprehensively. The book is indispensable to the students as it is exam-oriented and helpful in revision with features such as key points and self-assessment. The presentation of the book, with its short paragraphs and innumerable color images and illustrations, is reader friendly.

This book is invaluable not only as a textbook, but also as a reference book. I am sure the book will create interest and enthusiasm in dental students about general surgery as a subject. I have no hesitation in recommending this book to the dental students.

I greatly appreciate the efforts of the authors and wish them tremendous success.

Professor Abhinav Arun Sonkar
MS, FACS (USA), FUICC (Geneva), FRCS (England), FRCS (Ireland), FRCS (Glasgow)
Professor and Head
Department of Surgery (General)
King George's Medical University
Lucknow, Uttar Pradesh

Foreword

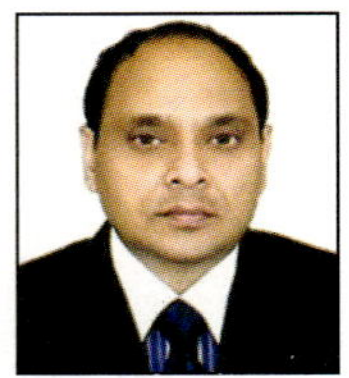

It is my proud privilege to write the foreword of the book *KGMU Textbook of General Surgery for Dental Students: Theory and Practical* by Professors TC Goel and Dr Apul Goel. It is true that there are volumes of general surgery books available which give exhaustive information or various aspects of surgical anatomy and etiopathophysiology and surgical treatment of diseases. But most of these books are helpful to those trainees who are desirous to do Masters in Surgery.

There is clearly a lacuna that needs to be filled up by a lucid yet comprehensive textbook for undergraduate students of dentistry giving basic tenets of surgery in general and surgical management of head and neck ailments in particular.

Prof. TC Goel, a teacher of teachers of the Department of General Surgery at King George's Medical University, Lucknow, UP, India, has oceanic experience in teaching surgery. As I was going through the manuscript I could see that he along with Dr Apul Goel left no stone unturned in making this book indispensable to the students. Not only this gem of the books will form an important addition in the arsenal of the dental undergraduates, it will also act as a ready reckoner for the medical graduates too.

I am certain that his work will go a long way in helping student's community and thank the authors on behalf of the medical fraternity for this endeavor.

Professor Shadab Mohammad
BSc, BDS (Gold Medalist), MDS (OMFS)
Dean-Faculty of Dental Sciences
Professor and Head
Department of Oral and Maxillofacial Surgery
King George's Medical University
Lucknow, Uttar Pradesh

Preface

In order to become a good dental surgeon, the students of BDS must gain a thorough knowledge of general principles of surgery, diagnosis and treatment of diseases of teeth, jaws, jaw joint, and oral cavity. They should also have a working knowledge of diseases of the head and neck. This book covers these topics with an exception of diseases of the teeth.

KGMU Textbook of General Surgery for Dental Students: Theory and Practical covers the theory, clinical, and practical aspects of surgery. It has four sections. The first three sections deal with the theoretical aspect and the section four deals with the clinical and practical aspects of surgery.

Each chapter ends with features such as key points and self-assessment including several objective type questions and their answers. These features are helpful in revision and preparation for exams.

Special emphasis is laid on the management of maxillofacial injuries, swellings of jaws, and swellings of neck. Management of causes of these conditions is also described.

In the clinical and practical part of the book, guidelines on preparation for clinical and nonclinical practical examinations are included. Representative clinical cases, pathology specimens, and images of diagnostic techniques are discussed in detail along with viva voce questions and their answers. The chapter on surgical instruments is especially made very useful by including the description and images of common surgical instruments and instruments of bone oral surgery and tracheostomy. Also included in this chapter are anesthesia and endotracheal equipment and rubber and polythene instruments. A sample of viva voce questions along with answers is also provided to help students understand what to expect. Thus, the chapter is complete and ready reckoner for surgical instruments.

We have made every effort to make this book an ideal resource for the dental students in learning the subject and preparing for exams and we hope the students as well as the faculty find it useful too. Any constructive criticism and suggestions for improvement for the next edition are welcome.

TC Goel
Apul Goel

Acknowledgments

Many of our colleagues, friends, juniors, and students helped in bringing out this book in a variety of ways, especially in providing images of clinical conditions, diagnostics, and therapeutic procedures. We thank them for their help and contribution. We are particularly indebted to the following institutions and the faculty mentioned below.

King George's Medical University, Lucknow, Uttar Pradesh

Professor MLB Bhatt, Vice Chancellor; Professor RM Mathur, Former Head of Department of Oral Pathology and Oral Medicine; Professor Ramesh Chandra, Former Head of Department of Plastic Surgery and Principal; Professor GN Agarwal (Late), Head of Department of Radiology and Radiotherapy; Professor (Mrs) PK Agarwal, Former Professor of Pathology; Professor UK Jain, Former Head of Department of Orthopedic Surgery; Professor KD Varma, Former Head of Department of Surgery; Professor Naresh Bhatia (Late), Head of Department of Otorhinolaryngology; Professor Sandeep Kumar, Former Professor of Surgery and Former Director, AIIMS, Bhopal, Madhya Pradesh; Professor GK Singh, Head of Department of Orthopedic Surgery, Former Director, AIIMS, Patna; Professor Sanjeev Misra, Department of Surgical Oncology, Director, AIIMS, Jodhpur; Professor Divya Mehrotra, Professor of Oral and Maxillofacial Surgery; Professor SP Agarwal, Head of Department of Otorhinolaryngology and Head and Neck Surgery; Professor Abhinav Arun Sonkar, Head of Department of General Surgery; Professor Ashish Wakhlu, Department of Pediatric Surgery; Professor JD Rawat, Department of Pediatric Surgery; Professor Sandeep Tiwari, Head of Department of Trauma Surgery; Professor Rajeev Gupta, Head of Department of Radiotherapy; Professor Brijish Mishra, Department of Plastic Surgery; Professor Sameer Gupta, Department of Surgical Oncology; Professor Arshad Ahmad, Department of Surgery; Professor Anupam Misra, Department of Otorhinolaryngology and Head and Neck Surgery; Professor Pallavi Aga, Department of Radiodiagnosis; Professor Divya Narain, Department of Plastic Surgery

Dr Ram Manohar Lohia Combined Hospital, Gomti Nagar, Lucknow, Uttar Pradesh

Dr RC Agarwal, Chief Medical Superintendent; Dr AC Dwivedi, Head of Department of Surgery; Drs Ravi Mishra, Alok, Imran Ahmad, and Vishal Bulla

RNT Medical College, Udaipur, Rajasthan

Professor RK Agrawal, Former Professor and Head of Department of Surgery; Professor AK Khare, Professor and Head of Department of Skin, VD and Leprosy

Sanjay Gandhi Postgraduate Institute of Medical Sciences, Lucknow, Uttar Pradesh

Professor Rajiv Agarwal, Head of Department of Plastic Surgery and Burns

Private Hospitals and Diagnostic Centers, Lucknow, Uttar Pradesh

Dr Surajit Bhattacharya, Plastic and Cosmetic Surgeon, Sahara Hospital, Lucknow; Dr Ashutosh Pandey, Pediatric Surgeon, Vivekananda Polyclinic, Lucknow; Dr RK Mishra, Sushrut Institute of Plastic Surgery, Burns and Trauma (SIPS), Lucknow; Drs Satyavan, Shiv Prabha Satyavan, and Saurabh Baiswar, Satya Shiv Hospital, Aliganj, Lucknow; Dr KN Singh, Mrs Madhulika Singh, and Dr MK Srivastava, Mayo Medical Centre, Gomti Nagar, Lucknow; Drs Amit Anand and Neha Dubey, Anand Dental Centre, Mahanagar, Lucknow; Dr MK Srivastava, Surgical Oncologist, Lucknow; Dr Sharad Kumar, Endocrinologist, Mahanagar, Lucknow; Dr Sushil Upadhyaya, Endocrinologist, Nirala Nagar, Lucknow; Dr Uttam Garg, Orthopedic Surgeon, Garg Orthopedic Clinic, Jankipuram, Lucknow; and Dr Prateek Mehrotra, Endocrinologist, Sahara Hospital, Lucknow

We thank Professor SN Sankhwar, Head of Department of Urology, where the computer work of this book was done.

Mr Shyam Kashyap has done the computer work with accuracy and proficiency and our driver, Mr Ram Sagar, has helped us remain in constant contact with Mr Kashyap; we are thankful to them.

We are thankful to Wolters Kluwer team, especially Mrs Vallika Devi Katragadda, for giving a shape to this work and bringing it out on time.

TC Goel
Apul Goel

Special Acknowledgment

I would like to specially thank my wife, Mrs Aruna Goel (my Bhamati) and my daughter, Alpana Goel, for diligently attending to my daily needs so that I can spend more time on writing.

TC Goel

Contents

Introduction

Surgery comprises the art and science of diagnosing and treating diseases, injuries or deformities through manual operation or by using instrumental appliances. It is a destructive (catabolic) method; in an attempt to cure or relieve disease symptoms, the tissues are incised or cut involving pain, blood loss, and risk of infection.

History of surgery: some important names

The art and science of surgery is as old as human civilization. For instance, people must have always tried to arrest the bleeding in a wounded person by applying pressure since time immemorial.

Sushruta (5th century BC) was an ancient Indian surgeon who lived near Varanasi. He wrote *Sushruta Samhita* which is a treatise of surgery of that time containing six sections (sthanum) and 8300 hymns.

Aulus Cornelius Celsus (30 AD) was a cultured Roman who described the four cardinal signs of inflammation, that is, pain (dolor), heat (calor), redness (rubor), and swelling (tumor). To these, a hundred years later, **Aelius Galenus** added functio laesa (loss of function).

Joseph Lister was a British surgeon who described his method of antisepsis using carbolic acid spray locally in 1867 (antiseptic surgery). Thus, he made the surgery safe as it reduced the wound infection rate markedly. Hence, he is known as the Father of Surgery.

Ernst **von Bergmann** from Berlin, in 1887, improved the matters further and devised the methods to make the operating environment germ-free by sterilization of instruments and equipment used during operation which is the current practice.

William Clark used ether for analgesia in 1842. **Hoarse Wells** used nitrous oxide for painless tooth extraction in 1844. A couple of years later **James Simpson Young** (1847) used chloroform for anesthesia.

The main effect of surgery is blood loss during operation which may be in excess sometimes. **Karl Landsteiner** discovered the blood groups in 1901 which made the safe blood transfusion possible.

Infection was a major problem and its cause, the bacteria, were discovered due to the efforts of **Louis Pasteur** (1856) and **Robert Koch** (1876). Thereafter the efforts to control the infection began which resulted in **Alexander Fleming** identifying penicillin in 1929 and Gerhard Johannes Paul Domagk in Germany discovering “pontosil” a sulfonamide in 1935. From then on search continued for more and more antibacterials and now hundreds of them are available.

From the World War II onwards, surgery made tremendous strides, and from the era of destructive surgery we entered into an era of reconstruction and replacements, minimal invasive techniques, endoscopic procedures, and robotics.

Dangers and risks of surgery

Surgery is a dangerous method of treatment. Hence, up to early 19th century surgical procedures were infrequently performed as they were painful and had a high complication rate. To face and deal with these problems a surgeon had to be a daring man of super strength who had to operate a crying patient with speed. Therefore, surgery was limited to chopping away diseased parts. There are three main dangers or problems caused by the surgical procedures:

1. Pain (and anxiety)
2. Hemorrhage (and shock)
3. Wound infection (and septicemia)

The developments and progresses made in the last 150 years have more or less solved these problems and made surgery convenient to the surgeon, and safe and comfortable to the patient. Pain (and anxiety) is no more a problem because of general and local anesthesia techniques. At present there are a number of drugs available to control anxiety and post-operative pain.

There are now methods available that can control intraoperative bleeding, replace the blood lost during operation and correcting fluid, electrolyte and nutritional balance to a reasonable extent.

The intraoperative contamination and infection of the wound is prevented by operating in a germ-free environment with the use of antisepsis, asepsis, and sterilization. Further, the wound infection is prevented by the prophylactic use of antibiotics.

Disease (dis+ease)

A disease is defined as a morbid process having symptoms affecting the whole body, many systems, one system or one organ of the body.

Classification of Diseases

Diseases can be congenital or acquired. The acquired diseases are of many types depending on the etiology (cause). A simple classification (etiological classification) of diseases is given below:

Congenital and Developmental Defects or Anomalies The organs and tissues of the body may be deficient or deformed due to developmental errors. The congenital diseases are present at the time of birth and developmental diseases may be present at the time of birth or may manifest later in life.

Infective or Inflammatory Diseases The body tissues may be invaded or infected by a variety of microorganisms and parasites such as viruses, bacteria, fungi, protozoa, and metazoa producing inflammation resulting in infective or inflammatory diseases. Some parasites live on the body surface (ectoparasites) or cavities without invading the tissues. It is called infestation.

Traumatic Diseases The body tissues and organs may be injured by a variety of traumatic forces such as mechanical (e.g., roadside accident), thermal (e.g., burns), chemical (e.g., acid and strong chemical burns), and electrical or irradiational leading to many types of problems.

Neoplastic Diseases These diseases are characterized by uncontrolled and purposeless proliferation of cells and tissues due to a number of known (e.g., alcohol, tobacco) and unknown factors producing a swelling or mass (oma, tumor) or a new growth (neoplasm). The most dreaded disease, that is, cancer comes under this heading.

Metabolic and Endocrinal Diseases Under this heading are included the diseases caused by anomalies of metabolism and hormonal secretion, for example, diabetes mellitus, Cushing's disease, and thyrotoxicosis.

Degenerative Disorders The body tissues, structures, or organs undergo wear and tear due to improper or incorrect use, and also with passage of time as a natural process manifesting with some symptoms and signs. They are known as degenerative diseases. The atrophy of lower jaw in elderly edentulous people, arteriosclerosis (hardening of arteries), and osteoarthritis (chronic inflammation of joints) are some of the examples of degenerative diseases.

Symptoms and signs

Symptoms These are the subjective complaints of the patient with which he/she comes to a doctor for treatment, for example, pain in the teeth or jaw, bleeding from the gums, swellings of the jaw, and offensive smell from the mouth (halitosis). A symptom or symptoms is or are the commonest manifestation of disease.

A patient may have a disease without symptoms (asymptomatic disease) which is detected or diagnosed by physical examination of the patient and/or investigations. It happens in the early stage of disease when it is difficult to diagnose but easy to treat, especially cancer. Hence, cancer-prone population is now periodically screened to detect early cancer.

Signs These are the abnormal findings detected on physical examination of the patient which is done under the headings of general examination and local examination. The general examination includes the examination of the patient as a whole including the general condition, palpebral conjunctiva for anemia, pulse, blood pressure, respiration, and temperature.

The local examination is the physical examination of a part or an area (e.g., oral cavity) where the patient has complaints or symptoms. It is done under the headings of inspection which means seeing carefully, palpation which includes touching and pressing, percussion which means hearing the sound produced by gentle striking, and auscultation which means hearing the natural sounds usually with a stethoscope.

Investigations

These are the special tests done to confirm a diagnosis, for example, biopsy in a clinical carcinomatous ulcer of oral cavity; or to make a diagnosis where a diagnosis is not made clinically, for example, orthopantomogram or CT scan to make a diagnosis of dentigerous cyst in a swelling of lower jaw.

Investigations are important to make a correct diagnosis but the clinical sense should never be overshadowed by too much dependence on investigations. They are of many types, for example, laboratory investigations, radiography, and endoscopy.

The laboratory investigations include examination of blood for hemoglobin, counts, ESR, sugar, urea, uric acid, calcium, and hormones as indicated; of natural secretions for example saliva; and excretions, for example, stool and urine; and FNAC (fine needle aspiration cytology) and biopsy.

The radiographic investigations include X-ray of jaws, orthopantomography, ultrasonography, CT scanning, and MRI. They are done to picturize the parts and organs of the body with the X-rays, sound waves, and magnetic waves.

The endoscopy is direct visualization of hollow organs and tubes from inside with the help of an endoscope. With the help of endoscopy all the hollow organs and tubes and body cavities can be seen from inside, biopsy can be taken and some therapeutic procedures can be done.

Evidence-based surgery

Evidence-based surgery is defined as a method of management of a surgical disease based on the clinical and investigative evidence of that particular disease.

Patient safety

Surgery is not a risk-free enterprise hence one should strictly adhere to the philosophy of "primum non nocere" that means "first do no harm." Hence, one should do even a minor procedure after taking informed consent and with full preparations.

Part I:

Theory

Pain

1

Introduction

Pain is the most common presenting symptom of disease for which humans have been searching for solutions from the very beginning of civilization. It is also the outcome of surgical procedures and hence is a challenging task for surgeons to alleviate postsurgical pain as well as chronic pain due to disease and debilitation. The cause of pain is multifactorial. Sometimes the cause can be identified easily and treated accordingly, whereas there are situations when the pain may occur in the absence of detectable physical, laboratory, or radiological abnormalities and may also be unresponsive to treatment. An interdisciplinary approach is often needed for establishing a diagnosis and treatment.

Definitions

The International Association for the Study of Pain (IASP) defines pain as "an unpleasant sensory and emotional experience associated with actual or potential tissue damage, or described in terms of such damage." Various terminologies are used to define the subjective nature of pain. They are enumerated in Table 1.1.

Considerations in defining pain

Pain is a protective mechanism. It occurs whenever there is a tissue damage causing the person to react to remove the pain stimulus. The following points are important to understand when dealing with the problem of pain:

- **Pain is a subjective symptom.** The pain and degree of suffering is an individual experience and may be influenced by physical, emotional, psychological, social, and pharmacological factors. So far there is no pain meter available by which we can judge the existence and severity of pain. Hence, one has to depend on the patient's expression and other associated symptoms and signs.
- **The expression of pain depends on the personality of the patient.** At one end there is a stoic who will admit to little pain and on the other end there is an expressionist who would communicate every nuance and variable.
- **Pain may be expressed in language or by nonverbal means.** It depends on the common set of values between the patient and the doctor.

Hence, the patient should describe his/her pain and express freely and the doctor must listen

Table 1.1 Various terminologies defining pain

Terminology	Definition
Allodynia	Perception of an ordinary non-noxious stimulus as pain
Analgesia	Absence of pain perception
Anesthesia	Absence of all sensations
Anesthesia dolorosa	Pain in an area that lacks sensation
Dysesthesia	Unpleasant or abnormal sensation with or without a stimulus
Hypoalgesia	Diminished response to noxious stimulus
Hyperalgesia	Increased response to noxious stimulus
Hyperesthesia	Increased response to mild stimulation
Hyperpathia	Presence of hyperesthesia, allodynia, and hyperalgesia usually associated with overreaction and persistence of the sensation after the stimulus
Hypoesthesia	Reduced cutaneous sensation, for example, light touch, pressure, or temperature
Neuralgia	Pain in the distribution of a nerve or group of nerves
Paresthesia	Abnormal sensation perceived without an apparent stimulus
Radiculopathy	Functional abnormality of one or more nerve roots

to him/her attentively and patiently and watch his/her expressions.

Physiology of pain

Nociceptive Receptor Nociceptive pain is pain produced by nociceptive receptors (free nerve endings). Somatic nociceptors respond to mechanical, thermal, and chemical stimuli. Visceral nociceptors respond to stretch, distension, and distortion of internal organs. Examples of nociceptive pain include musculoskeletal disorders, cancer-activating cutaneous receptors, and prolonged ischemia or inflammatory process.

Pain Transmission Pain is carried through the fast and slow fibers to the dorsal root of spinal cord. From the spinal cord, the fast pain passes through neospinothalamic tract and ends in the thalamus in the brain. It is sharp lancinating type and can be localized easily. Slow pain is transmitted through the paleospinothalamic tract to the brainstem and thalamus. It is chronic and its localization to a specific point is difficult. Usually slow pain is diffuse and this explains why patients have difficulty in localizing the source of chronic type of pain.

Classification of pain

Acute and Chronic Pain

The differences between acute and chronic pain are given in Table 1.2.

Other Types of Pain

Other types of pain include somatic, visceral, neuropathic, psychogenic, and phantom limb pain. The characteristics of somatic, visceral, and neuropathic pain are described in Table 1.3.

- **Somatic (somesthetic)**
  - *Superficial*: From skin and subcutaneous tissue, for example, superficial cuts or burns
  - *Deep*: From muscles/bone/fascia/periosteum, for example, fracture, arthritis, fibrositis, rupture of muscle belly
- **Visceral (from viscera)**: It is caused by ischemia, chemical stimuli, spasm of hollow organs, and overdistension of hollow organs, for example, angina pectoris, peptic ulcer, intestinal colic, and renal colic.
- **Neuropathic pain**: It is the pain caused by damage to peripheral nerves or spinal cord, for example, trigeminal neuralgia, postherpetic neuralgia, and diabetic neuropathy.

Table 1.2 Differences between acute and chronic pain

Characteristics	Acute pain	Chronic pain
Onset	Sudden	Gradual
Duration	Less than 3 months	Prolonged, persisting over 6 months or longer
Physiology	Ongoing nociceptive input	Nociceptive input has stopped but there is a persistent pain reaction without a biological cause
Symptoms	Sympathetic autonomic response such as pallor, sweating, hypertension	• No observable symptoms • Pain can be dull, throbbing • Patient may be withdrawn, isolated, display vegetative symptoms of anorexia, asthenia (weakness), and poor sleep
Examples	Postoperative pain, post-traumatic pain, acute infection, vascular obstruction	Past injuries or surgeries, fibromyalgia, arthritis, chronic infections, tumors, neuropathic pain
Treatment	Easily treatable	Difficult to recognize and treat

Table 1.3 Characteristics of somatic, visceral, and neuropathic pain

Characteristics	Somatic pain	Visceral pain	Neuropathic pain
Origin	Skin, subcutaneous tissue, bone, muscle, fascia, periosteum	Internal organs	Neural tissue due to damage to peripheral nerves or spinal cord
Clinical description	• Localized • Throbbing, aching, stabbing	• Generalized/diffuse • Cramping/gnawing	• Continuous, burning type • Spontaneous, lancinating/electric type
Associated factors	—	Associated with autonomic response such as nausea/vomiting	Associated with • Allodynia • Hyperalgesia • Hyperpathia

- **Psychogenic pain**: The pain is modified by mental state of the patient. Chronic pain and depression may exacerbate each other.
- **Phantom limb pain**: Amputation of a limb may result in phantom limb pain, especially if the limb was painful before surgery. Continuous local anesthetic blockade before and after surgery can reduce the incidence of phantom limb pain.

Referred Pain

The referred pain is the pain sensation produced in some part of the body and felt in other structures away from the place of development. The salient features of referred pain are given in Box 1.1.

Box 1.1 Features of referred pain

- Deep and visceral pain are referred to other areas. Superficial pain is not referred
- Examples:
  - Heart pain referred to inner aspect of left arm
  - Gallbladder pain referred to epigastric region
  - Pain from maxillary sinus referred to upper adjacent tooth
- Referred pain follows dermatomal rule
- Theories of referred pain: Convergence theory, facilitation theory

Etiology of pain

The etiological factors of generalized and localized pain are given as follows:

- **Generalized pain all over the body**
  - Acute febrile illness, for example, acute viral fevers
  - Musculoskeletal disorders, for example, osteoporosis, ankylosing spondylitis
  - Tumors, for example, multiple myeloma, metastatic disease
  - Psychogenic
- **Localized pain**
  - *Inflammations and infections*
    - Parietal, for example, boil, acute abscess (Fig. 1.1a), carbuncle, cellulitis, erysipelas, chancroid
    - Visceral
      - Solid organs, for example, hepatitis, thyroiditis, pancreatitis, sialadenitis, pyelonephritis
      - Hollow organs, for example, appendicitis, enteritis, colitis
      - Serous or mucous membranes lining the body cavities, for example, peritonitis, pleuritis, pericarditis, meningitis, aphthous ulcer (Fig. 1.1b)

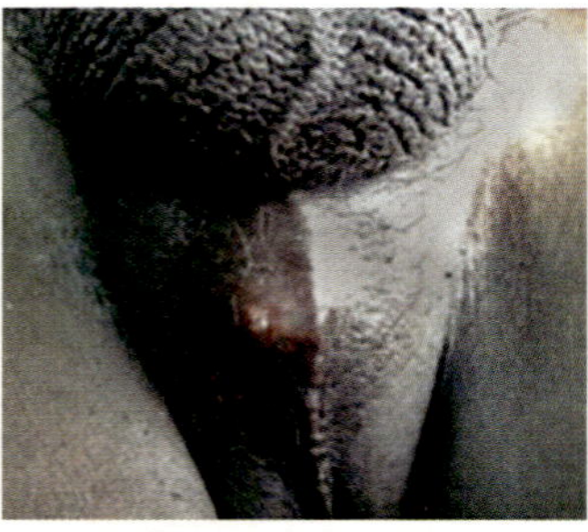

(a)

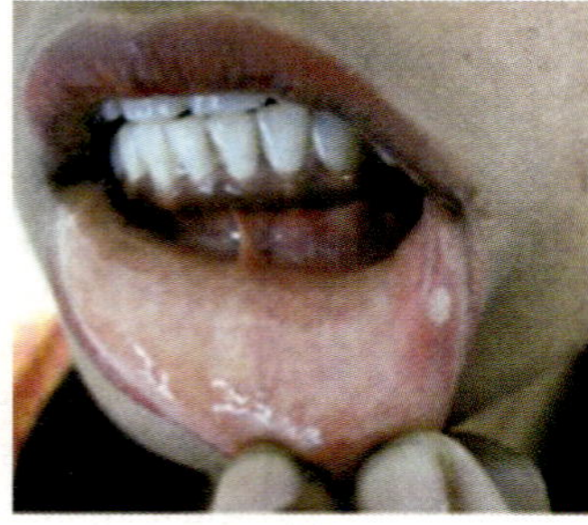

(b)

Figure 1.1 Pain due to (a) infection (acute abscess of perineum) and (b) inflammation (aphthous ulcer of lower lip).

  - *Trauma*
    - Accidental: Mechanical (abrasion, incision, laceration, stab, crush, fracture), thermal (burns and scalds), chemical (burns), cryogenic (frostbite, trench foot), and electrical (burns)
    - Iatrogenic, for example, invasive diagnostic and therapeutic procedures, operations, chemotherapy
  - *Ischemia*
    - Myocardial ischemia
    - Limb ischemia leading to claudication and rest pain
  - *Obstruction (colics)*
    - Intestinal obstruction: Intestinal colic
    - Ureteral obstruction: Ureteral colic
    - Biliary obstruction: Biliary pain
  - *Neurological disorders*
    - Nerve compression: Intervertebral disc prolapse producing root pain, costoclavicular compression
    - Nerve irritation/inflammation, for example, peripheral neuritis, herpes zoster
    - Neuralgias, for example, trigeminal neuralgia, glossopharyngeal neuralgia, intercostal neuralgia
  - *Tumors*
    - Painful benign tumors, for example, glomus tumor, osteoid osteoma
    - Painful malignant tumors, for example, osteosarcoma
    - Skeletal metastases
  - *Other causes*
    - Psychogenic pain
    - Physiological, for example, labor pain

Types of orofacial pain

The various types of orofacial pain are given as follows:

- **Typical orofacial pain of extracranial origin**
  - *Dental causes*: Pulpitis, dentin hypersensitivity, periapical lesions
  - *Periodontal causes*: Primary herpetic gingivostomatitis, acute necrotizing

ulcerative gingivitis, desquamative gingivitis
  - *Mucosal ulceration*: Aphthous, traumatic, herpetic
  - *Salivary gland disorders*: Sialadenitis due to any cause, salivary calculus
  - *Temporomandibular joint lesions*: Inflammation, dysfunction
  - *Paranasal sinus diseases*: Sinusitis, malignancy
- **Neuralgias**
  - Trigeminal neuralgia and its variants
  - Glossopharyngeal neuralgia
  - Ramsay Hunt syndrome
  - Postherpetic neuralgia
- **Vascular origin pain**
  - Migraine and its variants
  - Cluster headache
  - Giant cell arteritis
- **Referred pain**
  - Ocular pain
  - Anginal pain
  - ENT disorder pain
  - Myofacial pain dysfunction syndrome
- **Psychogenic pain**
  - Atypical facial pain
  - Burning mouth syndrome and others

Diagnosis and pain assessment

Pain is recognized as the "**fifth vital sign**" and hence efforts must be made to do a proper pain assessment with the aim of providing appropriate and correct treatment. The methods of evaluating pain are given in Box 1.2.

Pain History

A comprehensive pain history is taken by asking the patient to describe his/her pain. When the patient is unable to describe pain, observational tools to quantify pain can be used for assessment. A simple way to assess pain is by asking Ryle's 10 questions from the patient. The checklist includes characteristics of pain given in Box 1.3.

Box 1.2 Methods of evaluation of pain

- Pain history (Ryle's checklist), medical history, review of symptoms
- Psychological evaluation, for example, McGill Pain Questionnaire
- Psychometric testing, for example, Minnesota Multiphasic Pain Inventory
- Diagnostic imaging: X-rays, CT scan, MRI, bone scan to confirm pathology
- Diagnostic nerve blocks
- Electromyography and nerve conduction studies help to distinguish between neurogenic and myogenic pains
- Quantitative measurement of pain
  - Unidimensional tool, for example, Visual Analogue Scale, Verbal Rating Scale, Numerical Rating Scale
  - Multidimensional tool, for example, McGill Pain Questionnaire, Behavioral Pain Scale, Pain Disability Index
- Laboratory tests are of limited value

Box 1.3 Ryle's checklist for pain assessment

The checklist includes the following characteristics of pain:

- Site of pain
- Localization
- Radiation
- Character
- Severity
- Duration
- Frequency
- Relieving factors
- Aggravating factors
- Associated symptoms

Treatment of pain

Many emotional and cultural factors influence how the pain is perceived. The primary cause (infection, trauma), the pathogenesis (inflammation, ischemia, pressure, obstruction), and the contributory factors (recent changes in life situation, symbolic attributes of pain) must all be evaluated and corrected. Fortunately most of the pains can be managed effectively through relatively simple means. The therapeutic modalities of pain control include: pharmacological measures, physical/nonpharmacological measures, psychological measures, and invasive techniques.

A flowchart depicting the line of care in assessing and managing a patient with pain is given in Flowchart 1.1.

Pharmacological Measures

The pharmacological measures include the use of NSAIDs, opioids, and adjuvant drugs to alleviate pain.

WHO pain relief ladder

The World Health Organization (WHO) recommends a three-step hierarchy for the use of analgesic drugs (Box 1.4).

The WHO approach to analgesia has been summarized by Robert Twycross as follows:

- **By the clock**: The doses of drugs are scheduled regularly to maintain the drug level to abolish pain.
- **By the ladder**: Stepwise escalate analgesia.
- **By mouth**: Oral route is preferred.

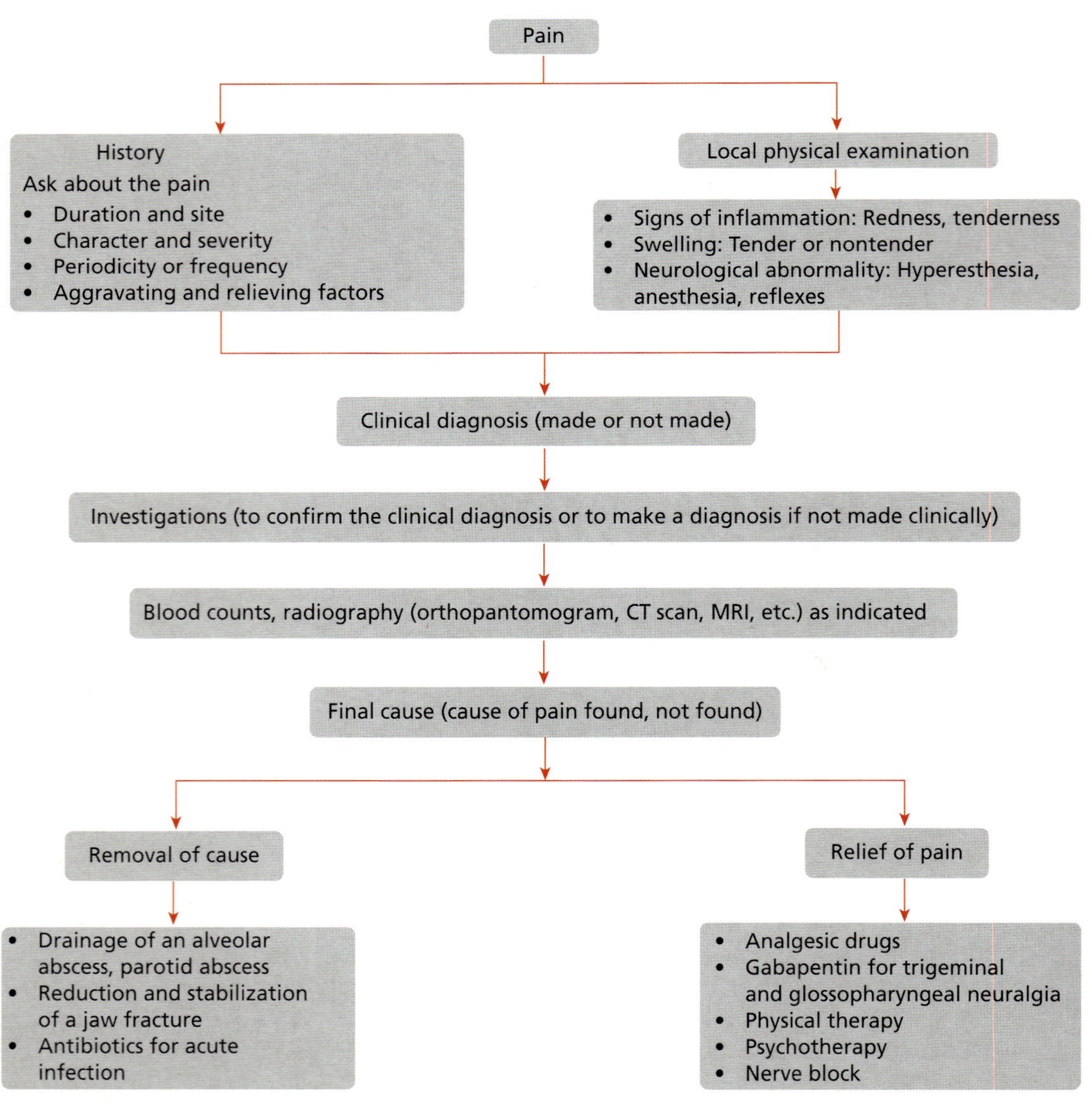

Flowchart 1.1 Diagnosis and treatment of pain.

Box 1.4 WHO recommendation for usage of analgesics

- **Step 1**: For mild pain, administer nonopioids such as aspirin, acetaminophen, or NSAIDs given with or without adjunctive agents
- **Step 2**: If the pain persists or increases, add an opioid, for example, morphine, meperidine, codeine, or tramadol, to the nonopioid with or without adjunctive agents
- **Step 3**: If the pain continues or increases, the potency or dosage of opioid is increased while continuing the nonopioid or adjunctive agents. Stronger opioids may be added

Box 1.5 Treatment of acute postoperative pain

- Expert team approach
- Regular assessment of pain levels
- Give analgesics before pain breaks through
- A combination of analgesics given for best results
- Not to withhold opioids
- Give adequate dose of analgesics
- Indwelling epidural catheter pain relief by infusion or intermittent injection (patient-controlled analgesia)

- **For the individual**: There is great individual variation in the doses required to control the pain.

Analgesics in WHO pain relief ladder

- **Simple analgesics**: NSAIDs, aspirin, paracetamol
- **Weak opioids**: Meperidine, codeine, tramadol
- **Strong opioids**: Morphine, diamorphine, oxycodine, fentanyl, hydromorphone
- **Adjuvant drugs**
  - Corticosteroids help in inflammatory pain and cancer pain. Dexamethasone 16–96 mg daily orally or intravenously, or prednisone 40–100 mg daily orally has a powerful anti-inflammatory effect.
  - Anticonvulsants, for example, phenytoin 300–500 mg daily orally, carbamazepine 200–1600 mg daily orally, or gabapentin 900–1800 mg daily orally, may be given.
  - Antidepressants, for example, amitriptyline or desipramine 20–50 mg daily orally, give relief in neuropathic pain.
  - Neuroleptics, for example, methotrimeprazine 40–80 mg daily IMI, help in chronic pain syndrome. Placebos may be used.
  - Other drugs include antiarrhythmics, antispasmodics, and bisphosphonates.

Treatment of acute postoperative pain

A joint working party report of the Royal College of Anesthetists and Surgeons to relieve postoperative pain recommends use of "**multimodal analgesia**" comprising local anesthesia and simple analgesics such as paracetamol and NSAIDs with opioid drugs. The techniques for postoperative pain relief and pain of acute trauma are outlined in Box 1.5.

Treatment of neuropathic pain

The neuropathic pain responds poorly to opioids. Monoaminergic, tricyclic antidepressants and anticonvulsants are standard drugs used for treatment.

Physical Measures

The physical measures are used as an adjunct and include the following:

- Bed rest
- Manipulation and immobilization
- Traction
- Massage
- Superficial heating modalities
- Ice packs/cryotherapy
- Exercise
- Ultrasound for deep pain
- Acupuncture or acupressure
- Transcutaneous electrical nerve stimulation (TENS)

Psychological Measures

The psychological modalities modify the patient's mental and emotional perceptions to pain. They include:

- Health education and reassurance
- Biofeedback

Box 1.6 Surgical removal of the cause of pain

- Inflammatory swellings
  - Pus removed by guided percutaneous needle aspiration or catheter drainage, or open drainage
  - Inflamed organs removed
    - Appendicectomy in acute appendicitis
    - Cholecystectomy in cholecystitis
- Trauma
  - Repair of injured structures and closure of wound (primary or delayed)
  - Reduction and stabilizations of fractures and dislocations
  - Skin grafting in burns
- Obstructions
  - Removal of obstructing stones and foreign bodies
  - Dilatation or repair of strictures
  - Untwisting or excision of a volvulus
  - Reduction or excision of an intussusception
  - Excision or bypass of a tumor
  - Angioplasty, endarterectomy, or stenting in arterial obstruction
- Perforation
  - Closure of peptic ulcer and small bowel perforation
  - Excision of perforated appendix or gallbladder
- Tumors
  - *Benign:* Excision
  - *Malignant:* Wide excision and/or chemotherapy and radiotherapy

- Relaxation and imagery techniques
- Cognitive distraction and farming
- Hypnosis
- Psychotherapy
- Structured support
- Prayer and pastoral counseling

Invasive Methods

The invasive methods include direct delivery of pain injections (nerve blocks), surgical procedures, surgically implanted electrotherapy devices (stimulators), and many other methods to alleviate chronic pain, restore function, and improve the quality of life.

Surgical removal of causative factor

Majority of pains in surgery are treated by surgical removal of the cause. Examples are outlined in Box 1.6.

Treatment of intractable pain

Treatment of intractable chronic pain due to metastatic cancer and neuropathic conditions is given in Box 1.7.

Box 1.7 Treatment of intractable pain

- Nerve block
  - *Somatic nerve block:* Trigeminal, cervical, thoracic, lumbar, paravertebral, facet, trans-sacral
  - *Sympathetic block:* Stellate ganglion, cervical plexus, thoracic/lumbar sympathetic chain block
- Epidural injections
- Spinal injection
- Spinal cord stimulation
- Intracerebral stimulation
- Neurolysis
  - Sympathectomy
  - Cordotomy
  - Thalamotomy
  - Prefrontal lobotomy
- Radiofrequency, rhizotomy, or ablative surgery

KEY POINTS

- Pain is the fifth vital sign and hence a systematic pain history and use of pain assessment tools are essential to identify the etiology of pain.
- The essence of treatment is removal of the cause and administering analgesic drugs.
- Pharmacological measures are successful in relieving pain. Side effects and overdose of medication must be carefully monitored and treated.

SELF-ASSESSMENT

Long answer questions

1. How do you define pain? What are the causes of pain? Described its treatment.
2. What are the types of orofacial pain. Describe WHO pain relief ladder.

Short answer questions

1. Ryle's check list
2. Methods of evaluation of pain
3. Definition of analgesia, anesthesia, neuralgia, dysesthesia, and paresthesia

Multiple choice questions

1. Anesthesia is defined as
   (a) Absence of pain perception
   (b) Increased response to noxious stimuli
   (c) Absence of all sensations
   (d) Abnormal sensation perceived without an apparent stimulation
2. Neuralgia is defined as
   (a) Pain in an area that lacks sensation
   (b) Pain in the distribution of a nerve or group of nerves
   (c) Abnormal sensation perceived without an apparent stimulation
   (d) Unpleasant or abnormal sensation with or without a stimulus
3. Analgesia is defined as
   (a) Pain in anal region
   (b) Absence of pain perception
   (c) Diminished response to a noxious stimulus
   (d) Absence of all sensations

Answers

1. (c) 2. (b) 3. (b)

Swelling, Nodule, and Lump

2

Introduction

A swelling (or swellings) is one of the commonest clinical presentations of disease in surgical practice. It can occur anywhere and can arise from any tissue, organ, or part of the body.

Definitions

Nodule A nodule is a small node or knuckle-like swelling (Fig. 2.1).

Lump A lump is a medium-sized swelling which appears to be heavy.

Bump A bump is a very large swelling (Fig. 2.2).

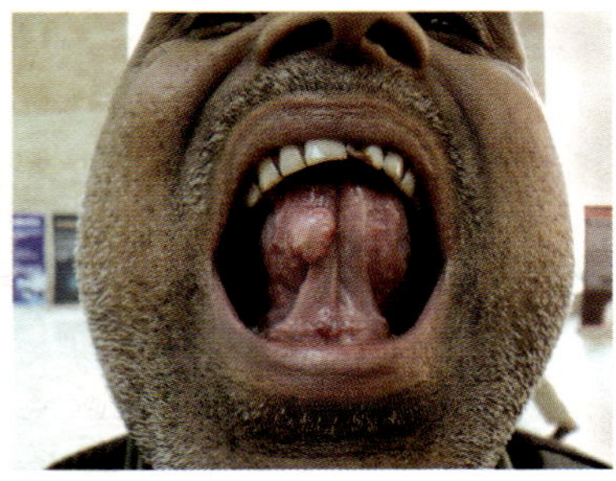

Figure 2.1 Nodule—a small carcinoma (nodule) of the undersurface of tongue.

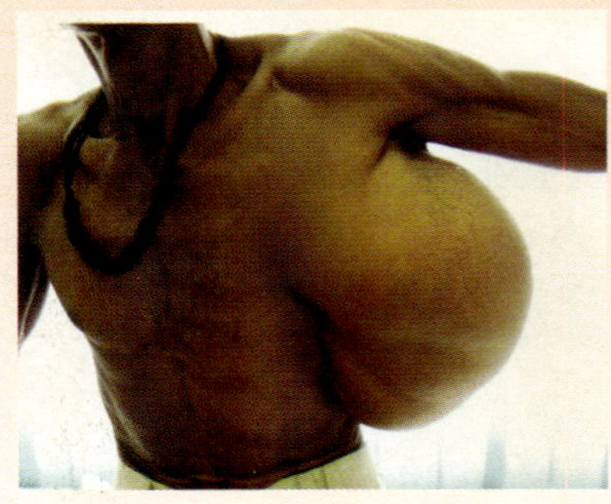

Figure 2.2 Huge lipoma of left axilla—a bump. (Courtesy: Dr. A.C. Dwivedi)

Organomegaly It is the enlargement of an organ as a whole; for example, thyromegaly is enlargement of the whole thyroid (Fig. 2.3) and splenomegaly is enlargement of spleen.

Etiology of swellings

The etiology of swellings is given as follows:

- Congenital and developmental
  - Meningocele
  - Cystic hygroma
  - Branchial cyst
  - Thyroglossal cyst
  - Dermoid cyst
- Infections

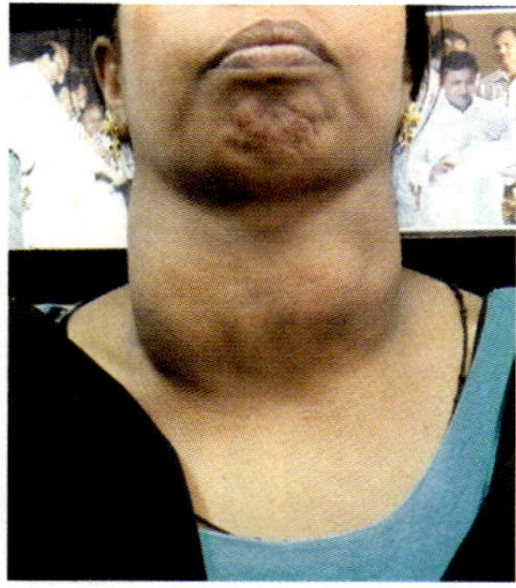

Figure 2.3 Nontoxic multinodular goiter—an example of organomegaly. (Courtesy: Dr. A.C. Dwivedi)

- Acute, for example, cellulitis, acute abscess, carbuncle
- Chronic, for example, cold abscess, granuloma, gumma

- Trauma
  - Acute, for example, hematoma, fracture, vesicles, and bullae of burns
  - Chronic or repeated trauma, for example, corn, chronic bursitis
  - Delayed effects of trauma, for example, hypertrophic scar, keloid, implantation dermoid, arteriovenous fistula
- Tumors
  - Benign, for example, lipoma, fibroma, osteoma, chondroma, adenoma, hemangioma
  - Primary malignant tumors, for example:
    - Carcinoma of skin, oral cavity, breast, thyroid, salivary glands, kidney, etc.
    - Sarcoma, for example, osteosarcoma, soft tissue sarcoma
  - Secondary malignant tumors, for example, metastatic lymph node
- Other swellings, for example, sebaceous cyst, arterial aneurysm, ganglion cyst, sternomastoid tumor

Clinical diagnosis

The diagnosis of a swelling consists of three components, that is, site of lesion, nature of lesion, and the functional disturbance caused by the swelling.

Site of Lesion

The site of lesion means from where and which structure or tissue the swelling is arising. It is decided by the following features:

Position or Site A swelling can arise from the structure or tissue present normally or abnormally in a particular area or region. Examples of site of some swellings are given in Box 2.1.

Box 2.1 Examples of position or site of swellings

- Thyroid swelling is situated in the lower front of neck
- Branchial cyst is situated in the upper neck near the angle of mandible
- Aneurysm is situated along the course of a large artery
- A jaw swelling is situated at the site of jaws
- Ranula is a swelling of floor of oral cavity
- Rhinophyma is a swelling of distal nose

Shape

- If the whole organ or structure is enlarged, the swelling usually assumes the shape of that organ, for example, a thyroid swelling has a butterfly-like shape and a gallbladder lump is pyriform in shape.
- A localized swelling of a part may have spherical, ovoid, or irregular shape.
- The benign swellings are usually smooth and regular while the malignant swellings are irregular and nodular.

Mobility Many organs or structures move with the natural activities of body while others can be made to move by manipulation. Examples of natural and passive mobility are given in Box 2.2.

Fixity The fixity and mobility are interrelated signs. A swelling of an organ or part can be moved or not according to the passive mobility of that organ. Hence, a swelling of the bone cannot be moved on that bone.

Consistency It depends on the consistency of the tissue of origin, for example, a lipoma is soft like fatty tissue, a fibroma is firm like fibrous tissue, and an osteoma is hard like bone.

Box 2.2 Swelling exhibiting natural and passive mobility

Swellings exhibiting natural mobility

- Thyroid swelling moves up with deglutition
- Thyroglossal cyst moves up with protrusion of tongue
- Gallbladder lump goes up and down with respiratory movements

Swellings exhibiting passive mobility

- Neurofibroma can be made to move across, and not along, the long axis of nerve from which it is arising
- Sternomastoid tumor can be made to move across the muscle but this mobility is lost if the muscle is made taut

Nature of Lesion

The nature of the swelling is found by history of disease and physical examination of swelling.

- A congenital swelling is present since birth, for example, meningocele and cystic hygroma.
- A developmental swelling appears later in life, for example, branchial cyst and dermoid cyst.
- An acute inflammatory swelling is of short duration and has pain, fever, redness, heat, tenderness, and loss of function.
- A chronic inflammatory swelling is of long duration, and may have mild pain and deep tenderness. Low-grade fever may be present.
- A traumatic swelling is of short duration, appears immediately following trauma, may be tender with soft (boggy) or variable consistency, and may have bruised (blood-stained) skin.
- A benign tumor grows slowly and painlessly, and is smooth or lobulated, uniform, well defined, and nontender.
- A malignant tumor grows rapidly, and is irregular and nodular, ill-defined, and hard or variable in consistency. It might have produced metastases.

Functional Effects

All the swellings do not produce functional effects but those produced by some are of two types.

Box 2.3 Local and general effects of a swellings

Local or distal effects (due to pressure)

- A thyroid swelling may cause respiratory obstruction or dysphagia due to pressure on trachea and esophagus, respectively
- Carcinoma of parotid may produce facial nerve palsy

General effects

- Multinodular goiter may produce symptoms of thyrotoxicosis
- Acute inflammatory swelling may cause pyrexia and toxemia (systemic inflammatory response syndrome)

Local or Distal Effects These are the local effects on the part or region of origin mainly due to mechanical pressure.

General Effects These include the systemic manifestations of the swellings.

Some examples of local or distal effects and general effects are given in Box 2.3.

Investigations

The various methods of investigation for diagnosing a swelling are given in the subsequent subsections.

Radiography

There are many methods of radiography which are employed to confirm or make the clinical diagnosis.

Plain Radiography It is very helpful in the diagnosis of bony swellings, for example, ameloblastoma is recognized by a multiloculated shadow and an Ewing's tumor by onion-peel appearance.

Contrast Radiography It helps in the diagnosis of swellings arising from hollow organs and tubes which are filled with an appropriate contrast. A benign lesion shows a regular filling defect while a malignant swelling casts an irregular shadow.

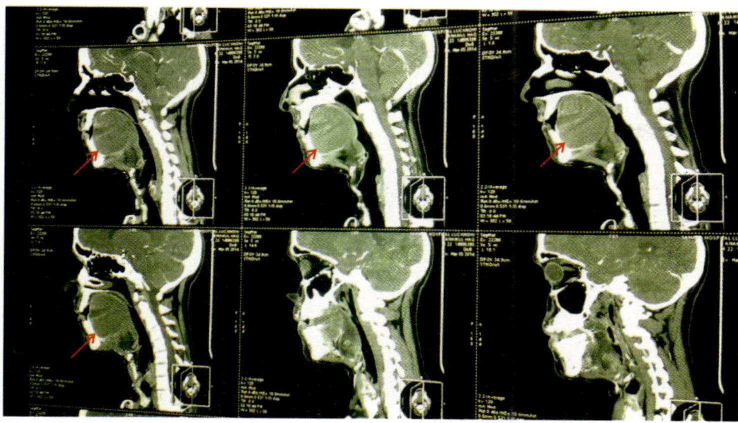

Figure 2.4 Sagittal CT scan of head and neck region showing soft-tissue shadow of a sublingual dermoid. (Courtesy: Professor Surajit Bhattacharya)

CT Scan It is a very helpful diagnostic investigation. The anatomical precision and multiorgan imaging capability of computed tomography is unmatched by any other investigation. It defines the exact extent and texture of the swelling (Fig. 2.4).

Ultrasonography It is a simple, cost-effective, and noninvasive method of imaging. It differentiates a solid from a cystic lesion and helps to guide needle puncture of the swelling for diagnostic aspiration or needle biopsy.

Magnetic Resonance Imaging (MRI) It images a swelling just like CT scan using magnetic waves. It gives better information about the vascular invasion and soft tissue extent.

Radioisotope Scanning It may be employed in the diagnosis of some swellings, for example, radioiodine in the diagnosis of a thyroid nodule.

Arteriography It is used to make the diagnosis of arterial swellings, for example, aneurysm and arteriovenous fistula. It is an invasive investigation. Now the vessels can be visualized by MRI and CT scan (MR angiography, CT angiography) without invasion. Hence, this method is less commonly employed.

Endoscopy

It is of tremendous use in visualizing the lesions of all hollow organs, tubes, and body cavities. Furthermore, biopsy can be taken at the same time under its guidance.

Laboratory

Blood studies of certain swellings show characteristic diagnostic features which are given in Table 2.1.

Biopsy

It is the final court of appeal for the diagnosis. There are many methods of taking tissue samples for this examination.

Table 2.1 Swellings and their laboratory findings

Type of swelling	Findings in blood studies
Acute inflammatory swellings	Polymorphonuclear leukocytosis
Tuberculous lesions	Lymphocytosis and elevated erythrocyte sedimentation rate (ESR)
Metastatic carcinoma of prostate	Elevated prostate-specific antigen (PSA)
Carbuncle	Sugar in urine/hyperglycemia
Hydatid cyst	Immunoblot positive

Fine Needle Aspiration Cytology (FNAC) It is a quick, convenient, minimally invasive, and simple method of diagnosis of a swelling, but it gives a cytological diagnosis and not a tissue diagnosis.

Needle Biopsy A core of tissue may be obtained by puncturing the swelling with a biopsy needle, for example, Vim Silverman needle or Trucut needle, and subjected to histopathological examination.

Open Biopsy It is required when other methods described above have failed or are not applicable. It is an invasive method but most reliable as it gives tissue diagnosis.

Symptoms and signs of some common swellings

Congenital Swellings

These swellings are present since birth.

Meningocele

- **Site**: It occurs in posterior midline or frontonasal region.
- **Other clinical features:** It is a spherical, smooth, soft cystic, and brilliantly transilluminant swelling seen in a neonate (Fig. 2.5). In a simple meningocele there is no neurological deficit. If nerve elements are present, it is associated with neurological deficit.

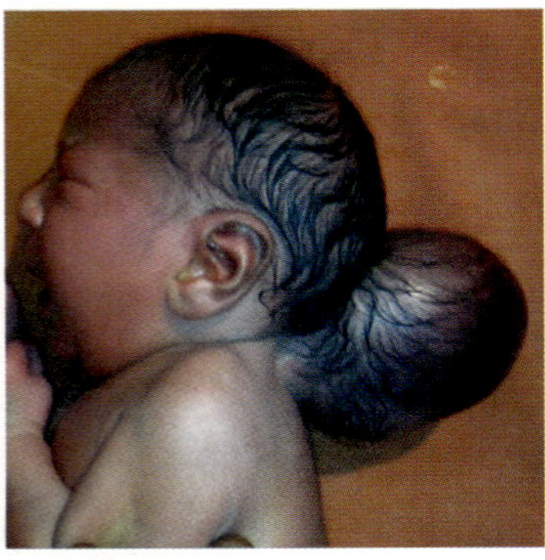

Figure 2.5 Cervical meningocele. (Courtesy: Professor J. D. Rawat)

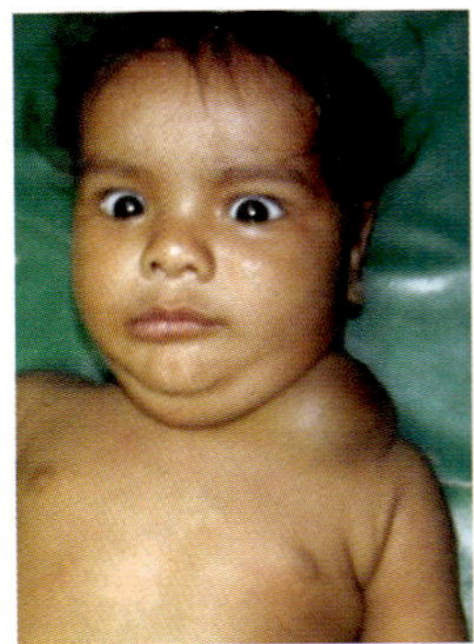

Figure 2.6 Cystic hygroma of left lower neck. (Courtesy: Professor J.D. Rawat)

Cystic hygroma

- **Site:** It occurs in the lower part of posterior triangle of neck (Fig. 2.6). It may occur in axilla, pectoral region, or groin.
- **Other clinical features**: Cystic hygroma is common in children and present since birth as a slow-growing, smooth or lobulated, soft, cystic, ill-defined, and brilliantly transilluminant swelling.

Developmental Swellings

These are developmental swellings which appear a little late in life and are not present at the time of birth.

Branchial cyst

- **Site:** It occurs near the angle of mandible, and is related to the upper one-third of sternomastoid partly covered by its anterior border.
- **Other clinical features:** Branchial cyst, which is a slow-growing, painless mass, and ovoid in shape with its long axis parallel with the long axis of sternomastoid, is common in an adolescent person. It is smooth, soft, cystic, and nontender and may be translucent.

Thyroglossal cyst

- **Site:** It occurs in anterior midline of neck a little to the left just below the hyoid bone (Fig. 2.7). It may be present above hyoid bone or at the level of thyroid cartilage.

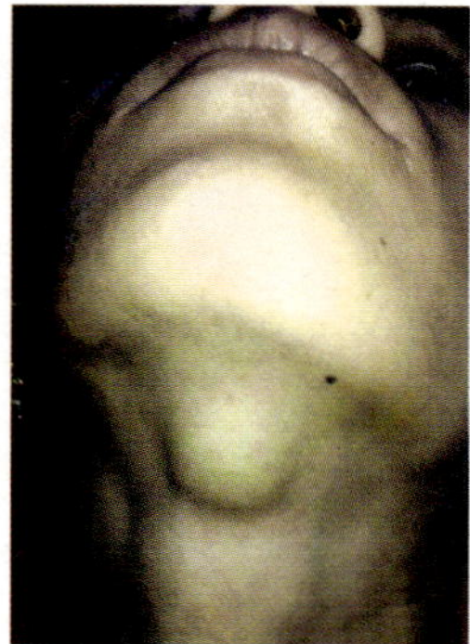

Figure 2.7 Thyroglossal cyst. (Courtesy: Dr. Ravi Mishra)

- **Other clinical features:** The patient is usually young and has a smooth, tensely cystic, nontender, and translucent swelling which moves up with the protrusion of tongue.

Dermoid cyst

- **Site**: It is situated at the lines of embryonic fusion, that is, above the outer canthus of eye, around the ear, root of nose, submental region (Fig. 2.8), lower front of neck, and midline of body.
- **Other clinical features**: It is a painless, slow-growing swelling, which is smooth, soft, and nontender and may be indented with digital pressure. The underlying bone may be indented due to its pressure.

Infective Swellings

Cellulitis

- **Site**: It can be present anywhere in the body but is common on face and submandibular region.

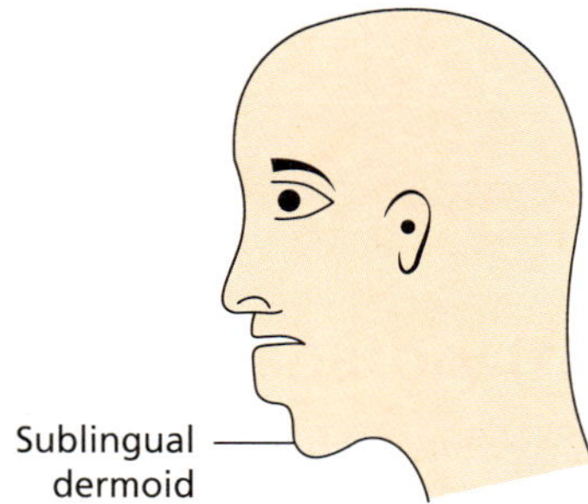

Figure 2.8 Sublingual dermoid giving a double chin appearance in lateral view.

- **Other clinical features:** Cellulitis is characterized by local pain and diffuse reddish swelling which is maximum in the center and reducing gradually toward the periphery till it merges imperceptibly into the normal tissues. It does not have an edge or limit. The skin is shiny, tender, and brawny. The regional lymph nodes may be enlarged and tender.

Acute abscess

- **Site**: It can be present anywhere in the body.
- **Other clinical features**: Acute abscess presents as a painful, red, hot swelling of short duration. The pain is throbbing type which increases if the part is made dependent. The swelling is tender and has brawny induration. Later, it becomes soft in the center or may be fluctuant or boggy.

Carbuncle

- **Site**: It occurs anywhere in the hairy areas but commonly on nape of neck and back.
- **Other clinical features**: Carbuncle is common in a middle-aged diabetic and presents as a painful swelling of recent onset. It may be bluish red in color or may appear red like fire. There are multiple openings on its surface showing thick pus or slough and giving a sieve-like appearance.

Cold abscess

- **Site**: It commonly occurs in the neck, paravertebral region, axilla (Fig. 2.9), groin, or chest wall.

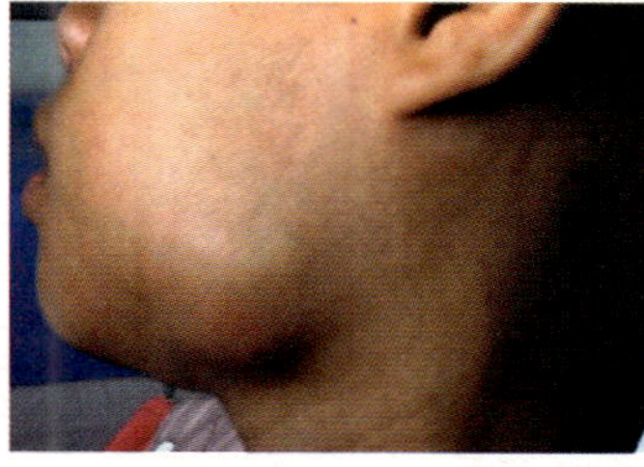

Figure 2.9 Cold abscess of left submandibular region. Note mild redness of overlying skin which indicates an impending rupture. (Courtesy: Professor Surajit Bhattacharya)

- **Other clinical features**: Cold abscess is a painless swelling of insidious onset which is soft, cystic or fluctuant, opaque, and nontender. The edge of the swelling is compressible and does not slip under the fingertip pressure. There may be an evidence of osteoarticular or lymph node tuberculosis.

Traumatic Swellings

Bruise or contusion

- **Site**: It occurs anywhere in the body, but is common on face and limbs.
- **Other clinical features**: Bruise or contusion presents as a minor swelling at the site of injury which is tender and ill-defined. It has blood staining on its surface. It changes its color with the passage of time.

Hematoma

- **Site**: It occurs anywhere in the body.
- **Other clinical features**: Hematoma is a swelling of variable size at the site of injury or operation. It is soft, boggy, ill-defined, and tender. The overlying skin may be discolored or abraded. The diagnosis can be confirmed by ultrasound and needle aspiration.

Fracture

- **Site**: It occurs anywhere in the body where there is a bone.
- **Other clinical features**: The swelling due to a fracture follows severe trauma. It is due to fracture hematoma and displaced fractured ends. Tenderness, step deformity, and crepitus are other signs.

Vesicles and bullae of burns

- **Site**: They occur anywhere in the body.
- **Other clinical features**: Vesicles and bullae usually follow injury by moist heat. They are thin-walled, small (vesicles) or large (bullae) swellings, translucent, and contain serous fluid.

Hypertrophic scar

- **Site**: It occurs anywhere in the body where there is a scar of recent injury.

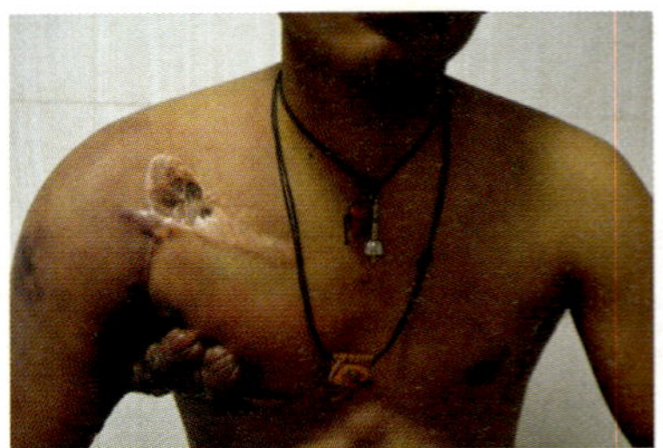

Figure 2.10 Keloids of right lower chest wall on a scar of operation.

- **Other clinical features**: Hypertrophic scar is a slow enlargement or hypertrophy of a scar of operation, burn, or trauma. It does not itch and does not grow into the neighboring tissues and stops growing after some time.

Keloid

- **Site**: It occurs anywhere in the body but is commonly present in the front of sternum or ear lobule.
- **Other clinical features**: Keloid is an enlargement of a scar which itches and grows into the neighboring normal skin with finger-like extensions (Fig. 2.10). It is tender. Its edge is pink and is more tender.

Arteriovenous fistula or aneurysm

- **Site**: It occurs at the site where an artery and a vein are going together.
- **Other clinical features:** Arteriovenous fistula or aneurysm is a pulsatile diffuse swelling with increased local temperature and distended superficial veins. A history of trauma is present. Branham's sign is a specific sign of this lesion. The salient features of arteriovenous fistula or aneurysm are given in Box 2.4.

Box 2.4 Salient clinical features of arteriovenous fistula or aneurysm

- A thrill is palpable at the site of communication
- The heart rate is increased (tachycardia)
- Branham's sign: If the artery proximal to the fistula is compressed, the heart rate comes down
- A continuous machinery murmur is present on auscultation

Implantation dermoid

- **Site**: It occurs on pulp of a finger, palm of hand, or ear lobule.
- **Other clinical features**: Implantation dermoid is a painless, slow-growing swelling which is smooth, soft or firm, and nontender. A history of thorn-prick (e.g., in a gardener) or needle-prick (e.g., in a tailor) may be present. It is a subcutaneous swelling.

Tumors

Tumors can occur anywhere in the body. Benign tumors grow slowly and painlessly. They are smooth and regular. They do not metastasize and do not harm the body. Malignant tumors grow rapidly and irregularly and produce metastasis. They usually kill the victim if not treated early.

Lipoma

- **Site:** It is a benign tumor that can occur anywhere in the body (universal tumor) but commonly occurs in subcutaneous plane of back of neck and trunk and shoulder region.
- **Other clinical features:** Lipoma is a painless, slow-growing swelling that is smooth or lobulated, soft, and nontender. It has an edge which slips under finger.

Fibroma

- **Site:** It is a benign tumor that can occur anywhere where there are subcutaneous nerves.
- **Other clinical features**: Fibroma is a painless, slow-growing, firm, and circumscribed swelling which moves on the underlying tissues. Neurofibroma is the commonest type of fibroma which arises from connective tissue sheaths of nerves (Fig. 2.11).

Osteoma

- **Site:** It is a benign tumor of a bone, more commonly a flat bone.
- **Other clinical features:** Osteoma is painless, very slow growing, smooth, hard, and fixed.

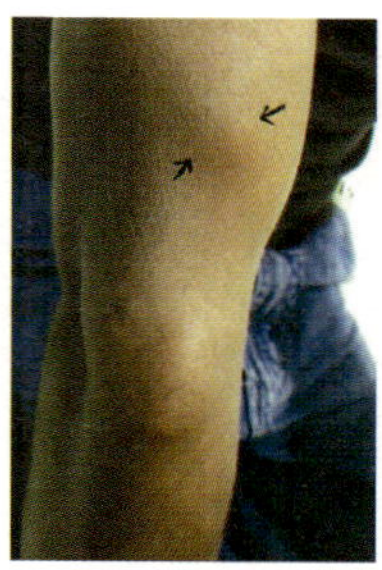

Figure 2.11 Subcutaneous neurofibroma of thigh.

Chondroma

- **Site**: It is a benign tumor that arises from flat bones, for example, sternum and ribs.
- **Other clinical features**: It presents as a painless, very slow-growing swelling of a bone. It is firm and nontender, and may be lobulated.

Adenoma

- **Site**: It is a benign tumor that arises from a gland, for example, thyroid and salivary glands.
- **Other clinical features**: It presents as a painless and slow-growing swelling which is firm, smooth or lobulated, and mobile.

Hemangioma (cavernous type)

- **Site**: It is a benign tumor that can arise anywhere in the body but occurs commonly in the lips, tongue, cheeks, and face (Fig. 2.12).
- **Other clinical features**: It presents as a painless and slow-growing swelling which is bluish in color, nontender, opaque, and compressible (empties on pressure).

Carcinoma

- **Site:** It is a malignant cancer that may occur in the skin, oral cavity, penis, vulva, vagina

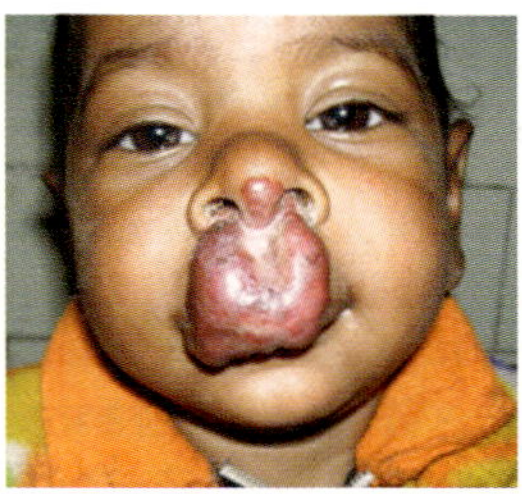

Figure 2.12 Hemangioma of upper lip and tip of nose. (Courtesy: Professor J.D. Rawat)

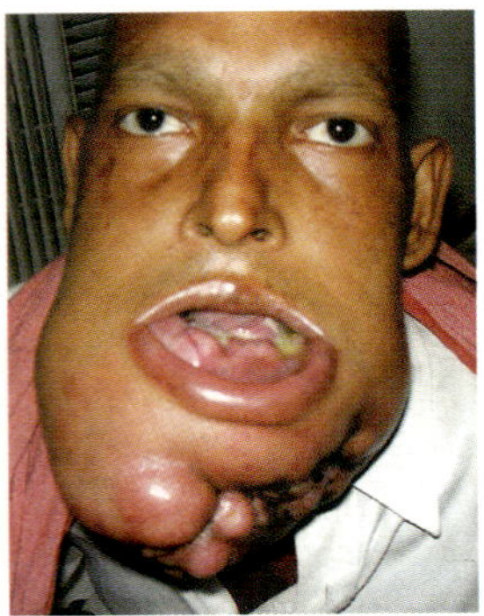

Figure 2.13 Advanced sarcoma of mandible with skin involvement.

(squamous cell carcinoma), breast, thyroid, salivary glands, kidney, colon, stomach, and other internal organs (adenocarcinoma).
- **Other clinical features:** Carcinoma usually affects middle-aged and elderly persons, is a little more common in males, and presents as a lump which is hard, irregular, nontender, and ill-defined. When present as an ulcer, it has a hard and an everted or raised edge.

Sarcoma

- **Site:** It is a malignant tumor of tissues of mesenchymal origin, that is, bone (osteosarcoma) (Fig. 2.13), cartilage, fibrous connective tissue, and lymphoid tissue.
- **Other clinical features:** There is a swelling of recent onset that grows rapidly, and occurs at any age but mostly in young people. Hence, it may attain a large size. It has a diffuse or ill-defined margin. The skin over the swelling may be stretched and glossy and may have engorged veins.

Metastatic cancer

- **Site**: It can occur anywhere.
- **Other clinical features**: Metastatic cancer can also present as a swelling which may be suspected to be metastasis by its clinical features, that is, hard, irregular, and nontender or tender. The primary cancer may be obvious or detected by investigations.

Other Swellings

It includes a miscellaneous group of swellings.

Sebaceous cyst

- **Site**: It occurs on skin of scalp, face, neck, trunk, and scrotum. It does not occur on the palm of hand and sole of foot.
- **Other clinical features**: Sebaceous cyst is a painless and slow-growing swelling which is smooth, hemispherical, soft or firm, and nontender. A black dot called punctum may be present on the top of swelling. It is mobile on deeper tissues but fixed to the skin at the punctum.

Ganglion cyst

- **Site**: It occurs on dorsum of wrist, and rarely in front of ankle.
- **Other clinical features**: Ganglion cyst is a small nodule or swelling which is smooth, firm but elastic, mobile, and nontender.

Arterial aneurysm

- **Site**: It occurs along the course of a large artery.
- **Other clinical features**: Arterial aneurysm is a pulsatile swelling of insidious onset which is smooth, nontender, and tensely cystic. It has expansile pulsation. It can be moved slightly across but not along the long axis of the artery (one must be careful during manipulation as it may rupture with massive bleeding).

Sternomastoid tumor

- **Site**: It occurs in the middle of sternomastoid muscle of neck.
- **Other clinical features**: Sternomastoid tumor is not a tumor but an organized hematoma of sternomastoid due to birth trauma. The patient is usually an infant 3–4 weeks' old who has a smooth, hard, nontender swelling nearly in the neck. If it is not treated in time, it results in shortening of sternomastoid leading to wry neck or torticollis.

Treatment

A flowchart depicting management of a swelling is given in Flowchart 2.1.

Removal of Cause For example, some of the infective swellings such as tuberculoma and gumma may disappear following antibiotic treatment.

Drainage A swelling due to collection of pus, that is, an abscess, is treated by drainage of pus which may be removed by open drainage or by a percutaneous catheter. In a tuberculous abscess the pus is removed by needle aspiration or by evacuation (open drainage and excision of necrotic tissue).

Excision It is the main method of treatment of swellings. Most of the swellings are excised, for example, dermoid cyst, sebaceous cyst, lipoma, cystic hygroma (Figs 2.14 and 2.15), fibroma, adenoma, meningocele, and branchial cyst. All these lesions should be excised completely to prevent recurrence. The malignant tumors are widely or radically excised. They may require radiotherapy and/or chemotherapy.

Repair The swelling of a hernia and an aneurysm are treated by repair—a hernia by herniotomy, herniorrhaphy, or hernioplasty and an aortic aneurysm by open or endovascular repair (EVR). An arteriovenous fistula is treated by ligation or reconstruction.

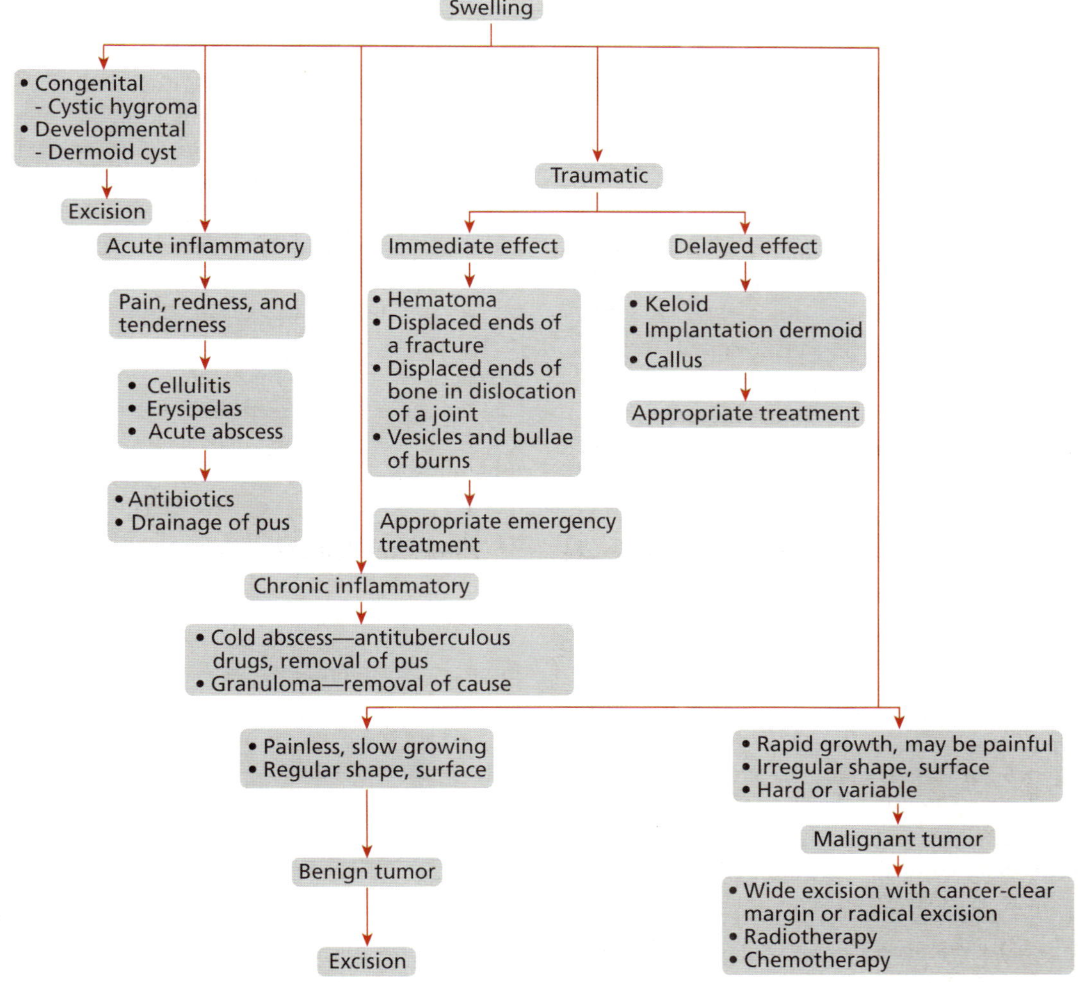

Flowchart 2.1 Management of a swelling.

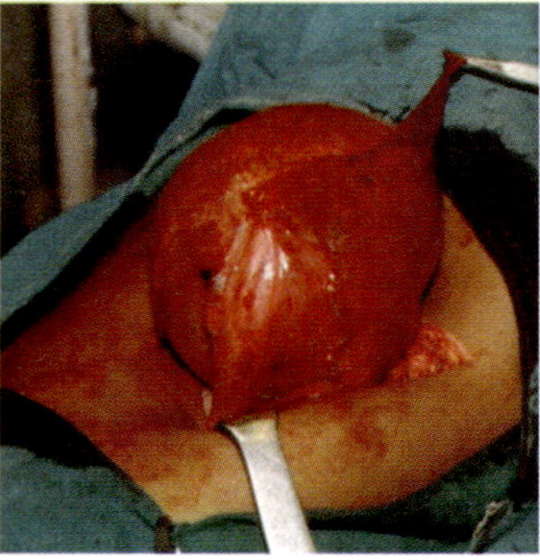

Figure 2.14 Cystic hygroma of lower neck being excised. (Courtesy: Professor Surajit Bhattacharya)

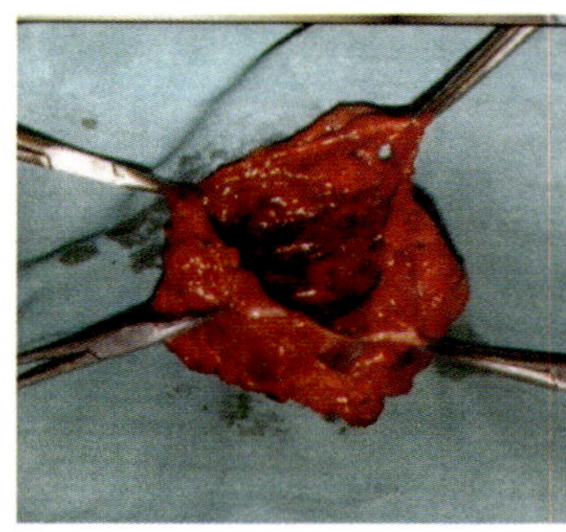

Figure 2.15 The wound left to be repaired after excision of a cystic hygroma. (Courtesy: Professor Surajit Bhattacharya)

KEY POINTS

- A swelling (or swellings) is one of the commonest clinical presentations of surgical disease.
- Swellings can be congenital, developmental, infective, traumatic, cystic, and tumorous.
- Clinical diagnosis is based mainly on inspection and palpation of the swelling. It includes site and nature of lesion and the functional disturbance caused by the swelling.
- Most important diagnostic investigations to picturize the lesion are radiography, ultrasonography, CT scan, and MRI.
- Biopsy is the most reliable method for arriving at a final diagnosis.
- Congenital swellings are present since birth and include meningocele and cystic hygroma.
- Developmental swellings appear later in life and include branchial cyst, thyroglossal cyst, and dermoid cyst.
- Carcinoma is a malignant neoplasm of epithelial origin. Sarcoma is a malignant neoplasm of mesenchymal origin.
- Principles of treatment include: removal of the cause, drainage (as in abscesses), excision of the swelling, and repair (as in hernia). Excision is the main method of treatment of most of the swellings.
- Malignant neoplasms require wide or radical resection and may be with adjuvant radiotherapy and chemotherapy treatment.

SELF-ASSESSMENT

Long answer questions

1. What are the causes of a swelling? How will you examine a case presenting with a swelling to reach a clinical diagnosis?
2. What are the investigations required to reach at a definitive diagnosis of a swelling? What are the methods of treatment?

Short answer questions

1. Acute abscess
2. Cold abscess
3. Lipoma
4. Fine needle aspiration cytology
5. Endoscopy

Multiple choice questions

6. Sign of emptying on pressure is typically seen in a
   (a) Lipoma
   (b) Branchial cyst
   (c) Cystic hygroma
   (d) Cavernous hemangioma

(CONTD...)

SELF-ASSESSMENT *(...CONTD)*

7. Indentation on digital pressure may be seen in a
   (a) Dermoid cyst
   (b) Lipoma
   (c) Thyroglossal cyst
   (d) Cystic hygroma
8. All of the following statements are true about a keloid, except
   (a) It is overgrowth of scar tissue
   (b) It grows into the normal skin present around it
   (c) Itching is a common symptom
   (d) It does not recur after excision
9. Implantation dermoid is usually found on
   (a) Fingertips
   (b) Face
   (c) Thigh
   (d) Anterior chest
10. The clinical signs of lipoma include all of the following, except
   (a) It is a slow-growing swelling
   (b) It has a definite edge which slips under finger
   (c) It is hard in consistency
   (d) It is smooth or lobulated
11. The clinical signs of a cold abscess include all of the following, except
   (a) It is a transilluminant swelling
   (b) It is smooth and soft
   (c) It is not hot and not tender
   (d) It is a fluctuant swelling
12. Expansile pulsation is seen in
   (a) Carcinoma of parotid
   (b) Arterial aneurysm
   (c) Branchial cyst
   (d) Adenoma of thyroid
13. The clinical signs of an acute abscess include all of the following, except
   (a) It is a swelling of short duration
   (b) It is red and hot
   (c) It is nontender
   (d) It may be soft or boggy in the center

Answers

1. (d) 2. (a) 3. (d) 4. (a) 5. (c) 6. (a) 7. (b) 8. (c)

Ulcers

3

Introduction

The external surface of the body and that of hollow organs and tubes is covered by epithelium, a part of which may be destroyed or lost due to many reasons leading to two types of clinical manifestations: ulcer and wound.

Anatomy of an ulcer

An ulcer is a breach in the continuity of the covering epithelium—skin or mucous membrane—due to molecular death mostly due to infection and trauma (Figs 3.1 and 3.2). An ulcer has many parts which are described below (Fig. 3.3):

- **Floor:** It is the surface of the ulcer which is visible on inspection. It contains slough (dead tissue with dirty looks) and red granulation tissue (healing tissue).
- **Base:** It is made up of tissues on which the ulcer is sitting. It is examined by palpation by lifting it up with fingers.
- **Edge or margin:** The junction of the ulcer with the normal tissue around is known as edge or margin. In a deep ulcer the edge is the

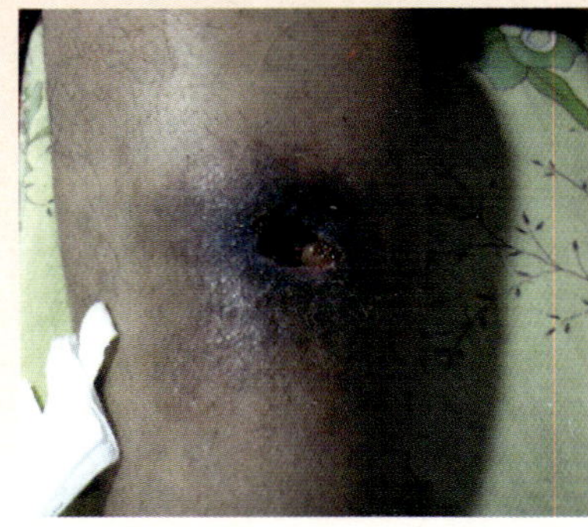

Figure 3.1 Deep ulcer of middle of leg on its anteromedial surface with pigmented undermined edge and thin watery discharge—tuberculous ulcer.

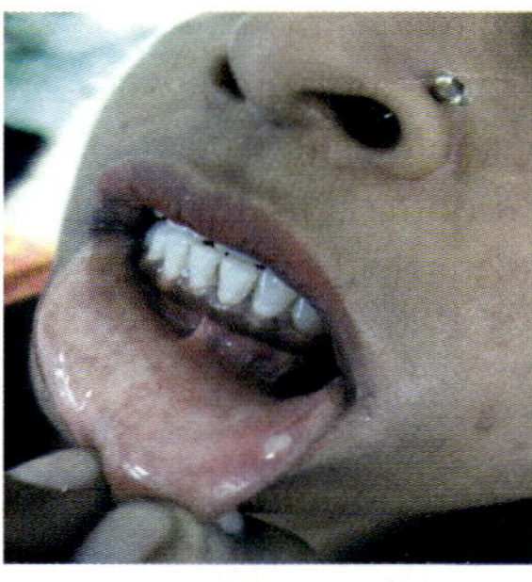

Figure 3.2 Aphthous ulcer of lower lip near left angle of mouth.

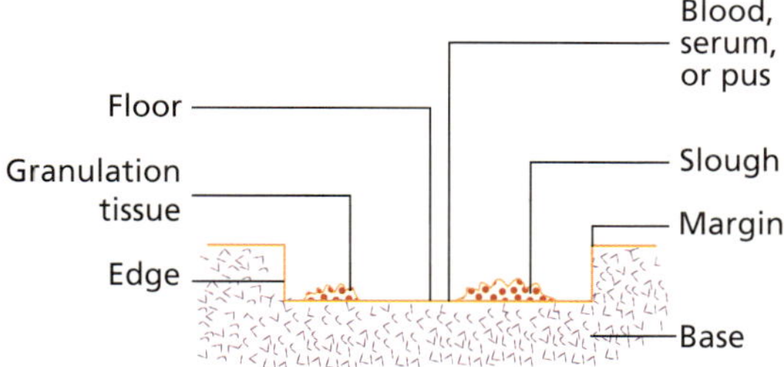

Figure 3.3 Anatomy of an ulcer.

side wall of the ulcer which has width, while in a shallow ulcer or healing ulcer the edge is a line and does not have width.

Wound

A wound is a traumatic discontinuity of tissues with or without contamination by bacteria.

- Most of the wounds produced by the surgeons are sterile or bacteria-free.
- All the accidental wounds are contaminated.
- Once the infection is settled and produces inflammatory reaction and necrosis of tissues, a contaminated wound becomes a traumatic ulcer.

The differences between an ulcer and a wound are given in Table 3.1.

Pathogenesis of an ulcer

Initiation An ulcer is usually caused or initiated by local trauma or infection resulting in loss of covering epithelium. In a normal person most of these ulcers heal by themselves or following simple treatment.

Maintenance In some patients, an ulcer fails to heal and becomes chronic because of any or many of the reasons given in Box 3.1.

Box 3.1 Factors leading to chronicity of an ulcer

General causes

- Diabetes mellitus
- Advanced malignancy, leukemia
- Anticancer drugs
- Prolonged corticosteroid therapy

Local causes

- Improper venous drainage, for example, venous ulcer
- Arterial insufficiency, for example, arterial ulcer
- Repeated trauma, for example, dental ulcer
- Local cancer, for example, carcinomatous ulcer, rodent ulcer
- Specific infection, for example, tuberculous ulcer
- Sensory loss, for example, neuropathic ulcer

Classification of ulcers

According to Site (or Visibility)

- **External ulcers:** These ulcers occur on the external surface of the body or in the superficial cavities such as oral cavity. Hence, they can be easily seen by the patient.
- **Internal ulcers**: They occur inside the hollow organs, for example, gastric ulcer in the stomach and tuberculous ulcer in the ileum.

In this chapter only the external ulcers are being described.

According to Etiology

- **Benign ulcers**
  - Traumatic—accidental, self-inflicted, dental ulcer
  - Infective—nonspecific, tuberculous, syphilitic, soft sore, tropical ulcer

Table 3.1 Differences between an ulcer and wound

Features	Ulcer	Wound
Etiology	Trauma, infection, malignancy	Trauma
Infection	Always infected	May be contaminated (accidental wound) or sterile (operative wound)
Signs of inflammation	Present	Absent
Discharge	Purulent or seropurulent	Blood or serosanguinous

- Arterial or ischemic ulcer
- Venous ulcer
- Diabetic ulcer
- Neuropathic ulcer

- **Malignant ulcers**
  - Rodent ulcer
  - Carcinomatous ulcer
  - Melanomatous ulcer

According to Clinical Course

- **Spreading ulcer**: It is an active or progressive ulcer having profuse purulent discharge with floor covered with necrotic tissue (slough) with hardly any evidence of granulation tissue.
- **Healing ulcer**: It is an ulcer which is reducing in size with minimal serous discharge, bright red granulation tissue in the floor, and iris-like growing epithelium at the edge.
- **Callus ulcer**: It is a type of nonhealing ulcer having pale, flat, and flabby granulation tissue in the floor and hard pale white edge.

Clinical features of an ulcer

- **Age and gender predilection**: An ulcer can occur at any age and in a male or a female.
- **Site:** It can occur anywhere on the body surface, the common sites being the lower limbs, external genitals, and oral cavity.
- **General clinical features**: The patient may present with varying degree of pain (e.g., herpetic and aphthous ulcers are painful and neuropathic ulcer is painless) and discharge.

Clinical examination of an ulcer

Site Rodent ulcer usually occurs on the upper part of the face, a dental ulcer and carcinomatous ulcer on the lateral border of tongue, a primary syphilitic sore on the penis or upper lip, and a venous ulcer around the ankle. The sitewise occurrence of ulcers including ulcers of head and neck region is given in Table 3.2.

Shape A Hunterian chancre is oval or circular in shape. All benign ulcers are regular while the malignant ulcers are irregular in shape.

Size Benign ulcers are usually small in size while a malignant ulcer may attain any size.

Edge Finding the type of edge is very important in making a clinical diagnosis. The diagnosis based on edges is given in Table 3.3 and illustrated in Figure 3.4.

Discharge It is an important feature of an ulcer. It may have any type of discharge as outlined in Table 3.4.

Floor It is the surface of the ulcer which is visible on inspection. It contains slough (dead necrotic tissue) in an acute ulcer and granulation tissue (red granular tissue) in a healing ulcer. The appearance of floor of various ulcers is described in Table 3.5.

Base The base of an ulcer is made by the tissues on which it is sitting. It is examined by palpation and by trying to lift it up between fingers and thumb. It is:

Table 3.2 Sites of occurrence of ulcers

Ulcer	Site of occurrence
Traumatic ulcer	Anywhere but commonly occurs in the leg, foot; lateral border of tongue and inside cheeks (dental ulcer)
Tuberculous ulcer	Anywhere but commonly in the neck, axilla or groin; near the tip of tongue
Lupus vulgaris	Face, rarely on arms
Primary chancre	External genitalia, rarely on lip and tip of tongue or nipple
Snail-track ulcers	Oral cavity in tonsillar area
Gummatous ulcer	Over tibia, sternum, skull, testis, dorsum of tongue
Carcinomatous ulcer	Lips, check, tongue, alveolus, floor of mouth, palate, penis, anus, vulva, and skin of head and face
Rodent ulcer	On the face above the line joining the angle of mouth with tragus of the ear (Ohngren line)

Table 3.3 Types of edges of ulcer

Types of edge of ulcer	Clinical diagnosis
Sloping or shelving edge	Nonspecific ulcer, healing ulcer
Undermined edge	Tuberculous ulcer
Punched-out edge	Gummatous ulcer
Raised and pearly edge	Rodent ulcer
Everted edge	Carcinomatous ulcer

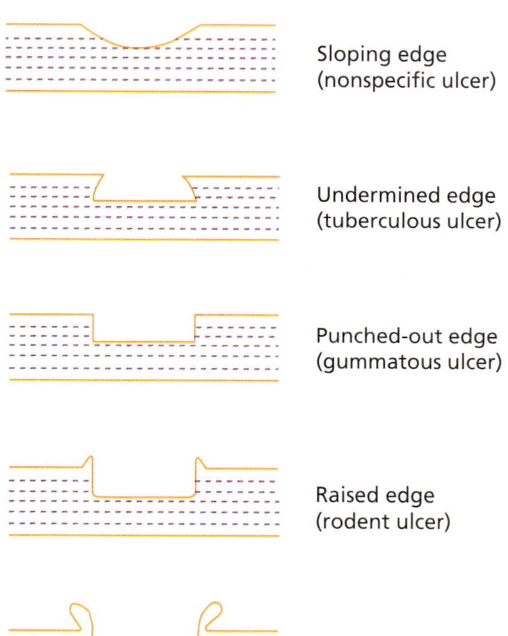

Figure 3.4 Types of edge of ulcers.

Table 3.4 Types of discharge in various ulcers

Type of discharge	Type of ulcer
Purulent discharge	Acute infective ulcer
Bluish green discharge	*Pseudomonas pyocyaneus* infection in the ulcer
Thin syrup-like or watery discharge with curdy flakes	Tuberculous ulcer
Scanty serous discharge	Healing ulcer
Serosanguinous or bloody discharge	Malignant ulcer

Table 3.5 Appearance of floor of ulcers

Appearance of floor of ulcer	Type of ulcer
Slough occupying whole floor	Acute infective ulcer
Watery or apple-jelly granulations	Tuberculous ulcer
Wash-leather slough	Gummatous ulcer
Bright red granulation tissue	Healing ulcer
Bluish green slough	Ulcer with *Pseudomonas pyocyaneus* infection

- Soft in a benign ulcer
- Indurated or hard in a carcinomatous ulcer
- Fixed to the underlying bone if it is invaded

Regional Lymph Nodes These are examined by inspection and palpation, the common findings of which are described in Table 3.6.

General Examination The general examination of the patient is done to find out if there is a systemic cause of ulceration, for example, diabetes mellitus, tuberculosis, syphilis, venous insufficiency, arterial disease, neurological deficit, or any other disease.

Grading of an ulcer

The grading of an ulcer (Table 3.7) is important in deciding the treatment (e.g., grade III and IV ulcers require a skin flap to cover them) and prognosis (e.g., grade I and II ulcers have a better prognosis).

Investigations

Laboratory Studies

- The blood is sent for hemoglobin, counts, sugar, and others depending on the etiology of ulcer, for example, serological tests for syphilis in a syphilitic ulcer and sugar in a diabetic ulcer.
- Urine is sent for detection of sugar.
- The examination of discharge (smear and culture) frequently gives the etiological diagnosis in infective ulcers.

Table 3.6 Characteristics of regional lymph nodes in ulcers

Type of ulcer	Characteristics of regional lymph nodes
Acute ulcers	Mildly enlarged and tender
Chronic nonspecific ulcer	Mildly enlarged, firm, nontender, and discrete
Tuberculous ulcer	Enlarged, firm, and matted
Rodent ulcer or basal cell carcinoma	Not enlarged
Hunterian chancre	Mildly enlarged, hard, mobile, and nontender (shotty nodes)
Carcinomatous ulcer	Enlarged, hard, and mobile or fixed

Table 3.7 Grading of an ulcer

Grading of ulcer	Features
Grade I	Involvement of skin only
Grade II	Involvement of skin and subcutaneous tissue
Grade III	Involvement of skin, subcutaneous tissue, deep fascia, muscles, and tendons
Grade IV	Involvement of the underlying bone

- In a tuberculous ulcer DNA–RNA amplification for tuberculosis may be done for rapid diagnosis.
- The discharge of a syphilitic chancre frequently shows Spirochetes in dark-field illumination.

Radiography

- In an ulcer near bone, radiography of the neighboring bone may be done to see its involvement.
- In an arterial ulcer color Doppler or arteriography may be done to see the condition of the related arteries.

Biopsy A small piece of tissue is taken from the edge of the ulcer under local anesthesia and sent for histological evaluation. It is the most important diagnostic investigation, especially in a malignant ulcer. For a quick diagnosis fine needle aspiration cytology (FNAC) may be done.

Clinical features of common ulcers

Nonspecific Ulcer or Traumatic Ulcer

- **Site:** It can occur anywhere but in the oral cavity on the lateral border of tongue or inside the cheek.
- **Other clinical features**: It is characterized by pain, seropurulent or purulent discharge, oval or round in shape, pale or pink floor, and a sloping edge.

Tuberculous Ulcer

- **Site:** It can occur anywhere but commonly occurs in the neck, on the face, and on the anterior part of tongue.
- **Other clinical features:** The patient presents with a chronic nonhealing ulcer which discharges thin syrup-like exudate and has a thin bluish and undermined edge. It has soft, pale, and feeble granulation tissue in the floor and the base is somewhat indurated. The regional lymph nodes may be enlarged and matted.

Lupus Vulgaris

- **Site:** It occurs on face and arms.
- **Other clinical features:** It is a rare type of cutaneous tuberculosis that occurs in children and young adults, and is characterized by superficial ulceration having apple-jelly granulation tissue.

Syphilitic Ulcers

Primary (Hunterian) Chancre

- **Site**: It occurs on the genitalia in primary syphilis usually 3 weeks after sexual contact.

It can occur on the upper lip or tip of tongue following kissing an infected person.

- **Other clinical features**: This ulcer is oval, slightly elevated from the surface with a sloping and well-defined edge. It exudes serosanguinous discharge. It is hard and nontender, and feels like a buried button when palpated through the prepuce. The inguinal lymph nodes are mildly enlarged, hard, discrete, and nontender (shotty). In cases of a lesion of upper lip, upper cervical lymph nodes are enlarged significantly.

Snail-Track Ulcers

- **Site:** They occur in secondary syphilis and appear as irregular wavy areas on the tongue, soft palate, and tonsils.
- **Other clinical features:** They are superficial and grayish with a well-defined edge and adherent mucus. Other features of secondary syphilis, for example, fever, generalized lymphadenopathy, and cutaneous rash, are present.

Gummatous Ulcer

- **Site:** It occurs over subcutaneous bones (e.g., sternum, tibia, ulna, and skull), dorsum of tongue, and sternomastoid.
- **Other clinical features:** It occurs in tertiary syphilis due to rupture of a gumma and has a punched-out and indurated edge. The floor is covered with yellowish-gray or wash-leather slough which may have one or more islands of healthy tissue escaping necrosis. It is round or crescentic in shape. The adjacent skin is congested and often pigmented to coppery color. The regional lymph nodes are usually not enlarged.

Venous Ulcer

- **Site:** It is the commonest ulcer of leg that occurs around the ankle just above medial malleolus.
- **Other clinical features:** It occurs in patients of chronic venous insufficiency of lower extremity. The surrounding area is hyperpigmented and the ulcer tends to ride a vein.

Arterial Ulcer

- **Site:** It commonly occurs on the tip of toes or fingers due to arterial insufficiency.
- **Other clinical features:** It is usually pale, multiple, and painful.

Neuropathic Ulcer

- **Site**: It usually occurs on sole of foot beneath the head of first metatarsal in patients with some neurological problem, for example, peripheral neuropathy.
- **Other clinical features:** It is a painless deep ulcer with punched-out callus edge and offensive slough in the floor.

Pressure (Bed) Sores

- **Site**: They occur on the bony prominences due to lying in the same position for prolonged periods. Hence, they occur at the site of iliac crest, greater trochanter, and ischial tuberosity.
- **Other clinical features:** They are very variable in size and depth and may have a bone exposed in the floor. They have all the features of a nonspecific ulcer, that is, sloping edge, purulent or seropurulent discharge, and a variable amount of slough in the floor.

Rodent Ulcer (Basal Cell Carcinoma)

- **Site:** It is common in an elderly person who has a nonhealing ulcer on the upper part of face above the line joining the angle of mouth with lobule of the ear (Fig. 3.5).
- **Other clinical features**: It starts as a small brownish-red nodule with shiny surface having fine capillaries. Later an ulcer develops which has a well-defined, hard, raised, and beaded

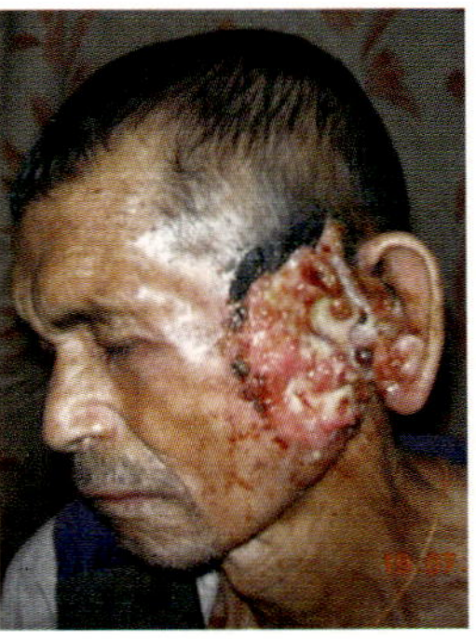

Figure 3.5 A large basal cell carcinoma (rodent ulcer) of left parotid region in an elderly male. (Courtesy: Professor Sandeep Kumar)

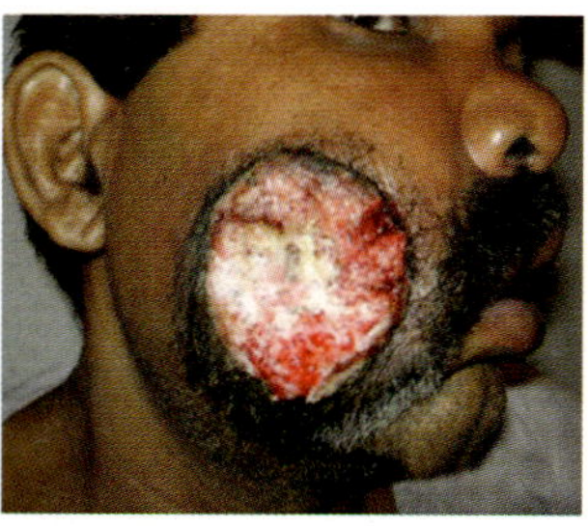

Figure 3.6 Carcinomatous ulcer of face. (Courtesy: Professor Sandeep Kumar)

edge like a motor car tire. The central part of the ulcer may heal and scab (pseudohealing) while it is spreading at the periphery like field fire. The regional lymph nodes are not enlarged.

Carcinomatous Ulcer (Squamous Cell Carcinoma)

- **Site:** It can occur anywhere but commonly seen on scalp, face (Fig. 3.6), hands, oral cavity, penis, and anus.
- **Other clinical features:** It may start as a fissure or nodule which progresses into a nonhealing ulcer with everted edge and hard indurated base. The regional lymph nodes may be enlarged, hard, and mobile or fixed.

Treatment of ulcers

Clinical diagnosis and treatment of ulcers are schematically presented in Flowchart 3.1.

Simple Ulcers

Removal of Cause

- Infective ulcers are treated with appropriate antibiotic or chemotherapeutic drugs, for example, tuberculous ulcer with antituberculous drugs orally and syphilitic ulcer with crystalline penicillin parenterally.
- Bed sores need a lot of attention and proper nursing care, a water bed, and frequent change of posture. They tend to heal soon if the patient is able to leave the bed.
- An arterial ulcer heals if the arterial supply is improved by stopping smoking, endarterectomy, or endoluminal angioplasty.
- A venous ulcer is treated by improving venous drainage by elevation of limb, centripetal massage, pressure garment, and treatment of varicosity.
- A diabetic ulcer heals following control of diabetes, avoidance of pressure on the ulcer site, and local care.
- A self-inflicted ulcer requires psychiatric support and local care. The self-mutilation is sometimes prevented by plastering the affected part.

Local Treatment

- The ulcer is dressed properly till it heals completely. If there is slough, it should be removed by dressing with eusol, or enzymatic or surgical debridement.
- Some modern dressing materials include hydrocolloid gels, alginates, and microporous polyurethane films. The hydrocolloid gels when come in contact with the exudates of the ulcer form a gel which expands to fill the wound. Microporous polyurethane films are good for shallow ulcers. They may be left in place for many days.
- Vacuum-assisted closure (VAC)—a large dirty ulcer may be made to heal rapidly by applying intermittent negative pressure of about −125 mm Hg to the ulcer surface by a closed system of dressing.

Skin Grafting

- A large ulcer is usually treated by skin grafting for rapid healing.
- A callus ulcer is managed by excision and skin grafting.
- Deep pressure sores are usually covered by a myocutaneous flap.

Malignant Ulcers

- They are mostly treated by wide excision and skin grafting.
- After excision the cancer-clear margin is confirmed by immediate microscopy of the excised tissue.
- A carcinomatous and rodent ulcer can be treated by radiotherapy.
- The use of chemotherapy, for example, 5-FU, methotrexate, and mitomycin, may improve

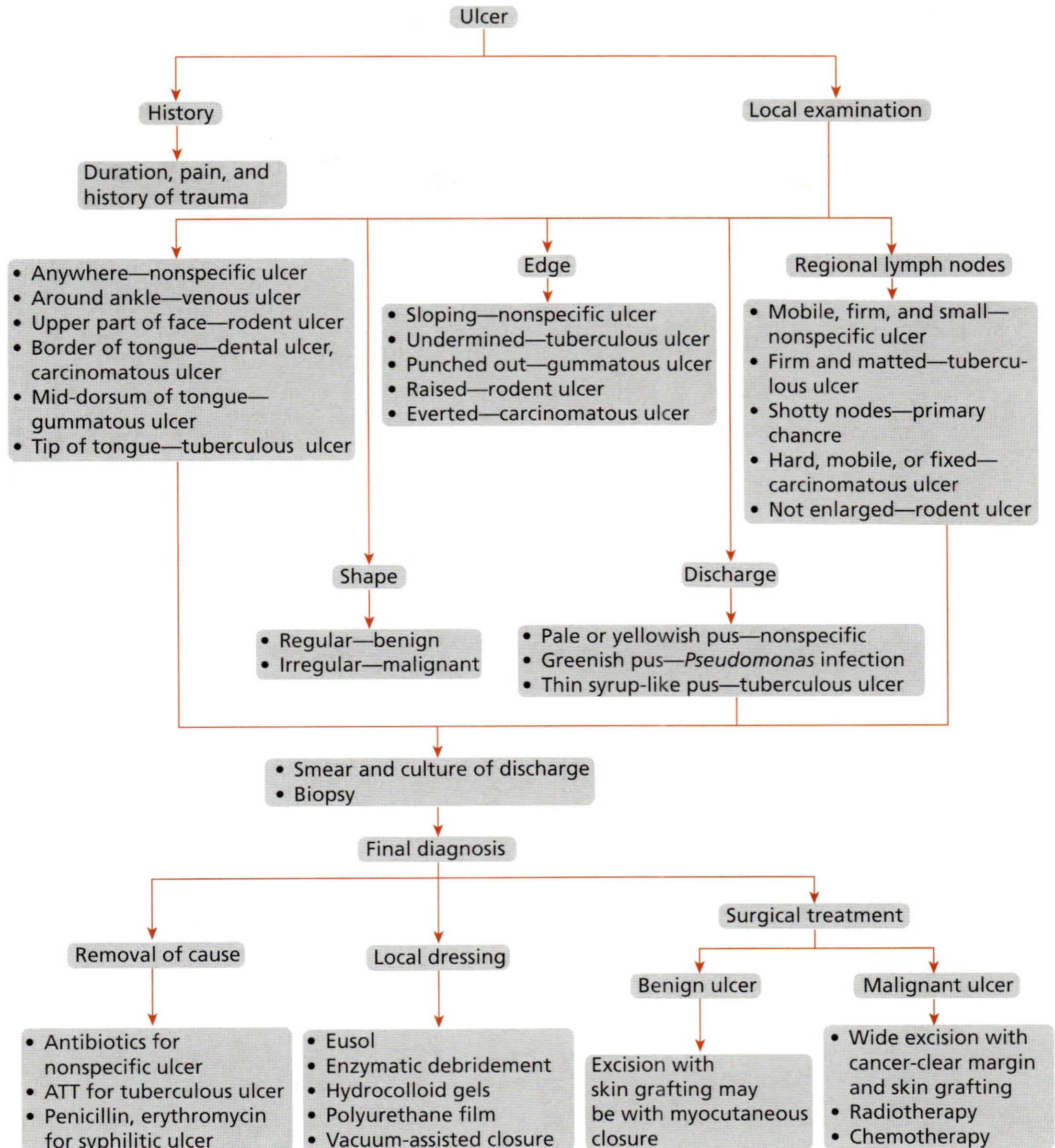

Flowchart 3.1 Clinical diagnosis and treatment of an ulcer. *ATT*, antituberculosis therapy.

the results in a carcinomatous ulcer. A small rodent ulcer may respond to local 5-FU cream.

Causes of nonhealing of an ulcer

The causes of nonhealing of an ulcer are:

- Repeated trauma
- Improper dressing
- Uncontrolled diabetes mellitus
- Arterial insufficiency
- Venous insufficiency
- Specific infection which is not identified and not treated, for example, tuberculosis
- Malignancy

KEY POINTS

- An ulcer is a breach in the continuity of skin or mucous membrane due to molecular death mostly due to infection and trauma.
- A wound is a traumatic discontinuity of tissues with or without contamination by bacteria.
- Most ulcers heal with minimum intervention. Local and systemic causes are responsible for chronicity of ulcers.
- A chronic nonhealing ulcer should be suspected as a malignant ulcer, hence must be biopsied.
- Clinical diagnosis of an ulcer is based on the site, size, shape, margin, floor and base, discharge, regional lymph node characteristics, and accompanying systemic manifestations.
- Biopsy is the main investigatory method especially in malignant ulcers.
- Treatment of simple ulcers includes removal of the cause, local dressing, and, in some cases, skin grafting.
- Treatment of malignant ulcers includes wide excision, radiotherapy, and chemotherapy.

SELF-ASSESSMENT

Long answer questions

1. What is an ulcer? Describe its etiology, clinical features, and treatment.
2. Describe the clinical features of syphilitic and tuberculous ulcers. How will you treat them?

Short answer questions

1. Rodent ulcer
2. Lupus vulgaris
3. Gummatous ulcer
4. Tuberculous ulcer
5. Carcinomatous ulcer
6. Primary chancre

Multiple choice questions

1. The commonest site of occurrence of a rodent ulcer is
   (a) Upper part of face
   (b) Around ankle
   (c) Inside cheek
   (d) On tongue
2. The commonest site of occurrence of a carcinomatous ulcer on the tongue is
   (a) Dorsum of tongue
   (b) Lateral border
   (c) Tip
   (d) Undersurface
3. Which of the following ulcers is painless?
   (a) Tuberculous ulcer of tongue
   (b) Gummatous ulcer
   (c) Aphthous ulcer
   (d) Traumatic ulcer
4. Undermined edge of the ulcer is typically seen in
   (a) Tuberculous ulcer
   (b) Carcinomatous ulcer
   (c) Gummatous ulcer
   (d) Rodent ulcer
5. Everted edge is a feature of
   (a) Gummatous ulcer
   (b) Tuberculous ulcer
   (c) Carcinomatous ulcer
   (d) Nonspecific ulcer
6. Wash-leather slough is seen in
   (a) Carcinomatous ulcer
   (b) Venous ulcer
   (c) Tuberculous ulcer
   (d) Gummatous ulcer
7. Bluish green slough in an ulcer is indicative of
   (a) Syphilitic infection
   (b) Tuberculosis
   (c) Staphylococcal infection
   (d) *Pseudomonas pyocyaneus* infection

Answers

1. (a) 2. (b) 3. (b) 4. (a) 5. (c) 6. (d) 7. (d)

Sinuses

4

Definition

A sinus is a blind-ending track usually lined by granulation tissue that leads from an epithelial surface into the tissues, usually into an abscess cavity (Fig. 4.1). It discharges pus continuously or intermittently. The sinus track may have branches. A sinus has to be differentiated from an ulcer. Their differences are given in Table 4.1.

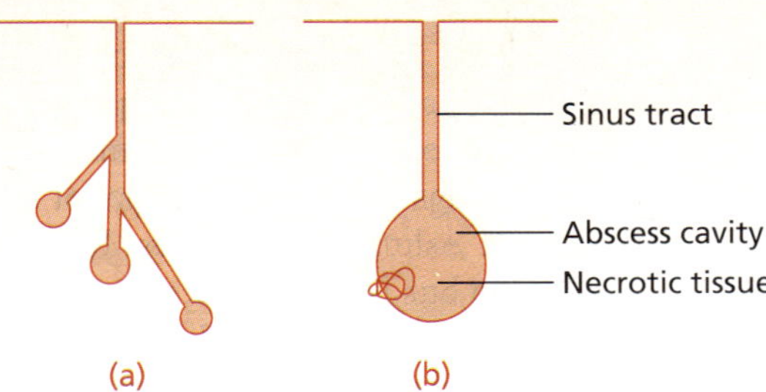

Figure 4.1 Sinus tract (a) with or (b) without branches.

Etiology of sinuses

Congenital Sinuses They are caused by some developmental problem. Examples include preauricular sinus, umbilical sinus, urachal sinus, and coccygeal sinus.

Acquired Sinuses They are usually due to infection or presence of necrotic tissue or foreign body in the tissues.

- Infective sinuses
  - Inadequate drainage of a pyogenic abscess
  - Failure of abscess cavity to collapse and obliterate after drainage, for example, chronic osteomyelitis, chronic empyema thoracis
  - Rupture or drainage of a tuberculous cold abscess
  - Actinomycosis
  - Hidradenitis suppurativa
- Retained necrotic tissue or a foreign body

Table 4.1 Differences between a sinus and an ulcer

Features	Sinus	Ulcer
Size	Small	Large
Depth	More	Less
Floor and extent	Cannot be seen ("blind" track)	Visible
Lining	Granulation tissue, may have epithelium	Granulation tissue

- Necrotic tissue, for example, sequestrum in an osteomyelitic sinus
- Foreign body, for example, pellet or bullet in a traumatic sinus; tuft of hair in a pilonidal sinus; drainage tube, swab, or unabsorbed suture in a postoperative sinus
- Epithelial lining, for example, rupture or drainage of an infected sebaceous cyst

Pathology of a sinus

- The sinus tract has a variable length and may have branches going into the tissues.
- It is usually lined by granulation tissue but in a long-standing sinus it may be partly lined by epithelium.
- A congenital sinus arises from the remnants of embryonic ducts that persist instead of disappearing during development. It is usually lined by epithelium.
- If the sinus has a retained foreign body or sequestrum, excessive granulation tissue forms which projects from its opening called "proud flesh."

Clinical features

- **Age and gender predilection:** A sinus can occur in anybody regardless of age and sex.
- **Site:** A sinus can occur anywhere in the body, the common sites being near the ends of bones, neck, axilla, and groin.
- **General clinical features:** The patient usually presents with an abnormal hole with recurrent or persistent discharge. There may be pain and swelling if the exudate is retained inside.

Clinical examination of a sinus

Site The location of some important sinuses is given in Table 4.2.

Table 4.2 Location of some important sinuses

Sinus	Site/location
Preauricular sinus	Root of helix or on the tragus of the ear
Osteomyelitic sinus	Near the ends of a long bone
Tuberculous sinus	Neck, axilla, groin, or near a bone or joint
Injection sinus	Gluteal region

Number

- Most of the sinuses are single.
- Tuberculosis, actinomycosis, and hidradenitis suppurativa may be associated with multiple sinuses.

Orifice

- A sinus containing a foreign body or sequestrum in depth may have pouting granulation tissue ("proud flesh") at the opening of the sinus.
- A tuberculous sinus is usually wide and has a thin blackish and undermined edge.

Discharge

- An osteomyelitic sinus discharges pus.
- A tuberculous sinus discharges thin watery pus that may have curdy flakes.
- The discharge of an actinomycotic sinus has "sulfur granules."

Fixity

- An osteomyelitic sinus is fixed to the underlying bone which is thickened and tender.
- A tuberculous sinus may be fixed to enlarged, matted lymph nodes or a bone (Fig. 4.2).

Regional Lymph Nodes

- In a tuberculous sinus, the regional lymph nodes are enlarged, firm, and matted.
- In an actinomycotic sinus, the lymph nodes are not enlarged.

Investigations

Laboratory Tests

- The blood is examined for hemoglobin, counts, and ESR.
- The discharge of the sinus is examined by smear and culture. Most of the organisms that are isolated are skin organisms or gut com-

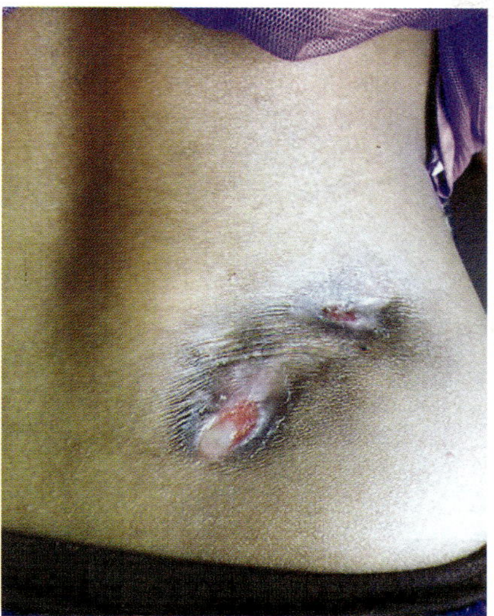

Figure 4.2 Two sinuses with pigmentation around the back of right sacroiliac joint region due to tuberculosis of right sacroiliac joint. The sinus is relatively large with undermined edge.

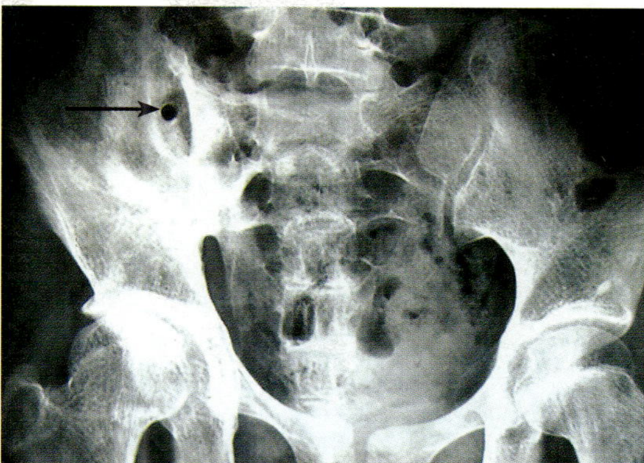

Figure 4.3 Anteroposterior radiograph of pelvis showing destruction of right sacroiliac joint with a hole in the affected bone due tuberculosis. The right part of pelvic brim in deformed. It is radiograph of the patient shown in **Figure 4.2**.

mensals, but the causative organism may also be found.
- In a suspected tuberculous sinus, if the culture is negative, then a DNA–RNA amplification for tuberculosis may be done.

Radiography
- Sinography is done by injecting Hypaque (angiographin 45) into the sinus. It reveals the depth, direction, and branching of the sinus tract. The pictures may be taken with image intensification. If a cavity is found, X-ray is taken in two planes.
- In an osteomyelitic sinus, the related bone is radiographed (Fig. 4.3).
- Sometimes a CT scan or MRI is required to study the total pathology of the lesion.

Biopsy For etiological diagnosis, biopsy of the sinus is required.

Probing Probing may be done with a malleable probe to know the depth and direction of the sinus, and the presence of a foreign body or a sequestrum. It must be done gently so as not to create a false passage. Instead of a probe, a very fine radio-opaque polythene catheter may be passed till its progress is halted and then a radiograph is taken to see its depth and direction. Ideally, probing should be avoided as far as possible.

Clinical features of common sinuses

Tuberculous Sinus

- **Site:** It can occur anywhere in the body, but the common sites are neck, axilla, groin, iliac fossa (Fig. 4.4), or near a bone or joint.
- **Other clinical features:** The patient is usually a young person who presents with a single or multiple openings that discharge thin syrup-like pus which may have curdy flakes. The openings are relatively wide with a thin bluish undermined edge. They are fixed to an enlarged lymph node or a bone which may be tender. The regional lymph nodes may be enlarged and matted.

Osteomyelitic Sinus

- **Site:** It occurs near the end of a long bone discharging pus.

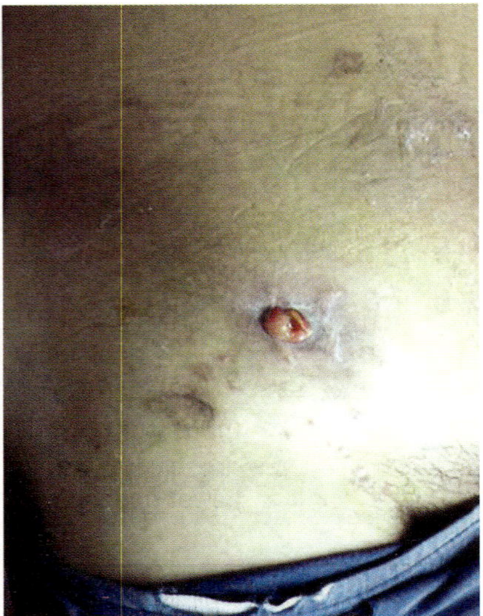

Figure 4.4 Sinus right iliac fossa just above the inguinal ligament following evacuation of a psoas abscess.

- **Other clinical features:** A history of discharge of small chips of bone from the sinus may be present. The sinus is fixed to the underlying bone which is thickened and tender. Pouting granulation tissue may be present at the mouth of the sinus.

Preauricular Sinus

- **Site:** The common site is preauricular region near the root of helix or tragus.
- **Other clinical features:** The patient is usually young and presents with a sinus, ulcer, abscess, or cyst in the preauricular region. A very tiny pit is present at the root of helix or tragus in which if a Prolene suture is passed it passes downwards and forwards for a short distance and then stops.

Median Mental Sinus

- **Site:** It occurs on or just below the chin in midline.
- **Other clinical features:** The patient is usually young and has a well-developed bifid type of chin. The sinus is usually nontender, is fixed to the mandible, and discharges a small amount of seropurulent fluid. Figure 4.5 depicts a median mental sinus of long duration with pouting granulation tissue at the sinus orifice. The sinus is fixed to the mandible which is tender on deep pressure (may be due to secondary infection).

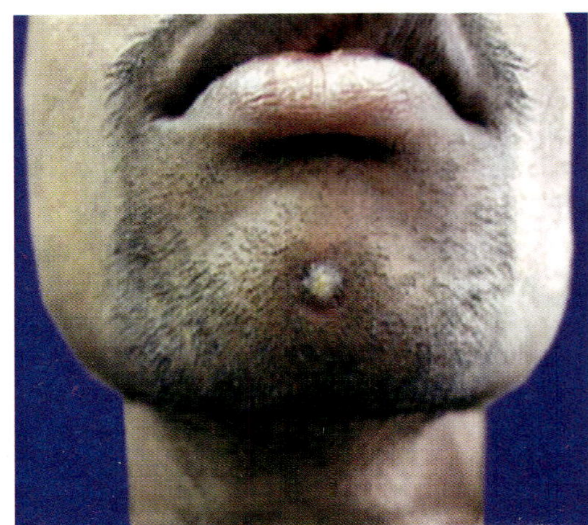

Figure 4.5 Median mental sinus with pouting granulation tissue.

Cervicofacial Actinomycotic Sinus

- **Site:** It occurs near the angle of the mandible, chest wall, or right lower abdomen.
- **Other clinical features:** It is characterized by a single or multiple sinuses with pus discharge containing sulfur granules. There is a mild swelling around the sinus or sinuses which is wooden hard in consistency. The regional lymph nodes are not enlarged.

Foreign Body Sinus

- **Site:** It occurs near the scar of a previous injury or operation.
- **Other clinical features:** It is a nonhealing sinus which discharges seropurulent or serosanguinous fluid. Pouting granulation tissue is usually present at the mouth of sinus ("proud flesh").

Injection Sinus

- **Site:** It occurs at the site of an injection, usually in the gluteal region or upper arm.
- **Other clinical features:** It is a complication that occurs usually in obese patients. There is single or multiple sinuses at the site of injection given some time ago. A history of spontaneous rupture or drainage of an injection abscess is present.

Treatment

The key to proper treatment of a sinus is detection of associated deep abscess cavity or complex deep extensions. Failure to do so results in persistence or recurrence of the disease at the same site or at an adjacent location.

Medical Treatment

- A tuberculous sinus may heal following antituberculous drug treatment (ATT).
- An actinomycotic sinus may heal following prolonged antibiotic therapy with penicillin, ampicillin, amoxicillin, or doxycycline.

Surgical Treatment

- Complete excision of sinus including the cavity or complex deep extensions and necrotic tissue is the treatment of choice in most of the sinuses. The excised tissue is sent for histopathological scrutiny. If the excision of total pathology is not possible, the sinus tract is laid open in its full course.
- In an osteomyelitic sinus the sequestrum is removed and the cavity is made shallow (saucerization).
- A foreign body sinus heals rapidly following removal of the foreign body.

The clinical features and management of some common sinuses are enumerated in Table 4.3 and schematically represented in Flowchart 4.1.

Table 4.3 Clinical features and treatment of common sinuses of head and neck region

Sinus	Site	Type of discharge	Clinical features	Treatment
Tuberculous sinus	Neck	Thin syrup-like and may have curdy flakes	May be fixed to enlarged, matted lymph nodes or underlying bone	• ATT • Excision of residual disease
Preauricular sinus	Root of helix or tragus of ear	Usually no discharge unless infected	May present as preauricular sinus, ulcer, abscess, or cyst	Symptomatic sinus is excised
Osteomyelitic sinus	At the end of a bone	Purulent, and may have bone chips	Fixed to underlying bone which is thickened and tender, and may have pouting granulation tissue	Sequestrectomy and saucerization
Cervicofacial actinomycotic sinus/sinuses	Near the angle of mandible	Thin pus with "sulfur" granules	• Bluish, wooden hard, and ill-defined swelling around the sinus/sinuses • No regional lymph node enlargement	• Penicillin G 10–20 million units parenterally for 4–6 weeks followed by oral penicillin V 500 mg four times daily • Pus drainage and excision of necrotic tissue
Median mental sinus	On or just below chin in midline	Small amount of seropurulent fluid	• Pouting granulation tissue at mouth of sinus • Usually nontender	Excision which may require extraction of lower incisors

ATT, antituberculous drug treatment.

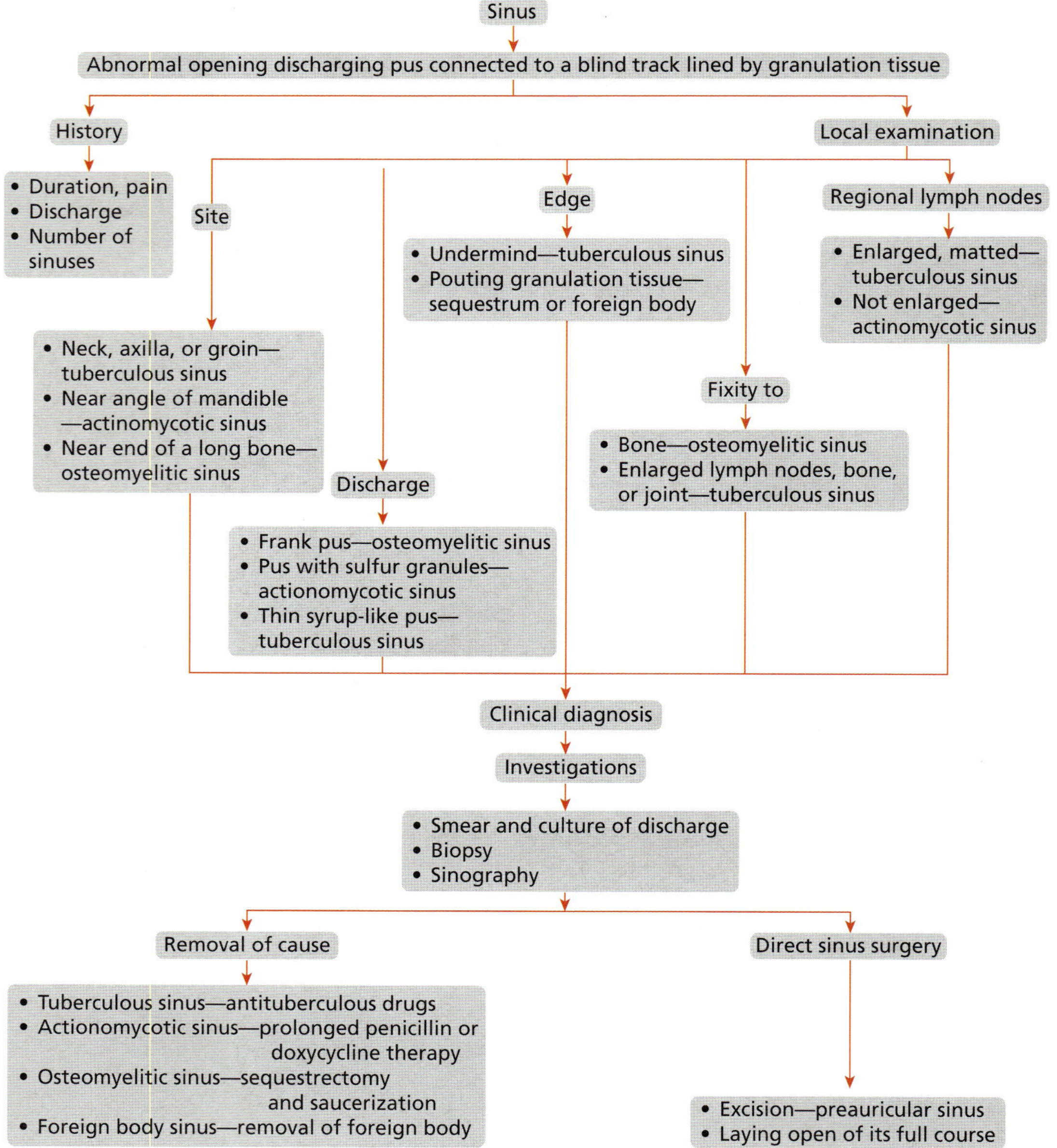

Flowchart 4.1 Clinical diagnosis and treatment of a sinus.

KEY POINTS

- Sinus is a blind-ending track usually lined by granulation tissue that leads from an epithelial surface into the tissues, usually into an abscess cavity with intermittent or continuous pus discharge.
- Sinuses can be congenital or acquired. Acquired sinuses are generally due to the presence of infection or a foreign body.
- A sinus containing a foreign body or sequestrum exhibits excessive granulation tissue projecting from sinus orifice called "proud flesh."

SELF-ASSESSMENT

Long answer question

1. What is a sinus? Describe its causes, diagnosis, and treatment.

Short answer questions

1. Sinus
2. Actinomycotic sinus
3. Preauricular sinus
4. Tuberculous sinus
5. Median mental sinus

Multiple choice questions

1. Which of the following is the commonest cause of multiple sinuses?
   (a) Tuberculosis
   (b) Hidradenitis suppurativa
   (c) Pyogenic osteomyelitis
   (d) Foreign body sinus
2. The edge of a tuberculous sinus is
   (a) Sharply cut
   (b) Sloping
   (c) Undermined
   (d) Everted
3. The discharge from an actinomycotic sinus is
   (a) Pus containing "sulfur granules"
   (b) Bluish green in color
   (c) Sanguinous
   (d) Thin syrup-like pus
4. Pouting granulation tissue from the mouth of a sinus is indicative of
   (a) Tuberculosis
   (b) Actinomycosis
   (c) Foreign body in the depth of sinus
   (d) Hidradenitis suppurativa
5. All of the following statements are true about a tuberculous sinus, except
   (a) It is a chronic sinus that has an undermined edge
   (b) It discharges pus having "sulfur" granules
   (c) It has a bluish pigmented edge
   (d) It may be fixed to underlying enlarged and matted lymph nodes
6. An adolescent patient presents with a recurrent small ulcer in front of tragus. In addition to this, there is a tiny shallow pit present at the root of helix or tragus. What is the clinical diagnosis?
   (a) Tuberculous sinus
   (b) Cervicofacial actinomycosis
   (c) Osteomyelitic sinus of mandible
   (d) Preauricular sinus
7. All of the following statements are true about actinomycotic sinus, except
   (a) The patient presents with a single or multiple sinuses near the angle of mandible
   (b) It/they discharges/discharge pus containing "sulfur" granules
   (c) There is mild diffuse local swelling which is wooden hard in consistency
   (d) The regional lymph nodes are enlarged and matted
8. All of the following facts are true about an osteomyelitic sinus of mandible, except
   (a) There is a sinus near the angle of mandible
   (b) It has an undermined pigmented edge
   (c) The sinus is fixed to the mandible which is thickened and tender on deep pressure
   (d) Pouting granulation tissue may be present at the mouth of the sinus
9. Sinography is defined as
   (a) Visualization of sinus tract by injecting methylene blue
   (b) Visualization by plain radiography
   (c) Radiographic visualization after injecting radio-opaque contrast into the sinus
   (d) MRI of sinus
10. All of the following statements are true about sinography, except
   (a) It is radiographic visualization of a sinus tract
   (b) Radiography is done after injecting contrast into sinus
   (c) It tells about the depth, direction, and branching of sinus tract
   (d) It always helps in the etiological diagnosis

Answers

1. (a) 2. (c) 3. (a) 4. (c) 5. (b) 6. (d) 7. (d) 8. (b) 9. (c) 10. (d)

Fistulae

5

Definition

A fistula is an abnormal communication between two epithelial surfaces. Its track may be lined by granulation tissue or epithelium.

Types of fistula

A fistula is of two types: external and internal.

- **External fistula**: An internal organ opens on the skin (Fig. 5.1).
- **Internal fistula**: Two adjacent hollow organs communicate contiguously or through a tube or cavity (Fig. 5.2).

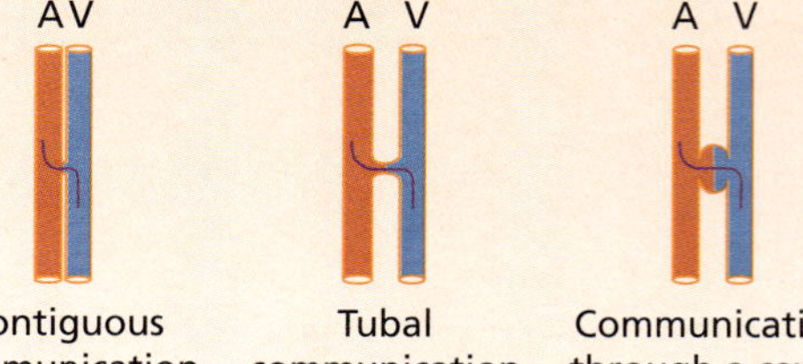

Figure 5.2 Internal fistulae: three types of arteriovenous fistula.

Etiology of fistula

- Congenital fistula
  - Tracheoesophageal fistula
  - Rectovesical fistula
  - Branchial fistula
  - Patent ductus arteriosus
- Traumatic fistula
  - Arteriovenous fistula following penetrating trauma
  - Vesicovaginal fistula following prolonged labor
- Infective or inflammatory fistula
  - Enterovesical fistula due to Crohn's disease
  - Bronchopleural fistula in empyema thoracis
  - Colovesical fistula in colonic diverticulitis
- Neoplastic fistula
  - Orocutaneous fistula in carcinoma of cheek
  - Tracheoesophageal fistula in carcinoma of esophagus
  - Gastrocolic fistula in carcinoma of stomach
  - Colovesical fistula in carcinoma of sigmoid colon

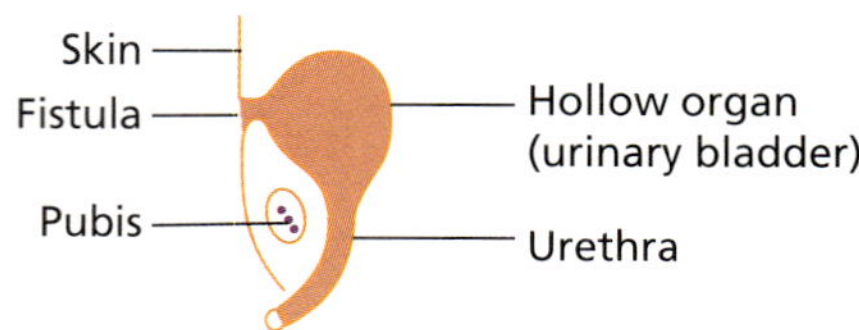

Figure 5.1 External fistula.

- Iatrogenic fistula
  - Intentional, for example, iliac colostomy for fecal diversion, ureterosigmoidostomy for urinary diversion, tracheostomy, feeding jejunostomy
  - Accidental, for example, salivary fistula following parotid abscess drainage, ureterovaginal fistula following hysterectomy, oroantral fistula following lateral maxillary teeth extraction

Clinical features

- A congenital fistula is present since birth.
- A traumatic fistula occurs following open or penetrating injuries.
- An external fistula is characterized by an abnormal opening on the skin which discharges the contents of the internal organ communicating with it. For example, an oroantral fistula is characterized by nasal regurgitation of swallowed liquids. The external fistula is visible on the body surface. It is mainly diagnosed by noting the site of external hole and the nature of discharge. Clinical features of some external fistulae of head and neck region are given in Table 5.1.
- In internal fistula, the abnormal communication is not visible but the patient has some symptoms of internal leak. The internal fistula cannot be clinically seen. Examples include leakage of urine from vagina in ureterovaginal and vesicovaginal fistulae, flatus and feces in urine in enterovesical and colovesical fistulae, and attacks of coughing and cyanosis following feeding in a neonate having congenital tracheoesophageal fistula.

Investigations

Laboratory Studies The blood is examined for hemoglobin, counts, and ESR. In an external fistula the discharge from the external opening is examined and in an internal fistula the discharge of communicating organs is examined. For example, if the intestine or rectum is joined to a urinary organ, the urine may contain traces of feces and is grossly infected with bowel bacteria such as *Escherichia coli*.

Radiography Fistulography may be done to image the anatomy of the fistulae. In an internal fistula, one of the affected organs or tubes is filled with contrast and X-rays are taken, for example, arteriovenous fistula by arteriography and colovesical fistula by cystography or barium enema. In the radiographs, the site, size, and nature of abnormal communication are seen. CT scan or MRI may be done to image the total pathology of fistula.

Biopsy Biopsy of the fistula is required to diagnose the cause of fistula. In an external fistula, it is easier to perform biopsy. In an internal fistula, endoscopic biopsy is performed.

Clinical features of common fistulae of head and neck region

Parotid Salivary Fistula

- **Site:** The common site is the parotid region.
- **Other clinical features:** It is an abnormal opening that discharges watery fluid which increases at the time of meals. A history of operation or trauma in the parotid region is usually present.

Table 5.1 Clinical features of some external fistulae of head and neck region

Type of external fistula	Location of fistula	Clinical features
Parotid salivary fistula	Parotid region	Discharges watery fluid especially during chewing tasty foods
Thyroglossal fistula	Midline of upper neck related to the body of hyoid bone	Discharges a small amount of mucoid fluid
Branchial fistula	Lower neck at the anterior border of sternomastoid	Discharges a small amount of mucoid or mucopurulent fluid

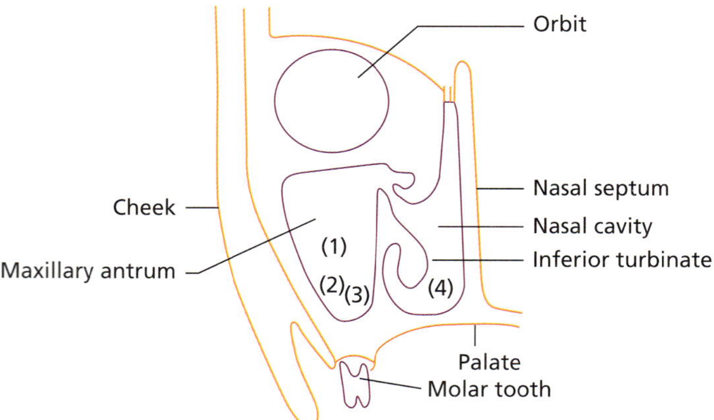

Figure 5.3 Line diagram of right midface showing various types of fistulae related to maxillary antrum, oral cavity, and nose.

Fistulae Related to Maxillary Antrum

They can be external (antrocutaneous fistula) or may be internal type. They are depicted in Figure 5.3.

Antrocutaneous fistula

- **Site:** The common site is the prominence of cheek.
- **Other clinical features:** Abnormal opening fixed to maxilla which discharges a small amount of mucoid fluid. A history of direct trauma is usually available.

Oroantral fistula

- **Site:** The common site is the floor of an extracted tooth.
- **Other clinical features:** The patient presents with nasal regurgitation of liquid food or recurrent attacks of unilateral maxillary sinusitis. A history of lateral maxillary tooth extraction or trauma may be present. The abnormal opening may be visible in the floor of a tooth socket. Air can be seen hissing out of the abnormal opening when the patient is asked to blow the closed nose.

Pharyngeal Fistula

- **Site:** It occurs in the lateral neck.
- **Other clinical features:** There is a history of neck trauma or operation. The abnormal opening in the side of neck discharges saliva all the time and foods and drinks immediately after swallowing. The patient loses weight rapidly and becomes anemic.

Tracheal Fistula

- **Site:** It occurs in the lower front of neck in midline.
- **Other clinical features:** It follows tracheostomy and cut-throat injury. It sucks in air during inspiration and discharges it during expiration. The voice of the patient is muffled.

Branchial Fistula

Branchial fistula is an abnormal communication between the pharynx and the exterior of neck due to persistence of second branchial cleft, the occluding membrane of which is broken.

Anatomy of branchial fistula

The fistula opening is present in the lower neck connected to fistulous tract surrounded by muscle fibers and is lined by ciliated epithelium. It passes between glossopharyngeal and hypoglossal nerves, stylopharyngeus and stylohyoid muscles, and two divisions of common carotid artery. It usually terminates in the lateral pharyngeal wall. Sometimes it may end up in the tonsillar fossa (Fig. 5.4).

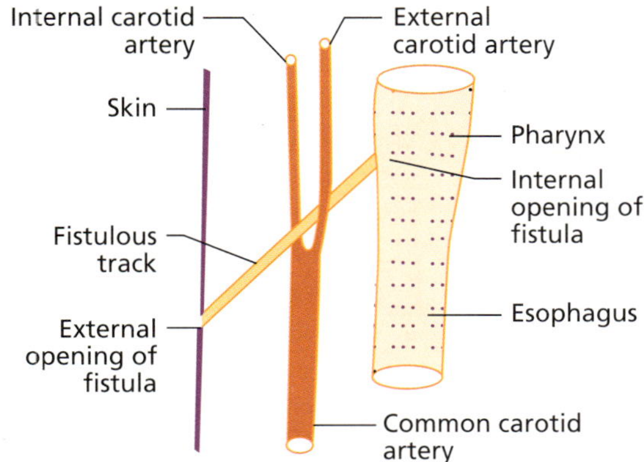

Figure 5.4 Anatomy of branchial fistula.

Clinical features

The patient is usually a child or an adolescent person who presents with an abnormal opening in neck situated at the anterior border of sternocleidomastoid (Fig. 5.5). It discharges a small amount of mucoid fluid (Fig. 5.6). If its orifice is lifted up and pulled, a cord-like structure appears to pass from it in upward direction.

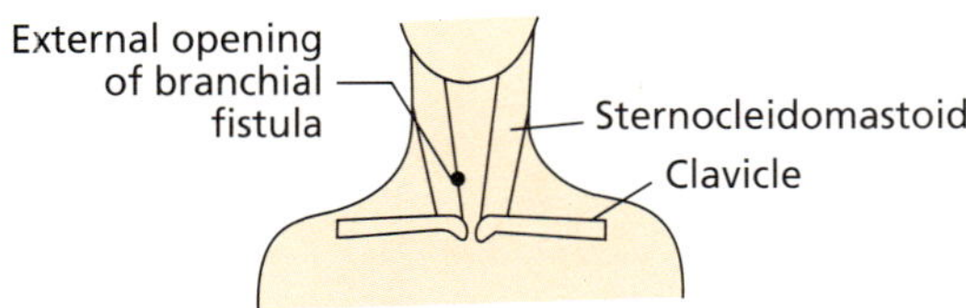

Figure 5.5 External orifice of right branchial fistula.

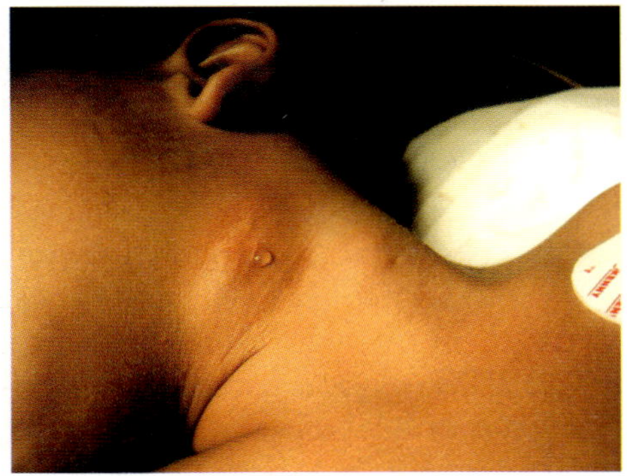

Figure 5.6 Branchial fistula: a drop of serous discharge visible at its opening. (Courtesy: Professor J.D. Rawat)

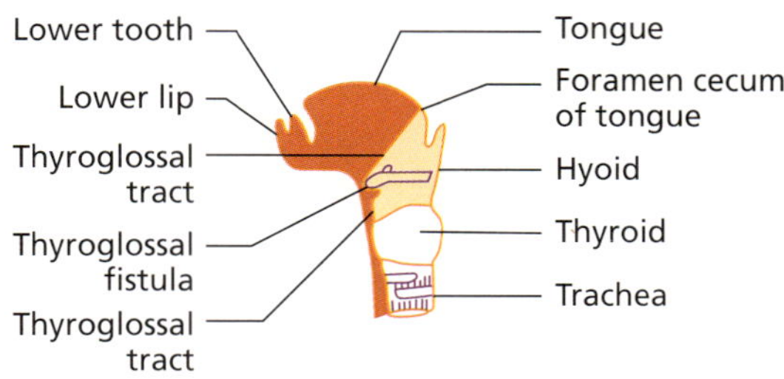

Figure 5.7 Anatomy of thyroglossal fistula.

Investigations

- The track may be visualized by fistulography and MRI.

Thyroglossal Fistula

Thyroglossal fistula is an abnormal opening in the neck connected to persistent embryonic thyroglossal duct. It is the result of rupture or incision into an infected thyroglossal cyst.

Anatomy of thyroglossal fistula

From the skin opening, the fistula track passes upwards behind the hyoid bone for a little way and then curves down its lower border to reach its anterior surface and to pass upwards in front of it and then upwards and backwards in midline to be lost in tissues or to open at foramen cecum of tongue (Fig. 5.7).

Clinical features

The patient is usually a young person who presents with an abnormal opening in the upper neck in the anterior midline, a little to the left (Fig. 5.8). Thyroglossal fistula discharges a small amount of mucoid or mucopurulent fluid. It has a semilunar hood of skin at the upper edge with concavity downwards. It moves up with deglutition and protrusion of tongue.

Investigation

Fistulography shows the fistula track going upwards and posteriorly toward the foramen cecum of tongue.

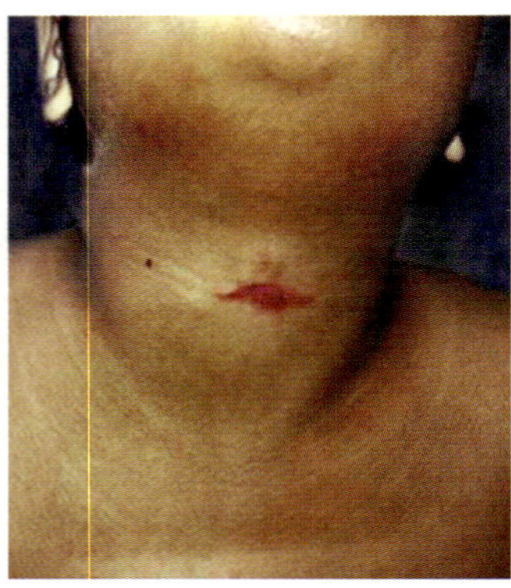

Figure 5.8 Thyroglossal fistula. (Courtesy: Professor Sandeep Tewari)

Treatment of fistulae

- **Congenital fistula**: It is usually treated by complete excision of tract and repair of defects.
- **Acquired acute fistula**: It may close without operation provided there is no distal obstruction, for example, a tracheostomy opening closes spontaneously soon after the tracheostomy tube is removed.
- **Acquired chronic fistula**: It usually does not heal spontaneously due to many reasons such as distal obstruction, epithelialization of fistula tract, tuberculosis, and malignancy. It requires removal of cause, that is, removal of distal obstruction, treatment of tuberculosis in a tuberculous fistula, and excision of epithelialized fistula tract and wide excision of a cancerous fistula.
- **Branchial fistula**: The complete fistula track is excised by two parallel transverse incisions in the creases of neck (stepladder operation). The complications of operation include bleeding, wound infection, scarring, recurrence, and injury to glossopharyngeal and hypoglossal nerves and carotid vessels.
- **Thyroglossal fistula**: The complete track is excised with the central part of hyoid bone in continuity (Sistrunk's operation) to prevent recurrence.

A comprehensive outline of the management of common fistulae of the head and neck is given in Table 5.2 and schematically represented in Flowchart 5.1.

Table 5.2 Management of common fistulae of head and neck region

Fistula	Site	Discharge	Other features	Treatment
Parotid salivary fistula	Abnormal opening in the parotid region	Watery fluid which increases during meals	Skin around the opening may be inflamed	• Saliva reduction • Duct fistula—repaired or parotidectomy
Antrocutaneous fistula	Abnormal hole of prominence of cheek fixed to maxilla	Mucoid fluid	May have features of maxillary sinusitis	Surgical repair
Oroantral fistula	Abnormal opening is molar tooth socket with air hissing during Valsalva maneuver	Cannot be appreciated	Nasal regurgitation of liquid food	Closure by a gum flap
Thyroglossal fistula	Abnormal opening in midline of neck below the body of hyoid bone	Small amount of serous or mucoid discharge	• Hood of skin in the upper part • Pulled up on protrusion of tongue • Seen in a young person	Excision of fistula with body of hyoid bone
Branchial fistula	Abnormal opening in lower neck at anterior border of sternomastoid	Mucoid or mucopurulent discharge	• May be bilateral • Seen in a child or a young person	Excision of fistula track by stepladder dissection

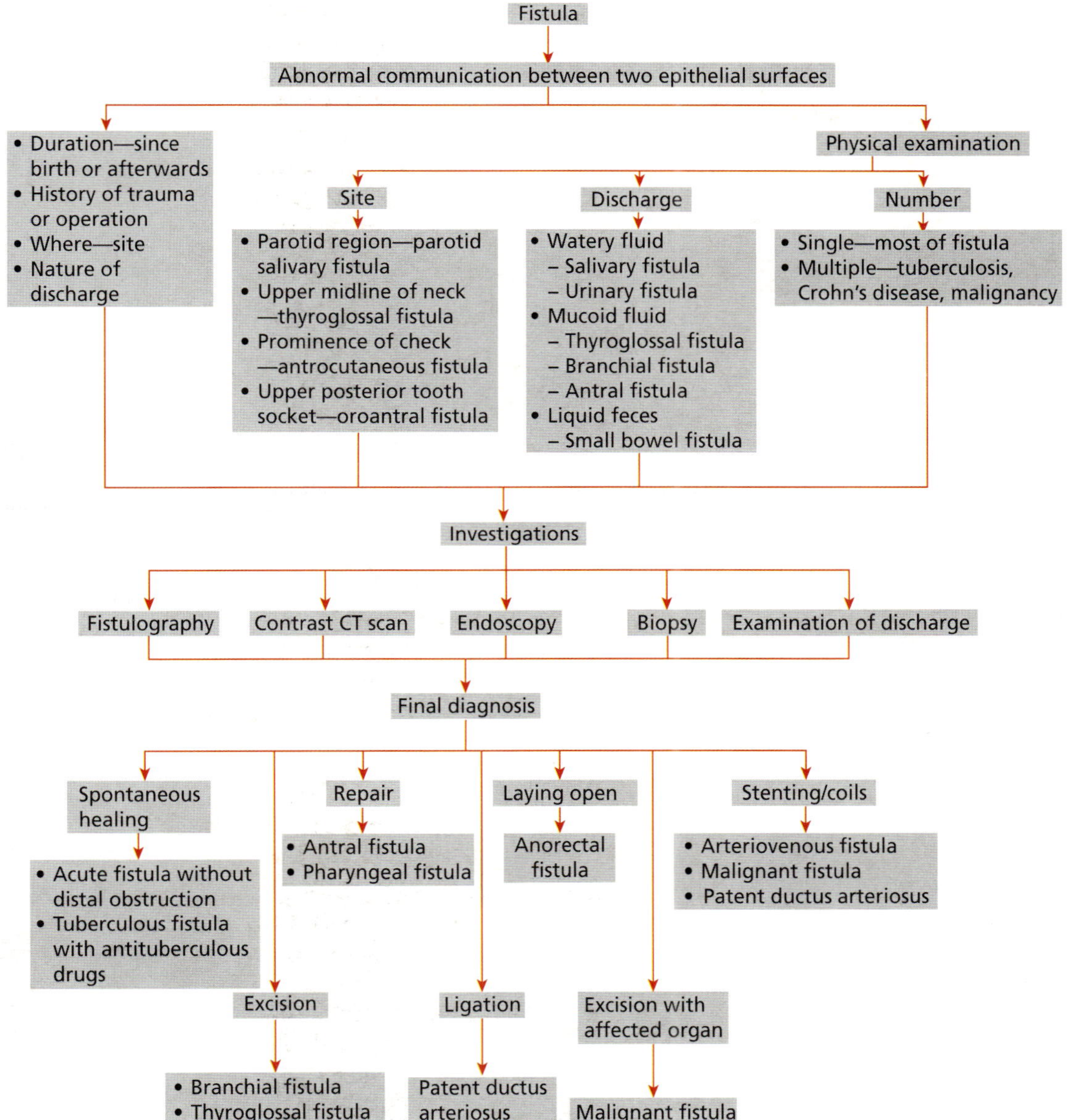

Flowchart 5.1 Management of a fistula.

Causes of persistence or nonclosure of a fistula

The treatment of a fistula may be very difficult and may result in repeated recurrences. Hence, one must know the causes of persistence or nonclosure so as to eliminate them while treating a fistula. The causes are:

- Fistula lined partially or completely by epithelium
- Presence of distal obstruction
- Infections such as tuberculosis or a fistula associated with malignancy
- Presence of a significant amount of irritating discharge, for example, bowel contents

KEY POINTS

- Fistula is an abnormal communication between two epithelial surfaces. Its track may be lined by granulation tissue or epithelium.
- Internal fistula is communication between two hollow organs. External fistula is communication with an internal organ and the skin.
- Fistulae can be congenital, traumatic, infective, neoplastic, and iatrogenic.
- External fistulae are diagnosed based on the location and the nature of discharge. Internal fistulae are difficult to diagnose as they are not clinically visible.
- Antrocutaneous fistula and oroantral fistula are the common fistulae associated with maxillary antrum. History of tooth extraction or trauma is a common feature in antral fistulae.
- Branchial fistula is an abnormal communication between the pharynx and the exterior of neck due to persistence of second branchial cleft. It presents as an abnormal opening in neck situated at the anterior border of sternocleidomastoid discharging mucoid fluid. Treatment is complete excision of the fistulous tract (stepladder operation).
- Thyroglossal fistula is an abnormal opening in the neck connected to persistent embryonic thyroglossal tract and presents as an abnormal opening in the upper neck in the anterior midline, a little to the left with mucoid or mucopurulent discharge. The fistula moves up with deglutition and protrusion of tongue. Sistrunk's operation is the treatment of choice.
- Fistulogram is performed to image a fistula. Biopsy of the fistula is important to diagnosis the cause of the fistula, for example, inflammatory or malignant.
- Treatment of fistula is removal of cause and complete excision of the fistulous tract.

SELF-ASSESSMENT

Long answer question

1. Define a fistula. Describe its etiology, pathology, clinical features, and treatment.

Short answer questions

1. Oroantral fistula
2. Branchial fistula
3. Thyroglossal fistula
4. Causes of nonhealing of a fistula

Multiple choice questions

1. Which of the following is the commonest cause of persistence or nonclosure of a fistula?
   (a) Persistent infection
   (b) Tuberculosis
   (c) Passing a significant amount of irritating discharge
   (d) Fistula tract lined by epithelium
2. The branchial fistula is a
   (a) Manifestation of cervical lymph node tuberculosis
   (b) Infective disease
   (c) Developmental defect
   (d) Manifestation of cervicofacial actinomycosis
3. A branchial fistula discharges
   (a) Greenish pus
   (b) Thin syrup-like pus in plenty
   (c) Small amount of mucoid fluid
   (d) Sanguinous fluid
4. The external opening of a branchial fistula is situated
   (a) In the midline of neck below the body of hyoid bone
   (b) At the anterior border of sternomastoid in the lower neck
   (c) Near the angle of mandible
   (d) In suprasternal notch
5. A thyroglossal fistula is a
   (a) Manifestation of cervical lymph node tuberculosis
   (b) Infective disease
   (c) Developmental defect
   (d) Manifestation of cervicofacial actinomycosis
6. The external opening of a thyroglossal fistula is situated
   (a) In midline of neck below the body of hyoid bone
   (b) At anterior border of sternomastoid in lower neck
   (c) Near the angle of mandible
   (d) In suprasternal notch

Answers

1. (d) 2. (c) 3. (c) 4. (b) 5. (c) 6. (a)

Inflammation and Surgical Infections

6

1. INFLAMMATION

Definition

Inflammation is the clinicopathological response of the body tissues to any type of injury which may be microbial, mechanical, thermal, electrical, or irradiational. It is the commonest of all the pathological processes of the body.

Causes of inflammation

Inflammation is essentially a microvascular phenomenon caused by microbial, mechanical, thermal, electrical, or irradiation insult to the tissues of the body.

Microbial Cause Invasion of tissues by microorganisms is the commonest cause of inflammation. It calls for much phagocytic activity by leukocytes, as well as large outpouring of fluid in the tissues due to interaction between powerful toxins produced by bacteria and the enzymes produced by leukocytes to dilute and neutralize them and subsequently to control infection.

Mechanical Cause Inflammation by mechanical cause is less intense and the predominant cell that is required will be for removal of dead tissue followed by its repair and replacement. The same happens in thermal, electrical, and irradiational inflammation.

Pathogenesis of inflammation

Inflammation is basically a defensive phenomenon which brings phagocytes, antibodies, and other mediators to the site of inflammation to neutralize and dilute the irritant or causative agent. The methods by which the host defense mechanism limits the progress of inflammation are given in Box 6.1.

Inflammation is more or less the same whether it occurs in the soft tissues or hard tissues, that is, bone. The inflammatory process in bone is given as a schematic representation in Box 6.2. It is nearly always due to infection.

Types of inflammation

Acute Inflammation It is of acute onset and short duration and is characterized by local vasodilatation, congestion, edema, and polymorphonuclear leukocyte infiltration.

Chronic Inflammation It is of long duration and gradual onset and is characterized by lymphocyte and plasma cell infiltration and fibrosis. It occurs when the injury is less severe, or the infection is of low virulence and the resistance of the host is good, or when the acute inflammation is subsiding.

Box 6.1 Methods by which host defense mechanism limits the progress of inflammation

- Inflammatory edema
- Limitation of spread of inflammation by fibrin formation
- Walling off with granulation tissue and fibrosis
- Completion of reparative process by scarring

The differences between acute and chronic inflammation are given in Table 6.1.

Granulomatous Inflammation It is a specific type of chronic inflammation characterized by granuloma formation with predominant proliferation of histiocytes. It is commonly seen in tuberculosis and syphilis.

Clinical features of inflammation

The classical local features of **acute inflammation** are:

- **Dolor (pain)**: There is pain at the local site which is usually associated with pain on touching or pressing (tenderness).
- **Tumor (swelling)**: The site of inflammation swells up to present as a swelling.
- **Rubor (redness)**: The site of inflammation becomes red due to increased vascularity.
- **Calor (heat)**: Due to increased vascularity, the local site feels warmer than normal.

Because of redness and increased temperature, this process is called inflammation which means burning.

- **Functio laesa (loss of function)**: Because of acute pain and swelling, the affected part loses its function.

Chronic inflammation may be asymptomatic or may have a variable combination of the above-mentioned features in a milder form.

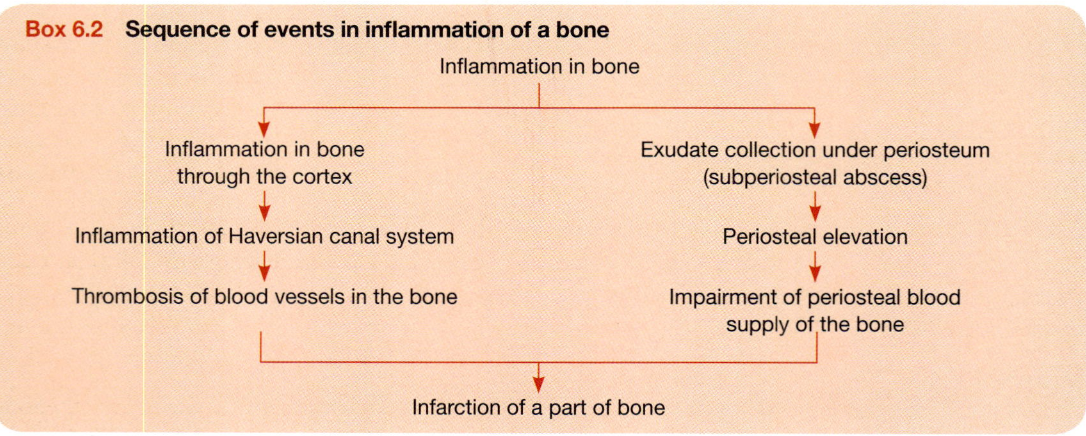

Table 6.1 Differences between acute and chronic inflammation

Characteristics	Acute inflammation	Chronic inflammation
Duration	Short—hours and days	Long—weeks and months
Onset	Acute	Gradual
Inflammatory cells	Polymorphonuclear leukocytes	Lymphocytes, plasma cells
Virulence	High	Low
Host resistance	Low	High
Host response	Local vasodilatation, congestion, edema	Plasma cell infiltration and fibrosis
Outcome	• Tissue destruction • Pus formation • Healing	• Tissue destruction • Granuloma formation • Healing

Outcome of inflammation

The inflammatory response may result in:

- Resolution: Spontaneous disappearance of the inflammation or following treatment with restoration of tissues to normal or near normal
- Tissue necrosis: The inflammation may result in local tissue necrosis which may lead to:
  - Liquefaction of necrotic tissue with pus formation
  - Sloughing of necrotic tissue followed by ulceration
  - Superadded putrefaction leading to gangrene of the affected part
  - Systemic response characterized by fever, toxemia, tachycardia, halitosis, and coated tongue, which is called systemic inflammatory response syndrome (SIRS)
- Acute inflammation turning into chronic inflammation
- Formation of an inflammatory granuloma

Treatment of inflammation

- **Removal of the cause:** The cause of inflammation must be removed or treated, for example, antibiotics are given to control infection.
- **Symptomatic treatment:** Anti-inflammatory analgesic drugs such as ibuprofen and diclofenac are given to relieve pain. The elevation of the affected part to relieve edema, local fomentation, and use of anti-inflammatory creams may be useful.
- **Surgical treatment**: If there is pus formation or necrosis of tissues, it usually requires drainage of pus or excision of necrotic tissue.

2. INFECTIONS

Definition

Infection is the invasion of body tissues by pathogenic microorganisms, and the reaction of tissues to their presence and toxins produced by them is called inflammation.

Risk factors for increased infection

These include hyperglycemia, corticosteroids, loss of general health, advanced cancer, acquired immune deficiency syndrome (AIDS), and use of anticancer drugs.

Microorganisms

We live in an ocean of bacteria in the environment around us with bacteria present in many body cavities, that is, oral cavity, gastrointestinal tract, nose, vagina, and external ear. Majority of these bacteria are harmless commensals and only a few are harmful or pathogenic. There is normally a bacteriological balance between commensals and pathogenic bacteria. Disturbance of this balance

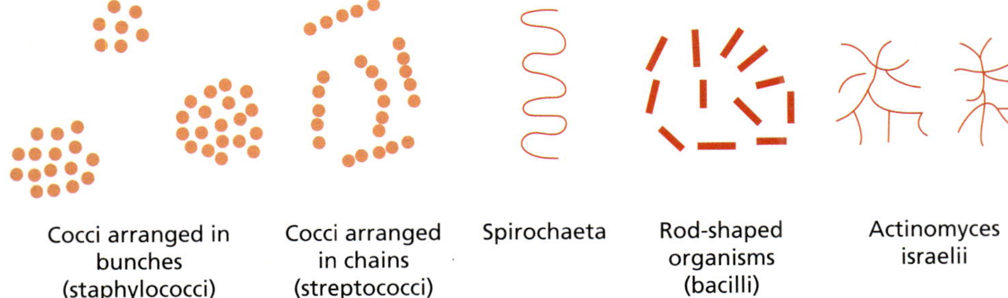

Figure 6.1 Common morphological types of bacteria.

is responsible for infective diseases. The common morphological types of bacteria are depicted in Figure 6.1.

Staphylococcus aureus

- *S. aureus* is a Gram-positive facultative anaerobe occurring in grape-like clusters. This bacterium is normally a commensal found in anterior nares, nasopharynx, and moist areas of skin.
- It produces:
  - Aflatoxin which is hemolytic, leukocidal, and cytotoxic
  - Enzyme coagulase which converts fibrinogen to fibrin and is responsible for localization of infection caused by this bacterium and pus formation
  - Enterotoxin, which if ingested with meat causes food poisoning
- Infections caused by *S. aureus* include furuncle, carbuncle, abscess, impetigo, paronychia, osteomyelitis, and wound infection.
- Antibiotics for treating *S. aureus* infection:
  - Empirical antibiotics: Pending the report of culture and sensitivity, the staphylococcal infection is treated with cloxacillin, flucloxacillin, or a first-generation cephalosporin.
  - For patients allergic to penicillin, the alternative drugs are gentamicin, vancomycin, clindamycin, fucidin, and erythromycin.
  - If the organism is sensitive to penicillin, benzyl penicillin can be given parenterally.
  - *S. aureus* has a tendency to develop resistance to antibiotics [methicillin-resistant *S. aureus* (MRSA)] due to production of β-lactamase. It destroys the β-lactam ring of penicillin molecule and makes it ineffective.

Staphylococcus epidermidis (Staphylococcus albus)

It is a harmless commensal residing in skin, anterior nares, and mouth. It does not produce aflatoxin or coagulase and is not pathogenic normally, but it may produce opportunistic infection such as central venous catheter–related sepsis.

Streptococcus haemolyticus (Streptococcus pyogenes)

- It is a Gram-positive facultative anaerobe.
- Virulence factors include hemolysin, streptokinase, and streptodornase. The latter two products are responsible for the characteristic spreading nature of streptococcal infections.
- Infections caused by *S. haemolyticus* include erysipelas, cellulitis, and acute tonsillitis.
- Antibiotic used for treating *S. haemolyticus* infection is penicillin (highly sensitive and there is no resistance to penicillin).

Streptococcus faecalis (Enterococcus)

It is a commensal of intestine of humans and animals. *Streptococcus faecalis* causes opportunistic infections of the urinary tract. It is resistant to many commonly used antibiotics.

Anaerobic *Streptococcus (Peptostreptococcus putridus)*

It is a Gram-positive obligate anaerobe that resides normally in vagina and intestine. Anaerobic

Streptococcus is responsible for synergistic bacterial gangrene and anaerobic streptococcal myositis. It is sensitive to penicillin.

Coliform Bacilli

Escherichia coli It is Gram-negative aerobe and a commensal of ileum and colon. *E. coli* is the commonest cause of urinary tract infection and infections related to intestinal tract such as appendicitis, peritonitis, and cholecystitis. It is sensitive to ampicillin, cephalosporins, and co-trimoxazole.

Klebsiella pneumoniae It is present in water supplies and intestine. It causes opportunistic infection. The hospital strains of this bacterium are multidrug resistant.

Proteus mirabilis It is a Gram-negative aerobe that is found in putrefying matter and water. *Proteus mirabilis* is a secondary invader of surgical wounds and bed sores, already infected by pyogenic cocci. It splits urea into ammonia. It is sensitive to aminoglycosides, third-generation cephalosporins, and quinolones.

Pseudomonas aeruginosa (Pseudomonas pyocyaneus)

- It is a Gram-negative strict aerobe.
- *Pseudomonas aeruginosa* is a hardy organism which may grow even in cetrimide and chloroxylenol. It is present in soil, sewage, and contaminated water.
- It infects the wounds and then produces a pigment pyocyanin which gives a bluish green tinge to slough and pus.

Bacteroides

- They are Gram-negative, strict anaerobic, nonsporulating coccobacilli which reside in colon, vagina, and oropharynx.
- *Bacteroides fragilis* is the main microorganism of this group which is commonly encountered in infections with anaerobic streptococci. It causes Vincent's angina, appendicitis, peritonitis, wound infection after intestinal operations, bacteremia, septicemia, and pyemia.
- It is sensitive to metronidazole and clindamycin, but resistant to aminoglycosides.

Clostridia

They are Gram-positive obligate anaerobes that produce resistant spores. Two bacteria of this group are *Clostridium perfringens* and *Clostridium tetani* that produce gas gangrene and tetanus, respectively.

Actinomyces israelii

- It has a central Gram-positive filamentous mass and radiating clubs which are Gram-negative. It grows on tissues as colonies which attain a size visible to naked eye as sulfur granules.
- *Actinomyces israelii* is present in the normal mouth as a harmless commensal, but may cause actinomycosis.
- It is sensitive to penicillin and tetracyclines.

Candida albicans

- It is a fungus and a part of normal flora of the mouth, intestine, and vagina.
- *Candida albicans* is an endogenous cause of opportunistic infections.
- It is sensitive to amphotericin B, 5-fluorocytosine, and clotrimazole.

Treatment of bacterial infections

As soon as the diagnosis is made, the infection must be treated to prevent complications, and the mainstay of the treatment is to use antibacterial drugs.

Selection of Antibacterial Drugs

- **Identification of the causative organism:** The treatment of surgical infections depends on identification of the causative organism and its sensitivity to various antibacterial drugs. It takes 24–48 hours for these data to be available. Hence, the initial treatment is started on the clinical impression of the causative organism and the prevailing sensitivity pattern in that hospital, and the status of the patient as a host. Subsequently when the report is available, the same antibiotic is continued or changed.

- **Immune status of the patient:**
  - The patient's status as a host is important in determining the choice of the antibiotic. Immunocompromised patients require immediate administration of parenteral bactericidal antibiotics.
  - In hepatic and renal diseases, the antibiotic has to be carefully chosen and the dosage should be modified to avoid toxicity.
  - One has to select an appropriate antibiotic when it has to be given during pregnancy, lactation, and childhood.
  - Drug allergy and toxicity also modify the choice of antibiotics.
- When more than one antibiotic is available to treat an infection, the cheaper and simpler drug should be selected.

Antimicrobial Drugs

These are the drugs which kill or stop the growth and proliferation of bacteria.

Sulfonamides

They are the earliest antibacterials that act by inhibiting the folic acid synthetase which converts para-aminobenzoic acid (PABA) to folic acid. Now they have a very limited use. Uses include:

- Silver sulfadiazine is used for dressing wounds, especially burns.
- Co-trimoxazole is a combination of trimethoprim and sulfamethoxazole (1:5), and is used to treat otitis media, sinusitis, and urinary tract infections. It is a drug of choice for *Pneumocystis carinii* infection in immunocompromised patients.

These drugs may cause pancytopenia, hypersensitivity, and hemolysis in patients with G6PD deficiency.

Penicillin

It is highly bactericidal against *S. pyogenes* and anaerobic *Streptococcus*. Only 25% of strains of staphylococci are sensitive to it. Penicillin is effective against Gram-positive anaerobes such as clostridia but not against *B. fragilis*. It has been used with success in the treatment of anthrax, actinomycosis, and syphilis.

Isoxazolyl penicillins

This group includes cloxacillin, methicillin, and flucloxacillin. They are penicillinase resistant, hence are active against β-lactamase–producing *S. aureus*. They are less effective against streptococci and ineffective against clostridia.

Aminopenicillins

This group includes ampicillin and amoxicillin. They are effective against Gram-negative organisms such as *E. coli*, *P. mirabilis*, and *S. faecalis*.

Carboxypenicillins and *ureidopenicillins*

They include carbenicillin, piperacillin, and ticarcillin. *Carboxypenicillins* and *ureidopenicillins* are specifically active against *Pseudomonas*, *Enterobacter*, *P. mirabilis*, and *B. fragilis*. They are used in combination with aminoglycosides to prevent emergence of resistant strains.

Adverse effects of penicillins

The commonest toxicity of penicillin and its derivatives is anaphylaxis. Methicillin can cause cholestatic jaundice and interstitial nephritis. The carboxypenicillins can cause bleeding due to platelet dysfunction.

Cephalosporins

- Structurally they are similar to penicillin. Hence, they share its hypersensitivity reactions.
- These antibiotics are excreted by kidneys. Hence, their doses have to be modified in renal insufficiency.
- They have a greatly extended activity against Gram-negative rods including many resistant strains. They act on Gram-negative bacilli and staphylococci. *S. faecalis* (*Enterococcus*) is resistant to them.
- Their successive generations have increasing efficacy against Gram-negative bacilli at the expense of staphylococcal coverage.

First-generation cephalosporins

The first generation includes cephalexin, cefradine, cephaloridine, cephalothin, and cefadroxil.

- They are very effective against MRSA, streptococci, and pneumococci.
- They are also effective against most strains of *E. coli*, *Klebsiella*, and *Proteus*.
- They are also effective against *Pseudomonas* and anaerobes.
- They are useful in surgical wound prophylaxis, urinary tract infections, and pneumonitis.

Second-generation cephalosporins

The second generation consists of cefoxitin, cefamandole, and cefuroxime. They have a broader Gram-negative coverage which includes *Haemophilus influenzae* and *Enterobacter*. Cefoxitin is also effective against *B. fragilis*.

Third-generation cephalosporins

The third generation includes cefsulodin, ceftazidime, cefoperazone, cefotaxime, moxalactam, and ceftriaxone. They have a long half-life requiring 8- to 12-hourly doses. The first three are strictly anti-*Pseudomonas*. Cefoperazone achieves high concentration in bile. Moxalactam is effective against *Bacteroides*.

Fourth-generation cephalosporins

The fourth generation consists of cefepime and cefpodoxime. They are given in twice-daily doses.

Aztreonam

It is a monocyclic β-lactam antibiotic (monobactam) which is effective against Gram-negative bacteria including *Pseudomonas* and *Serratia*. It is inactive against Gram-positive cocci and anaerobes.

Imipenem

It is a β-lactam antibiotic with a broad-spectrum activity against Gram-positive and Gram-negative bacteria and anaerobes. It is provided only in combination with enzyme inhibitor cilastatin which prevents its hydrolysis in kidneys and resultant nephrotoxic action. Meropenem is another drug in this group (carbapenems).

β-lactamase inhibitors

- Included under this group of drugs are sulbactam, clavulanate, and tazobactam.
- They inhibit the β-lactamase produced by *S. aureus*, *E. coli*, *Klebsiella*, and *B. fragilis*.
- The enzymes produced by *Pseudomonas*, *Serratia*, and *Enterobacter* are resistant to these drugs.
- Sulbactam is combined with ampicillin, clavulanic acid with amoxicillin, ticarcillin with ampicillin, and tazobactam with piperacillin.

Aminoglycosides

- This group includes gentamicin, amikacin, tobramycin, netilmicin, and streptomycin.
- They are effective against Gram-negative bacilli including *Pseudomonas* and inhibit most isolates of *S. aureus*.
- Aminoglycosides are susceptible to breakdown by plasmid-encoded bacterial enzymes.
- They are predominantly excreted by kidneys. Hence, their dose has to be adjusted (reduced) in renal insufficiency.
- They are otovestibulotoxic and nephrotoxic.

Macrolides

- This group includes erythromycin, roxithromycin, azithromycin, clarithromycin, and clindamycin.
- Erythromycin, roxithromycin, and azithromycin are substitutes of penicillin for streptococcal infections. They are also effective against most of the strains of *S. aureus*.
- Clindamycin is as effective as erythromycin. In addition, it is effective against anaerobes, especially *B. fragilis*. It can cause pseudomembranous colitis.
- Clarithromycin is used to control *Helicobacter pylori* in the treatment of peptic ulcer.
- The side effects include allergy, gastric irritation, and cholestasis.

Tetracyclines

They include chlortetracycline, oxytetracycline, demeclocycline, minocycline, and doxycycline. Tetracyclines are bacteriostatic and less commonly used now except doxycycline which is given 100 mg twice daily for 10–14 days.

Quinolones

This group includes nalidixic acid, norfloxacin, ciprofloxacin, pefloxacin, ofloxacin, lomefloxacin, sparfloxacin, levofloxacin, and gatifloxacin. They are effective against most strains of *S. aureus*, *Enterobacter*, and *Pseudomonas*.

Oxazolidinones

The first representative of this class is linezolid. It is a broad-spectrum antimicrobial and is available in both oral and parenteral forms.

Vancomycin

It inhibits synthesis of bacterial cell wall and is active against a variety of bacteria, especially staphylococci (methicillin resistant) and streptococci. It is absorbed poorly after oral administration, hence given parenterally, but can be given orally to treat pseudomembranous colitis.

Metronidazole

Besides its antiprotozoal action, it is active against Gram-negative anaerobes, especially *B. fragilis*. It has no activity against any aerobic or facultative pathogens. Hence, it must always be combined with a suitable antibiotic for full coverage. It leaves a metallic taste in mouth.

3. PREVENTION OF INFECTION DURING OPERATION

One of the very important dangers of an operation is wound infection. Hence, a substantial effort and vigilance is required to prevent this complication of surgery. It requires attention to meticulous details of sterilization of instruments and equipment, aseptic practices, and control of environment in the operating room and the wards. Definitions of important terminologies related to surgical infections are given in Box 6.3.

Box 6.3 Definitions related to surgical infections

- **Sepsis:** It is the presence of pathogenic microorganisms in the blood or other tissues, for example, bacteremia, septicemia, abscess, and carbuncle
- **Antisepsis:** It is the prevention of infection by inhibiting the growth of microorganisms. A chemical capable of doing antisepsis is called antiseptic
- **Asepsis:** It is the freedom from infection or prevention of contact of bacteria. Asepsis is the technique which is followed in doing all operative procedures
- **Sterilization:** It is the process of completely removing or destroying all microorganisms including spores from an object. Sterilization is the most essential requirement to do all operations
- **Antibiosis:** It is microbial antagonism in which one type of bacteria harms or kills another type through the production of a chemical known as antibiotic
- **Disinfection:** It refers to the act of freeing an object from pathogenic organisms
- **Surgical site infection (SSI):** It is the infection of an operative wound due to intraoperative contamination by bacteria. SSI is a major contributor to postoperative morbidity. It must be prevented by all possible measures

Sources of surgical infection

To prevent wound infection, it is important to know the sources of infection which may be either within the patient's body (endogenous) or outside environment (exogenous).

Endogenous Infection It is caused by the organisms which normally live in or on the human body as harmless commensals, for example, *S. epidermidis* in the skin, *S. aureus* in the nasopharynx, pneumococci in the oropharynx, and *E. coli* and fecal bacteria in the perineum. These organisms may infect the wound by direct contamination.

Exogenous Sources of Infection They include other patients, hospital personnel, instruments and equipment, dressing materials, and hospital environment (operating room and wards).

Nosocomial Infection It is a hospital-acquired exogenous infection. It is caused by bacteria which have acquired a degree of resistance to

Box 6.4 Mithicillin-resistant *Staphylococcus aureus*

- It is resistant to methicillin and other common antibiotics
- Vancomycin and linezolid are the drugs of choice to treat it

antibiotics and antiseptics in use in the hospital. MRSA (methicillin resistant staphylococcus aureus) is an example of nosocomial infection (Box 6.4). The infection is transmitted from one patient to another by airborne dust particles, by infected blankets and hospital linen, and by doctors, nurses, and other paramedical staff.

Factors contributing to surgical infections

- Diabetes mellitus, obesity, and immunocompromised due to any cause
- Prolonged hospital stay
- Bad personal hygiene
- Duration of operation—longer the duration, more the chances of infection
- Use of drainage tubes

Prevention of surgical infections

Prevention of infection of an operative wound is possible if the preventive measures vis-à-vis the patient, hospital personnel, and instruments and equipment are taken from the very beginning.

Prevention at the Patient's Level

- The patient's medical conditions such as diabetes mellitus and malnutrition are identified and well controlled before surgery.
- The part to be operated upon is shaved without cuts and scratches. The patient is given a bath on the morning of operation, and sent to the operating room in clean clothes.
- On the operating table, the part to be operated upon is cleaned with HiBiScrub or iodophor scrub (Hibitane or povidone–iodine + detergent, e.g., cetrimide) and then painted with povidone–iodine and allowed to dry for 2 minutes. Then the part is draped with sterile linen and covered with Steri-Drape.
- Antibiotic prophylaxis is given just before operation intravenously, if indicated.
- Endocarditis prophylaxis in dental surgery:
  - Some patients with cardiac conditions who undergo some dental procedure have an increased risk of infective endocarditis due to bacteremia during the manipulation of gingival tissues, periapical region of teeth, and perforation of oral mucosa. The cardiac conditions associated with high risk for infective endocarditis are given in Box 6.5. In these patients, to prevent infective endocarditis, antibiotics are given as a prophylactic measure (Table 6.2).

Box 6.5 Cardiac conditions associated with high risk of infective endocarditis

- Prosthetic cardiac valves or prosthetic material used for cardiac valve repair
- Previous infective endocarditis
- Repaired or unrepaired congenital heart disease
- Cardiac transplantation

Prevention at Treating Team's Level

- The personnel working in the operating room should change into operating room clothes and footwear.
- The hair is covered with a cap, and a mask covers the nose and mouth.
- The hands and forearms are scrubbed with HiBiScrub or iodophor followed by wearing a sterile gown and gloves. Important protocols to be observed when scrubbing are given in Box 6.6.
- Good operating technique is important to prevent infection, that is, gentle tissue handling, perfect hemostasis, bringing the drainage tube out through a separate incision, and closed system of drainage.

Table 6.2 Antibiotic regimen for infective endocarditis prophylaxis

Situation	Antibiotic	Regimen—single dose (30–60 minutes before the procedure)	
		Adults	Children
Oral route	Amoxicillin	2 g	50 mg/kg
Unable to take oral medication	Ampicillin or cefazolin or ceftriaxone	2 g IM or IV	50 mg/kg IM or IV
Allergic to penicillin or ampicillin (alternative oral drugs)	• Cefalexin • Clindamycin • Azithromycin	• 2 g • 600 mg • 500 mg	• 50 mg/kg • 20 mg/kg • 15 mg/kg
Allergic to penicillin or ampicillin (unable to take oral medication)	• Cefazolin or ceftriaxone • Clindamycin	• 1 g IM or IV • 600 mg IM or IV	• 50 mg IM or IV • 20 mg/kg IM or IV

Box 6.6 Protocol of surgical scrubbing

- Remove wrist watch, ring, and jewelry from hands and forearms
- Wear a head cap, mask, and eye protection
- Scrub hands and forearms, especially nails and deep skin creases, with 2% chlorhexidine or 5% povidone–iodine with a brush for 1–2 minutes
- Hands and forearms should be washed systematically three times, and then the hands held above the level of elbows
- Wet parts should be dried with a sterile towel from distal to proximal
- The top of the folded gown is held and allowed to unfold with inside facing the wearer
- Hands are inserted in the armholes and the gown is worn. It is tied at the back by an assistant
- Gloves are worn after catching everted cuff, without touching their outer surface
- Hands must remain above waist level at all times

- Aseptic no-touch technique should be used when changing dressing in the ward.
- Infection-prone patients are nursed in a separate cubicle (barrier nursing). Whatever is being used on the patient, for example, catheters, drip sets, tubes, syringes, and needles, should all be disposable, and must be properly disposed of after use.

Prevention at the Instruments and Equipment Level

At this level the infection is prevented by sterilization of all the instruments, equipment, and material used during the operation which means complete eradication of all microorganisms including spores.

Autoclaving

Autoclaving is the principal method of sterilization of surgical instruments, operating room linen, and many other items.

An autoclave (Fig. 6.2a and b) is a closed rectangular chamber of metal with a steam jacket surrounding it which uses pure steam under pressure for sterilization of instruments and linen. As higher steam pressures are used, higher temperatures (more than 100°C) are obtained when a shorter time is required for sterilization. Table 6.3 shows the temperature, pressure, and time relationship during autoclaving.

Table 6.3 Autoclave: temperature, pressure, and time relationship

Temperature (°C)	Pressure of steam (lb/in^2)	Time required (minutes)	Holding time (minutes)
132	27	2	3
121	15	12	18
115	10	30	45

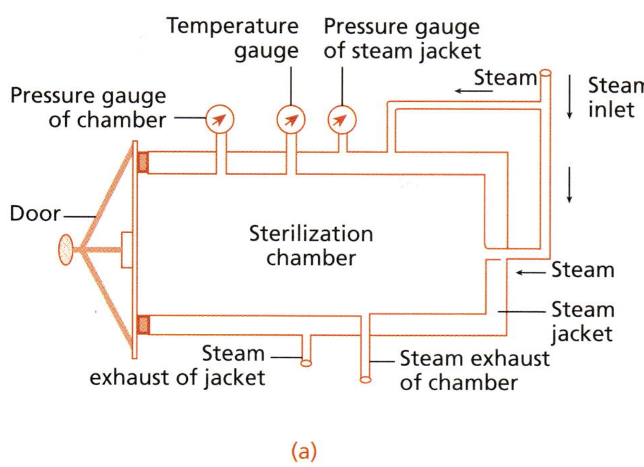

(a)

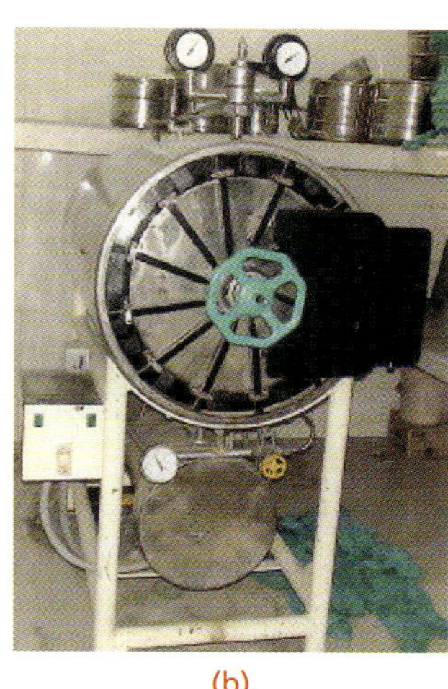

(b)

Figure 6.2 (a) Line diagram of an autoclave; (b) autoclave.

Autoclave is an apparatus for performing sterilization by steam under pressure. It is fitted with a gauze which automatically regulates pressure, and thereby the temperature, to which the contents are subjected.

Procedure for autoclaving of linen and instruments

Before autoclaving, the linen and instruments are washed, cleaned, and dried and then packed in a manner so as to permit free circulation of steam between them. The autoclave is then heated by letting steam into the jacket and then loaded with the items to be sterilized. The door is then closed and the air is removed by vacuum extraction. The steam is then allowed to enter the chamber and the desired pressure and temperature allowed to be attained and maintained for 1.5 times of that required for sterilization (holding time). At the end of the period, the steam is evacuated, and the steam jacket is heated again to dry the contents of the chamber.

Monitoring the efficacy of autoclave

To monitor the efficacy of autoclaving, two systems are in use.

Chemical Indicator It is contained in a sticky paper tape which is applied to the packets. It changes its color after the required temperature is attained and maintained for the holding time.

Spore Indicator It uses spores of *Bacillus stearothermophilus* which are destroyed at a temperature of 121°C for 12 minutes. A test tube containing the spores is placed in the center of the load. It is cultured at the end of autoclaving.

Boiling

Boiling in soft water at 100°C for 5 minutes is a very convenient and simple method of disinfection. But it does not kill the spores.

Irradiation

In this method gamma rays or accelerated electrons are used for sterilization. It is an industrial process. Hence, it is appropriate for sterilizing large batches of similar products such as syringes, needles, cannulas, catheters, and gloves. The delivery of a dose in excess of 25 cGy is accepted as providing adequate sterility assurance.

Glutaraldehyde

Two percent glutaraldehyde solution is nonirritant, bactericidal, sporicidal, and viricidal. It is much more active but less stable in an alkaline solution. Glutaraldehyde is used to sterilize endoscopes, anesthetic equipment, plastic materials, and thermometers which cannot be sterilized by heat. It can cause allergic reactions.

Ethylene oxide

It is a highly penetrative noncorrosive gas that has a broad-spectrum germicidal action. Ethylene oxide is used to sterilize heat- and moisture-sensitive materials including electrical equipment. It is not recommended for soiled instruments because organic debris including serum has a deleterious effect.

Hot air

It is inefficient as compared to steam under pressure. Hot air is used to sterilize nonaqueous liquids and grease/ointments and closed (airtight) containers.

Low-temperature steam and formaldehyde

The main advantage of this combination is that the sterilization is achieved at a low temperature (73°C). This method is therefore suitable for heat-sensitive materials and equipment with integral plastic components.

Peracetic acid (STERIS)

This system includes a table-top microprocessor working at 50–56°C for 12 minutes with constant fluid circulating during the sterilizing and rinsing cycles. It is particularly suitable for sterilizing flexible endoscopes.

Nowadays plasma sterilizer is used for sterilizing endoscopes and endoscopic equipment (Fig. 6.3).

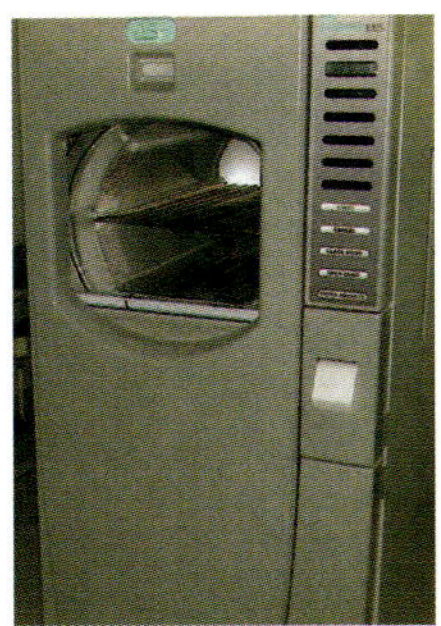

Figure 6.3 Plasma sterilizer for sterilization of endoscopes and endoscopic instruments.

Control of Environment

The environment including air around us has a large number of bacteria. They may directly contaminate an operative wound. Hence, the environment around the patient to be operated upon must be controlled.

Ultraviolet light

It has been used to reduce the number of bacteria in the atmosphere. Ultraviolet light can harm the skin and eyes; hence, its use has been restricted.

Bacterial filters

The bacterial filters are used to prevent entry of dust particles carrying bacteria. The air entering the operating room should pass through 5-μm dust filters. Air filters are not an absolute requirement, but about 10 air changes per hour should be achieved as it keeps a low bacterial count in the operating room.

Disinfection

Disinfection of furniture and cleanliness of linen and blankets should be ensured.

Restricted entry

The number of visitors to the ward should be restricted to reduce the movements of dust particles.

Hepatitis B infection

It is preventable by hepatitis B vaccination which must be done in high-risk healthcare workers such as surgeons, dentists, operating room staff, and technicians working in dialysis units and oncology services.

AIDS

All the patients should be screened for AIDS. A positive patient should be kept in isolation. All sharps used in these patients must be carefully disposed off. Exposure to blood and body fluids of these patients must be carefully avoided. Surgeons and endoscopists should use protective goggles to prevent conjunctival transmission.

4. SURGICAL INFECTIONS

Surgical infections are very common. These are the diseases which may require some sort of surgical procedure for treatment. Hence, some of the common infections are being described here.

Abscess

An abscess is a localized collection of pus in the tissues in a cavity having granulation tissue in its walls. It is of three types: acute (hot), cold, and pyemic.

Acute Abscess (Hot Abscess)

An acute abscess is of short duration and caused by pyogenic organisms.

Pathogenesis

- Acute abscess is mainly caused by *S. aureus* and *S. pyogenes*.
- The infection leads to tissue necrosis followed by liquefaction and pus formation.
- Apart from liquefied necrotic tissue, the pus contains dead and dying leukocytes that release damaging cytokines, oxygen free radicals, and other molecules.
- It is surrounded initially by acute inflammatory response and a pyogenic membrane composed of fibrinous exudates.
- Later on, granulation tissue (macrophages, angiogenesis, and fibroblasts) forms around the pus.
- The pus and necrotic tissue are hyperosmolar, hence they draw fluid inside increasing intracavitary pressure which causes pain.

Clinical features

- An abscess can occur anywhere in the body and in anybody—male or female and child, adult, or elderly.
- The patient presents with a swelling of acute onset which is red, hot, and tender (Fig. 6.4).
- The presence of pus makes the swelling soft, boggy, or fluctuant.

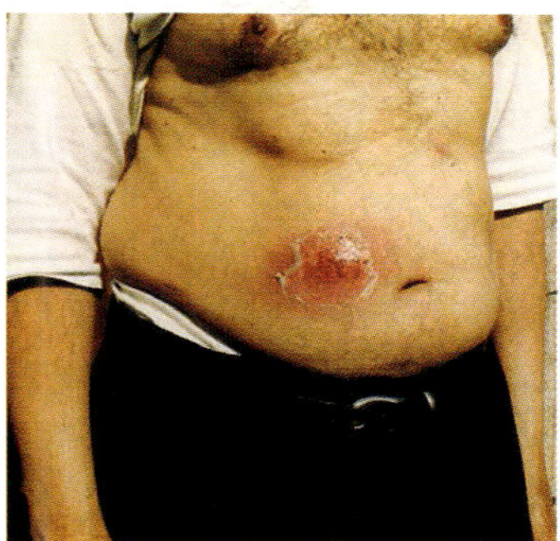

Figure 6.4 Acute abscess of anterior abdominal wall with marked redness and pus.

Investigations

- The blood shows polymorphonuclear leukocytosis. It may be sent for sugar and culture.
- A deep-seated abscess can be seen by imaging methods, for example, a lung abscess by radiography, liver abscess by ultrasonography, and brain abscess by CT scan or MRI.

Complications

Pyemia It is one of the complications of an acute abscess in which the pus enters the blood and emboli of pus circulate in the blood. Pyemia is a serious condition as it may lead to formation of multiple abscesses in the body. It is treated by removal of the cause and intravenous antibiotics.

Treatment

Removal of Pus (Drainage) It is the most important part of treatment. The pus can be removed by open drainage by giving an incision on the top of abscess parallel to the axis of main local nerves and blood vessels (Hilton's method). At the site of large vessels, before giving an incision one must make sure that the swelling is not an arterial aneurysm by aspirating with a needle. Primary closure may be done but delayed primary closure or secondary suture is safer. Deep-seated abscesses may be treated by needle aspiration or catheter drainage under ultrasonographic or CT guidance.

Antibiotics Antibiotics are mandatory to forestall the spread of infection, although a school of thought is against it. They are usually given if there are signs of spreading infection and to diabetics. The drugs of choice are flucloxacillin, co-amoxiclav, and cephalosporins.

Fate of an abscess

- Resorption and resolution
- Spontaneous rupture followed by healing, or sinus formation
- Surgical drainage and healing
- Antibioma (if the abscess is not drained but treated by long-term antibiotics, it may be partly sterilized and solidified to become an antibioma; it commonly occurs in a breast abscess)
- Progress to chronic abscess which is very rare these days

Cold Abscess

Cold abscess is a collection of pus in the tissues without the signs of acute inflammation, that is, there is no heat, no redness, and no tenderness like in an acute (hot) abscess. Hence, it is called "cold abscess."

Etiology

It is usually caused by tuberculosis. Other causes include actinomycosis, leprosy, and fungal infections. Lymph node tuberculosis and osteoarticular tuberculosis are two common types of tuberculosis that result in a cold abscess.

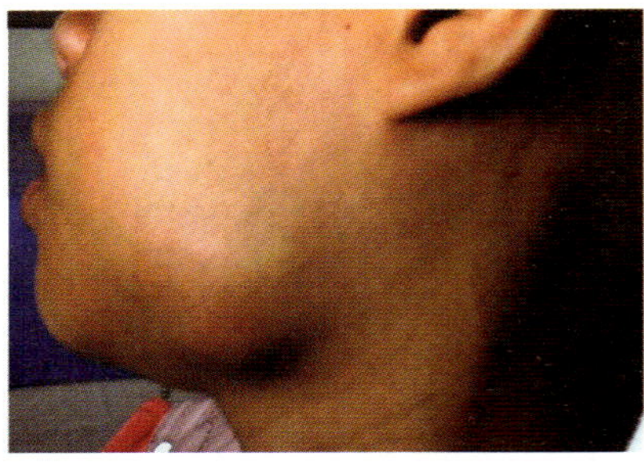

Figure 6.5 Cold abscess of left submandibular region. (Courtesy: Professor Surajit Bhattacharya)

Clinical features

- The patient is usually a young person, more commonly a female, who presents with a painless swelling of insidious onset anywhere in the body. Figure 6.5 shows a cold abscess of left submandibular region with mild redness of overlying skin which may rupture.
- The common sites include neck, axilla, groin, near a bone or joint, and paravertebral region.
- A cold abscess may track along the nerves or anatomical planes from the site of origin to far-off places and present there clinically.

A cold abscess should be differentiated from an acute abscess as described in Table 6.4.

Table 6.4 Differences between a cold abscess and an acute abscess

Features	Cold abscess	Acute abscess
Definition	Localized collection of pus in the tissues due to tuberculous destruction and liquefaction of tissues	Localized collection of pus in the tissues due to infection by pyogenic bacteria
Causative organisms	*Mycobacterium tuberculosis*	Commonly *Staphylococcus aureus* and *Streptococcus pyogenes*
Duration	Long	Short
Onset	Insidious	Acute
Signs of acute inflammation	Not present	Present
Treatment	• Antituberculous drugs • Removal of pus by aspiration or evacuation	• Removal of pus by open drainage, or ultrasound-guided needle aspiration or catheter drainage • Antibiotics

Investigations

- The blood usually shows lymphocytosis and elevated ESR.
- The aspirate of the abscess is sent for bacteriological examination and DNA/RNA amplification for tuberculosis.
- In osteoarticular tuberculosis, X-ray, CT scan, or MRI is required to see the suspected source of pus.

Complications

The complications of a cold abscess include rupture, ulceration, and single or multiple sinus formation.

Treatment

Medical Treatment The patient is given a full course of antituberculous drugs. A small abscess may heal with this treatment.

Surgical Treatment A large abscess or a persistent abscess is surgically evacuated of pus and necrotic material. For evacuation, the abscess cavity is opened, the pus and necrotic tissue are removed, and the wound is suture closed with or without a drain.

Pyemic Abscess

A pyemic abscess is a secondary abscess produced at some distance from the site of primary infection by transportation of bacteria in pus emboli circulating in blood.

Clinical features

- The patient develops high fever with chills and rigors followed by a crop of multiple swellings. They are usually small, diffuse, and nontender (nonreactive abscess).
- This problem may prove fatal if the vital organs such as brain are involved.

Investigation

The blood is sent for bacterial culture and antibiotic sensitivity.

Complications

The complications of pyemic abscess include toxemia [multiple organ dysfunction syndrome (MODS)] and its consequences.

Treatment

The patient is given antibiotics and the pus is drained. An effort is made to find the source of pyemia and if it is found it is also treated. Usually it is not found.

Cellulitis

Cellulitis is an acute nonsuppurative spreading inflammation of subcutaneous cellular tissue. This tissue contains many small enclosed spaces like the cells in a beehive, hence the name "cellulitis."

Causative Organisms

Cellulitis is caused by β-hemolytic streptococci which enter the tissues through a puncture, scratch, or cut. Apart from streptococci, *C. perfringens* and many other bacteria can also cause this disease.

Predisposing Factors

Cellulitis is common in diabetics, immunosuppressed people, and the elderly.

Clinical Features

- **Site:** The common sites are face, floor of mouth and sublingual region, limbs, and scrotum.
- **Local symptoms:** The patient presents with local pain, diffuse swelling and redness without edge or limit (Fig. 6.6), tenderness, and tender regional lymphadenopathy.
- **Systemic symptoms:** Chills, fever, and rigors can occur and it is called SIRS. It occurs due to release of organisms (bacteremia), exotoxins (toxemia), and cytokines in general circulation. But the blood culture is usually negative.

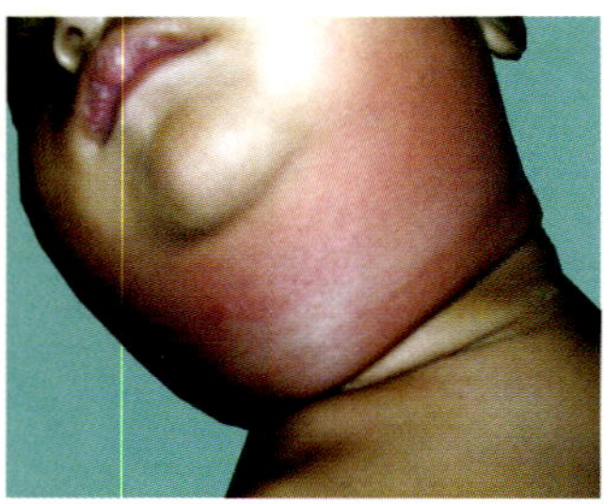

Figure 6.6 Cellulitis of neck. (Courtesy: Professor J.D. Rawat)

The differences between cellulitis and an acute abscess are enumerated in Table 6.5.

Investigations

Apart from routine investigations including blood sugar, the extent of the disease can be imaged by MRI.

Complications

- Pyogenic abscess due to localization of infection
- Ulceration due to progressive inflammation caused by release of streptokinase, hyaluronidase, and other proteases
- Gangrene especially in diabetic cellulitis of lower extremity
- Systemic spread leading to SIRS, MODS, and multiple systemic organ failure (MSOF)

Treatment

Medical Treatment Antibiotics, for example, crystalline penicillin 1 million units intravenously or intramuscularly 6 hourly for 5–7 days or cephalosporins, are the main line of treatment.

Symptomatic Treatment The affected part is kept elevated. It reduces swelling and pain. Local magnesium sulfate cream dressing also reduces edema. In a diabetic patient, the diabetes is controlled by diet control and insulin.

Ludwig's angina

It is the cellulitis of sublingual, submental, and submandibular spaces due to spread of infection from decaying mandibular teeth or submandibular salivary gland.

Predisposing Factors

It may be precipitated by tooth extraction, uncontrolled diabetes, and oral cancer and its chemotherapy and radiotherapy.

Pathogenesis

The infection from the first lower molar spreads to sublingual space while the infection from second and third molars spreads to submandibular space and infection from anterior mandibular teeth to submental space.

Clinical Features

- If the infection is above the mylohyoid muscle, it causes edema of floor of mouth pushing the

Table 6.5 Differences between cellulitis and acute abscess

Features	Cellulitis	Acute abscess
Definition	Acute spreading infection of subcutaneous cellular tissue by *Streptococcus haemolyticus* (*S. pyogenes*)	A localized collection of pus in the tissue caused by pyogenic bacteria, for example, *Staphylococcus aureus*, *S. pyogenes*, and others
Swelling type	Diffuse, spreading	Localized
Edge	No edge, no limit	Well defined
Pus formation	Does not occur	Occurs
Systemic response	More likely	Less likely
Treatment	• Antibiotics, for example, penicillin, cephalosporins • Surgical decompression–debridement in cellulitis of closed spaces	• Antibiotics • Removal of pus by incision and drainage

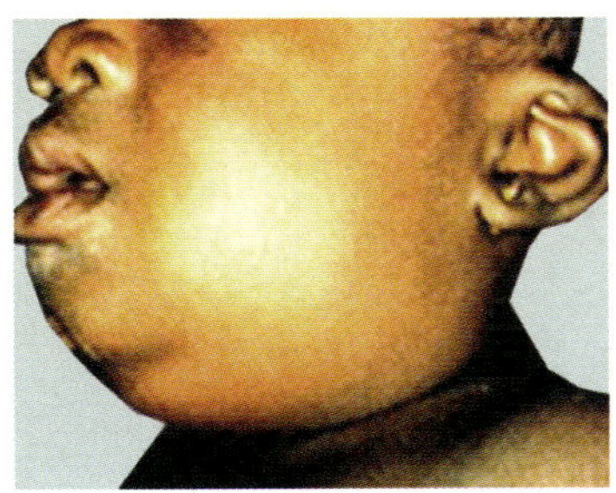

Figure 6.7 Ludwig's angina: cellulitis of upper neck including submandibular region. (Courtesy: Professor Surajit Bhattacharya)

tongue upwards to the palate causing difficulty in speaking and swallowing (Fig. 6.7).

- If the infection is below the mylohyoid, it affects submandibular, submental, and parapharyngeal spaces.
- The edema of this disease may spread to the laryngeal opening to cause airway obstruction; hence, the name angina (strangling) is given.
- Other features of this disease include high fever, putrid halitosis, trismus, and tachycardia.

Investigations

The edema can be imaged by ultrasound or CT scan. The blood should be sent for counts, sugar, and bacterial culture and sensitivity.

Complications

The complications of this disease include septicemia, laryngeal edema, thrombosis of internal jugular vein, and mediastinitis.

Treatment

- **Treatment of precipitating factors:** Diabetes must be controlled with insulin.
- **Medical treatment:** Intravenous antibiotics are started immediately with supportive treatment.
- **Surgical treatment**: Usually early surgical decompression is required to prevent complications. Under general anesthesia a curved incision is given in the submandibular region extending on both sides. It divides the deep fascia and mylohyoid muscle to open and drain the infected spaces. After cleaning the cavity the wound is closed with loose sutures around a drain. Airway obstruction may require endotracheal intubation (short run) or tracheostomy.

Lymphangitis

Lymphangitis is an acute nonsuppurative spreading inflammation of lymphatics (cuticular lymphangitis) of skin usually caused by *S. haemolyticus*. Filarial infection is one of the common causes in coastal India.

Causative Organisms

These include β-hemolytic streptococci, staphylococci, and clostridia.

Clinical Features

- Lymphangitis presents as painful red streaks due to inflamed lymphatics (which are difficult to appreciate in dark-pigmented people) and swelling due to lymphedema.
- The regional lymph nodes are enlarged and tender.
- In upper extremity, the lymphatics are mainly located on the dorsum of hand; hence, redness and edema occur on the dorsum.
- The infection of thumb and index finger affects axillary nodes, that of little and ring finger affects epitrochlear nodes, and that of middle finger affects deltopectoral nodes. The nodes may eventually suppurate to form an abscess.
- Lymphangitis is always associated with SIRS, that is, chills, high-grade fever, rigors, and tachycardia.

Investigations

Investigations include blood for counts, culture, and sugar.

Complications

Recurrent attacks of lymphangitis may result in adenolymphatic obstruction leading to acquired lymphedema.

Treatment

Treatment of lymphangitis is like that of cellulitis.

Erysipelas

Erysipelas is a nonsuppurative spreading (acute) inflammation of skin and subcutaneous tissue with associated lymphangitis.

Causative Organism

Erysipelas is caused by *S. pyogenes* which enters through a minor scratch.

Clinical Features

- The patient presents with local pain and diffuse swelling and redness which has a border or limit unlike cellulitis.
- The affected skin has a roseolar rash. Soon the redness becomes brown and later yellow with vesicles which rupture, discharging serous fluid.
- It is always associated with toxemia characterized by chills, high-grade fever, and rigors (SIRS).
- Milian's ear sign: The erysipelas of face can spread to involve pinna unlike cellulitis as the pinna has skin but no subcutaneous connective tissue.
- Butterfly lesion: Erysipelas of nasal skin and both the adjacent areas of cheek look like a butterfly, hence known as butterfly lesion.

Treatment and Complications

- The treatment and complications are similar to those of cellulitis. The antibiotics of choice include penicillin, amoxicillin, and first-generation cephalosporins. The erysipelas has to be differentiated from cellulitis which is described in Table 6.6.

Boil (furuncle)

- It is an acute staphylococcal infection of hair follicle containing a bead of pus with perifolliculitis.
- Site of occurrence: It is common in head, neck, back, thigh, and other hairy areas.
- Clinical features: It is characterized by short-duration pain and a small red swelling (Fig. 6.8) with yellowish top.
- Complications: Cellulitis, regional lymphadenitis, and a boil of dangerous area of face may cause cavernous sinus thrombosis.

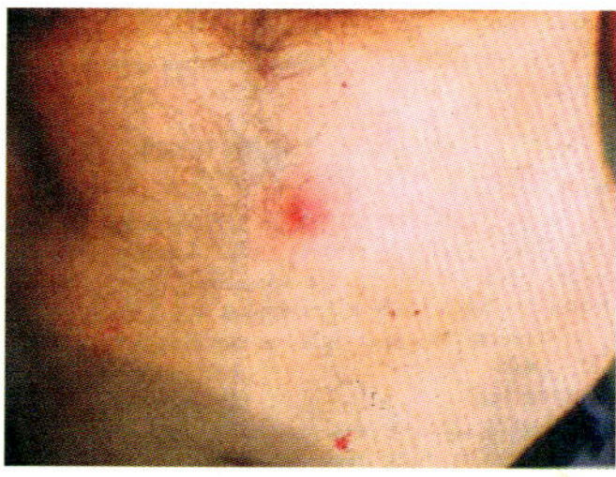

Figure 6.8 Boil of anterior abdominal wall showing marked erythema (rubor).

Table 6.6 Differences between erysipelas and cellulitis

Features	Erysipelas	Cellulitis
Etiology	Acute nonsuppurative spreading inflammation of skin (cuticular lymphangitis) caused by *Streptococcus haemolyticus*	Acute nonsuppurative spreading inflammation of subcutaneous cellular tissue caused by *S. haemolyticus* and other bacteria
Tissues involved	Skin with cuticular lymphatics	Subcutaneous cellular tissue (and of fascial planes)
Edge or limit	Well defined and above skin level	No edge or limit
Roseolar rash	Present	Absent
Vesicles	May be present	Absent
Facial disease (Milian's ear sign)	Facial erysipelas can spread into the pinna of ear	Facial cellulitis cannot spread into the pinna of ear

Box 6.7 Pathogenesis of a carbuncle

Causative organism: *Staphylococcus aureus*

Predisposing factor: Diabetes mellitus

↓

Hair follicle infection with perifolliculitis (small pustules)

↓

Slow liquefaction necrosis with pus formation at many points with intercommunication

↓

Rupture of small abscesses at many points with discharge of pus, giving a sieve-like (cribriform) appearance

- Treatment: It may subside by itself or with suitable antibiotics, for example, amoxicillin. Occasionally it requires drainage.

Carbuncle

Carbuncle is a type of infective gangrene of subcutaneous tissue.

Pathogenesis

The pathogenesis of a carbuncle is described in Box 6.7.

Clinical Features

- The patient is usually a middle-aged diabetic who presents with severe pain and swelling of acute onset.
- Site: It commonly occurs on the nape of neck, back of trunk (Fig. 6.9), and dorsum of hand and fingers.
- It is red, hot, tender, indurated, and ill-defined, and discharges pus from many small openings, giving a cribriform appearance.

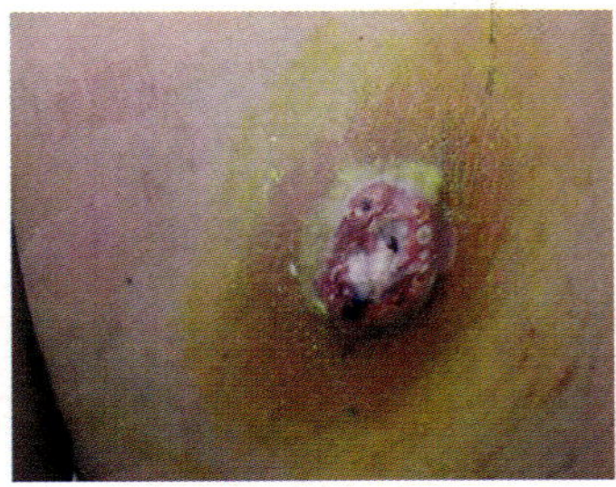

Figure 6.9 Sieve-like appearance of a carbuncle of back of chest near midline.

Investigations

The pus is sent for culture and sensitivity and blood for hemoglobin, counts, sugar, and bacterial culture. The extent and the texture of the lesion can be imaged by ultrasonography.

Complications

The complications of a carbuncle include diabetic ketoacidosis, extensive necrosis of local tissues, and septicemia.

Treatment

- Diabetes is controlled by diet control and insulin.
- Medical treatment: Antibiotics are given to control infection and they include flucloxacillin, co-amoxiclav, some of the cephalosporins, and gentamicin. Vancomycin may have to be given to control MRSA.
- Surgical treatment: If there is pus and the lesion is not responding to the above-mentioned treatment, it is opened by a cruciate incision and the pus is drained and the slough is excised with a cautery. After a few days following dressing, the wound may require skin grafting.

Bacteremia and septicemia

- Bacteremia is defined as the presence of bacteria in circulating blood.
- Bacteremia is usually transient and commonly follows procedures undertaken through infected tissues, for example, dental extraction and instrumentation in infected bile and urine.
- It can be dangerous in patients with prosthetic implants in the body as they may get infected. Hence, surgery should be done under antibiotic cover in these patients.
- Bacteremia and septicemia are complications of wound infection (e.g., burn wounds) and spreading or extensive infections of the body (erysipelas, cellulitis, and peritonitis).

Sequelae of severe septicemia

Systemic Inflammatory Response Syndrome

- SIRS is a manifestation of established infection affecting the whole body. In secondary peritonitis, SIRS may occur through the release of lipopolysaccharide endotoxin from the walls of dying Gram-negative bacilli, mainly *E. coli* or other bacteria or fungi.
- SIRS is characterized by two or more of the findings given in Box 6.8.
- Bacteremia, septicemia, SIRS, MODS, and MSOF are closely related problems and follow one after the other. The main investigation is blood culture which is done repeatedly apart from other investigations depending on the clinical features.

Box 6.8 Characteristics of SIRS

SIRS is characterized by two or more of the following findings:

- Temperature more than 38°C or less than 35°C
- Heart rate more than 90 beats/minute
- Respiratory rate more than 20 breaths/minute or $PaCO_2$ more than 32 mm Hg
- WBC count more than 12,000 or less than 4000 mm^3

Multiple Organ Dysfunction Syndrome

In severe sepsis, systemic organs are affected by the release of proinflammatory cytokines, for example, interleukin-1 (IL-1) and tumor necrosis factor alpha (TNF-α), and a series of other changes. It leads to cellular damage within the organs which become dysfunctional (MODS).

Multiple System Organ Failure

If the problem of multiple organ dysfunction is severe and continues, the affected organs start failing, that is, respiratory, cardiac, intestinal, renal, and hepatic failure ensue in combination with circulatory failure and shock. In this phase the patient is likely to die despite modern intensive care and organ support. The mainstay of treatment is antibiotics, intravenous fluids, and intensive care unit support of stressed organs.

5. SPECIFIC INFECTIONS

Tuberculosis

Tuberculosis is a specific infective disease caused by *Mycobacterium tuberculosis* which can affect any organ or tissue of the body, with the lungs, lymph nodes, bones and joints, and intestine being the commonest.

Causative Organism

It is caused by *M. tuberculosis hominis* or *bovis*. It is a slow-growing obligate intracellular rod. Now many strains of this bacterium have developed resistance to commonly used antituberculous drugs (MDR-TB).

Mode of Spread

Inhalation and ingestion of bacteria are the usual methods of entry into the body:

- **Inhalation**: It is the commonest mode of entry of infection into the lungs.
- **Ingestion**: It is the commonest mode of entry of infection into the gastrointestinal tract.
- **Inoculation**: It may be inoculated into the skin by touching infected lesions or pathological tissues.

Risk Factors

- Close contact with infected individuals
- Malnutrition
- Repeated pregnancies
- Urban homeless people, usually migrants to large cities from rural areas
- Postgastrectomy
- Silicosis
- Any cause of immune deficiency including AIDS

Pathogenesis

- As the mycobacteria enter the tissues, they cause inflammatory reaction characterized by caseous necrosis surrounded by epithelioid histiocytes and giant cells, in turn surrounded by lymphocytes and fibrocytes. Acid-fast bacillus (AFB) stains show red rods in phagocytes in the necrotic areas.
- The bacteria in the primary lesions that are not successfully killed by cell-mediated immunity can spread through lymphatics and blood or into the contiguous tissues to other areas of body to produce secondary lesions.
- The mycobacteria can thrive for many years in inactive foci of disease, and the recrudescent postprimary disease may become manifest with pregnancy, stress, old age, and many other illnesses.
- Reactivation most commonly occurs in the apices of lungs (85%). The highest risk of active disease is within the first 2 years of exposure.

Clinical Features

- **Age**: It commonly affects the young people but all age groups are vulnerable to this disease.
- **Sex**: It is slightly more common in females.
- **Symptoms**:
  - General symptoms: These include low-grade evening pyrexia, night sweats, weight loss, weakness, loss of appetite, fatigue, and anemia.
  - Pulmonary tuberculosis: The pulmonary disease is characterized by cough, hemoptysis, and chest pain.
  - Tuberculous lymphadenitis: The lymph node disease is characterized by local or regional lymphadenopathy usually affecting the cervical lymph nodes. The lymph nodes are firm, nontender, and matted (fused with each other). Later on, the patient may present with single or multiple cold abscesses, sinuses, or ulcers.
  - The osteoarticular disease presents with pain, local tenderness, restriction of movements, deformity, cold abscess, and a sinus.
  - The patient may present with intestinal, urinary tract, or central nervous system disease and disease of other organs and tissues, and also a widespread disease known as miliary tuberculosis.

Investigations

Laboratory Studies

- The blood may reveal anemia, lymphocytosis, elevated ESR, and hypergammaglobulinemia.
- Sputum, pus, pleural or peritoneal aspirate, gastric aspirate in small children (as they swallow sputum), bone marrow, and CSF may be studied by Ziehl–Neelsen (Fig. 6.10) or auramine-rhodamine staining method, or culture on a special (Lowenstein–Jensen) medium. The culture takes 3- to 6-week time, but it is required to test the antituberculous drug sensitivity.
- In urinary tract involvement, the urine is acidic and may have sterile pyuria.

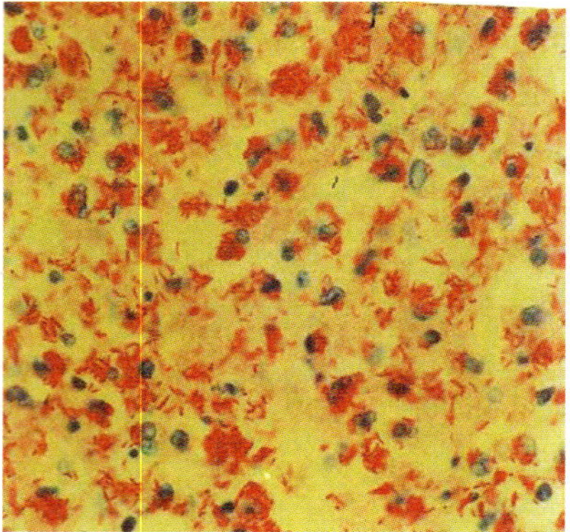

Figure 6.10 Smear of pus of a tuberculous sinus showing a large crowd of acid-fast bacilli (Ziehl–Neelsen stain).

Radiography

- X-ray of chest may show infiltrates with or without effusion in primary disease (Fig. 6.11). Cavitary lesions and upper lobe disease with hilar adenopathy are the common findings. Diffuse miliary pattern with millet seed-like appearance may be seen.
- In primary infection of lungs in children, right upper lobe atelectasis with hilar adenopathy is a common finding.
- In osteoarticular tuberculosis, radiography shows rarefaction, erosion or destruction of bone, and reduction of joint space.

Nucleic Acid Amplification Tests (NAATs) In recent times, DNA and RNA amplification for tuberculosis is being done which confirms the diagnosis within a few hours. This testing not only detects *M. tuberculosis* (NAAT-TB) but also identifies resistance markers (NAAT-R).

Biopsy Biopsy of the enlarged lymph node or from an ulcer or sinus can be taken for histopathological diagnosis. Fine-needle aspiration cytology may be used for rapid diagnosis. Cytological appearance of fine-needle aspirate from a tuberculous lymph node includes epithelioid cells, lymphocytes, and Langhans type of giant cells (Fig. 6.12).

Tuberculin Test and Mantoux Test

- These are the old methods of diagnosis. They are based on immunological response.
- Tuberculin test is a multiple puncture test. It has a 10–20% false-positive rate.

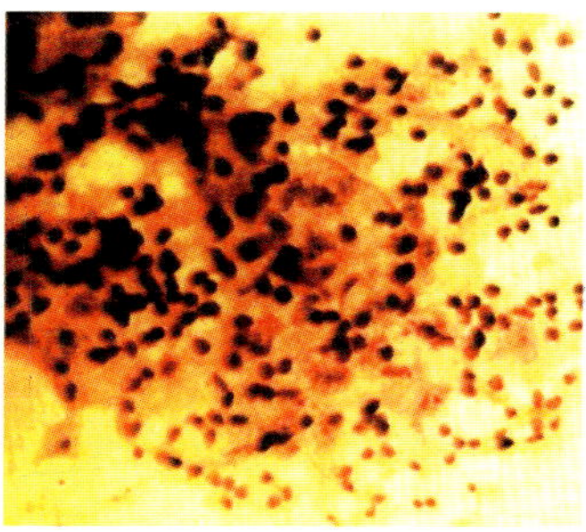

Figure 6.12 Cytological appearance of fine-needle aspirate from a tuberculous lymph node. (Courtesy: Professor P.K. Agarwal)

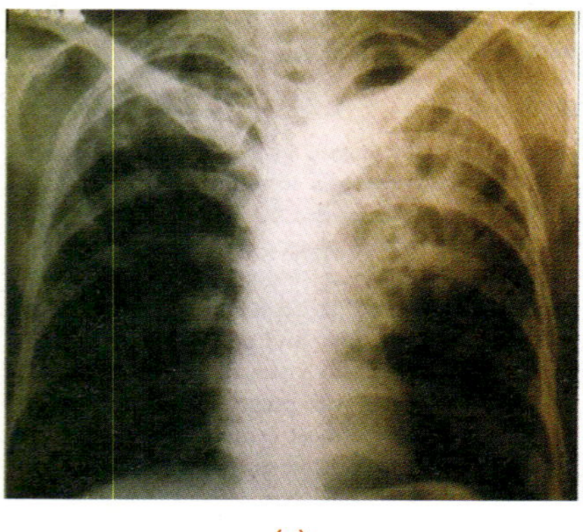

(a)

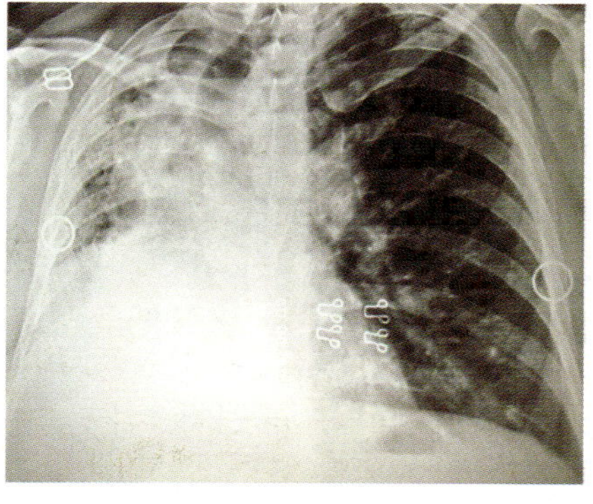

(b)

Figure 6.11 Radiograph of chest PA view in pulmonary tuberculosis. (a) Bilateral disease especially of left upper lung; (b) right destroyed lung with fibrosis and shift of mediastinum ipsilaterally.

- Mantoux test is done by giving 0.1 mL of purified protein derivative (PPD) containing 5 tuberculin units by an intradermal injection in volar forearm. It is read for swelling and redness after 48–72 hours. If the reaction (local redness and swelling) is larger than 10 mm, it is positive, but a positive test does not differentiate between active and latent infections.

Complications

Nearly any organ or tissue of the body can be affected by tuberculosis which may be destroyed completely or partially with pus formation and later with single or multiple sinus formation.

Treatment

The patients are given a diet that is rich in proteins, minerals, and vitamins. Patients are advised to take sunbath daily which is helpful in early cure of this disease. Smear-positive patients are treated in isolation till they become smear-negative.

Medical management

- The basic principles of drug treatment include to use multiple drugs to which the organism is susceptible, to provide the safest and most effective treatment for the shortest period of time, and to ensure adherence to therapy.
- The drug treatment includes the use of a minimum of two drugs, for example, rifampicin and isoniazid for 9 months, or three to four drugs (rifampicin, isoniazid, pyrazinamide, ethambutol) for the first 2 months and then two drugs to complete 6 months (Table 6.7).
- Nonadherance to treatment can be avoided by Directly Observed Therapy (DOT) which requires a healthcare worker to see the patient ingest the drugs.
- In children three drugs are given for 2 months and then two drugs are given for 4 months.
- In human immune deficiency virus (HIV)-positive patients a minimum of three drugs are used.

Surgical treatment

Majority of patients heal with proper medication, but some patients require surgical treatment. The indications for surgery are:

- Cold abscess
- Destroyed organs and tubes
- Obstruction of hollow organs and tubes

Table 6.7 Antituberculous drugs

Drug	Dose	Comments	Common toxicity
Isoniazid	5 mg/kg, maximum 300 mg/day	• Bactericidal to both extracellular and intracellular bacteria • Add pyridoxine 10 mg daily to prevent neuritis	Peripheral neuropathy, hepatitis, rash, mild CNS toxicity
Rifampicin	10 mg/kg, maximum 600 mg/day	• Bactericidal to all types of tubercle bacilli • Stains urine and other secretions orange	Hepatitis, fever, rash, flu-like symptoms, gastrointestinal upset, bleeding problems, renal failure
Pyrazinamide	15–30 mg/kg, maximum 2 g/day	Bactericidal to intracellular mycobacteria	Hyperuricemia, hepatotoxicity, rash, gastrointestinal upset, joint pain
Ethambutol	5–25 mg/kg, maximum 2.5 g daily	Bacteriostatic. Use with caution in renal disease or when eyes are not healthy	Optic neuritis, rash
Streptomycin	15 mg/kg, maximum 1 g/day	Bactericidal to extracellular microorganisms. Use with caution in elderly and in renal disease; never use for more than 12 weeks	Auditory nerve damage, nephrotoxicity

Treatment includes:

- The cold abscesses are aspirated or evacuated (operative removal of pus and necrotic tissue).
- The destroyed organs and tissues are excised.
- Obstruction of hollow organs and tubes is removed by stricturoplasty, excision with end-to-end anastomosis, or bypass.

Prevention

It is a preventable disease, being prevented by a healthy living (good diet, fresh air, and sun exposure) and BCG vaccination.

Syphilis (lues)

Syphilis is a venereal disease caused by *Treponema pallidum* which is transmitted by sexual intercourse with an infected partner and is characterized by the appearance of a series of symptoms and signs in sequential stages.

Etiology

T. pallidum is a spirochaete which is capable of infecting almost any organ or tissue. The infection enters the body through sexual intercourse (including oral sex) with an infected partner. It may be transmitted by contact with infected body fluids. During pregnancy it may be transmitted transplacentally to the fetus from the infected mother after the 10th week. The risk factors include multiple sexual partners, intravenous drug use, and male homosexuality.

Natural History

The natural history of acquired syphilis is generally divided into two major clinical stages: early (infectious) syphilis and late (noninfectious) syphilis. They are separated by a symptom-free latent phase.

Clinical Features

- **Age and sex**: It is predominantly seen during sexually active years, more in males than in females.

Infectious (primary) syphilis

- The incubation period is 9–90 days with an average of 3 weeks.
- The patient develops a sore or chancre on the genitalia at the site of exposure, which starts as a papule. It soon erodes to a 0.3- to 2-cm-sized nontender ulcer with a hard edge and clean yellow floor (Hunterian chancre). The ulcer heals by itself in 3–6 weeks with 75% of patients having no symptoms.
- The regional lymph nodes are mildly enlarged, hard, mobile, and nontender (shotty).

Infectious (secondary) syphilis

- Two to six weeks after exposure, 25% of patients enter this stage.
- It is characterized by fever, rash with generalized lymphadenopathy, malaise, anorexia, and headache.
- The rash is bilaterally symmetrical, polymorphic, and nonpruritic, and frequently occurs on palms and soles.
- Patchy alopecia of scalp, eyebrows, and beard is common.
- Mucous patches (thin gray smears) may be present on mucosal surfaces, and condylomata (moist, flat, pink warty lesions) may be present at mucocutaneous junctions, for example, glans, vulva, oral orifice, and anus. Linear shallow ulcers may occur in the tonsillar region (snail-track ulcers). The disease may resolve or pass into latent or late syphilis.

Latent syphilis

This phase is characterized by positive serology but no signs and symptoms. The patient is usually noninfectious after 1 year.

Late syphilis (tertiary syphilis)

It is characterized by one or more system involvement with the following features:

- Late benign syphilis characterized by granulomatous lesions (gummata) involving skin, mucous membranes, bones, and other organs
- Cardiovascular syphilis which includes aortic aneurysm and coronary ostial stenosis

- Neurosyphilis which includes meningovascular syphilis, tabes dorsalis, and general paresis

Congenital syphilis

- It is acquired by the fetus in uterus.
- Congenital syphilis is characterized by wasting, coryza (running nose), rashes, and osteitis in the first few months of life (early congenital syphilis).
- In later childhood, it is characterized by interstitial keratitis, deafness, orchitis, Clutton's joints, and notches in the cutting edge of permanent incisor teeth (Hutchinson's teeth). The first three features are collectively called Hutchinson's triad (late congenital syphilis).

The clinical features of syphilis are schematically given in Flowchart 6.1.

Oral Manifestations of Syphilis

See Table 6.8.

Investigations

Dark-Field Microscopy The causative organism in the fresh exudates from the primary lesion or the aspirate from regional lymph nodes can be seen in dark-field microscopy. The organism is not found in late syphilitic lesions. It cannot be cultured. An immunofluorescent staining technique for demonstrating *T. pallidum* in dried smears of fluid from early lesions is now available.

Serological Tests They are the mainstay of diagnosis of syphilis and are of two types:

1. Nontreponemal tests, for example, Venereal Disease Research Laboratory (VDRL) and rapid plasma reagin (RPR) tests. They usually become positive 4–6 weeks after infection.

2. Treponemal tests, for example, *T. pallidum* hemagglutination (TPHA) test and *T. pallidum* particle agglutination (TPPA) test. The latter test has supplanted the fluorescent treponemal antibody absorption (FTA-ABS) test because of ease of performance.

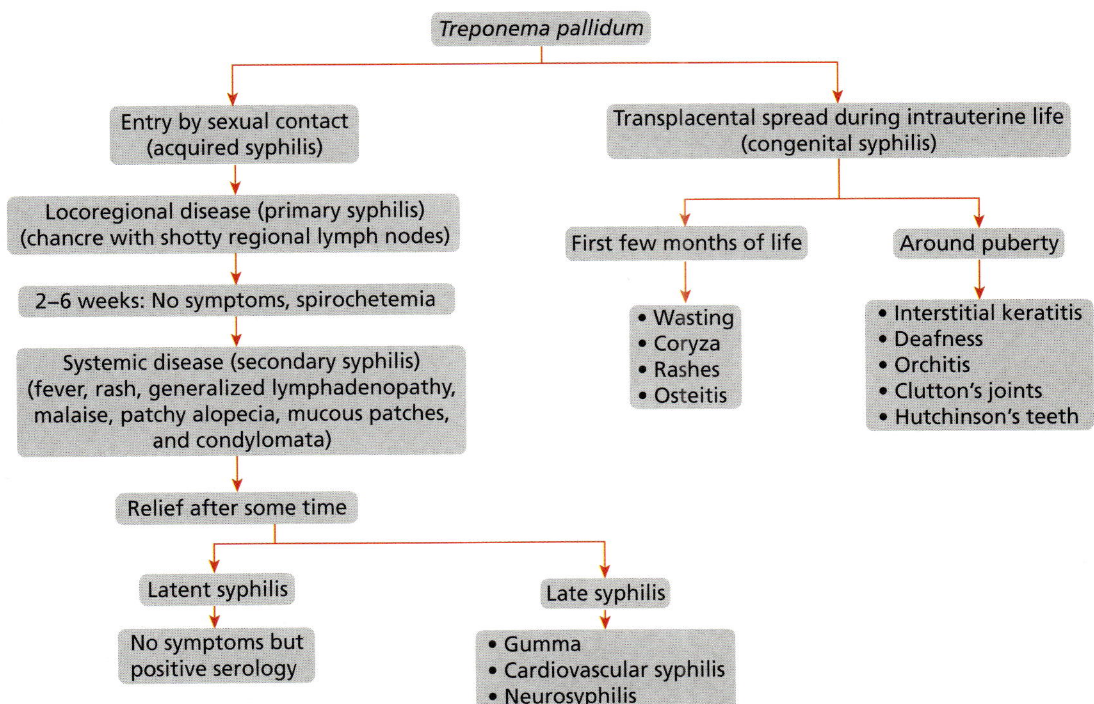

Flowchart 6.1 Clinical features of syphilis.

Table 6.8 Oral manifestations of syphilis

Primary syphilis	Secondary syphilis	Tertiary syphilis	Congenital syphilis
Chancre of lip or tongue • Occurs following kissing an infected person • The neck nodes are enlarged, often markedly	• Mucous patches on tongue • Snail-track ulcers in tonsillar region • Condylomata at the angles of mouth	• Gumma of dorsum of tongue • Gummatous ulcer of dorsum of tongue • Syphilitic leukoplakia	• Mucous patches of tongue • Hutchinson's teeth (deformed upper central incisors of second dentition) • Moon's molars (deformed cusps) • Perforation of palate in midline

Polymerase Chain Reaction (PCR) PCR is also used, but it is not freely available.

Treatment

Antibiotic therapy

- Primary, secondary, and early latent diseases are treated with benzathine penicillin 2.4 million units intramuscularly once. The alternative drugs are doxycycline 100 mg orally twice daily for 14 days (not during pregnancy), tetracycline 500 mg orally four times daily for 14 days, or ceftriaxone 1 g intramuscularly or intravenously daily for 8–10 days.
- Late latent and tertiary syphilis without neurosyphilis are treated with benzathine penicillin G 2.4 million units intramuscularly weekly for 3 weeks.
- There is no specific treatment of orodental manifestations of syphilis except antisyphilitic antibiotic (benzathine penicillin), maintenance of oral hygiene, and repair or reconstruction of structural defects (teeth and palate).

Other measures

Other measures include full activity but no sexual activity till declared cured, and treatment of sexual contacts. No local antiseptic on the primary chancre should be used till investigations are done.

Jarisch–Herxheimer reaction

It manifests by fever and aggravation of existing clinical picture in the hours following treatment, and ascribed to the sudden massive destruction of spirochaetes. It is blunted by simultaneous administration of antipyretics.

Prognosis

The prognosis is good in stage I and stage II. It is bad in tertiary and congenital syphilis.

Prevention

Avoidance of sexual contact is the most reliable method of prevention, but it is an impractical public health measure. Hence, use of latex or polyurethane condoms is recommended, but they protect the covered areas only. Early acquired syphilis (primary and secondary) is infectious.

Gonorrhea

Gonorrhea is a purulent inflammation of urethra and other mucosal surfaces caused by *Neisseria gonorrhoeae* transmitted by sexual intercourse.

Risk Factors

The risk factors include sexual exposure to an infected sex partner without proper protection, multiple sex partners, delivery of fetus through infected birth canal, sexual abuse of children by infected individuals, and autoinoculation, for example, infected fingers to eyes.

Pathogenesis

- In a male the infection from urethra may spread to prostate, epididymis, and testis.
- In a female it may spread from endocervical canal to fallopian tubes (salpingitis) with extension to ovaries. It may result in local abscess formation.

Hematogenous dissemination may occur. It may lead to endocarditis, septic arthritis, meningitis, and other lesions. When the acute phase passes away, the patient may pass into asymptomatic carrier stage.

Clinical Features

- **Incubation period**: It is 2–8 days.
- **Age and sex**: This infection can occur at any time in life, but most commonly at 15–29 years of age. It occurs more commonly in males than in females.

Disease in adolescent and adult males

The patient presents with dysuria (burning or scalding pain during micturition) and a variable amount of urethral discharge (yellow, creamy). Testicular pain is present in a few patients. Acute retention of urine may occur due to acute urethritis. Later on, chronic urethral obstruction may occur due to urethral stricture.

Disease in homosexual males (passive)

The patient presents with purulent or bloody rectal discharge, tenesmus, and rectal burning or itching (gonococcal proctitis).

Females without pelvic inflammatory disease (PID)

The patient may present with vaginal discharge, urinary frequency, urgency, and discharge. Later on, bartholinitis and abscess formation may occur. There may be asymptomatic cervicitis.

Females with pelvic inflammatory disease

It is characterized by dysmenorrhea, menometrorrhagia, lower abdominal or pelvic pain and tenderness and rebound tenderness, fever, cervical traction tenderness, and palpable and tender fallopian tubes and/or ovaries. The chronic disease presents with chronic pelvic pain and infertility.

Infants and children

The fetus may get infected during passage through infected birth canal. The common presentations are:

- Eye infection (ophthalmia neonatorum) is characterized by purulent discharge, chemosis, and eyelid edema (conjunctivitis, corneal ulceration).
- Pneumonia in newborn is characterized by fever, cough, and pulmonary infiltrates on X-ray.
- The patient may present with fever, headache, neck rigidity, and altered mental state (meningitis).
- A female child may be brought with vaginal discharge and inflammation of vulva (vulvovaginitis).

Other presentations

- Pharyngitis may occur following oral sex when a girl/woman sucks on the penis of her sexual partner. The patient may be asymptomatic or may present with sore throat and discharge.
- Disseminated syndromes characterized by fever, chills, arthralgias (small joints), synovial sheath swelling (hands, feet), painful red and pustular skin lesions, and septic arthritis may occur.

Investigations

Gram Staining Gram staining of exudates from infected mucosal surfaces, for example, urethra, shows Gram-negative, kidney-shaped diplococci in polymorphonuclear leukocytes.

Culture Culture of discharge, blood in disseminated disease, joint aspirate in septic arthritis, or fluid obtained from culdocentesis is done on selective medium (Thayer–Martin or Martin–Lewis containing antibiotics to inhibit other microorganisms). Then the isolate is confirmed as gonococcus by standard fermentation tests, enzymatic tests, or DNA probes.

Nucleic Acid Amplification Tests NAATs of endocervical swabs, vaginal swabs, urethral swabs (men), and urine (both men and women) for *N. gonorrhoeae* have excellent sensitivity and specificity.

Differential Diagnosis

Gonococcal urethritis and cervicitis must be differentiated from nongonococcal urethritis, cervicitis, or vaginitis which occurs due to *Chlamydia trachomatis*, *Gardnerella vaginalis*, *Trichomonas*, and *C. albicans*.

Complications

The main complication of gonorrhea is urethral stricture. Others include arthritis, endocarditis, cervicitis, and blindness in neonates.

Treatment

Uncomplicated Gonococcal Infection For uncomplicated gonococcal infection of cervix, urethra, and rectum, ceftriaxone 250 mg intramuscularly plus either azithromycin 1000 mg orally as a single dose or doxycycline 100 mg twice daily for 7 days is given.

In patients in whom an oral cephalosporin is the only option, cefixime 400 mg orally as a single dose can be combined with azithromycin or doxycycline as above, but a "test of cure" should be performed 1 week after treatment. Pharyngeal gonorrhea is also treated in the similar manner.

Disseminated Infection Disseminated infection is treated with ceftriaxone 1 g intravenously daily, until 48 hours after improvement begins when the treatment can be switched to cefixime 400 mg orally daily to complete at least 1 week of treatment. Ciprofloxacin 500 mg twice daily or levofloxacin 500 mg once daily for 7 days is also effective.

For endocarditis, ceftriaxone 2 g intravenously is given daily for at least 3 weeks. Post-gonococcal urethritis and cervicitis which are usually caused by *Chlamydia* are treated with a regimen of erythromycin, doxycycline, or azithromycin.

Prognosis

Early gonorrhea treated properly in time has a good prognosis. Late disease with urethral stricture is bad, because once a stricture always a stricture is still true to some extent.

Chancroid (soft sore)

Chancroid is a sexually transmitted disease caused by a Gram-negative bacillus, *Haemophilus ducreyi*. It produces a lesion at the site of inoculation after an incubation period of 3–5 days.

Clinical Features

The initial lesion is a vesicopustule which breaks down to produce a painful soft sore with a necrotic floor, undermined edge, and surrounding erythema. Subsequently, multiple sores may develop started by autoinoculation (Fig. 6.13).

The inguinal lymph nodes of one side are enlarged to a moderate size, tender, and matted with overlying erythema. They may become fluctuant (bubo) and may rupture spontaneously to discharge pus. The lymph node involvement is associated with fever, chills, and malaise.

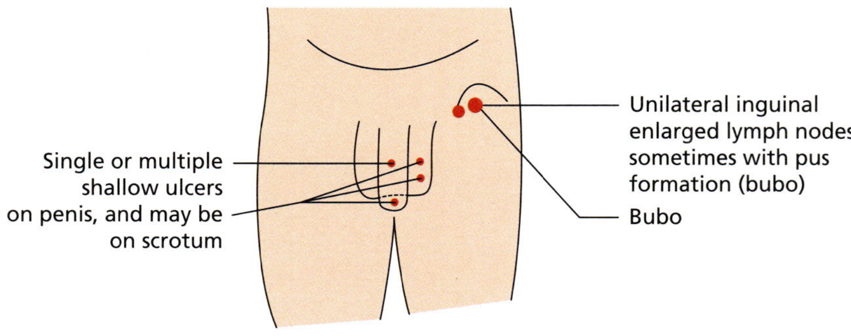

Figure 6.13 Chancroid (soft sore).

Investigation

The diagnosis is confirmed by culturing a swab of the lesion on to a special medium.

Treatment

A single dose of either azithromycin 1 g orally or ceftriaxone 250 mg intramuscularly cures this infection. Erythromycin 500 mg orally twice a day for 3 days is another effective regime.

Prognosis

It is good. There are hardly any notable complications.

Anthrax

Anthrax is an infective disease caused by *Bacillus anthracis* which is a Gram-positive spore-forming aerobic rod. Spores and not the vegetative bacteria are the infectious form of this organism.

Etiology

Anthrax is a disease of cattle which is likely to occur in people who handle carcasses, wool, hides, hair, and bone meal. The infection is transmitted by inoculation of broken skin or mucosa, by inhalation of aerosolized spores, or rarely by ingestion resulting in cutaneous, inhalational, or gastrointestinal forms of anthrax, respectively.

Clinical Features

Cutaneous Anthrax

- It is the common human variety that has an incubation period of 3–4 days, may be up to 2 weeks.
- The initial lesion is an erythematous itchy papule often on an exposed area of skin (hands or face).
- It vesiculates and then ulcerates and undergoes necrosis, ultimately progressing to a purple to black eschar.

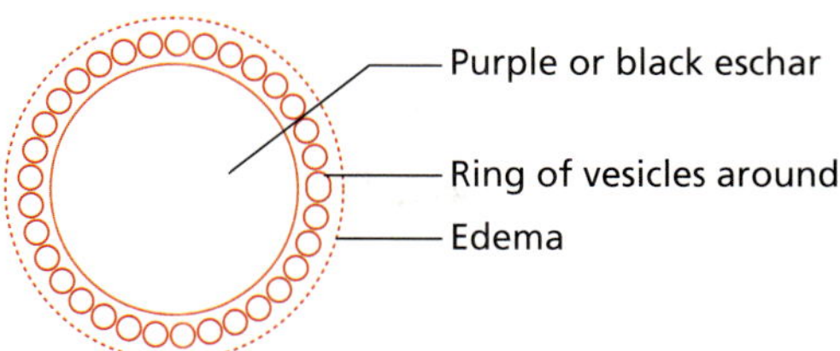

Figure 6.14 Malignant pustule of cutaneous anthrax.

- A ring of vesicles appears on the surrounding indurated area. It is now called "malignant pustule" (Fig. 6.14).
- Regional lymphadenopathy, fever, malaise, headache, nausea, and vomiting may be present.

Inhalational Anthrax or Woolsorter's Disease

- It begins usually 10 days after exposure and occurs in two stages:
  - The initial stage is characterized by fever, malaise, headache, cough, dyspnea, and congestion of upper airway.
  - The next stage is characterized by anterior chest pain due to mediastinitis followed by symptoms and signs of overwhelming sepsis.

Gastrointestinal Anthrax It is characterized by fever, abdominal pain and tenderness, vomiting, constipation, and diarrhea 2–5 days after swallowing the spores. The vomitus and stool may be blood-stained. Bowel perforation can occur.

Investigations

Bacteriological Tests The causative organism can be isolated from the culture of skin lesion, blood, or pleural fluid. It is invariably positive. In patients on antimicrobial therapy the culture may be negative. In these patients immunohistochemical tests, PCR, and serological tests may be used.

Imaging Studies X-ray of the chest is done in inhalational disease where mediastinal widening is found due to hemorrhagic lymphadenitis which is a specific sign of this disease. Pleural effusion is another finding. CT scan is done in gastrointestinal disease.

Treatment

First-Line Drugs

- Ciprofloxacin 500 mg twice daily orally or 400 mg every 12 hours intravenously
- Doxycycline 100 mg every 12 hours orally or intravenously

Second-Line Drugs

- Amoxicillin 500 mg three times daily orally
- Penicillin G 2–4 million units every 4 hours intravenously

Other Drugs Rifampicin, clindamycin, clarithromycin, erythromycin, vancomycin, and imipenem are other effective drugs.

The duration of treatment for cutaneous disease is 7–10 and 14 days or more for other types.

Prevention

There is a vaccine available for persons at high risk for exposure to anthrax spores. Multiple injections are given over 18 months and an annual booster dose is required for protection. A person exposed to contaminated meat is given antibiotics for 100 days.

Prognosis

Prognosis of cutaneous anthrax is excellent. Eighty-five percent of patients of other two types are likely to die.

Tetanus

Tetanus is a specific infective disease due to exotoxins produced by *C. tetani* which stimulates the nervous system. This disease is now rarely seen.

Pathogenesis

- The spores of these bacteria are ubiquitous in soil, especially in highly manured (biological manure) soil or roadside dust.
- Any wound may be infected by this bacterium but the punctured wounds are particularly prone to cause tetanus.
- After entry into the wound the spores germinate into vegetative bacteria which produce tetanospasmin which is a zinc metalloprotease that cleaves synaptobrevin, a protein essential for neurotransmitter release. It interferes with neurotransmission at spinal synapses of inhibitory neurons.
- As a consequence of this, minor stimuli result in uncontrolled spasms and exaggerated reflexes.

Clinical Features

- Incubation period: It varies from 5 days to 15 weeks with an average of 8–12 days.
- It occurs mostly in unvaccinated persons and the people at risk are elderly persons, migrant workers, neonates, and injection drug users.
- The first symptom may be pain and tingling at the site of infection followed by spasticity of muscles in the vicinity. Stiffness of jaw and neck, dysphagia, and irritability are early signs. Later on, spasm of jaw muscles (trismus) and facial muscles (risus sardonicus) and rigidity and spasm of muscles of neck, back (opisthotonus), and abdomen develop. The types of tetanus include acute tetanus, delayed tetanus, chronic tetanus, postoperative tetanus, postpartum tetanus, facial tetanus, tetanus neonatorum, and cephalic tetanus.
- Finally the patient develops painful tonic convulsions which are precipitated by minor stimuli. The spasm of glottis and respiratory muscles may cause acute asphyxia and death. The patient is awake and alert throughout this disease. The sensory system is normal. The temperature is normal or slightly raised.

The head and neck manifestations of tetanus are given in Box 6.9.

Box 6.9 The head and neck manifestations of tetanus

- Trismus due to stiffness or spasm of muscles of jaws
- Painful facial smile (risus sardonicus)
- Stiffness of neck or neck rigidity
- Twitching of muscles of face in facial tetanus

Differential Diagnosis

This disease may require to be differentiated from meningitis, strychnine poisoning, and phenothiazine toxicity.

Investigations

The diagnosis of tetanus is clinical. Hence, no investigations are required.

Complications

The complications of tetanus include airway obstruction, retention of urine, constipation, respiratory arrest, and cardiac failure.

Treatment

- Human tetanus immune globulin (TIG) 500 units is given intramuscularly within 24 hours of presentation. In addition, it may be given intrathecally, with a total dose of 4000 units.
- Penicillin 20 million units is given intravenously daily in divided doses to eradicate the causative bacteria.
- The patient is given bed rest in a quiet environment and sedatives. To control tetanic spasms, curare-like agents are given to paralyze the muscles and the patient is put on mechanical ventilation.
- If a wound is present, it may be debrided but it may be difficult in a serious patient.

Tetanus Prophylaxis

- Tetanus is a preventable disease by active immunization which is done by administering Td (tetanus and diphtheria) vaccine as two doses 4–6 weeks apart, with a third dose after 6–12 months. One dose should be substituted by Tdap (tetanus toxoid, reduced-dose diphtheria toxoid, acellular pertussis vaccine). Active immunization is a permanent preventive measure of tetanus.
- Booster doses are given every 10 years or at the time of injury if it occurs more than 5 years after the last dose.
- Nonimmunized persons are given passive immunization by giving TIG 250 units intramuscularly.
- Immunization can be done during pregnancy in nonimmunized women.

Prognosis

The overall mortality is about 40%. The high mortality is associated with short incubation period, early onset of convulsions, and delay in treatment. Contaminated wounds of head and face region are more dangerous than those in other parts of body.

Actinomycosis

Actinomycosis is a granulomatous inflammation of tissues caused by *A. israelii* which is an anaerobic, Gram-positive, branching, filamentous bacterium.

Etiopathogenesis

The causative organism of this disease is normally present in the mouth in caries teeth and tonsillar crypts. It directly invades the traumatized tissues and produces a suppurative lesion. From the local site the infection spreads by local infiltration or by bloodstream. It does not spread by lymphatics. It can infect any part or organ of the body, but three anatomical types are common: cervicofacial (65%), thoracic (15%), and abdominal (20%).

Clinical Features

Cervicofacial Actinomycosis

- Trauma and carious teeth are the main predisposing factors.
- The infection produces a lesion in the lower jaw adjacent to a carious tooth. The local gums swell and become indurated like bone. Further progress of the disease produces osteomyelitis with appearance of hard nodules.
- The overlying skin of the face and neck becomes bluish and indurated.
- Later softening occurs in patches which burst, discharging pus-containing "sulfur granules" through multiple sinuses.

Thoracic Actinomycosis The infection reaches the lung and pleura either by aspiration or by direct spread from pharynx or neck and produces pneumonitis and empyema. As the disease progresses, the chest wall is invaded producing multiple sinuses discharging pus.

Abdominal Actinomycosis

- The infection reaches the ileocecal junction by ingestion that directly invades the traumatized bowel, for example, the site of appendicectomized bowel.
- It produces a suppurating inflammation but does not cause narrowing of the lumen of bowel as happens in tuberculosis.
- The patient presents with discomfort or pain in right lower abdomen and a hard, tender, and immobile mass or multiple sinuses.
- The ipsilateral hip may have fixed flexion deformity.

Investigations

- **Gram staining:** Pus shows Gram-positive organism in a granule or as scattered branching filaments (Fig. 6.15).
- **Culture:** Anaerobic culture is required to distinguish it from *Nocardia*.
- **Imaging methods**: X-ray of the affected part is required to assess the lesion in cervicofacial and thoracic actinomycosis. CT scan/MRI may be done to find the extent of disease.

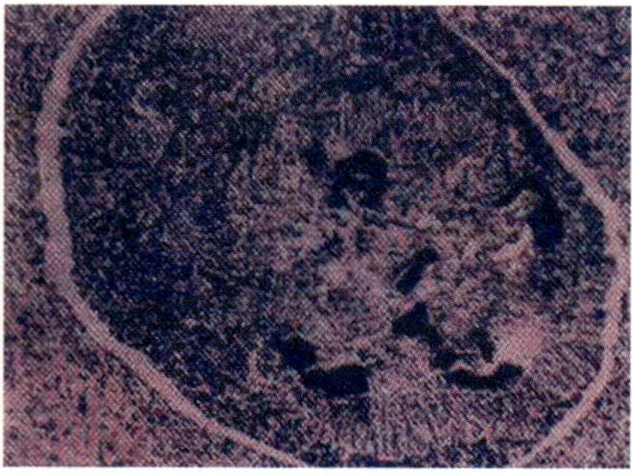

Figure 6.15 Microphotograph showing a sulfur granule of actinomycosis having radiating clubs of the causative organism. (Courtesy: Professor P.K. Agarwal)

Treatment

- **Medical treatment**: Penicillin G 10–20 million units is given intramuscularly for 4–6 weeks followed by oral penicillin V 500 mg four times daily till the disease is cured. Alternative drugs include ampicillin 12 g daily intravenously for 4–6 weeks followed by oral amoxicillin 500 mg three times daily, or doxycycline 100 mg twice daily intravenously or orally.
- **Surgical treatment:** Surgical treatment may be required to drain pus and remove the necrotic tissue.

Prognosis

With modern antibiotic treatment supplanted by surgery, the prognosis is good.

Hepatitis B

Hepatitis B is a diffuse inflammation of liver caused by hepatitis B virus which is a 42-nm hepadnavirus with a partially double-stranded DNA genome, inner core protein [hepatitis B core antigen (HBcAg)], and outer surface coat [hepatitis B surface antigen (HBsAg)].

Pathogenesis

- It enters the body through infected blood and blood products. Hence, it is also called transfusion hepatitis.
- It can also spread through sharing of infected needles and syringes (syringe hepatitis in drug users).
- The hepatitis B virus may produce an acute self-resolving hepatitis which is more serious than hepatitis A.
- After the resolution of acute disease the virus is often not cleared and may continue to damage the liver, producing hepatic cirrhosis and primary hepatic carcinoma.

Clinical Features

- The clinical picture varies from asymptomatic disease to fulminant hepatitis with a fatal outcome.

- It starts with prodromal symptoms of anorexia, nausea, vomiting, malaise, and aversion to smoking, followed by fever, right upper abdominal pain, enlarged tender liver, and jaundice.
- The acute disease usually subsides over 2–3 weeks with complete recovery by 16 weeks.
- It may become chronic which usually presents with complications of cirrhosis, most commonly ascites and variceal hemorrhage and primary hepatic carcinoma.

Investigations

Blood shows normal to low leukocyte count, markedly elevated aminotransferases early in disease, and several antigens and antibodies as well as HBV DNA that relate to HBV infection, for example, HBsAg, anti-HBs, anti-HBc, HBcAg, and HBV DNA.

Complications

The complications of chronic hepatitis B, especially if the infection is acquired in early life, are cirrhosis and hepatocellular carcinoma (up to 25–40%).

Treatment

- The treatment is symptomatic and supportive with palatable meals as tolerated without overfeeding.
- Antiviral therapy is usually not required but given to patients of fulminant hepatitis B and spontaneous reactivation of chronic hepatitis B presenting as acute-on-chronic liver failure. The drugs include lamivudine, interferon, and ribavirin.

Prevention

- HBV vaccination should be done in all infants and children and all adults who are at a higher risk of infection such as doctors, nurses, and pathology lab workers. The standard regime for adults is 10–20 μg repeated again at 1 and 6 months.
- The medical staff should handle disposable needles and blades carefully.
- The donated blood must be properly screened for HBsAg, anti-HBc, and anti-HCV. HBV-infected persons should practice safer sex.

Acquired immune deficiency syndrome

AIDS is an infective disease caused by HIV characterized by acquired immunosuppression with CD4 lymphocyte count $<0.2 \times 10^6$L with symptoms.

Pathogenesis

- It is a blood-borne infection transmitted to a susceptible host after a percutaneous or mucous membrane exposure to infected blood or body fluids.
- The virus attaches to specific receptors on the CD4 lymphocytes and is internalized releasing RNA.
- The reverse transcriptase of the virus incorporates into the chromosomal configuration of the host cells and initiates synthesis of new viral particles.
- All this process gradually depletes CD4 depressor cells with dominance of CD8 cells and immunosuppression of the host.
- The immune deficiency is a direct result of the effects of HIV on immune cells.

Risk Factors

The risk factors include sexual contact with an infected person, receptive anal intercourse, infected blood transfusion, needle sharing or needlestick injury, and perinatal exposure.

Clinical Features

- Systemic symptoms: Sweats, weight loss more than 10%, diarrhea of more than 1 month, fever, and lymphadenopathy
- Opportunistic infections due to diminished cellular immunity: Tuberculosis, herpes, candidiasis (especially oral and esophageal), pneumocystosis, and toxoplasmosis which are often life-threatening

- Aggressive cancers, especially Kaposi's sarcoma and extranodal lymphoma [other cancers include cervical cancer, CNS lymphoma, anogenital squamous cell carcinoma, and testicular tumors (germ cell types)]
- Neurological manifestations including dementia, aseptic meningitis, and neuropathy

The oral manifestation of AIDS is given in Box 6.10.

Box 6.10 Oral manifestations of AIDS

- Oral candidiasis or hairy leukoplakia
- Two types of oral candidiasis: pseudomembranous and erythematous
- Aphthous ulcers

Phases of AIDS

- **First phase**: Acute viral infection characterized by fever, malaise, and pharyngitis
- **Second phase**: A sustained period of asymptomatic disease during which active viral replication occurs resulting in reduction of CD4 cells
- **Third phase**: AIDS-related complex in which the patient is asymptomatic with regional lymphadenopathy
- **Fourth phase:** Clinical AIDS with the presence of indicator condition or a CD4 cell count of less than 200

Investigations

- Blood may show anemia, leukopenia (particularly lymphopenia), thrombocytopenia, and elevated ESR.
- HIV antibody testing is done by ELISA. Positive result is then confirmed by Western blot.
- Absolute CD4 lymphocyte count provides prognostic information and guides therapy decisions.

Treatment

It is a difficult problem to treat. The principles of treatment include the following:

- Prevention of opportunistic infections and other complications, for example, trimethoprim–sulfamethoxazole given for pneumocystis pneumonia and toxoplasmosis, and isoniazid for tuberculosis
- Treatment of opportunistic infections, malignancies, and other complications, for example, amphotericin B for cryptococcal meningitis and combination chemotherapy (modified CHOP, M-BACOD, with or without G-CSF or GM-CSF) for lymphoma
- Treatment of HIV infection by antiretroviral therapy which includes a combination of agents from:
  - *Nucleoside reverse transcriptase inhibitors*: Zidovudine, didanosine, abacavir, lamivudine, stavudine
  - *Non-nucleoside reverse transcriptase inhibitors*: Nevirapine, delavirdine
  - *Protease inhibitors*: Ritonavir, indinavir, fosamprenavir

Prophylaxis

So far no vaccine is available to prevent this disease. The preventive measures for the common people are health education and practice of safe sex. The use of condom reduces the risk of transmission.

Prevention

HIV infection can be transmitted to healthcare people including surgeons by skin puncture with a hollow needle containing HIV-infected blood or a cut during operation. If contamination occurs, the area is washed under running water and the following agents are given for 1 month: zidovudine 250 mg twice daily, lamivudine 150 mg twice daily, and indinavir 800 mg thrice daily. The preventive precautions given in Box 6.11 should be followed at all times.

Opportunistic Infections

These are the infections that occur in patients with immune deficiency.

Box 6.11 Prevention of AIDS

Universal precautions

- Routine use of barriers (such as gloves and/or goggles) when anticipating contact with blood or body fluids
- Washing of hands and other skin surfaces immediately after contact with blood or body fluids
- Careful handling and disposal of sharp instrument, during and after use

Detailed precautions

- Wearing safety spectacles and a face mask
- Wearing a gown that provides waterproof protection
- Wearing boots rather than open-toed shoes to protect the feet when something sharp is dropped
- Wearing two pairs of gloves to check skin contamination from punctures in the gloves
- Carrying out the operation in an orderly manner and passing sharp instruments in a dish
- Putting used needles in puncture resistant containers and never trying to place them back in protective sheath
- Disposing of the contaminated disposables, excreta, fluids, discharge, pus, and other materials properly (e.g., incinerated)

Immune deficiency may be due to diabetes mellitus, HIV infection, corticosteroid therapy, radiotherapy, starvation, and old age.

The causative organisms include *E. coli*, *Pseudomonas*, *Klebsiella*, *Proteus*, *Serratia*, *S. epidermidis*, and *Streptococcus pneumoniae* (bacteria); herpes, CMV, and *varicella zoster* (viruses); *Candida*, *Aspergillus*, and yeast (fungi); and *Cryptosporidium* and *Pneumocystis carinii*.

Investigations

These include culture of swab, urine, and others depending on the manifestation.

Treatment

These infections are difficult to treat as they are usually multidrug resistant. Hence, a combination of broad-spectrum antibiotics, for example, cephalosporins, aminoglycosides, and metronidazole, is required. Critical care including ventilatory support may be necessary.

KEY POINTS

- Inflammation is a clinicopathological response of the body tissues to any type of injury which may be microbial, mechanical, thermal, electrical, or irradiation.
- Acute inflammation is of short duration and occurs when virulence of the microorganism is high and the host resistance is low. Predominant cell in acute inflammation is polymorphonuclear leukocytes.
- Chronic inflammation is of long duration and the predominant cells include lymphocyte and plasma cells.
- Granulomatous inflammation is a specific type of chronic inflammation characterized by granuloma formation with predominant proliferation of histiocytes. It is commonly seen in tuberculous and syphilitic infections.
- Classic features of acute inflammation include dolor (pain), tumor (swelling), rubor (redness), calor (heat), and functio laesa (loss of function). Chronic inflammation may be asymptomatic or may have a variable combination of the above-mentioned features in a milder form.
- Sequelae of inflammation include resolution, tissue necrosis, systemic inflammatory response syndrome (SIRS), and healing by scarring.
- Management of inflammation includes removal of cause and effect by antibiotics or surgery, and relieving pain.
- Infection is the invasion of body tissues by pathogenic microorganisms and the reaction of tissues to their presence and toxins produced by them.
- The common bacteria that produce surgical infections include *Staphylococcus aureus*, *Streptococcus haemolyticus*, *Escherichia coli*, *K. pneumoniae*, *Proteus mirabilis*, *Pseudomonas aeruginosa*, *Clostridium perfringens*, *Clostridium tetani*, and *Actinomyces israelii*, and fungus *Candida albicans*.
- *S. aureus* and *S. haemolyticus* are the two common pus-forming bacteria. *P. aeruginosa* produces bluish or greenish pus.
- *S. aureus* produces localized infections such as furuncle or acute abscess and *S. haemolyticus* produces spreading inflammation such as cellulitis and erysipelas.
- *S. aureus* has a tendency to develop resistance to antibiotics [methicillin-resistant *S. aureus* (MRSA)] due to production of β-lactamase.

(CONTD...)

KEY POINTS *(...CONTD)*

- *E. coli* is a Gram-negative aerobe and is the commonest cause of urinary tract infection. It is sensitive to ampicillin, cephalosporins, and co-trimoxazole.
- *C. perfringens* and *C. tetani* produce gas gangrene and tetanus, respectively.
- Common antibacterials used to control surgical infections include penicillin, co-trimoxazole, cloxacillin, methicillin, flucloxacillin, carbenicillins, piperacillin, ticarcillin, cephalosporins, β-lactamase inhibitors (sulbactam, clavulanate, and tazobactam), erythromycin, roxithromycin, azithromycin, and metronidazole.
- Inflammation is a clinicopathological response of the body tissues to any type of injury which may be microbial, mechanical, thermal, electrical, or irradiation.
- Acute inflammation is of short duration and occurs when virulence of the microorganism is high and the host resistance is low. Predominant cell in acute inflammation is polymorphonuclear leukocytes.
- Chronic inflammation is of long duration and the predominant cells include lymphocyte and plasma cells.
- Granulomatous inflammation is a specific type of chronic inflammation characterized by granuloma formation with predominant proliferation of histiocytes. It is commonly seen in tuberculous and syphilitic infections.
- Classic features of acute inflammation include dolor (pain), tumor (swelling), rubor (redness), calor (heat), and functio laesa (loss of function). Chronic inflammation may be asymptomatic or may have a variable combination the of above-mentioned features in a milder form.
- Sequelae of inflammation include resolution, tissue necrosis, systemic inflammatory response syndrome (SIRS), and healing by scarring.
- Management of inflammation includes removal of cause and effect by antibiotics or surgery, and relieving pain.
- Infection is the invasion of body tissues by pathogenic microorganisms and the reaction of tissues to their presence and toxins produced by them.
- The common bacteria that produce surgical infections include *Staphylococcus aureus*, *Streptococcus haemolyticus*, *Escherichia coli*, *K. pneumoniae*, *Proteus mirabilis*, *Pseudomonas aeruginosa*, *Clostridium perfringens*, *Clostridium tetani*, and *Actinomyces israelii*, and fungus *Candida albicans*.
- *S. aureus* and *S. haemolyticus* are the two common pus-forming bacteria. *P. aeruginosa* produces bluish or greenish pus.
- *S. aureus* produces localized infections such as furuncle or acute abscess and *S. haemolyticus* produces spreading inflammation such as cellulitis and erysipelas.
- *S. aureus* has a tendency to develop resistance to antibiotics [methicillin-resistant *S. aureus* (MRSA)] due to production of β-lactamase.

- *E. coli* is a Gram-negative aerobe and is the commonest cause of urinary tract infection. It is sensitive to ampicillin, cephalosporins, and co-trimoxazole.
- *C. perfringens* and *C. tetani* produce gas gangrene and tetanus, respectively.
- Common antibacterials used to control surgical infections include penicillin, co-trimoxazole, cloxacillin, methicillin, flucloxacillin, carbenicillins, piperacillin, ticarcillin, cephalosporins, β-lactamase inhibitors (sulbactam, clavulanate, and tazobactam), erythromycin, roxithromycin, azithromycin, and metronidazole.

- Penicillin is highly bactericidal against *S. pyogenes* and anaerobic *Streptococcus*. Only 25% of strains of staphylococci are sensitive to it. It is effective against Gram-positive anaerobes such as clostridia but not against *B. fragilis*.
- Cloxacillin, methicillin, and flucloxacillin are penicillinase resistant, hence are active against β-lactamase–producing *S. aureus*.
- Metronidazole has antiprotozoal action and it is active against Gram-negative anaerobes, especially *B. fragilis*.
- Some patients with cardiac conditions who undergo some dental procedure have an increased risk of infective endocarditis due to bacteremia during the manipulation of dental tissues. In these patients, antibiotics are given as a prophylactic measure.
- Autoclaving is the principal method of sterilization. Other methods include irradiation, 2% glutaraldehyde, ethylene oxide, hot air, low-temperature steam, formaldehyde, and peracetic acid.
- An abscess is a localized collection of pus in the tissues caused by staphylococcal infection. It is treated by removal of pus and appropriate antibiotics.
- Cold abscess is without the signs of acute inflammation mostly caused by *Mycobacterium tuberculosis*.
- Cellulitis is an acute nonsuppurative spreading inflammation of subcutaneous cellular tissue (no limit) caused by β-hemolytic *Streptococcus*.
- Ludwig's angina is the cellulitis of sublingual, submandibular, and submental spaces due to spread

(CONTD...)

KEY POINTS *(...CONTD)*

of infection from decaying mandibular teeth or submandibular salivary gland. The edema may spread to the laryngeal opening to cause airway obstruction which is fatal. Management includes intravenous antibiotics, surgical decompression, and maintenance of a patent airway.

- Lymphangitis is an acute nonsuppurative spreading inflammation of lymphatics of skin caused by *S. haemolyticus*.
- Erysipelas is a nonsuppurative spreading (acute) inflammation of superficial skin with associated lymphangitis caused by *S. haemolyticus*.
- Facial erysipelas can spread to involve pinna, while cellulitis cannot spread to involve pinna (Milian's ear sign).
- Furuncle (boil) is an acute staphylococcal infection of hair follicle containing a bead of pus with perifolliculitis. A boil of dangerous area of face may cause cavernous sinus thrombosis.
- Carbuncle is a type of infective gangrene of subcutaneous tissue seen in an uncontrolled diabetic. It presents with an inflammatory swelling having multiple holes discharging pus to give a sieve-like appearance. It is treated by control of diabetes, antibiotics, and removal of pus and necrotic tissue by a cruciate incision.
- Bacteremia is defined as bacteria in circulating blood. It is usually transient and commonly follows procedures undertaken through infected tissues, for example, dental extraction.
- Systemic inflammatory response syndrome (SIRS) is the systemic inflammatory response to severe infection. Multiple organ dysfunction syndrome (MODS) is the effect of SIRS on systemic organs. Multiple system organ failure (MSOF) is the end-stage failure of multiple system organs.
- Tuberculosis is a granulomatous disease caused by *Mycobacterium tuberculosis* and characterized by destruction of tissue with pus formation. It may affect any tissue or organ but lungs, lymph nodes, intestine, and bones and joints are commonly affected.
- Pulmonary tuberculosis is characterized by cough, hemoptysis, and chest pain. Lymph node tuberculosis is characterized by enlarged matted lymph nodes, which may later on present as a cold abscess followed by sinus/sinus formation.
- Syphilis is a venereal disease caused by *Treponema pallidum* which has many stages. Primary syphilis is characterized by Hunterian chancre on the genitalia; secondary syphilis by nonpruritic symmetrical skin rash, mucous patches, snail-track ulcers, and condylomata; and tertiary syphilis by gummatous inflammation.
- Early congenital syphilis is characterized by wasting, coryza (running nose), rashes, and osteitis in the first few months of life, and late syphilis by interstitial keratitis, deafness, orchitis, Clutton's joints, and notches in the cutting edge of permanent incisor teeth (Hutchinson's teeth).
- Primary, secondary, and early latent diseases are treated with benzathine penicillin 2.4 million units intramuscularly once. Late latent and tertiary syphilis without neurosyphilis are treated with benzathine penicillin G 2.4 million units intramuscularly weekly for 3 weeks.
- Gonorrhea is a purulent inflammation of urethra and other mucosal surfaces caused by sexually transmitted diplococci, *Neisseria gonorrhoeae*. Urethritis is the presenting symptom and urethral stricture is the commonest complication. Treatment includes cefixime 400 mg orally as a single dose.
- Anthrax is caused by *Bacillus anthracis*. It is a disease of cattle which is likely to occur in people who handle carcasses, wool, hides, hair, and bone meal. It is of three types. The cutaneous anthrax presents with a malignant pustule on the face. Other types are pulmonary and intestinal.
- Tetanus is caused by exotoxins of *Clostridium tetani* which stimulates the whole body, especially the muscles with trismus, neck rigidity, risus sardonicus, and convulsions. It is a preventable disease by immunization. Hence, it is seen rarely now.
- Actinomycosis is a granulomatous inflammation of tissues caused by *Actinomyces israelii*. The cervicofacial actinomycosis is characterized by a single or multiple sinuses near the angle of mandible which discharge pus-containing "sulfur granules." The overlying skin of the face and neck becomes bluish and indurated.
- Hepatitis B is a diffuse inflammation of liver caused by hepatitis B virus. It may recover by itself or may become chronic with cirrhosis and primary hepatic carcinoma. It is a preventable disease by HBV vaccination.
- Acquired immune deficiency syndrome (AIDS) is a viral disease caused by human immune deficiency virus (HIV) characterized by acquired immunosuppression with CD4 lymphocyte count $<0.2\times10^6$/L with symptoms. It is a transmissible disease to healthcare workers which has serious consequences. It must be prevented by observing "universal precautions."

SELF-ASSESSMENT

Long answer questions

1. Name the two most common pus-forming bacteria. Describe their main features, mechanism of production of pus, and its clinical features.
2. What is an abscess? Describe its etiology, pathology, clinical features, complications, and treatment.
3. Describe the etiology, pathology, clinical features, and treatment of tuberculosis.
4. What is the causative organism of syphilis and how is it transmitted? Describe the clinical features and treatment of acquired syphilis.
5. What are the orodental lesions caused by various clinical types of syphilis? How will you treat them?
6. Describe the etiology, clinical picture, investigations, complications, and treatment of gonorrhea.
7. Discuss the etiology, clinical features, investigations, and treatment of chancroid.
8. Discuss the etiology, pathology, clinical features, and treatment of anthrax.
9. Describe the etiology, clinical features, types, and treatment of tetanus.
10. What are the causes of trismus? Describe the etiology, clinical features, and treatment of tetanus.
11. Discuss the etiology, pathology, clinical features, investigations, and treatment of actinomycosis.

Short answer questions

1. *Escherichia coli*
2. *Pseudomonas pyocyaneus*
3. Co-trimoxazole
4. Aminoglycosides
5. Sterilization
6. Autoclave
7. Cold abscess
8. Cellulitis
9. Ludwig's angina
10. Lymphangitis
11. Erysipelas
12. Milian's ear sign
13. Boil
14. Carbuncle
15. Septicemia
16. Pyemia
17. SIRS, MODS, MSOF
18. *Mycobacterium tuberculosis*, radiographic signs of tuberculosis, tuberculin test, antituberculous drugs
19. Hunterian chancre, snail-track ulcers, gummatous ulcer, dark-field illumination
20. Gonococcus, gonococcal stricture, pharyngitis, urethritis
21. Soft sore, *Haemophilus ducreyi*, bubo
22. *Bacillus anthracis*, malignant pustule, cutaneous anthrax, woolsorter's disease
23. Tetanospasmin, risus sardonicus, TIG, tetanus prophylaxis
24. Cervicofacial actinomycosis, sulfur granules, treatment of actinomycosis
25. Hepatitis B, complications of hepatitis B
26. AIDS, HIV infection, CD4 lymphocytes, opportunistic infections, AIDS-related cancers

Multiple choice questions

1. Which one of the following facts about *Staphylococcus aureus* is not true?
   (a) It is a Gram-positive facultative anaerobe
   (b) It occurs in grape-like clusters
   (c) It produces an aflatoxin, a coagulase, and an enterotoxin
   (d) It is the main causative organism of erysipelas
2. Which among the following is not true about hemolytic *Streptococcus*?
   (a) It is a Gram-positive facultative anaerobe
   (b) It produces hyaluronidase
   (c) It is responsible for spreading inflammation such as erysipelas and cellulitis
   (d) It has developed resistance against penicillin
3. The β-lactam ring of penicillin molecule is destroyed by
   (a) Coagulase
   (b) Hemolysin
   (c) Penicillinase
   (d) Streptokinase

(CONTD...)

SELF-ASSESSMENT *(...CONTD)*

4. Which among the following enzymes is responsible for localization of infection with pus formation?
   (a) Hemolysin
   (b) Streptokinase
   (c) Hyaluronidase
   (d) Coagulase
5. The spreading nature of streptococcal infection is due to
   (a) Coagulase
   (b) Streptokinase and hyaluronidase
   (c) Aflatoxin
   (d) Hemolysin
6. The commonest causative organism of urinary tract infection is
   (a) *Staphylococcus aureus*
   (b) *Streptococcus pyogenes*
   (c) *Escherichia coli*
   (d) *Pseudomonas aeruginosa*
7. Which one of the following bacteria splits urea into ammonia?
   (a) *Proteus mirabilis*
   (b) *Staphylococcus aureus*
   (c) *Pseudomonas aeruginosa*
   (d) *Streptococcus pyogenes*
8. Which among the following facts is not true about penicillin?
   (a) It is stabilized by penicillinase
   (b) It was discovered by Sir Alexander Fleming
   (c) It is highly bactericidal for *Streptococcus pyogenes*
   (d) It is the antibiotic of choice for treating syphilis
9. Which among the following facts is true about moxalactam?
   (a) It belongs to first-generation cephalosporins
   (b) It belongs to second-generation cephalosporins
   (c) It belongs to third-generation cephalosporins
   (d) It is not a cephalosporin
10. All of the following drugs are aminoglycosides, except
   (a) Gentamicin
   (b) Amikacin
   (c) Tobramycin
   (d) Aztreonam
11. Nosocomial infection is
   (a) Infection of the nose
   (b) Community-acquired infection
   (c) Endogenous infection
   (d) Hospital-acquired exogenous infection
12. Infection of the wound during operation is prevented by taking measures at
   (a) Patient's level
   (b) Operating team level
   (c) Instruments, equipment, and dressing material level
   (d) All three levels
13. The hands are scrubbed up to
   (a) Hands only
   (b) Hands and half forearm
   (c) Hands and forearms
   (d) Hands, forearms, and half upper arms
14. Autoclaving is usually done at
   (a) 100°C for 0.5 hour
   (b) 120°C at 15 lb pressure for 20 minutes
   (c) 134°C at 30 lb pressure for 5 minutes
   (d) 115°C at 10 lb pressure for 45 minutes
15. All of the following facts about glutaraldehyde are correct, except
   (a) It is much more active but less stable in acidic solution
   (b) It is bactericidal, sporicidal, and viricidal
   (c) It is used to sterilize endoscopes and plastic materials
   (d) It can cause allergic reaction
16. The causative organism of cold abscess is
   (a) *Mycobacterium tuberculosis*
   (b) *Treponema pallidum*
   (c) *Neisseria gonorrhoeae*
   (d) *Streptococcus pyogenes*
17. Cellulitis is caused by
   (a) *Treponema pallidum*
   (b) *Neisseria gonorrhoeae*
   (c) *Streptococcus haemolyticus*
   (d) *Actinomyces israelii*
18. A patient presents with acute spreading swelling and redness of facial skin following a minor scratch. It has spread to involve the pinna. The skin has roseolar pink rash. What is the diagnosis?
   (a) Erysipelas

(CONTD...)

SELF-ASSESSMENT *(...CONTD)*

(b) Boil
(c) Carbuncle
(d) Cellulitis

19. A middle-aged diabetic presents with an acute inflammatory swelling on the nape of neck discharging pus from many openings (sieve-like appearance). What is the diagnosis?
(a) Cold abscess
(b) Cellulitis
(c) Erysipelas
(d) Carbuncle

20. What is the causative organism of tuberculosis?
(a) *Clostridium tetani*
(b) *Mycobacterium tuberculosis*
(c) *Streptococcus pyogenes*
(d) *Staphylococcus aureus*

21. Hemoptysis is a specific symptom of
(a) Pulmonary tuberculosis
(b) Intestinal tuberculosis
(c) Tuberculosis of bones
(d) Renal tuberculosis

22. The most important clinical diagnostic sign of tuberculous lymphadenitis is
(a) Tender nodes
(b) Soft nodes
(c) Enlarged matted nodes
(d) Hard nodes

23. The dose of isoniazid is
(a) 0.5 mg/kg of body weight
(b) 5 mg/kg of body weight
(c) 7.5 mg/kg of body weight
(d) 10 mg/kg of body weight

24. Which one of the following is a quick and reliable diagnostic investigation for tuberculosis?
(a) Tuberculin test
(b) Culture on Lowenstein–Jensen medium
(c) DNA–RNA amplification
(d) ESR

25. The most important toxicity of ethambutol is
(a) Hepatotoxicity
(b) Optic neuritis
(c) Skin rash
(d) Nephrotoxicity

26. Which among the following is the causative organism of syphilis?
(a) *Treponema pallidum*
(b) *Nocardia*
(c) *Chlamydia trachomatis*
(d) *Haemophilus ducreyi*

27. What is the usual mode of transmission of infection of syphilis?
(a) Inhalation
(b) Ingestion
(c) Sexual intercourse
(d) Skin contact

28. *Treponema pallidum* is a
(a) Spirochaete
(b) Coccus
(c) Fungus
(d) Protozoa

29. The lymph nodes of primary syphilis are
(a) Shotty
(b) Matted
(c) Tender
(d) Soft

30. The most important clinical manifestation of primary syphilis is
(a) Cutaneous rash
(a) Alopecia
(c) Hunterian chancre
(d) Generalized lymphadenopathy

31. The most common orodental manifestation of congenital syphilis is
(a) Notch at cutting edge of permanent incisors
(b) Condyloma
(c) Chancre of lip
(d) Gumma of tongue

32. The diagnostic investigation of primary syphilis is
(a) Seeing the spirochaete by dark-field microscopy
(b) Culture of exudate
(c) VDRL
(d) Skin reaction

33. Which of the following is the antibiotic of choice for treating syphilis?
(a) Streptomycin
(b) Penicillin
(c) Chloromycetin
(d) Rifampicin

(CONTD...)

SELF-ASSESSMENT *(...CONTD)*

34. Which among the following is the causative organism of gonorrhea?
    (a) *Neisseria gonorrhoeae*
    (b) *Treponema pallidum*
    (c) *Chlamydia trachomatis*
    (d) *Haemophilus ducreyi*
35. *Neisseria gonorrhoeae* is a
    (a) Spirochaete
    (b) Bacillus
    (c) Diplococcus
    (d) Protozoa
36. The gonococcal infection is usually transmitted by
    (a) Ingestion
    (b) Inhalation
    (c) Skin contact
    (d) Sexual intercourse
37. The incubation period of this disease is
    (a) 2–8 hours
    (b) 2–8 days
    (c) 2–8 weeks
    (d) 2–8 months
38. Which among the following is the earliest clinical lesion?
    (a) Arthritis of temporomandibular joint
    (b) Urethritis
    (d) Urethral stricture
    (d) Endocarditis
39. The culture of gonococcal discharge is done on
    (a) Thayer–Martin medium
    (b) Dorset egg medium
    (c) Lowenstein–Jensen medium
    (d) Agar gel
40. Which among the following is the drug of choice for gonorrhea?
    (a) Streptomycin
    (b) Chloromycetin
    (c) Cefixime
    (d) Doxycycline
41. Which among the following is the causative organism of chancroid?
    (a) *Neisseria gonorrhoeae*
    (b) *Treponema pallidum*
    (c) *Chlamydia trachomatis*
    (d) *Haemophilus ducreyi*
42. The infection of chancroid is usually transmitted by
    (a) Ingestion
    (b) Inhalation
    (c) Skin contact
    (d) Sexual intercourse
43. The incubation period of this disease is
    (a) 3–5 days
    (b) 8–10 days
    (c) 10–15 days
    (d) 15–21 days
44. The edge of ulcer of chancroid is
    (a) Sloping
    (b) Punched out
    (c) Everted
    (d) Undermined
45. The drug of choice for treatment of chancroid is
    (a) Azithromycin
    (b) Streptomycin
    (c) Doxycycline
    (d) Rifampicin
46. What is the causative organism of anthrax?
    (a) *Staphylococcus aureus*
    (b) *Streptococcus haemolyticus*
    (c) *Bacillus anthracis*
    (d) *Candida albicans*
47. All of the following are the features of *Bacillus anthracis*, except
    (a) It is a Gram-positive bacterium
    (b) It is an anaerobic organism
    (c) It is spore forming
    (d) Spores and not the vegetative bacteria are the infectious form of the organism
48. Which among the following is the causative organism of tetanus?
    (a) *Clostridium perfringens*
    (b) *Clostridium septicum*
    (c) *Clostridium tetani*
    (d) Anaerobic *Streptococcus*
49. The usual portal of entry of tetanus bacteria is
    (a) By ingestion
    (b) By inhalation
    (c) By skin contact
    (d) Through a wound

(CONTD...)

SELF-ASSESSMENT *(...CONTD)*

50. The average incubation period of tetanus is
    (a) 8–12 hours
    (b) 8–12 days
    (c) 8–12 weeks
    (d) 8–12 months
51. Which among the following is the earliest clinical manifestation?
    (a) Trismus
    (b) Opisthotonus
    (c) Toxic convulsions
    (d) Hyperpyrexia
52. The permanent preventive measure of tetanus is
    (a) Administration of TIG
    (b) Administration of tetanus toxoid
    (c) Antibiotics
    (d) Prevention of injury
53. Which among the following is the causative organism of actinomycosis?
    (a) *Haemophilus ducreyi*
    (b) *Candida albicans*
    (c) *Actinomyces israelii*
    (d) *Staphylococcus aureus*
54. This organism spreads in the body by all of the following routes, except
    (a) Local invasion
    (b) Hematogenous spread
    (c) Lymphatic
    (d) Inhalation
55. The discharge from actimycotic sinus is
    (a) Blue-green pus
    (b) Bloody fluid
    (c) Pus having "sulfur granules"
    (d) Thin syrup-like pus
56. The drug of choice for treating actinomycosis is
    (a) Penicillin
    (b) Streptomycin
    (c) Rifampicin
    (d) Gentamicin
57. The causative organism of hepatitis B is a
    (a) Virus
    (b) Coccus
    (c) Bacillus
    (d) Fungus
58. The infection enters the body
    (a) By ingestion
    (b) By inhalation
    (c) Through cut, puncture, or transfusion of infected blood
    (d) By skin contact
59. Hepatitis B is a preventable disease and prevented by
    (a) Antibiotics
    (b) Antiviral serum
    (c) Vaccination
    (d) Dietary hygiene
60. The causative organism of AIDS is
    (a) *Staphylococcus aureus*
    (b) *Treponema pallidum*
    (c) *Actinomyces israelii*
    (d) HIV virus
61. The infection enters the body by
    (a) Ingestion
    (b) Inhalation
    (c) Skin or mucous membrane exposure to infected blood and body fluids
    (d) Touching a patient of AIDS
62. Which among the following is the commonest tumor that occurs as a complication?
    (a) Carcinoma of cheek
    (b) Basal cell carcinoma
    (c) Carcinoma of maxillary antrum
    (d) Kaposi's sarcoma
63. Which among the following statements about AIDS is not true?
    (a) It is a viral infection
    (b) It causes depletion of CD4 depressor cells
    (c) One of the etiological risk factors is sexual contact with an infected person
    (d) It can be prevented by vaccination

Answers

1. (d) 2. (d) 3. (c) 4. (d) 5. (b) 6. (c) 7. (a) 8. (a) 9. (c) 10. (d) 11. (d) 12. (d) 13. (c) 14. (b) 15. (a) 16. (a) 17. (c) 18. (a) 19. (d) 20. (b) 21. (a) 22. (c) 23. (b) 24. (c) 25. (b) 26. (a) 27. (c) 28. (a) 29. (a) 30. (c) 31. (a) 32. (a) 33. (b) 34. (a) 35. (c) 36. (d) 37. (b) 38. (b) 39. (a) 40. (c) 41. (d) 42. (d) 43. (a) 44. (d) 45. (a) 46. (c) 47. (b) 48. (c) 49. (d) 50. (b) 51. (a) 52. (b) 53. (c) 54. (c) 55. (c) 56. (a) 57. (a) 58. (c) 59. (c) 60. (d) 61. (c) 62. (d) 63. (d)

Tumors

7

Definitions

Tumor A tumor or neoplasm is a swelling or mass (oma) produced by uncontrolled and purposeless proliferation of a clone of cells. In tumorigenesis there is loss of body control on the growth and proliferation of cells, and the newly formed cells are without any useful function.

Hypertrophy It is the enlargement of an organ without any increase in the number of cells.

Hyperplasia It is the enlargement of an organ due to an increased number of cells.

Metaplasia It is the change in the characteristics of epithelium due to prolonged irritation. A malignant tumor may arise from this changed or metaplastic epithelium. Examples of metaplasia are given in Box 7.1.

Anaplasia It is the loss of differentiation of cells (dedifferentiation) and of their orientation to one another.

Box 7.1 Examples of metaplasia

- Transitional epithelium of the urinary bladder may change into squamous epithelium
- Columnar epithelium of gall bladder and bronchial tubes may change into squamous epithelium
- Squamous epithelium of esophagus may change into columnar epithelium (Barrett's esophagus)

Dysplasia It includes the alterations in intracellular organization, size and shape of the nucleus, size and shape of cell, and the intracellular three-dimensional organization. Salient features of dysplasia are given in Box 7.2.

Carcinoma In Situ It is the earliest type of cancer in which the cellular, nuclear, and three-dimensional architecture resembles cancer but without invasion into extracellular matrix. It usually follows severe dysplasia.

Box 7.2 Salient features of dysplasia

- Alteration in intracellular organization, size and shape of nucleus, size and shape of cell, and intracellular three-dimensional organization
- Represents the earliest change of neoplastic transformation which can be detected by microscopy
- May be mild, moderate, or severe
- May revert to normal following elimination of the neoplastic clone, but is least likely with severe dysplasia

Genotype It is the molecular structure of any cell. A malignant genotype has losses and mutations of tumor suppressor genes and the presence of oncogenes.

Phenotype It is the appearance of a cell at microstructural level (microscopic phenotype) and its functional state (biological phenotype). A changed genotype precedes a particular phenotype. The cell may appear normal for some time even though it has already acquired a malignant genotype.

Teratoma It arises from embryonic stem cells containing representative cells from all three embryonic layers (ectoderm, mesoderm, and endoderm). A teratomatous dermoid contains hair, nails, teeth, muscle, and gland tissue.

Blastoma It develops from "unipotent" cells and arises from any one of the three embryonic layers, for example, neuroblastoma.

Benign Tumor It grows slowly and does not disseminate, and does not recur after complete excision. It is usually encapsulated (Fig. 7.1).

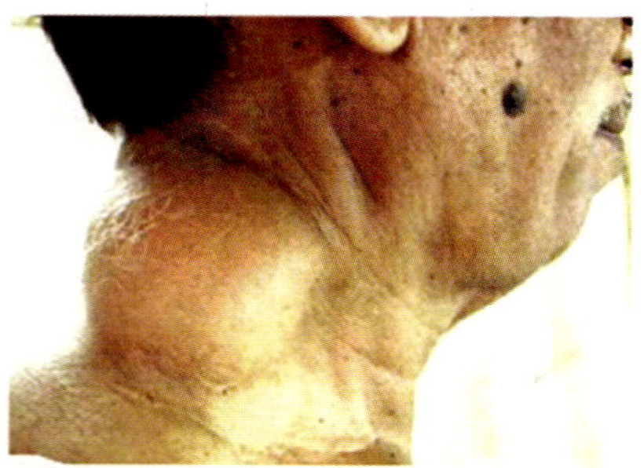

Figure 7.1 Lipoma of nape of neck—an example of a benign tumor.

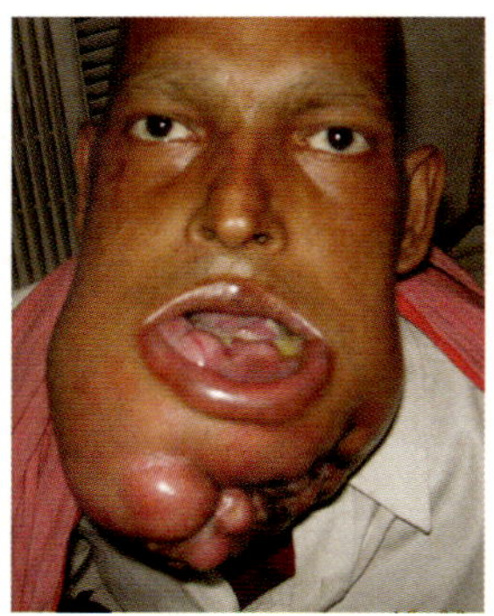

Figure 7.2 Osteosarcoma of lower jaw—an example of a malignant tumor.

Malignant Tumor (Fig. 7.2) It grows rapidly and has a tendency to spread locally or to other parts of body by lymphatics or bloodstream. It has pleomorphism of cells and nuclei. A malignant tumor is what is called cancer. Many cells of cancer have an abnormal number of chromosomes which is not a multiple of the usual haploid number (aneuploidy). The differences between a benign and a malignant tumor are given in Table 7.1.

Locally Malignant Tumor It is an intermediate type of tumor which invades the local tissues but is less inclined to lymphatic or vascular dissemination. The examples of locally malignant tumors are pleomorphic adenoma of salivary glands, osteoclastoma, and basal cell carcinoma.

Nomenclature

The word "oma" means a tumor. To give a name to the tumor, it is suffixed with the name of the tissue from which the tumor is arising. Thus, fibroma is a benign tumor of fibrous tissue, lipoma of fatty tissue, myoma of muscle tissue, osteoma of bone, chondroma of cartilage, and adenoma of glandular tissue.

Regarding the nomenclature of malignant tumors, carcinoma is a malignant tumor of ectodermal and endodermal cells and accordingly it is classified as squamous cell carcinoma, basal cell carcinoma, and adenocarcinoma. Sarcoma is a malignant tumor of tissues of mesodermal

Table 7.1 Differences between a benign and a malignant tumor

Features	Benign tumor	Malignant tumor
Rate of growth	Slow	Rapid
Surface	Smooth or lobulated	Irregular or nodular
Shape	Regular	Irregular
Consistency	Uniform	Hard or variable
Number	May be multiple	Usually single
Pattern	Uniform	Irregular
Capsule	Encapsulated	Nonencapsulated
Cut surface	Uniform	Variegated
Similarity to normal tissues	Corresponds very closely to the normal structures from which it has arisen	• Deviates markedly from the normal tissue from which It has arisen • Shows anaplasia
Nucleus	Normal size, shape, and staining	Large, variable in shape and size, hyperchromatic
Local invasion	Absent	Present
Metastasis	Absent	May be present
Recurrence	Does not recur	Recurrence is common

origin, for example, fibrosarcoma from fibrous tissue, osteosarcoma from bone, chondrosarcoma from cartilage, and liposarcoma from fatty tissue.

Etiology

The full etiology of tumorigenesis is not known, but many causative factors are known which are different for different types of tumors. Some of the etiological factors are described in the subsequent text.

Genetic Factors

The genes may be inherited or acquired. Inherited cancers are caused by specific DNA mutation of a tumor suppressor gene inherited in all cells. In the cells of the affected organ the homologous (second) gene is lost, initiating a sequence of genetic mutations culminating in cancer (Box 7.3).

There are three important classes of genes involved in cancer.

Tumor Suppressor Genes They control the cell cycle by slowing down the cycle or triggering apoptosis. The examples of these genes include *p53*, *P16*, *APC*, and *RB1*.

Box 7.3 Examples of inherited cancer

- Familial adenomatous polyposis (FAP)
- Hereditary nonpolyposis colonic cancer (HNPCC)
- Familial breast cancer
- Familial breast–ovarian cancer
- Familial retinoblastoma
- Neurofibromatosis

Oncogenes They promote cell proliferation by increasing signaling activity from the cell surface to the transcription apparatus or gene promotors. The examples of oncogenes include *k-ras*, $ERB\text{-}B_2$, and *C-myc*.

Growth Factors Growth factors and their receptors are switched on by oncogenes or switched off by tumor suppressor genes. The examples are EGF, TGF-α, IGF, and FGF. They are also involved in the etiology of cancer.

Chemical Carcinogens

Chemical carcinogens probably account for the majority of sporadic (acquired) cancers. Some examples of cancers of chemical carcinogenesis are bronchogenic carcinoma (tobacco-associated nitrosamines), vesical carcinoma (aromatic amines), and mesothelioma (asbestos). Kashmiris are prone to squamous cell carcinoma of thigh and lower abdomen due to the habit of keeping them warm by squatting and hugging kangri (earthenware pot) containing glowing charcoal. It causes irritation of skin by heat and fumes.

Some examples of cancers of chemical carcinogenesis are given in Table 7.2.

Ultraviolet and Ionizing Radiation

DNA strand breaks are induced by ultraviolet and ionizing radiation which if not repaired lead to cancer. The examples of cancers caused by ultraviolet and ionizing radiation are malignant melanoma and basal cell carcinoma. Some examples of tumors etiologically related to ionizing radiation are cancer of thyroid, skin, and bone marrow.

Viruses

Some cancers are etiologically related to viruses, for example, nasopharyngeal carcinoma, endemic Burkitt's lymphoma, Hodgkin's disease (40%), post-transplant lymphomatous proliferation disease (PTLPD), Kaposi's sarcoma, carcinoma of cervix, adult T-cell leukemia-lymphoma (ATLL), and carcinoma of liver. At least 2% of cancers are caused by viruses. However, most of these tumors do not have features of a transmissible disease. Hence, they are unlikely to be caused by infective agents.

Cellular Instability and Senescence

Cellular instability from ageing of stem cell lines (many common cancers) or chronic inflammation leads to increased cell proliferation and reduced apoptosis. It causes malignant transformation, the examples of which are squamous cell carcinoma in a chronic ulcer or scar (Marjolin's ulcer) and a fibrosarcoma in a scar.

Other Factors

Environmental cofactors are also important. For example, *Helicobacter pylori* is linked to gastric carcinoma. A diet rich in calories and saturated fats (red meat) is responsible for many cancers including those of colorectum and pancreas.

Methods of spread

Benign Tumors These do not spread and remain localized to the place of origin for many years.

Malignant Tumors These have a tendency to spread in the body. The methods of spread are described as follows:

- **Direct spread (local spread)**: It occurs readily along connective tissue planes, but it may spread by local invasion, and any tissue or structure may be infiltrated.
- **Bloodstream**: The cancer cells are present frequently in the venous blood draining the organ having cancer. They may be arrested or implanted in the lungs, bones, liver, brain, and other areas producing metastases or second-

Table 7.2 Malignancies due to chemical carcinogens

Chemical carcinogens	Malignancy
Tobacco-associated nitrosamines	Bronchogenic carcinoma
Tobacco chewing, alcohol drinking	Carcinoma of oral cavity, esophagus, and liver
Aromatic amines	Vesical carcinoma
Asbestos	Mesothelioma
Wood dust	Carcinoma of paranasal sinuses
Vinyl alcohol	Angiosarcoma
Arsenic	Carcinoma of skin

ary cancer. The spread by bloodstream is the usual method of spread of a sarcoma.

- **Lymphatic spread**: Carcinomas usually spread by lymphatic permeation or embolism. Permeation is an active process where the cancer cells grow along the lymphatic vessels ahead of reactionary fibrosis. In embolism, the cancer cells are carried by lymph circulation (passive process) into the draining lymph nodes.

Histological grading

Histological grading is important as it tells about the prognosis. It depends on the degree of differentiation of the tumor based on pleomorphism of cells, and in an adenocarcinoma attempt at gland formation. The grades of a malignant tumor are given in Box 7.4.

Box 7.4 Histological grading of malignant tumors

- **Gx**: Grade cannot be assessed
- **G1**: Well differentiated
- **G2**: Moderately differentiated
- **G3**: Poorly differentiated
- **G4**: Undifferentiated

Clinical features

Age and Sex Anybody—child, young, or elderly and male or female—may suffer from this disease.

Site of Occurrence Based on the site of occurrence, the tumors are of two types:

1. **Surface tumor**: As the tumor is visible and/or palpable, the patient may present early for treatment.
2. **Internal or deep-seated tumors**: This tumor is not visible and is without symptoms in early stage. Hence, frequently a delay of approximately 2 years between the onset of disease and its detection is very common. This loss of useful time frequently proves dangerous as it delays treatment.

Clinical Features of a Benign Tumor

- The patient has a painless and slow-growing swelling or a nodule of insidious onset.
- The swelling is smooth or lobulated, uniform, soft or firm, well defined, and mobile.
- These tumors are usually not harmful (benign means kind), but sometimes may present with symptoms of pressure on the structures in the vicinity, or of production of hormones, for example, a pituitary adenoma producing acromegaly.

Clinical Features of a Malignant Tumor

- An early malignant tumor usually does not have any symptoms. As the disease advances, some symptoms appear which should make one suspect the presence of cancer (Box 7.5). If any of these symptoms is present, it must be thoroughly evaluated.

Box 7.5 Symptoms that may be of malignancy

- An ulcer which refuses to heal with 3 weeks' treatment
- Any swelling, nodule, or lump, especially of recent origin or growing rapidly
- Abnormal nontraumatic hemorrhage from anywhere in the body, that is, vagina, rectum, urethra, oral cavity, nose, nipple, or gum
- Persistent indigestion or loss of appetite in a middle-aged or elderly person
- Any recent pathological change, that is, pigmentation, ulceration, bleeding, sudden enlargement, or appearance of pain in a mole or wart
- Difficulty in swallowing (dysphagia)
- Persistent hoarseness of voice
- Recent change in the bowel habit
- Persistent cough, breathlessness, and segmental wheezing in the lungs
- Unexplained loss of body weight
- Loss of general health, pyrexia of unknown origin, and fatigue, especially if they are present in a middle-aged or elderly person, must be investigated for cancer

- The swelling of a malignant tumor is irregular, hard or variable, and ill-defined, and may be fixed to the underlying structures. Malignant ulcers have an everted or raised edge and indurated base.

Clinical Features of Metastasis

A malignant tumor may metastasize to the lymph nodes, lung, liver, bones, and brain, presenting with lymphadenopathy, hemoptysis and/or breathlessness, hepatomegaly and/or jaundice, bone pain or a pathological fracture, or focal neurological deficit, respectively.

Features of Malignant Transformation of a Benign Tumor

Some benign tumors are likely to change into a malignant tumor as time passes, for example, pleomorphic adenoma of parotid into carcinoma and mole into a malignant melanoma. It is very important to recognize this change for the purpose of early treatment. Some signs of malignant transformation are given in Box 7.6.

Box 7.6 Signs of malignant transformation of a benign tumor

- **Increase in size**: A recent rapid rate of growth being an important sign of malignant change
- **Increased vascularity** as indicated by dilated cutaneous veins, surrounding anger and, probably expansile pulsation
- **Fixity**: A tumor which was previously mobile getting fixed to the superficial or deep structures
- **Involvement of neighboring structures**: For example, recurrent laryngeal nerve in a thyroid swelling and facial nerve in a parotid swelling
- **Spread**: Evidence of local or general spread
- **Ulceration and/or bleeding**

Staging of tumors

No staging is required in benign tumors. Staging is required in malignant tumors for the purposes of planning treatment and predicting the prognosis.

Box 7.7 Clinical staging of malignant tumors

- **Stage I:** The tumor is small and limited to a part of the affected organ
- **Stage II:** The tumor is small with limited or early regional (lymphatic) spread
- **Stage III:** The tumor has become large and the regional spread has grown to become extensive or fixed
- **Stage IV:** Distant spread has occurred

There are many methods of staging a malignant tumor.

Clinical Staging In this staging only the clinical factors are taken into account. It is the simplest method of staging in which a tumor is described to have four stages (Box 7.7).

TNM Staging It is an accurate modern method of clinical staging in which numerical values are given to the character of primary tumor (T), lymph nodes (N), and the presence of distant metastases (M). The T and N stages are defined differently for each type of tumor while M is the same for all cancers.

Investigations

The main aim of the investigations in tumors is to make or confirm the diagnosis and to find the extent of spread of disease. They are important in deciding the treatment and predicting the prognosis.

Laboratory Studies

The blood is sent for hemoglobin, counts, ESR, sugar, urea, creatinine, and other tests depending on the nature of tumor, for example, PSA in carcinoma of prostate. Hemoglobin is usually low in most of the cancers.

Radiology

Plain Radiography Radiography of the bone helps in the diagnosis of most of bone tumors. For the diagnosis of lesions of the jaws, orthopantomography is the modern method which provides good images of jaws. X-ray of the chest helps in the diagnosis of both primary and secondary tumors of the lungs.

Contrast Radiography These studies are done to image the lesions of hollow organs and tubes by filling them with a contrast and taking appropriate pictures. A tumor is recognized by a filling defect—regular filling defect in a benign tumor and irregular in a malignant tumor. Thus, barium studies (meal and enema) are done to diagnose tumors of gastrointestinal tract and cystography for tumors of urinary bladder.

Mammography It is soft-tissue radiography of breast and done to picturize the breast for early detection of cancer. The carcinoma of breast is diagnosed by irregular speculated border and punctate calcification of the lesion.

Ultrasonography One can "see" inside the body with the help of high-frequency sound waves and draw pictures. Thus, ultrasound helps in the diagnosis of tumors of internal organs.

CT Scan Combining X-ray equipment with a TV cathode ray tube and a computer, a CT scanner can see and record inside the body to detect cancer and to find its exact site, size, and extent by studying the desired cross-sections of the body.

MRI It is more or less similar to CT scan. Here the magnetic waves are used for scanning. It gives better pictures of soft tissues than a CT scan, especially angioinvasion. It is the investigation of choice for tumors of brain and spinal cord.

Biopsy

Any suspicious lesion must be subjected to biopsy for making a histological or tissue diagnosis. Hence, it is rightly said "when in doubt cut it out." The biopsy is the best and reliable method to confirm the diagnosis of a tumor.

- The biopsy procedure is easy in surface lesions (incisional, excisional, or punch biopsy).
- The lesions having depth or of internal organs are biopsied by a needle (Tru-Cut needle) which may be inserted under US or CT guidance.
- Biopsy from lesions of hollow organs can be taken through an endoscope (endoscopic biopsy) by a long delicate forceps or by brushing (brush biopsy).
- Sometimes biopsy from internal organs requires an open operation.

Fine-Needle Aspiration Cytology or Biopsy (FNAC or FNAB)

It is done by inserting a 23-gauze needle into the lesion, maintaining suction, and making several passes of the needle through the tumor. The material obtained from the needle is studied cytologically. IFNAC/FNAB gives a cytological diagnosis, not a tissue diagnosis. It is a rapid method of diagnosis.

Other Methods

Endoscopy Nearly all the hollow organs, tubes, and body cavities can be seen from inside by endoscopy and the nature of the lesion can be diagnosed by its gross appearance and then confirmed by endoscopic biopsy. The endoscopy has reduced the importance of some of the radiocontrast studies. For example, the gastric tumors are now mostly diagnosed by gastroscopy and not by barium meal.

Radioisotope Scanning It also helps in the diagnosis of some cancers, for example, ^{131}I thyroid scan to find a "cold" nodule and later on functioning metastases in the bones after thyroidectomy in a follicular carcinoma of thyroid. Similarly bone scanning is done to detect bony metastases of carcinoma of prostate.

Screening for early detection of cancer

It involves detection of disease in asymptomatic prone population when curative treatment is possible because of early stage of disease, for example, carcinoma of breast, cervix, and colon. The criteria for screening are:

- The tumor must be sufficiently common to warrant screening, and must be recognizable

at an early stage when it can be better treated than at a later stage.
- The screening test must be sensitive and effective, acceptable to people, and safe and inexpensive, for example, mammography for carcinoma of breast and Pap smear for carcinoma of cervix.
- The program must have adequate diagnostic and therapeutic facilities for those with a positive test result.

Treatment

The main aim of the treatment is complete removal of the disease. Even if one live cancer cell is left, the disease is likely to recur frequently with increased momentum.

Treatment of a Benign Tumor

A small asymptomatic benign tumor may be left as such with appropriate instructions given to the patient or it may be excised with its capsule, for example, lipoma, a benign mole, and subcutaneous neurofibroma.

Treatment of a Malignant Tumor

Malignant tumors are treated by a multidisciplinary team comprising surgeons, oncologists, radiotherapists, pathologists, and often specialist nurses. There are three major methods of treatment of cancer: surgery, radiotherapy, and chemotherapy. These treatment modalities are complementary to one another.

Surgery

Surgery is the most powerful and reliable method of treatment of malignant tumors. It has several roles including diagnosis by doing biopsy or exploration, removal of primary tumor, excision of metastatic disease, palliation, and reconstruction.

The main aim of surgery is local control which equates to cure when the disease is localized. Many types of operations are done for controlling the disease or to palliate some of the disturbing symptoms.

Wide Excision It implies removal of a tumor 2–3 cm beyond the visible and/or palpable limit of the tumor through the healthy tissue in all the three dimensions (three-dimensional excision). The margin of the removed specimen is studied histologically for absence of cancer cells or complete clearance of disease. It is the usual treatment of sarcomas and early carcinomas without local spread.

Radical Excision This operation includes wide excision of the primary combined with en bloc excision of draining lymph nodes. Radical excision is usually employed in the treatment of carcinomas which spread to regional lymph nodes.

Resection of Distant Metastasis Localized or one or two distant secondaries, for example, in liver in colonic carcinoma and in lung in renal cell carcinoma, can also be excised with many satisfactory results, after the successful treatment of the primary tumor.

Palliative Procedures In advanced cancer it may not be possible to do curative resection but some of its disturbing effects can be controlled or relieved by surgery described as follows:
- **Obstruction:** It can be controlled by providing a bypass or alternative route for the flow of contents, for example, tracheostomy for carcinoma of larynx. One of the modern methods of relieving obstruction includes vaporization of obstructing tumor with laser, and stent insertion.
- **Fungation:** It can be relieved by excision of tumor (as much as possible) and thermocoagulation.
- **Bleeding:** It can be controlled by ligation or percutaneous embolization of feeding artery, for example, ligation of external carotid artery in bleeding orofacial tumors.
- **Pathological fracture:** It is treated by open reduction, internal fixation, and radiotherapy.

Radiotherapy

Radiotherapy is the second most powerful method of treatment. Under favorable circumstances, radiation is lethal to cancer cells and sublethal to normal cells. Different tumors have differing

Box 7.8 Tumors and their degree of sensitivity to radiation

- **Very sensitive to radiation:** Lymphoma, Ewing's tumor
- **Sensitive to radiation:** Squamous cell carcinoma, basal cell carcinoma
- **Resistant to radiation:** Chondrosarcoma, malignant melanoma

degree of sensitivity to radiation damage which makes it possible to divide them roughly into very sensitive, sensitive, and resistant (Box 7.8).

Principles of radiotherapy

- The cells are irradiated at the most sensitive phase of the cell cycle to have the maximum effect.
- Delays in cell division are induced frequently in G2 phase or less frequently in G1 or S phase. They are most likely to be due to changes in the expression of genes such as *p53* and *bcl-2*.
- Radiation is given in multiple fractions.
- The mechanism of radiation-induced cell damage is given in Box 7.9.

Delivery of high-dose radiation therapy

Technical developments over the past two decades have made incremental improvements in the delivery of high-dose radiation therapy for cure through linear accelerators. The high-energy X-ray beams emitted from a linear accelerator spare superficial normal tissues and organs adjacent to the tumor which often receives large volumes of high-dose radiation that is required to control cancer.

Box 7.9 Mechanism of radiation-induced cell damage

- Radiotherapy affects cell differentiation, proliferation, and maturation
- DNA is the most sensitive target
- Gene transcription is induced
- Cell membranes are damaged due to lipid peroxidation
- Apoptosis (programmed cell death) is induced

If too small radiation fields are used to prevent exposure of normal tissues, there is a risk of inadequate treatment. Thus, this "extra" radiation dose to the normal tissues has to be accepted to assure adequate coverage of target volume.

The "extra" radiation is partly responsible for the side effects and complications that accompany high-dose curative radiotherapy. Hence, in order to keep the complication rate at an acceptable level, the total dose should be kept in a moderate or safe range.

Techniques of radiotherapy

Planning the Radiation Dose Cross-sectional imaging modalities (CT, MRI) help the clinicians in planning the dose and the method of giving radiation, that is, to visualize therapy targets and direct the radiation beam directly at the tumor and the tissues at risk of having cancer while sparing adjacent critical structures. They help in delivering a precise dose to the exact volume by using linear accelerators with devices called multileaf and micromultileaf collimator which make it possible to cure more tumors with minimal radiotoxicity.

Brachytherapy In this method the radiation source is placed on the surface of the tumor or in the tumor. One type of therapy is intracavitary which is used in many gynecological and oral tumors, dose being 3500–5000 cGy in a fractionated fashion over 4–6 weeks.

Modern Techniques of Radiotherapy The modern techniques have the advantages of high cure rates and reduced toxicity but the infrastructure is expensive and requires a lot of physician's and physicist's time, and machine time. The techniques are:

- Stereotactic radiation therapy
- Three-dimensional conformal radiation therapy
- Intensity-modulated radiation therapy (IMRT)

Novel Modalities

- **Gamma knife radiosurgery** allows focused radiation for limited brain metastasis and is associated with fewer long-term complications.

- **Cyber knife** is designed to perform tumor ablation anywhere in the body. It combines robotics and advanced image guidance to deliver radiosurgery to tumors at critical locations previously considered untreatable by surgery or radiation.
- **Radiolabeled antibodies** are under investigation as a means of delivering high levels of radiation locally to the tumor bed avoiding systemic toxicity.

Complications of radiotherapy

The complications of radiotherapy can be classified as local and systemic (Table 7.3).

Table 7.3 Complications of radiotherapy

Local complications	Systemic complications
• Epilation of hair • Wet and dry epidermatitis • Radiation ulcer	• Malaise, nausea, vomiting, and loss of weight • Immunosuppression • Mutagenesis

Chemotherapy

Surgery and radiotherapy are mainly the local methods of treatment. But many cancers have a systemic spread and manifestations. Hence, a systemic method of treatment is also required. Chemotherapy fills this gap. Hence, these three methods of treatment, that is, surgery, radiotherapy, and chemotherapy, are not competitive but supplementary to each other.

Mechanism of action of chemotherapeutic agents

All anticancer drugs act on cell metabolism at various stages of cell cycle of a dividing cell. The phases of cell cycle are G1 (presynthesis phase), S (DNA synthesis phase), G2 (premitosis phase), and M (phase of mitosis) (Fig. 7.3). The duration of G1 is very variable, of S is 8–30 hours, of G2 is 1 hour, and of M phase is 30–90 minutes. In G0 phase the cells are not in the cycle but can be recruited into it.

Chemotherapeutic agents

The anticancer drugs are of many types.

Polyfunctional Alkylating Agents They act by forming covalent bonds with nucleic acid and thus chemically interact with DNA. Some examples of these drugs are mechlorethamine, chlorambucil, melphalan, busulfan, and cyclophosphamide.

Antimetabolites They have a structural similarity to physiological intermediates of metabolism and thus enter vital biochemical reactions and interfere with normal cell survival. The common examples of drugs of this group are methotrexate and 5-fluorouracil.

Antibiotics They are derived from different species of the fungus *Streptomyces*. The examples of antibiotics are doxorubicin, bleomycin, and dactinomycin. They appear to act by binding with double-stranded DNA preventing its replication.

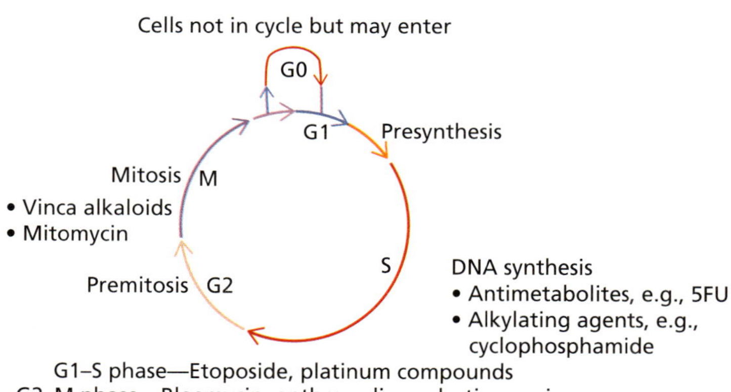

Figure 7.3 Phases of cell cycle with names of some anticancer drugs for that phase.

Hormones and Related Compounds Many cancers are hormone dependent, for example, carcinoma of prostate and breast. Hence, estrogens are given to treat carcinoma of prostate and antiestrogens, for example, tamoxifen and aromatase inhibitors in carcinoma of breast.

Prednisone It does not have any antimitotic property but it is used as a potentiator in many protocols containing combination of drugs.

Other Drugs In this group are included vinca alkaloids (e.g., vincristine and vinblastine), nitrosoureas (e.g., BCNU and CCNU), and platinum-based compounds (e.g., cisplatinum).

Types of chemotherapy

Neoadjuvant Chemotherapy

- Here the anticancer drugs are given before surgery or radiotherapy.
- This treatment gives better cure rates in osteogenic sarcoma, Wilms' tumor, neuroblastoma, and rhabdomyosarcoma.
- Advantage: The tissues are not scarred by surgery and radiotherapy and the vascular supply of the area is good, facilitating adequate local delivery and concentration of drugs.
- Disadvantage: As the tumor shows regression, the patient may not complete the treatment.

Perioperative Chemotherapy Here the drugs are given during or in the immediate postoperative period, the object being to kill the circulating cancer cells released by operative manipulation.

Adjuvant Chemotherapy It involves the use of anticancer drugs in the postsurgical or postradiation period. Multiple drugs are usually used. This therapy results in improved survivals in osteogenic sarcoma, certain pediatric tumors, testicular tumors, and carcinoma of breast and ovary.

Combination Chemotherapy Different cytotoxic drugs act at different sites of the cycle of a dividing cell. Hence, if drugs acting on different sites and having different toxicities are used, the effectivity of treatment improves with reduced resistance and less doses to obtain a better result.

High-Dose Chemotherapy Increasing the dose over the conventional dose results in a better response but with a higher toxicity. The latter can be countered by the use of an antidote at the same time or bone marrow transplantation. For example, in the treatment of osteosarcoma, 8–10 g of methotrexate may be given with leucovorin factor or folic acid rescue. While most of the drug is fixed to the tumor, the leftover drug in the blood is mostly neutralized by folinic acid (a derivative of folic acid). Most of the anticancer drugs cause bone marrow depression which is being managed by bone marrow transplantation. This method of chemotherapy is used to treat leukemias.

Clinical response to chemotherapy

- The best results of chemotherapy as the principal method of therapy are obtained in gestational trophoblastic tumors, acute lymphoblastic leukemia, and lymphoma. Many patients of these cancers are cured by chemotherapy.
- Chemotherapy as an adjuvant to surgery has dramatically improved the cure rates of testicular tumors, osteogenic sarcoma, Wilms' tumor, and rhabdomyosarcoma.
- Significant but less dramatic improvement in the survivals has occurred when chemotherapy is used alone or as an adjuvant in myeloblastic leukemia, carcinoma of breast and prostate, and small cell carcinoma of lung.
- Multiple myeloma, ovarian and endometrial cancer, neuroblastoma, and squamous cell carcinoma of aerodigestive tract show a very good response to chemotherapy.
- The carcinomas of gastrointestinal tract including liver and pancreas, non-small cell lung cancer, and carcinoma of uterine cervix and adrenal cortex show no significant response, and melanoma and chondrosarcoma do not show any response to chemotherapy.

Toxicity of chemotherapy

- **Immediate toxicity**: Nausea, vomiting, phlebitis at injection site and tissue reaction if the drug leaks out, and hyperuricemia

- **Early toxicity**: Myelosuppression leading to thrombocytopenia, leucopenia, oral ulceration, and diarrhea
- **Late toxicity**: Anemia, aspermia, hepatocellular damage, and pulmonary fibrosis

Other Treatment Modalities

Immunotherapy

It is a weak method of treatment. It aims at restoration of proper balance between tumor growth and destruction and inducing protective immunity. Some methods currently in use are as follows.

Bacterial Vaccines These include, for example, BCG.

Cytokines These include, for example, interleukins, especially IL-2, and interferon-alpha.

Strategies to Target Acquired Immunity

- Active immunization, for example, alteration of tumor cell immunogenicity by infection with certain viruses, genetic vaccines
- Passive immunization, for example, administration of antibodies against growth factors or growth factor receptors such as HER-2/neu receptors in epithelial cell malignancies and IL-2 receptor in cells
- Transfer of immune effector cells, for example, lymphokine-activated killer cells

Gene therapy

It involves the transfer and expression of genes or oligonucleotides that restore, add, or block the cellular function.

Prognosis

The results of treatment are assessed by regular follow-up of all the treated patients to find out the number of surviving patients after a definite period (3-year survival rate, 5-year survival rate, and 10-year survival rate).

Tumor markers

Definition

A tumor marker is a molecule, the expression or altered level of expression of which is associated with the development or progression of a malignant tumor.

Types of Tumor Markers

Tumor markers may be of the nature of proteins, enzymes, carbohydrates, DNA/RNA, gangliosides, immunoglobulins, and glycoproteins. Some common tumor markers are given in Table 7.4. The information about tumor markers is used both in the diagnosis and in the prognosis.

Table 7.4 Tumor markers for various malignancies

Classification	Subtypes	Tumor markers	Malignancy
Tumor-specific marker	Mutated	MUM-1, Cdk4, β-catenin	Melanoma
		Human leukocyte antigen A2	Renal cell carcinoma, bladder carcinoma
		KIAA 0205	Squamous cell carcinoma
	Viral	EBNA (EBV)	Lymphoma
		E6/E7 (HPV 16)	Carcinoma cervix
Tumor-associated markers	Differentiation	HER-2/neu	Carcinoma of breast
		PSA	Carcinoma of prostate
	Oncofetal	CEA	Colonic carcinoma
		RAGE	Renal cell carcinoma
	Clonal		Immunoglobulin idiotype—lymphoma

KEY POINTS

- A tumor or neoplasm is a swelling or mass produced by uncontrolled and purposeless proliferation of a clone of cells.
- Anaplasia is the loss of differentiation of cells (dedifferentiation) and of their orientation to one another. Dysplasia refers to alterations in intracellular organization, the size and shape of the nucleus and size and shape of cell, and the intracellular three-dimensional organization.
- A benign tumor grows slowly and does not disseminate, and does not recur after complete excision. It is usually encapsulated. The cells correspond very closely to the normal structures from which they have arisen. The tumor does not recur after surgical excision.
- A malignant tumor grows rapidly and has a tendency to spread locally or to other parts of body by lymphatics or bloodstream. The swelling of a malignant tumor is irregular, hard or variable, and ill-defined, and may be fixed to the underlying structures. Malignant ulcers have everted or raised edge and indurated base.
- Malignant tumors have pleomorphism of cells and nuclei. The cells deviate markedly from the normal tissue from which they have arisen. This rumor is likely to recur after surgical excision.
- A locally malignant tumor invades the local tissues but does not spread, for example, pleomorphic adenoma of salivary glands, osteoclastoma, and basal cell carcinoma.
- The causes of tumorigenesis include genes, chemical carcinogens, ultraviolet and ionizing radiation, viruses, cellular instability and senescence, and environmental cofactors.
- Benign tumors do not spread and remain localized to the place of origin for many years. Malignant tumors have a tendency to spread in the body by direct spread (local invasion), hematogenous route (sarcomas), and lymphatic spread (carcinomas).
- Histological grading of a malignant tumor (Gx, G1, G2, G3, G4) depends on the degree of differentiation of the tumor based on pleomorphism of cells. Prognosis of cancer is based on the histological grades.
- Features of malignant transformation of a benign tumor include an increase in the size of the tumor, increased vascularity, fixity to underlying structures, involvement of neighboring structures, evidence of local or distal spread, ulceration, or bleeding.
- Staging is required in malignant tumors for the purposes of planning treatment and predicting the prognosis. Clinical staging and TNM staging are the commonly used methods.
- Biopsy is the gold standard for confirming the diagnosis of tumors. CT and MRI are used to find the extent of the disease.
- Benign tumors are excised along with the capsule. Malignant tumors are treated with a combination of surgery, radiotherapy, and chemotherapy.
- The main aim of surgery is local control which equates to cure when the disease is localized. The types include wide excision, radical excision, resection of distal metastasis, palliative procedures such as removal of obstruction caused by tumors, excision of fungated growth, control of bleeding in tumors by ligation of feeding artery, and treatment of pathological fracture of bones caused by tumors.
- Radiotherapy is the second most powerful method of treatment. Different tumors have differing degree of sensitivity to radiation damage. Lymphoma and Ewing's sarcoma are very sensitive to radiation while chondrosarcoma and melanoma are resistant to radiation.
- Chemotherapeutic drugs act on cell metabolism at various stages of cell cycle of a dividing cell. Gestational trophoblastic tumors, acute lymphoblastic leukemia, and lymphoma respond to chemotherapy.
- A tumor marker is a molecule, the expression or altered level of expression of which is associated with the development or progression of a malignant tumor. It may be of the nature of proteins, enzymes, carbohydrates, DNA/RNA, gangliosides, immunoglobulins, and glycoproteins. The information about tumor markers is used both in the diagnosis and in the prognosis.

SELF-ASSESSMENT

Long answer questions

1. What are the differences between a benign and a malignant tumor? Describe the modes of spread of malignant tumors.
2. What do you understand by a tumor? Describe the pathology and clinical features of a tumor.
3. What are the methods of confirming the diagnosis of a malignant tumor? Discuss the principles of treatment of tumors.

Short answer questions

1. Nomenclature of tumors
2. Malignant transformation of a benign tumor
3. Biopsy
4. FNAC
5. Tumor markers

Multiple choice questions

1. Hyperplasia is defined as
   (a) Change in the character of epithelium
   (b) Enlargement of an organ without increase in the number of cells
   (c) Enlargement of an organ due to an increased number of cells
   (d) Alteration in the intracellular organization
2. Dysplasia is defined as
   (a) Loss of architecture of tissues
   (b) Alteration in the intracellular organization
   (c) Change in the architecture of epithelium
   (d) Enlargement of an organ due to increase in the number of cells
3. All of the following facts about a benign tumor are correct, except
   (a) It grows slowly
   (b) It does not produce metastasis
   (c) It does not recur after complete excision
   (d) It always transforms into a malignant tumor
4. Carcinoma is
   (a) A malignant tumor of cartilage
   (b) A benign tumor
   (c) A malignant tumor of cells of ectodermal and endodermal origin
   (d) Also known as cancrum oris
5. All of the following facts about a malignant tumor are true, except
   (a) It grows rapidly
   (b) It produces metastasis
   (c) It can recur after surgical excision
   (d) All types of malignant tumors are sensitive to therapeutic radiation
6. All of the following facts about the pathology of a benign tumor are correct, except
   (a) It is usually encapsulated
   (b) The cut surface is variegated in appearance
   (c) There is no local invasion
   (d) There are no mitotic figures
7. All of the following facts about the pathology of a malignant tumor are true, except
   (a) It does not have a capsule
   (b) The cut surface is variegated
   (c) There is no anaplasia
   (d) Mitotic figures may be present
8. Which of the following is true about a locally malignant tumor?
   (a) It does not spread
   (b) It spreads by local invasion
   (c) It spreads by hematogenous route
   (d) It spreads by lymphatic permeation
9. An osteosarcoma most commonly spreads by
   (a) Bloodstream
   (b) Lymphatic permeation
   (c) Local infiltration
   (d) It does not spread at all
10. G2 in histological grading of a malignant tumor is indicative of which type of tumor?
    (a) Well differentiated
    (b) Moderately differentiated
    (c) Poorly differentiated
    (d) Undifferentiated
11. The most definitive diagnostic investigation for a tumor is
    (a) Plain radiography
    (b) Biopsy
    (c) Isotope scanning
    (d) Contrast radiography
12. The local extent of a tumor is determined by
    (a) Plain X-ray
    (b) MRI

(CONTD...)

SELF-ASSESSMENT (...CONTD)

(c) Isotope scanning
(d) Biopsy

13. Metastases in the skeleton are most commonly detected by
    (a) Isotope bone scan
    (b) Radiographic survey
    (c) Bone marrow smear
    (d) Bone biopsy

14. Mobile metastatic nodes are usually treated by
    (a) Radiotherapy
    (b) Chemotherapy
    (c) En bloc excision
    (d) Chemoradiation

15. Which of the following is the most radiosensitive tumor?
    (a) Chondrosarcoma
    (b) Neurofibrosarcoma
    (c) Ewing's tumor
    (d) Malignant melanoma

16. The S phase of cell cycle is indicative of
    (a) Presynthesis
    (b) DNA synthesis
    (c) Premitosis
    (d) Mitosis

17. Cyclophosphamide belongs to which of the following groups?
    (a) Antimetabolites
    (b) Polyfunctional alkylating agents
    (c) Anticancer antibiotics
    (d) Vinca alkaloids

18. Methotrexate belongs to which of the following groups?
    (a) Polyfunctional alkylating agents
    (b) Anticancer antibiotics
    (c) Antimetabolites
    (d) Nitrosourea

19. In neoadjuvant chemotherapy the anticancer drugs are given
    (a) Before surgery or radiotherapy
    (b) During operation
    (c) In the immediate postoperative period
    (d) Sometime after the operation (after healing of the wound)

20. EBNA (EBV) is a viral tumor-specific marker of
    (a) Squamous cell carcinoma
    (b) Lymphoma
    (c) Melanoma
    (d) Osteosarcoma

Answers

1. (c) 2. (b) 3. (d) 4. (c) 5. (d) 6. (b) 7. (c) 8. (b)
9. (a) 10. (b) 11. (b) 12. (b) 13. (a) 14. (c) 15. (c)
16. (b) 17. (b) 18. (c) 19. (a) 20. (b)

Cysts

8

Definition

Cyst Cyst is fluid containing a closed cavity lined by epithelium, fibrous tissue, or degenerating, inflamed, or neoplastic tissue. It presents as a soft spherical swelling. It is of two types: true and false (Fig. 8.1).

True Cyst True cyst is lined by epithelium. Epidermoid, dermoid, and branchial cysts are examples of a true cyst.

False Cyst False cyst (pseudocyst) has a fibrous lining. Examples of a false cyst are traumatic cyst, pseudopancreatic cyst, and cystic tumors.

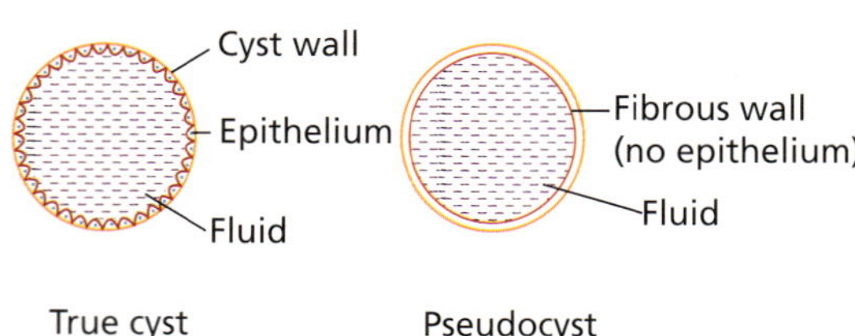

Figure 8.1 True and false cysts.

Pathogenesis

A true cyst is the accumulation of secretion of the lining which has nowhere to go. A false cyst is the accumulation of pathological fluids in the tissues which may be surrounded by a reactionary fibrotic wall.

Types of cysts

Cysts can be congenital and acquired (Table 8.1). The congenital cysts are due to some developmental defect and may be present at birth or appear a little late in life. The acquired cysts are due to some disease occurring later in life.

Congenital Cysts

Sequestration Dermoid Cyst It develops from the dermal cells buried during fusion of embryogenic clefts. It is lined by epidermis and contains dirty toothpaste-like material. The

Table 8.1 Types of cysts

Classification	Types	Examples
Congenital cyst	Sequestration dermoid	• Sublingual dermoid • External angular dermoid • Postauricular dermoid • Branchial cyst
	Tubulodermoid cyst	Thyroglossal cyst
	Cysts of embryonic remnants	• Retroperitoneal cyst • Cysts from urachus and vitellointestinal duct remnants
Acquired cysts	Retention cyst	• Sebaceous cyst • Retention cyst of salivary glands, breast, and epididymis
	Distension cyst	• Cystic hygroma • Lymphatic cyst • Lymph varix
	Exudation cyst	• Scrotal hydrocele • Chylocele • Housemaid's and Clergyman's knee
	Implantation cyst	Implantation dermoid
	Traumatic cyst	Unabsorbed hematoma inside a muscle of a limb may resolve into a cyst (pseudocyst)
	Degeneration cyst	• Ganglion cyst of dorsum of wrist • Apoplectic cyst of brain
	Cystic tumors	• Cystic teratomas of gonads, mediastinum, retroperitoneum, and pancreas • Serous and pseudomucinous cystadenomas of ovary
	Granulomatous cyst	• Encysted ascites • Dental cyst
	Parasitic cyst	• Hydatid cyst • Cysticercosis • Trichinosis

examples of sequestration dermoid include sublingual dermoid, external angular dermoid, and postauricular dermoid. Branchial cyst is also an example of sequestration dermoid.

Tubulodermoid Cyst It is a dermoid cyst arising from fetal tubular structures or ducts. An example of this cyst is thyroglossal cyst which arises from thyroglossal tract.

Cysts of Embryonic Remnants The examples of these cysts are retroperitoneal cysts arising from urogenital remnants, and cysts from urachus and vitellointestinal duct remnants.

Acquired Cysts

Retention Cyst It develops from retention of secretion caused by obstruction of the duct of a gland, the classic example being a sebaceous cyst which can occur in the skin of scalp, face, and other areas. Other sites of retention cyst are salivary glands, breast, and epididymis.

Distension Cyst It is caused by dilatation of duct of a gland which can occur in thyroid or ovary due to dilatation of follicles. Cystic hygroma, lymphatic cyst, and lymph varix are examples of a distension cyst.

Exudation Cyst It develops from collection of exudate caused by subclinical infection or inflammation. Examples include scrotal hydrocele, chylocele, and housemaid's and clergyman's knee.

Implantation Cyst It follows minor punctures when a part of skin epithelium is implanted or driven inside the tissues beneath the skin. Implantation dermoid on the palm of hand or fingers is an example of this type of cyst.

Traumatic Cyst It is also known as blood cyst and characterized by a cavity arising from softening of clot and absorption of blood pigment. An unabsorbed hematoma inside a muscle of limb may resolve into a cyst. It may contain cholesterol-rich straw-colored fluid. It is an example of a pseudocyst.

Degeneration Cyst It is a cyst formed within the normal tissues through softening and degeneration. Examples include ganglion cyst of dorsum of wrist and apoplectic cyst of brain.

Cystic Tumors They may occur primarily as cystic tumors (e.g., cystic teratomas of gonads, mediastinum, retroperitoneum, and pancreas) or may follow cystic degeneration of a tumor (e.g., serous and pseudomucinous cystadenomas of ovary).

Granulomatous Cyst It has granulomatous inflammation in the cyst wall, for example, encysted ascites and dental cyst.

Parasitic Cyst It is a cyst which is either a stage in the life history of a parasite or the result of parasitic activity in the tissues such as hydatid cyst, cysticercosis, and trichinosis.

- Hydatid cyst is produced by *Echinococcus granulosus* infection which mainly affects liver and lungs. Other organs and tissues may also be affected.
- Cysticercosis is caused by *Taenia solium* and may affect any organ including brain when it presents as focal epilepsy.
- Trichinosis is caused by *Trichinella spiralis* and affects mainly the muscles.

General clinical features of cysts

- The patient presents with a painless, slow-growing swelling of insidious onset.
- It is variable in size and is usually soft, smooth, and nontender.
- The specific physical signs of a cyst include fluctuation, transillumination, and fluid thrill which are not present in all the cysts.
- Transillumination depends on the nature of fluid of the cyst and thickness of its wall. Thus, a cystic hygroma is brilliantly transilluminant while a dermoid cyst is opaque.
- A cyst may produce symptoms by compressing a hollow organ or a tube in the vicinity, for example, a choledochal cyst may produce obstructive jaundice by obstructing the bile duct.
- Majority of cysts do not have any systemic effects on the body but a cyst inside the brain may have pressure symptoms. A hydatid cyst may have urticaria and may cause anaphylaxis if it ruptures.

Investigations

Radiology

- Ultrasonography for seeing the cysts in the abdomen and neck, for example, hydatid cyst of liver
- X-ray of chest for imaging the cysts of chest, for example, hydatid cyst of lung
- Orthopantomography for imaging cysts of jaws
- CT scan and MRI for imaging cysts of deeper organs and structures (Fig. 8.2)

Other Investigations These include immunoblot for a hydatid cyst.

If an ovarian cyst harbors a tumor, tumor markers of an ovarian cancer may be sought.

Treatment of cysts

Removal of Cause An example is albendazole in a hydatid cyst and cysticercosis but this treatment is not reliable.

Excision of the Cyst Examples include excision of a dermoid, a sebaceous, and a branchial cyst. The lining of the cyst must be completely excised to prevent recurrence.

Anastomosis A large cyst of abdomen which cannot be excised may be treated by anastomosing it to the nearest part of gastrointestinal tract, for example, a pseudopancreatic cyst is anastomosed with stomach (cystogastrostomy).

Marsupialization Sometimes a cyst which is difficult to excise is deroofed and its edges are sutured with the lining epithelium. This procedure is called marsupialization. It is sometimes done in a ranula.

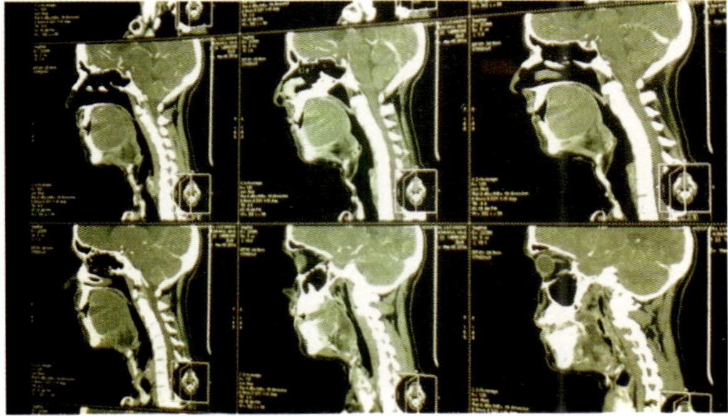

Figure 8.2 Sagittal CT scan of head and neck region showing soft tissue shadow of a sublingual dermoid. (Courtesy: Professor Surajit Bhattacharya)

Complications in a cyst

- Infection: A sebaceous cyst may present as an abscess.
- Torsion: An ovarian cyst may undergo torsion on its pedicle.
- Hemorrhage may occur in a cyst.
- Rupture: Rupture may follow trauma. It may lead to disappearance of a cyst. In a hydatid cyst it may produce anaphylactic shock which may kill the patient if not managed urgently, and may produce diffuse hydatid disease (hydatidosis).
- Calcification: A long-standing cyst may get calcified.

Sebaceous cyst (epidermal cyst)

It is a cyst of skin containing sebaceous material which occurs probably due to blockage of orifice of a sweat/sebaceous gland and its consequent distension (Fig. 8.3).

Clinical Features

- Site: It can occur anywhere in the skin except the palm of hand and sole of foot.
- The patient presents with a painless, slow-growing swelling of scalp, face, and neck.
- It is hemispherical, single or multiple, smooth, soft, nontender, and fixed to skin.
- It may have a dark spot on its top called punctum which is the site of orifice of obstructed sweat or sebaceous gland.

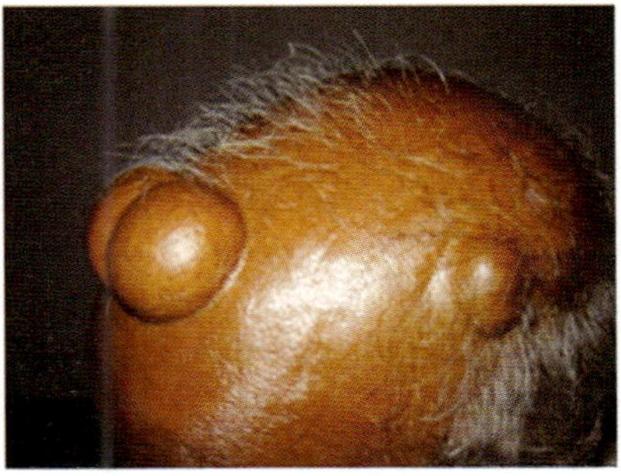

Figure 8.3 Sebaceous cysts of scalp (multiple). (Courtesy: Professor Surajit Bhattacharya)

Complications

- Infection resulting in abscess formation which may discharge offensive material
- Ulceration (the ulcer of the scalp of a sebaceous cyst that looks like a squamous cell carcinoma but not a carcinoma; hence, it is called Cock's peculiar tumor)
- Sebaceous horn and calcification rarely

Treatment

A small asymptomatic cyst may be left as such. Otherwise it is removed by enucleation making sure that whole of its lining is removed.

Dermoid cyst

It is a cyst lined by skin with hair follicles, and sebaceous and sweat glands which contain sebaceous material and hair.

Box 8.1 Sequestration dermoids of head and neck

- External angular dermoid
- Dermoid of root of nose
- Periauricular dermoid
- Implantation dermoid of ear lobule
- Sublingual dermoid
  - Supramylohoid
  - Inframylohoid
- Anterior midline dermoid of neck
- Suprasternal dermoid

Types of Dermoid Cyst

It is of two types: sequestration dermoid and implantation dermoid, which are described in the subsequent text (Box 8.1).

Sequestration dermoid

- **Site:** It occurs at the sites of closure of embryonic fissures, that is, outer and inner angles of orbit, midline of neck or back or abdomen, or the site of union between ectoderm and another germinal layer, for example, pituitary, floor of mouth, pharynx, mediastinum, and retroperitoneum.
- **Subcutaneous dermoid**: It presents as a firm or elastic swelling more deeply placed than a sebaceous cyst and not attached to the skin. It is nontender, soft, smooth, and opaque to transmitted light, and may be indented by a finger.

Implantation dermoid

Etiology It develops from epidermal cells implanted in subcutaneous tissue by minor pricks. Hence, it commonly occurs in tailors and gardeners and occurs in the palm of hand and fingers and occasionally on the sole of foot.

Clinical features It is a smooth, firm, nontender, and mobile subcutaneous swelling.

Investigation It can be imaged by ultrasonography.

Treatment It is treated by complete excision.

Sublingual dermoid

It is a dermoid cyst of floor of mouth that occurs under the tongue.

Etiology This cyst arises from the residual epithelium thought to originate from the embryonic branchial arches.

Histology It is a thick-walled cyst lined by squamous epithelium that contains varying amounts of keratin and dermal appendages.

Types Depending on its relationship with the mylohyoid muscle, it may be supramylohyoid or inframylohyoid.

Clinical features

- **Supramylohyoid type**: It presents as an opaque cystic swelling of the floor of mouth lifting the tongue up.
- **Inframylohyoid type**: It presents as a swelling below the mandible to give a double chin appearance (Fig. 8.4). The cyst enlarges slowly and may extend up to the hyoid bone.

Teratomatous dermoid

It is a dermoid cyst of ovary which is actually a benign cystic teratoma. It can occur in the testis also.

Investigations

Apart from routine investigations, the cyst can be imaged by ultrasonography, CT scan, or MRI as required.

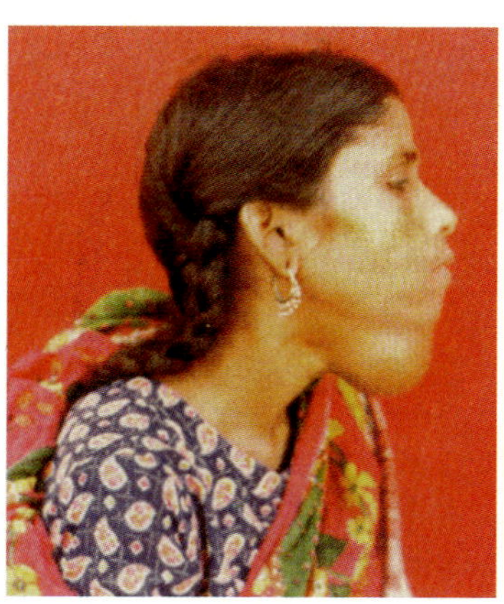

Figure 8.4 Sublingual dermoid giving double chin appearance.

Complications

The complications of a dermoid cyst include infection, rupture and pressure on neighboring structures, for example, brain in an intracranial dermoid.

Treatment

It is usually excised by intraoral approach by dissecting between the muscle layers. Large cysts and those adherent because of infection are excised by the cervical approach by giving an incision along the lower border of mandible.

A subcutaneous dermoid cyst must be differentiated from a sebaceous cyst. Their differences are given in Table 8.2.

Ranula

Ranula is a cystic swelling of floor of mouth which occurs due to submucosal extravasation of saliva from sublingual salivary gland. It resembles the belly of a small frog ("rana" means a small frog), hence this name. It is of two types: simple and plunging.

Clinical Features

- It is a thin-walled cyst that commences unilaterally and then enlarges slowly to form a bluish, dome-shaped, fluctuant, and transilluminant swelling in the floor of mouth usually on one side of frenulum linguae (Fig. 8.5).

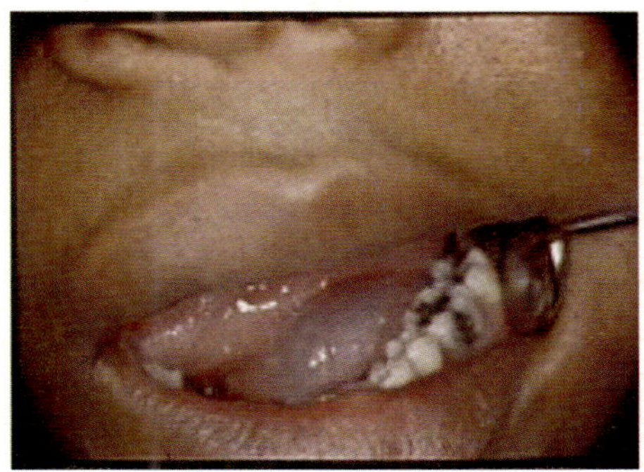

Figure 8.5 Ranula: bluish translucent swelling of left side of floor of mouth. (Courtesy: Professor Surajit Bhattacharya)

- Sometimes the cyst becomes large when it extends into the neck between muscle layers and is called plunging ranula. It has cross-fluctuation between the oral and neck swellings.

Complication

It may rupture and then reform.

Treatment

It is treated by excision of the cyst including the sublingual salivary gland. In a plunging ranula the submandibular salivary gland is also excised. The operation may be difficult due to thin wall of the cyst which frequently ruptures during operation.

Table 8.2 Differences between a dermoid cyst and a sebaceous cyst

Features	Dermoid cyst	Sebaceous cyst
Etiology	Sequestration of dermal cells in the subcutaneous tissue	Retention cyst due to accumulation of sebaceous material
Site	• Midline of body • Lines of embryonic fusion	• Can occur anywhere in the skin except palm and sole • Face, scalp, scrotum, and back are common sites
Indentation, molding	May be present	Usually absent
Punctum	Absent	Present in 50%
Skin fixation	Absent	Present at the site of punctum
Bony defect	Present in most of the cases	Absent
Intracranial extension	May be present in cysts around head	Absent
Treatment	Excision	Excision

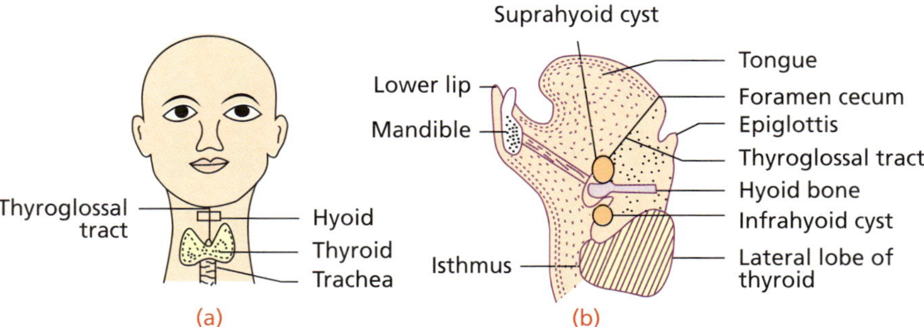

Figure 8.6 (a) Thyroglossal tract and (b) cyst.

Thyroglossal cyst

It is a cyst of upper neck which develops from the remnants of thyroglossal tract (Fig. 8.6).

Histology The cyst is usually small and contains mucoid material often with cholesterol crystals. The lining of the cyst may be cubical, columnar, or transitional.

Types Anatomically, it is of two types: suprahyoid and infrahyoid.

Features of Suprahyoid Cyst It lies above the body of hyoid bone in midline in the base or substance of tongue. It may interfere with speech, swallowing, and breathing. It can be best imaged by CT scan or MRI.

Features of Infrahyoid Cyst It usually lies just below the body of hyoid bone in midline, may be slightly to the left (Fig. 8.7). It may lie at a lower level. It is spherical, smooth, soft, and nontender.

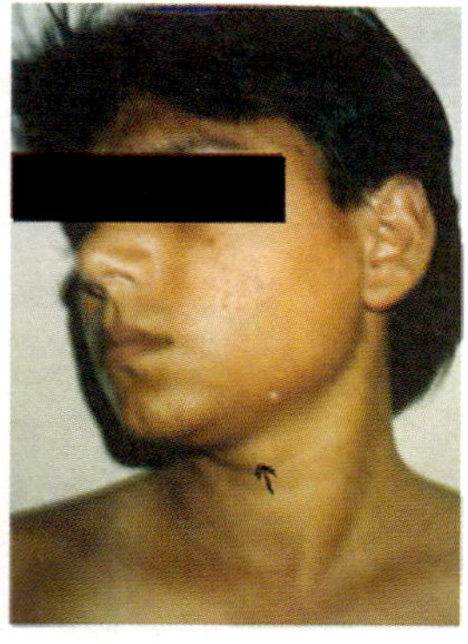

Figure 8.7 Thyroglossal cyst. (Courtesy: Dr. Sharad Kumar)

It moves vertically upwards during swallowing and protrusion of tongue.

Complications These include rupture, fistula formation, and secondary infection resulting in an abscess.

Treatment The cyst is excised completely in continuity with the central part (body) of the hyoid bone (Sistrunk's operation).

Branchial cyst

It is a developmental defect which develops from the second branchial cleft.

Anatomy The cyst is usually deep to posterior belly of digastric muscle but superficial to glossopharyngeal and hypoglossal nerves.

Histology It is lined by squamous epithelium and contains a thick clear or toothpaste-like material full of cholesterol crystals. The microscopic examination of the excised cyst usually shows a layer of lymphoid tissue in its wall. Hence, it is now considered that this cyst arises as a result of branchial epithelium entrapped within a local lymph node.

Clinical Features The patient is an adolescent person who presents with a painless, slow-growing cystic swelling of insidious onset in the upper neck. It protrudes at the anterior border of sternomastoid in the upper one-third. It is smooth, soft, and nontender, and may be translucent.

Complications The complications include secondary infection with abscess formation and rupture resulting in a fistula.

Treatment Treatment is excision.

Cystic hygroma

It is a developmental defect that occurs due to sequestration of lymph sacs from the lymphatic system characterized by a cystic swelling.

Pathology

It contains multiple thin-walled lymph vesicles giving a soap-bubble appearance. The vesicles or cysts do not communicate with each other. The larger cysts are on the surface, whereas the smaller ones are deep inside going into various local tissue planes. They are filled with lymph and lined by a single layer of epithelium with a mosaic appearance.

Clinical Features

- The patient is usually a neonate or infant who is brought with a swelling in the neck may be since birth.
- Site: It may be present in the lower part of neck (posterior triangle) or may involve the parotid and submandibular region, tongue, and floor of the mouth (Fig. 8.8). It may occur in the axilla, groin, and mediastinum.
- It is smooth or lobulated, soft, cystic, and non-tender. It is brilliantly transilluminant. It may be so large as to cause obstructed labor as it may be impacted in birth canal.

Investigations

The investigation of cystic hygroma includes ultrasound or CT scan to find out its nature and extent.

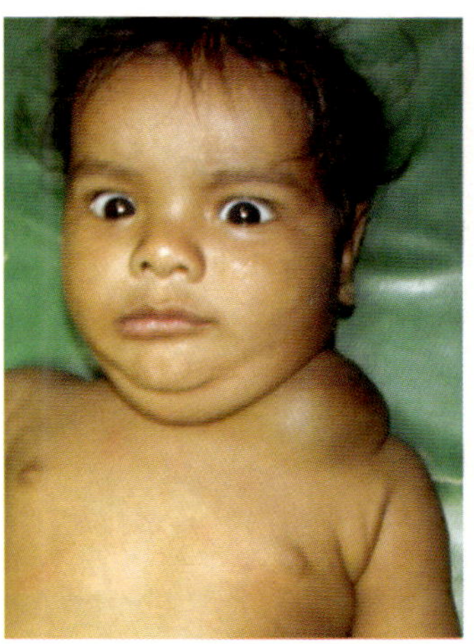

Figure 8.8 Cystic hygroma of left lower neck. (Courtesy: Professor J.D. Rawat)

Complications

The complications include compression of trachea and rupture with leakage of lymph (lymphorrhea).

Treatment

Excision It is treated by excision which may be difficult because of its frequent extension in various tissue planes. Postoperatively there is significant lymphorrhea from the wound which may cause fluid and electrolyte imbalance.

Sclerotherapy Local injection of Picibanil (OK432) may reduce the size of the lesion but cannot cure as these lesions are frequently multicystic and extensive. Furthermore, it may make subsequent excision difficult because of inflammatory fibrous adhesions.

KEY POINTS

- Cyst is fluid containing a closed cavity lined by epithelium, fibrous tissue, or degenerating, inflamed, or neoplastic tissue. A true cyst is lined by epithelium while a false cyst has a fibrous lining. Cysts can be congenital or acquired.
- In general, cysts present as a painless, slow-growing, soft, smooth, and nontender swelling of insidious onset.
- Treatment includes excision of the cyst, anastomosis of large cysts of abdomen which cannot be excised with bowel in the vicinity, and marsupialization (deroofing) of cysts which are difficult to excise due to their proximity to vital structures. Complications of a cyst include infection, torsion, hemorrhage, rupture, and calcification.

(CONTD...)

KEY POINTS (...CONTD)

- Sebaceous cyst is a cyst of skin containing sebaceous material. It can occur anywhere in the skin except the palm of hand and sole of foot. It can be single or multiple, smooth, soft, nontender, and fixed to skin with a punctum on the top.
- An ulcerated sebaceous cyst of scalp looks like a squamous cell carcinoma but it is not a carcinoma, hence called Cock's peculiar tumor.
- Dermoid cyst is a cyst lined by skin which contains sebaceous material, teeth, and hair. Sequestration dermoid occurs at the sites of closure of embryonic fissures.
- Subcutaneous dermoid presents as a firm or elastic swelling more deeply placed than a sebaceous cyst and not attached to the skin. It is nontender, soft, smooth, and opaque to transmitted light, and may be indented by a finger.
- Implantation dermoid develops from epidermal cells implanted in subcutaneous tissue by minor pricks.
- Sublingual dermoid cyst arises from the residual epithelium thought to originate from the embryonic branchial arches. It is present in the floor of the mouth.
- Ranula is a cystic swelling of floor of mouth which is bluish, dome-shaped, and transilluminant. A large cyst may extend into the neck called plunging ranula. It has cross-fluctuation between the oral and neck swellings. It is treated by excision of the cyst including the sublingual salivary gland. In a plunging ranula the submandibular salivary gland is also excised.
- Thyroglossal cyst is a cyst of upper neck which develops from the remnants of thyroglossal tract. It can be suprahyoid or infrahyoid, the latter being more common. The first one may lie in the substance of tongue. The latter cyst lies just below the body of the hyoid bone a little to the left. It moves vertically upwards during swallowing and protrusion of tongue. The treatment is complete excision with the central part (body) of the hyoid bone (Sistrunk's operation).
- Branchial cyst is a developmental defect which is now considered to arise from branchial epithelium entrapped within a local lymph node. It protrudes at the anterior border of sternomastoid in the upper one-third of neck. It is smooth, soft, and nontender, and may be translucent. It is excised.
- Cystic hygroma is a developmental defect that occurs due to sequestration of lymph sacs from the lymphatic system characterized by a cystic swelling in lower neck which is smooth or lobulated, soft, and brilliantly transilluminant. Excision and sclerotherapy are the methods of treatment.

SELF-ASSESSMENT

Long answer questions

1. What is a cyst and what are its types? Describe the clinical features, types, and treatment of a dermoid cyst.
2. Describe the clinical features, complications, and treatment of a cystic hygroma.

Short answer questions

1. True cyst
2. Pseudocyst
3. Retention cyst
4. Dermoid cyst
5. Sublingual dermoid
6. Ranula
7. Thyroglossal cyst
8. Branchial cyst
9. Cystic hygroma

Multiple choice questions

1. Sebaceous cyst is a
   (a) Sequestration dermoid
   (b) Retention cyst
   (c) Cyst of embryonic remnants
   (d) Pseudocyst
2. All of the following facts about a sebaceous cyst are correct, except
   (a) It is a retention cyst
   (b) It commonly occurs on the palm of hand or sole of foot

(CONTD...)

SELF-ASSESSMENT *(...CONTD)*

(c) It may have a punctum
(d) It is hemispherical, soft, and nontender

3. A sebaceous cyst may have all of the following complications, except
(a) Infection
(b) Rupture
(c) Ulceration
(d) Malignant change

4. Cock's peculiar tumor is a
(a) Benign tumor
(b) Malignant tumor
(c) Ulceration of a sebaceous cyst of scalp
(d) Ulceration of a dermoid cyst

5. Dermoid cyst is a
(a) Retention cyst
(b) Exudation cyst
(c) Degeneration cyst
(d) Congenital cyst due to sequestration of dermal cells

6. All of the following are true about sequestration dermoid, except
(a) It is lined by skin
(b) It contains sebaceous material and hair
(c) It can occur anywhere
(d) It presents with a soft opaque swelling which may be indented by digital pressure

7. A dermoid cyst is treated by
(a) Drainage
(b) Aspiration
(c) Complete excision
(d) Marsupialization

8. Thyroglossal cyst is a
(a) Sequestration dermoid
(b) Tubulodermoid
(c) Retention cyst
(d) Exudation cyst

9. All of the following facts about thyroglossal cyst are correct, except
(a) It arises from thyroglossal tract
(b) It is lined by cubical or columnar epithelium
(c) It contains dirty toothpaste-like material
(d) It moves up with protrusion of tongue

10. Branchial cyst is a
(a) Sequestration dermoid
(b) Tubulodermoid
(c) Retention cyst
(d) Distension cyst

11. All of the following facts about a branchial cyst are correct, except
(a) It is a developmental defect of second branchial cleft
(b) It is lined by columnar epithelium
(c) It contains fluid rich in cholesterol crystals
(d) It presents as a cystic swelling of upper neck

12. Cystic hygroma is a
(a) Tubulodermoid
(b) Sequestration dermoid
(c) Distension cyst
(d) Exudation cyst

13. All of the following facts about cystic hygroma are correct, except
(a) It is a distension cyst
(b) It contains multiple thin-walled lymph vesicles
(c) It presents with a swelling in the neck in a neonate or infant
(d) It is opaque to transmitted light

14. Hydatid cyst is a
(a) Degeneration cyst
(b) Exudation cyst
(c) Parasitic cyst
(d) Retention cyst

Answers

1. (b) 2. (b) 3. (d) 4. (c) 5. (d) 6. (c) 7. (c) 8. (b) 9. (c) 10. (c) 11. (b) 12. (c) 13. (d) 14. (c)

Injuries

9

Introduction

Injury or trauma is the most primitive or natural disease of living beings. It is one of the commonest killers of humans and other living beings. It causes pain and may result in bleeding and respiratory obstruction threatening life.

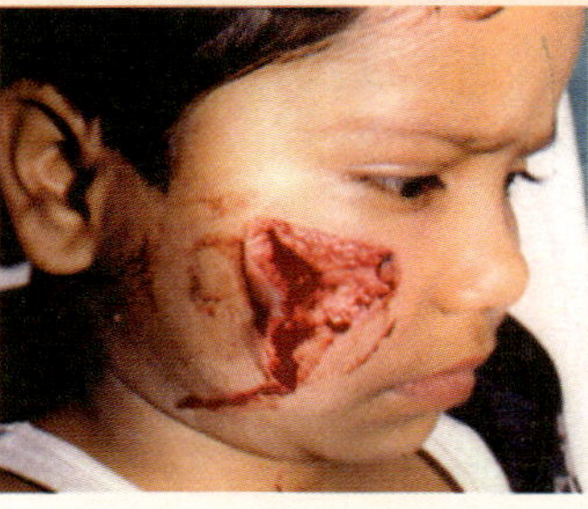

Figure 9.1 Soft-tissue trauma with clean edges and retraction and eversion of skin flap of right cheek. (Courtesy: Professor Surajit Bhattacharya)

Effects of trauma

The main effects of trauma/injury are production of a wound and bleeding (Fig. 9.1). The other effects are secondary depending on the site (head, face, neck, chest, abdomen, or extremities), type (blunt or sharp, crushing, penetrating, thermal, missile, or blast), and severity of injury.

Etiology of trauma

The injuries may be accidental or intentional, the first being more common. The intentional injuries may be suicidal or homicidal, the latter being more common. The common causes of injuries are:

- Sharp-edged weapon, for example, knife and sword injury
- Sharp-pointed weapon such as dagger
- Blunt weapon, for example, hockey-stick injury
- Crush injury under a falling wall or roof or wheels of a vehicle
- Fall from a height or in the bathroom
- Road traffic accidents
- Industrial accidents
- Firearm injury
- Blast injury
- Bull horn injury
- Bites and stings
- Thermal burns
- Chemical injury
- Radiation injury

Wounds

Definition

A wound is a traumatic discontinuity of tissues mainly of the skin and related tissues.

Types of Wounds

Locally, the injury damages the local tissues producing a wound, which may be a closed wound, an open wound, or a complicated wound. Classification of wounds is given in Box 9.1.

Box 9.1 Classification of wounds

- Closed injury wounds
  - Abrasion or scratch
  - Contusion
  - Hematoma
- Open injury wounds
  - Incised wound or incision
  - Lacerated wound or laceration
  - Stab or punctured wound
  - Penetrating and perforating wounds
- Complicated wounds

Closed Injury Wounds

In these wounds the local skin is not torn or disrupted as in a simple fracture. Hence, there is no risk of environmental contamination of the wound.

Abrasion or scratch

- **Cause:** It is the most minor injury in which the superficial layers of skin (epidermis) are denuded due to frictional injury as occurs in roadside accidents.
- **Clinical features:** Following injury droplets of blood ooze out from multiple points with local pain and burning. The roadside dirt or grit may stick to the wound and may result in tattooing of the skin later on. As the time passes, the droplets of blood dry up and form a scab which falls by itself after the wound heals leaving a depigmented scar.

Contusion or bruise

- **Cause:** It is caused by a blunt impact. When the weapon strikes (acceleration), the local tissues are suddenly compressed and then the layers suddenly separate on deceleration, which tears the small blood vessels leading to minor hemorrhages in between the layers.
- **Clinical features**: Locally, there is a mild diffuse swelling and discoloration due to edema and extravasation of blood. Initially it is red but as it loses oxygen it becomes dark blue. Soon it shades into greenish yellow due to biliverdin and then fades to yellow color. Finally the pigment is absorbed with return to normal color in 7–10 days.

Ecchymosis

If the hemorrhage extends from deeper structures to discolor the overlying skin, an ecchymosis is produced (Fig. 9.2).

Hematoma

- Cause: It is due to tearing or rupture of blood vessels. If the bleeding is more, the blood accumulates in tissues, tissue spaces, and body cavities producing a hematoma.
- Types: Depending on the size of injured vessels the hematoma may be small or large, and depending on the site of accumulation of blood a hematoma can be subcutaneous, intermuscular, intramuscular, subperiosteal, extradural, subdural, and retroperitoneal.
- It may accumulate in the body cavities, that is, hemoperitoneum in peritoneal cavity,

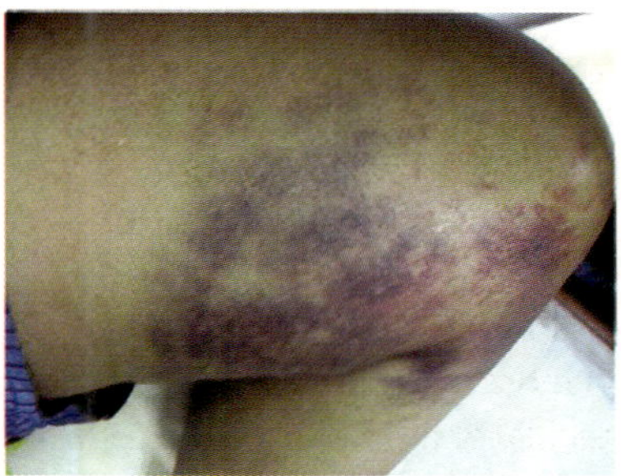

Figure 9.2 Extensive ecchymosis of lower part of thigh and knee region following a fall (blunt injury).

Box 9.2 Fate of a hematoma

- Resolution (initially the blood is in fluid state; then coagulation starts from the periphery followed by fibrosis, and finally the whole hematoma heals by fibrosis)
- Secondary infection with pus formation
- Rupture
- Absorption of blood and its replacement by tissue fluid as occurs in a chronic subdural hematoma
- Calcification

hemopericardium in pericardial cavity, hemarthrosis in a joint cavity, hematocele in tunica vaginalis, and hematometra in uterus.

- Fate of a hematoma: The fate of a hematoma is enumerated in Box 9.2.
- Complications of hematoma: This abnormal collection of blood may not cause any problem, but collection of blood in the cranial cavity (extradural hematoma), pericardium, and pleural cavity may cause serious problem by pressure or interference in the function of brain, heart, and lungs, respectively. It may get infected.

Open Injury Wounds

In these wounds the local skin is disrupted resulting in exposing the tissues to environmental contamination.

Incised wound or incision

- **Cause:** It is produced by horizontal movement of a sharp-edged weapon with pressure on the body surface or skin. Such wounds are produced during open operations. Broken glass pieces can also produce such wounds.
- **Clinical features**: Such a wound tends to gape with protrusion of subcutaneous tissue. The edges are clean cut and bleed freely. The tissue injury is only that much which is visible. There is no injury to the tissues around. There is severe pain when the injury is occurring. Subsequently, there is no pain unless the wound is touched or pressed.

Stab and punctured wounds

- **Cause:** These wounds are produced by vertical movement of a knife or dagger on the body surface.
- **Clinical features:** They are deep but short in length and width. Hence, the structures in the depth, for example, blood vessels, nerves, and internal organs such as heart, lungs, and liver, may be injured depending on the site and depth of stab or puncture. The infection may also be carried into the depth of tissues.

Penetrating and perforating wounds

- **Cause:** These wounds are produced by vertical movement of injuring force on the body by a sharp-pointed weapon, or a bullet penetrating or perforating a body cavity such as thorax or abdomen.
- **Clinical features:** In a perforating wound the body cavity is perforated through and through with a wound of entry and a wound of exit. In these injuries the internal organs of these cavities may be injured. If the injury is caused by a bullet and there is only a wound of entry and no wound of exit, the bullet must be inside the body.

Lacerated wound or laceration

- **Cause:** Such wounds are caused by blunt objects or weapons, road traffic accidents, shell fragments, and industrial accidents.
- **Clinical features:** In this wound not only the surface is broken but also the tissues around are crushed and devascularized, and liable to subsequent infection. Thus, the injury is many times more than whatever is visible. The wound is irregular and does not bleed freely.

Complicated Wounds

In these wounds the important deeper structures are injured, for example, large nerves, blood vessels, bones, and internal organs; hollow organs such as small bowel may perforate; and solid organs such as liver may rupture.

Other effects of trauma

Bleeding

Bleeding is the second most common manifestation of trauma. The severity or degree of bleeding depends on the size and number of injured vessel or vessels. For example, if heart, aorta, or venae cavae are injured or perforated, the bleeding may be so severe, sudden, and quick that there is hardly any time available for treatment. It may be trivial bleeding from a minor cut or laceration without any effect on body physiology.

Effects of bleeding

Hypovolemic Shock If the blood loss is significant, there is reduction of blood volume (hypovolemia), fall of blood pressure (hypotension), and increase in heart rate (tachycardia). It may result in hypovolemic shock which causes reduction of tissue perfusion and hypoxia of tissue which damages the brain at the earliest. If the brain does not get oxygen for 3 minutes, it is irreversibly damaged.

Effect of Bleeding in a Closed Cavity If the bleeding occurs in a closed cavity, for example, cranial, pericardial, or pleural cavity, the vital organs contained in these cavities may be compressed. Thus, in the cranium an extradural hematoma may decerebrate and/or kill its victim if urgent decompression is not done.

Effect of Bleeding on Heart The pressure on the heart due to hemopericardium (cardiac tamponade) prevents diastolic filling of the heart which results in reduced cardiac output, fall in blood pressure, and increased central venous pressure.

Effect of Bleeding on Lung In hemothorax the lung of the affected side cannot expand fully during inspiration, disturbing the respiratory function.

Compartment Syndrome The accumulation of blood in the closed fascial compartments of forearm and leg may cause compartment syndrome due to increased intracompartmental pressure.

Respiration

The effects of various types of trauma on respiration are given as follows:

- In head injury, if brainstem is damaged and the respiratory center is affected, it may result in arrest of breathing.
- In cervical spinal injury, if the cord is injured above C3 segment, all the muscles of respiration are paralyzed and the patient dies of lack of breathing unless put on immediate ventilatory support.
- In maxillofacial injury, the airway may be obstructed due to falling back of tongue, blood, oropharyngeal secretions, and vomitus.
- In thoracic injuries, if many ribs are fractured with a flail chest, or in pulmonary atelectasis due to tension pneumothorax, the patient may die due to anoxia.
- In blast injury, the airway may be damaged or burnt from inside by inhaling smoke, hot gases, and steam. It results in burns of airway with edema causing obstruction. The pulmonary alveoli may be filled with blood.

Wound Infection

The main risk of open wounds is wound infection which must be prevented or treated promptly. The classification of wounds depending on wound infection is given in Table 9.1.

Table 9.1 Types of wounds depending on contamination/infection

Etiological type of wounds	Subtypes depending on contamination/infection
Accidental wounds	• Tidy wounds • Untidy wounds
Operative wounds	• Clean wounds • Clean-contaminated wounds • Contaminated wounds • Infected or dirty wounds

Accidental wound infection

Accidental wounds are heavily contaminated by the dirt and dust of the environment of injury. Hence, there is every chance of infection resulting in cellulitis, pus formation, tissue necrosis, tetanus, and gas gangrene. Hence, all these wounds need prompt treatment. Depending on the extent of tissue damage and contamination, the accidental wounds are of two types.

Tidy Wounds They are incised wounds which are relatively clean without much tissue damage. The chances of infection in such wounds are less.

Untidy Wounds Crush injury wounds and lacerated wounds which are usually associated with contamination and tissue loss are untidy wounds. The chances of infection in these wounds are significant.

Operative wound infection

The operative wounds are of four types depending on the extent of contamination and chances of wound infection (Table 9.2).

Clean Wounds These are the wounds of clean elective surgery where the gastrointestinal, respiratory, and urinary tracts are not entered, for example, thyroidectomy, hernioplasty, and vascular operations. The chances of infection in these wounds are 2% and the commonest infecting organism is *Staphylococcus aureus*.

Clean-Contaminated Wounds These wounds are produced during elective operations of respiratory, genitourinary, and gastrointestinal tracts. These patients are well prepared before operation and operated in such a manner that there is minimal contamination or "spillover" during operation. The infection rate in these wounds is 7–10% and the infecting organism is related to the viscus opened.

Contaminated Wounds These are the wounds which are grossly contaminated during operation, for example, spillage of stool during colonic operation and removal of ruptured appendix. Accidental lacerated wound is also a contaminated wound. The infection rate of these wounds is 15–20%.

Infected or Dirty Wounds These are the wounds of operation for established infection, for example,

Table 9.2 Types of operative wounds

Type of wound	Definition	Examples	Wound infection rate (%)	Infective organism
Clean wound	Wounds of elective surgery where gastrointestinal, biliary, or genitourinary tracts are not entered	• Thyroidectomy • Hernioplasty • Vascular operations	2	*Staphylococcus aureus*
Clean-contaminated wound	Wounds of operation where gastrointestinal, biliary, or genitourinary tracts are entered with no or minimal contamination	• Cholecystectomy • Open ureterolithotomy • Oral surgery wounds	7–10	Related to organ system entered
Contaminated wound	Wounds with major contamination during operation, for example, spillage of feces during colonic surgery, spillage of infected bile or urine during operation of these systems	• Removal of ruptured appendix • Lacerated wound • Colonic resection	15–20	Related to underlying organ entered
Infected or dirty wound	Wounds made for operation of established infection	Drainage of a parotid abscess	30–40	Depends on underlying cause

wound of drainage of a parotid or neck abscess. The infection rate of these wounds is 30–40% and the infecting organism depends on the underlying cause.

Clinical features of trauma

Age

- Anybody, that is, male or female, child, adult, or elderly, can be injured.
- Young adults are more likely to be injured outside the house in road traffic accidents or workplace injuries, elderly are more likely to have a fall in bathroom, and the adult females are more likely to be injured in the kitchen.

Symptoms The common symptoms of injury are pain, bleeding, swelling, wound or wounds, and loss of function.

Systemwise Manifestation of Injury Other manifestations depend on the region, structure, or organ injured (Table 9.3).

Physical Examination The whole body of the patient is exposed and examined from top to toe in good light and comfortable environment, as the injuries may be multiple. No injury should be missed.

- The general examination includes level of consciousness, pulse, blood pressure, respiration, and temperature.
- Local examination includes examining the local area of trauma for wound/wounds, swelling, and deformity.

Investigations

- **Laboratory studies:** The blood is sent for hemoglobin, counts, packed cell volume, blood gases, sugar, urea, creatinine, and electrolytes.
- **Radiology:** It depends on the part injured, for example, plain X-ray of part in fractures, examples being orthopantomography in lower jaw trauma (Fig. 9.3), CT scan in head and neck injury and faciomaxillary trauma (Fig. 9.4), and MRI in spinal injury. The

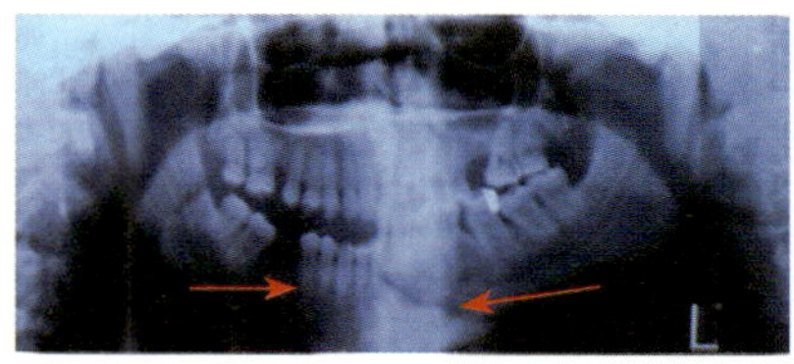

Figure 9.3 Orthopantomogram showing fractures of mandible. (Courtesy: Professor Surajit Bhattacharya)

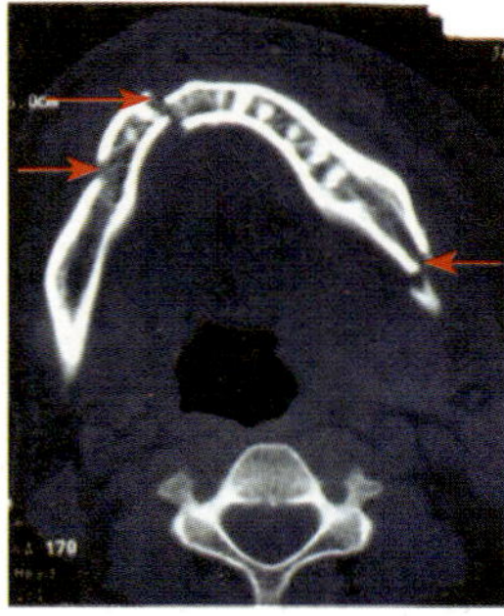

Figure 9.4 Axial CT scan of lower face showing multiple fractures of mandible. (Courtesy: Professor Surajit Bhattacharya)

Table 9.3 Sitewise symptoms of injuries

Region/organ injured	Symptoms
Head injury	Unconsciousness
Lung injury	Breathlessness
Abdominal injury	Abdominal pain and distension
Nerve injury	Sensory and/or motor loss
Arterial injury	Bleeding, pain, pallor, puffiness, pulselessness, and paralysis
Fracture	Tenderness, deformity, abnormal mobility, and crepitus

patient must be stabilized by life-supportive treatment before sending for investigations.

Treatment

The management of a trauma patient requires a team of trained workers who are prompt, quick, and calculative in all their movements.

Treatment at the Site of Accident

- **Assessing consciousness of the patient:** First, it is seen whether the patient is alive: breathing, heart is beating, moving hands and feet, or wincing or crying due to pain.
- **Assessment of airway:** If the airway is obstructed as detected by labored noisy breathing, the obstruction must be removed. If there is something in the throat, it must be sucked and removed. If available, an oropharyngeal airway is inserted. If the patient is not breathing, mouth-to-mouth respiration may be given (Fig. 9.5). The air-sucking wound of the chest must be sealed.
- **Assessment of bleeding:** Bleeding is controlled by pressure or any other method which is available and applicable. If the heart has stopped beating, external cardiac massage is given (Fig. 9.6).
- **Positioning the patient:** The patient is made to lie on his/her side and transferred to the hospital. The limbs must not hang or dangle around. If there is suspicion of injury to the vertebral column, the patient is transferred as he/she is lying without any change or movement in the vertebral column.

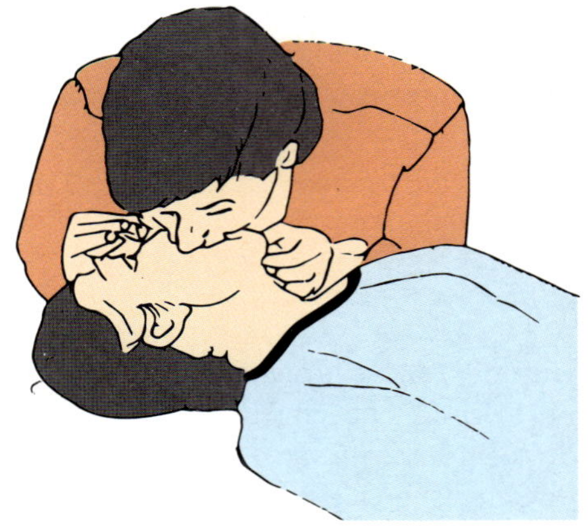

Figure 9.5 Mouth-to-mouth breathing.

Treatment in the Hospital

Triage

This term is derived from the French word "trier" which means sorting. It is a method of sorting out (or classification) the injured persons, depending on the severity and type of injury. It is especially required during mass casualties. The patient gets treatment according to the severity of injury. Triage is a skilled activity. The patients are sorted

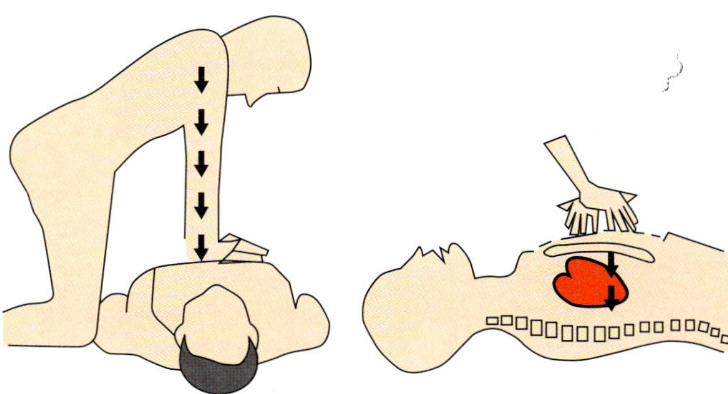

Figure 9.6 Method of external cardiac message where heart is massaged to activity by sudden repeated thrusts with overlapping heels of palm of both hands keeping the limbs straight at elbows at lower end of sternum of the patient.

Table 9.4 Categories of triage

Category	Color code	Description	Example
Critical	Red	This patient will die in a few seconds if no immediate treatment is given	Acute obstruction of larynx or trachea
Immediate	Red	This patient has to be treated within minutes	Tension pneumothorax and severe bleeding
Urgent	Yellow	This type of patient has to be treated within the golden hour	Within an hour in head injury with extradural hematoma, chest injury, and severe burns
Deferred (nonurgent)	Green	This patient does not have a serious or life-threatening injury. Hence, the treatment can be deferred	Simple fracture, for example, fracture of clavicle
Unsalvageable	Black	—	—

out into four categories and may be color coded (Table 9.4).

Emergency treatment

The initial treatment is done according to the mnemonic ABCDEF which stands for airway, breathing, circulation, disability, exposure, and fluid resuscitation.

- **Airway (A)**: The airway must be patent. If there is a cause of obstruction, it must be promptly removed. It may need endotracheal intubation or tracheostomy.
- **Breathing (B)**: If the patient is not breathing, mouth-to-mouth breathing may be given till the patient is shifted to a ventilator.
- **Circulation (C)**: The circulation is maintained by arresting bleeding and restoring the blood volume. If there is cardiac tamponade or tension pneumothorax, it is managed by decompression. The external cardiac massage may be required.
- **Disability (D)**: The disability caused by trauma must be assessed. There are many methods of assessment depending on the region or system injured, for example, Glasgow Coma Scale (GCS) for head injury.
- **Exposure (E)**: The patient is fully exposed to do complete head-to-toe examination to see for total injures, for example, in burns to assess the extent of burn by "rule of nine."
- **Fluid resuscitation (F)**: The main effect of most of the injuries is blood or fluid loss. Hence, the patient needs intravenous replacement of lost fluid. Furthermore, the intravenous route helps in administration of the drugs as and when needed.

Other measures

The other measures include relief of pain, administration of antibiotics, and performing tetanus prophylaxis. A seriously injured patient is admitted to ICU and his/her basic parameters, for example, blood pressure, pulse, and oxygen levels, are monitored. A Foley's catheter may be passed in the bladder to keep a record of urinary output.

Wound Care

Wound is the basic effect of trauma. Hence, it also needs attention with general care.

Hemostasis

Hematoma is evacuated and the bleeding is controlled by compression (packing), ligation, clipping, and electrocoagulation. In bleeding disorders it is controlled by packing and pressure and correction of coagulopathy. The wound is irrigated with sterile saline. No antiseptics are used on the raw tissues.

Treatment of a tidy wound

- A clean incised wound may be suture closed—skin with skin and fascia with fascia. The divided blood vessels, nerves, and tendons are suture repaired. The fractured bones are reduced and immobilized.

- The nerves are repaired with 8-0 or 10-0 monofilament nylon (may be done under loupe magnification or using a microscope), arteries by 6-0 polypropylene, and tendons by 3-0 or 4-0 polypropylene.
- The sutured wound can be covered by polymeric films such as Opsite or Tegaderm which are adhesive transparent dressings or a stretchable adhesive dressing.
- If there is a doubt regarding cleanliness of the wound, it may be kept covered by a sterile gauze for 3–4 days. If the wound remains clean, it is closed by sutures. This is called delayed primary closure. If after 3–4 days the wound looks dirty, it is treated like an untidy wound.

Treatment of an untidy wound

- If the wound is dirty with lacerated or crushed tissues, it is cleaned and excised.
- The presence of nonviable tissue can be determined by intravenous fluorescein, tissue oxygen determination, and blood flow studies. These methods are cumbersome; hence, the clinical judgment is the best.
- Sometimes the questionable tissue is left and the wound is kept open and inspected again after 24 hours.
- In a clean and viable wound the inflammatory phase is short with quick healing with a good scar.
- After excision wound is cleaned with 0.9% saline under pressure. After that the wound is managed in three ways (Table 9.5).

Methods of wound closure

Methods of wound closure include:

- Suturing with needle and suture material
- Approximating with tapes, staples, and adhesives
- Coverage with split-thickness or full-thickness grafts or flaps

Wound dressing

The best and natural dressing of a wound with skin loss is the patient's own skin but till it can be put or made available the wound is dressed by alternative methods.

Dressing for a Sutured Wound The wound is sealed by epithelial migration in about 48 hours. If the wound is dry, it can be left open if it is not inconvenient or uncomfortable to the patient. If the wound is discharging, it is dressed with an absorbent dressing.

Dressing for Open Wounds

- An open wound with necrotic debris is covered with a gauze moistened with Eusol and absorbent material, for example, cotton wool. It removes the slough by oxidation. The gauze dries up and sticks to the necrotic tissue. When the dressing is removed, it may take away necrotic tissue with it and may be a part of newly growing epithelium. Furthermore, its removal is painful. Hence, the dressing is moistened and soaked well before removal.
- For removal of slough, debriding agents such as benzoylbenzoic acid or enzymatic agents, for example, Varidase (streptokinase-streptodornase), may be used. Subsequently, the

Table 9.5 Types of wound closure based on wound contamination

Type of wound closure	Type of wound	Description
Primary closure	A relatively clean wound with a low risk of infection	It can be closed by suture after cleaning
Delayed primary closure	If there is doubt regarding cleanliness	Left open for 3–5 days
	If it remains clean after 3–5 days	It is closed by suture. It is likely to heal nearly similar to primary closure
No closure	• If the wound is dirty after 3–5 days • Wound with a high risk of infection	Left open to heal with granulation tissue, contraction, and epithelialization. A large granulating surface may be skin grafted to expedite healing

wound may be dressed by hydrogels such as Geliperm or Intrasite which maintain moist environment, allow gas exchange, and absorb exudates; or hydrocolloids such as Comfeel or Granuflex which promote epithelialization and granulation tissue formation.

- Large dermal wounds, for example, donor sites of split skin grafts, require epithelialization only. They are dressed with scarlet red which forms a scab under which the epithelium migrates. They may be dressed with alginate mesh.

Treatment of Different Types of Wounds

Abrasion and Contusion Apart from application of a local antiseptic paint, for example, povidone-iodine, nothing else is needed. One or two doses of a painkiller, for example, diclofenac or indomethacin, may be indicated.

Hematoma A small asymptomatic hematoma may be left as such. A large or a compressing hematoma, for example, extradural hematoma, is treated by urgent evacuation.

Incised Wound The wound is irrigated, bleeding is stopped, and then closed by suture.

Lacerated Wound The wound is explored and the crushed and damaged tissue is excised. The damaged muscle is excised since the devitalized muscle offers the most attractive pabulum for the anaerobic organisms to grow. Hence the excision must continue till the bleeding cut edge of the healthy muscle.

- If the underlying bone is fractured, completely detached and grossly contaminated fragments are removed. The clean fragments still attached by periosteum are put in position and the fracture is reduced. All the foreign bodies are removed and their removal may be confirmed by intraoperative radiography. The fracture is immobilized by external fixation.
- A clean wound may be closed by loose sutures or may be skin grafted. If the cleanliness is doubtful, it may be kept open for daily inspection and dressing till it is fit for closure. The patient is given appropriate antibiotics with metronidazole to control anaerobic infection.
- Stab, puncture, penetrating, and perforating wounds are opened widely up to the floor to examine every structure in the depth, removing foreign body/bodies and dead tissue, and repairing the wound from the floor up in layers.

A schematic representation of management of trauma is given in Flowchart 9.1.

Wound healing

Some important facts about the healing response are:

- All injured tissues pass through the same series of events during healing.
- The phases of healing overlap in both time and activity.
- The greater the injury, the more is the reparative process and more is the scarring.
- All injuries heal by scarring with loss of parenchyma. Regeneration is seen only in liver, nerves, and bones (fracture). The brain tissue does not regenerate.

Phases of Healing

The healing of wounds is a natural and normal process. All the wounds tend to heal spontaneously unless there is a cause or factor that prevents or delays it. The healing of a wound occurs in three phases. The schematic representation of wound healing is given in Flowchart 9.2.

Stage 1: inflammatory phase (1–4 days)

It is the immediate response following injury, the aim of which is to prevent further injury and to limit the extent of damage. It is also called lag or preparatory phase when little seems to be occurring in the wound while there is intense enzymatic and leukocytic activity in the wound.

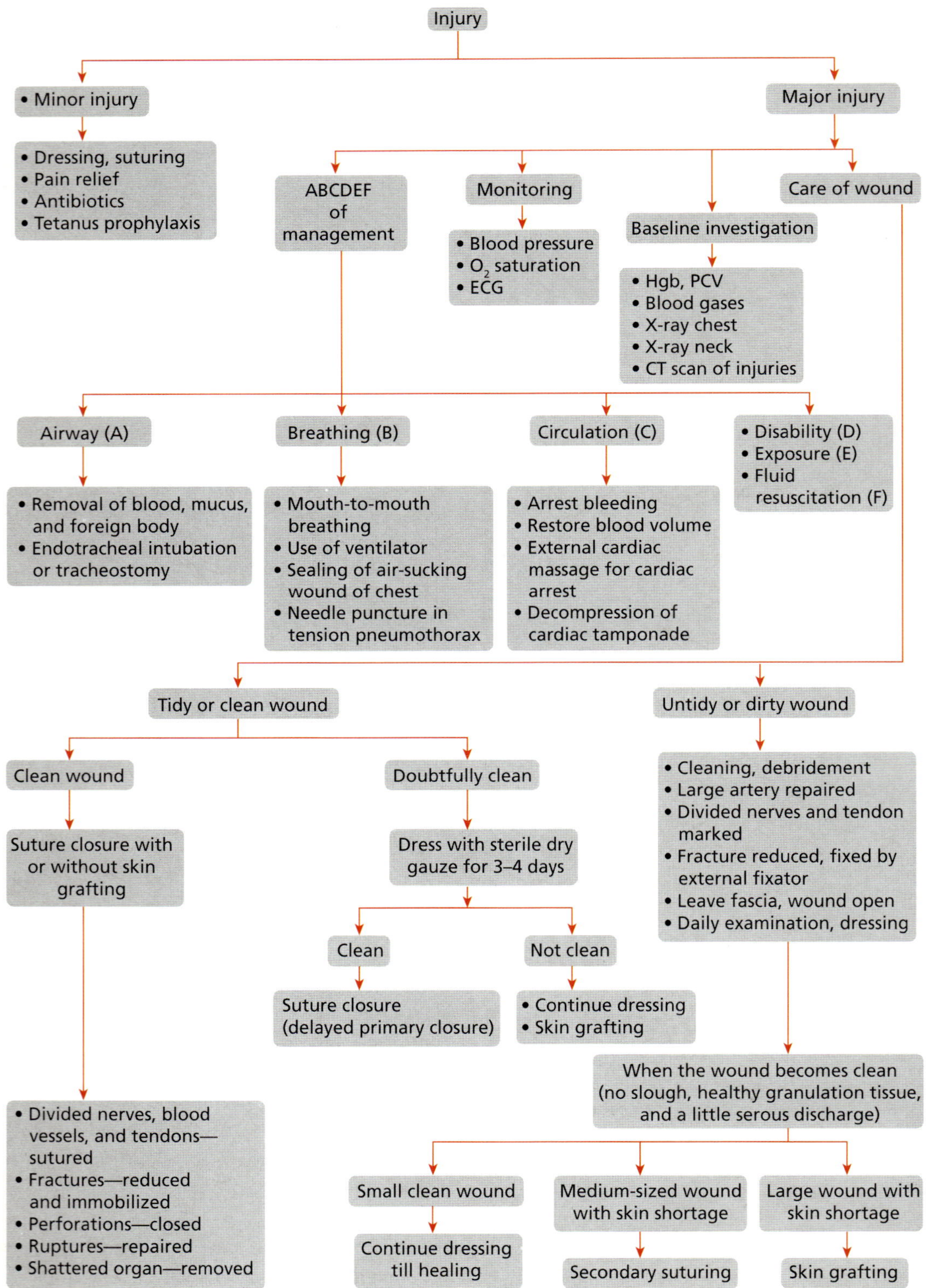

Flowchart 9.1 Management of trauma.

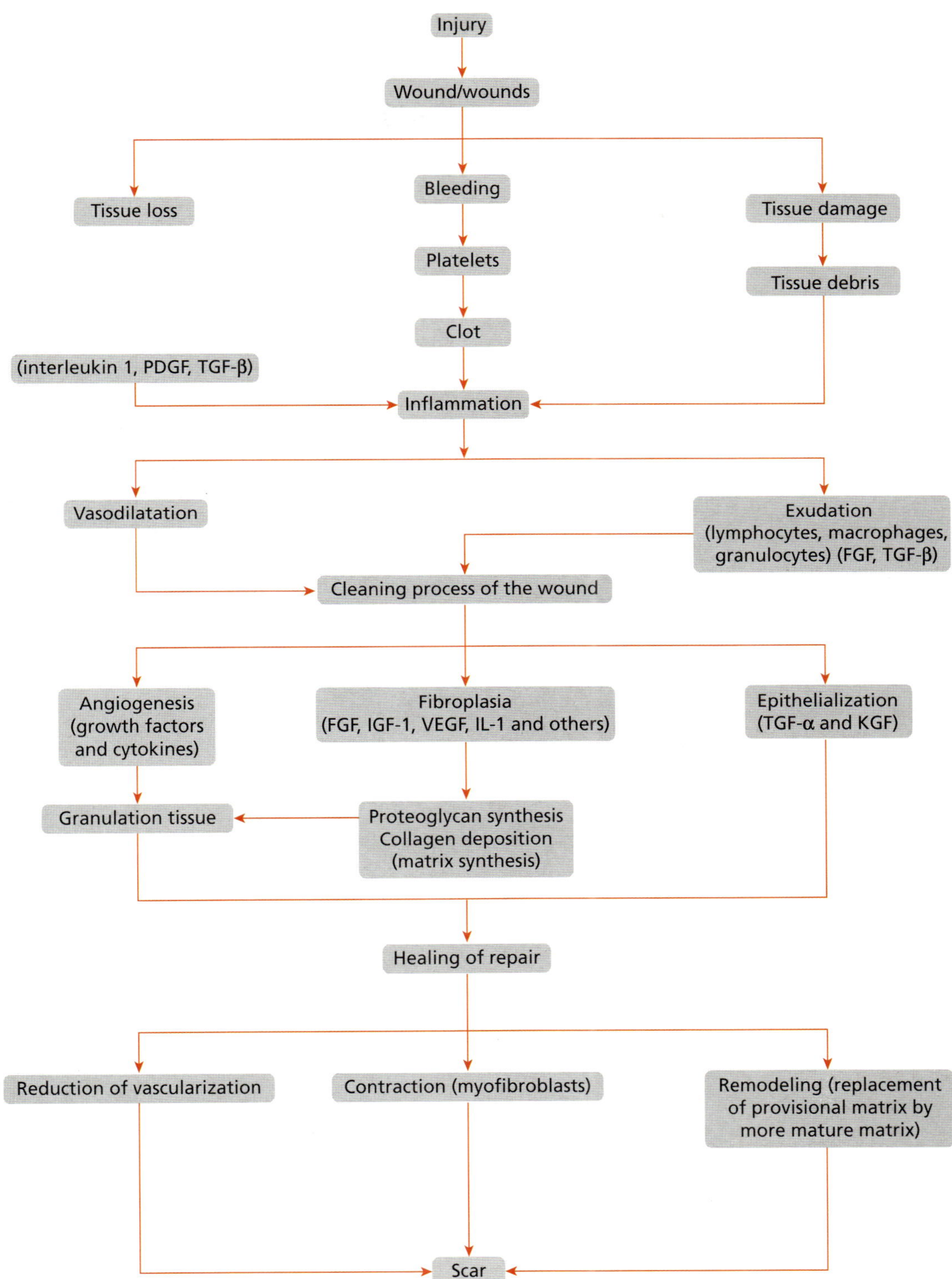

Flowchart 9.2 Wound healing. *FGF*, fibroblast growth factor; *KGF*, keratinocyte growth factor; *PDGF*, platelet derived growth factor; *TGF-β*, transforming growth factor-β; *VEGF*, vascular endothelial growth factor.

When the tissues are injured, the bacteria enter the wound, bleeding occurs, cellular contents are liberated, and tissue debris is deposited which initiates the clotting cascade resulting in deposition of fibrin to form clot. This leads to an inflammatory reaction with release of inflammatory cytokines that continues till the white cells clear all the debris.

Initial vasoconstriction is followed by vasodilatation which causes erythema or redness. The capillary permeability is increased which allows the red cells, leukocytes, and platelets to migrate into the wound. The leukocytes are chemoattracted by injured tissues and bacteria. The exudation of fluid and migration of cells into the wound leads to local swelling or "tumor."

With passage of time, the acute inflammation subsides when the macrophage becomes more dominant which continues to clear tissue debris and bacteria. Also, it releases growth factors required for wound healing.

Stage 2: proliferative phase (5–12 days)

It is also called regenerative or reparative phase. It is characterized by angiogenesis (neovascularization), matrix synthesis (fibroplasia), and epithelialization.

The wound is hypoxic. The hypoxia along with growth factors (VEGF, TNF-alpha) stimulates angiogenesis from existing capillaries. The activated endothelial cells divide to form capillary loops.

The fibroblasts are chemoattracted and divide to produce components of extravascular matrix, the main component of which is collagen. The mass of capillaries, fibroblasts, and collagen collectively is known as granulation tissue which is called so because of its visual appearance in an open wound.

The epithelial cells from the edge of the wound migrate in an effort to cover the wound. They move as an intact sheet until edges of the wound establish contact. The migrating cells release collagenase and plasminogen activator. The proteases assist the epithelial cells in migration.

Stage 3: maturation phase (3 weeks to many months)

The production of collagen continues for about 3 weeks. During this phase myofibroblasts (derived probably from fibroblasts) multiply and start contracting, thereby reducing the size of the wound.

When a wound is produced, the cut edges retract immediately making the wound look larger than what it is. When healing starts, the wound contracts by which the edges of the wound come closer. It occurs more readily in areas where the skin is loose such as buttocks and back of neck. It is a physiological process and different from the pathological process of scar contracture.

Initially the collagen is laid in a haphazard manner. Later on, it is replaced by new collagen which is laid down along the lines of stress (remodeling). The new collagen has more cross-links between collagen strands increasing the tensile strength of scar which reaches approximately 90% of the original tissue strength in 6 weeks to many months.

Inhibitors of Wound Healing

Wound healing is inhibited or delayed due to local and general factors.

Local factors

- Wound infection: Wound infection delays healing by further tissue damage and prolonging the inflammatory phase.
- Wound hypoperfusion and hypoxia: It may be due to peripheral vascular disease, excessive tissue tension to achieve closure, or secondary to infection.
- Foreign body: It may keep the tissues separated. If it is contaminated, it acts as a focus of persistent infection and inflammation.
- Hematoma or seroma in the depth of wound also leads to inhibition or delay in wound healing.
- Neoplasia: The tissue affected by neoplasia does not heal. Irradiation also has an adverse effect on wound healing.

- Repeated trauma also leads to inhibition or delay in wound healing.

General factors

- **Malnutrition**: Nutrition is an important requirement for wound healing but wounds do heal in patients with severe malnutrition. If a malnourished patient needs an urgent operation, a short preoperative course of total parenteral nutrition improves wound healing. The nutritional support must continue in the postoperative period.

Specific deficiencies such as vitamin C (necessary for collagen synthesis and cross-linkage), zinc (an enzyme cofactor), and vitamin A delay the healing process.

- **Diabetes mellitus**: Hyperglycemia inhibits all aspects of inflammatory response of wound healing and the immune system resulting in increased susceptibility to infection and delayed wound healing. Diabetes is often associated with microvascular disease which reduces tissue perfusion and oxygenation.

If the diabetes is kept under control, preferably on insulin, wound healing is nearly normal.

- **Steroids**: They are the powerful inhibitors of all phases of wound healing. This effect is potentiated by malnutrition.
- **Cytotoxic drugs**: All these drugs have an inhibitory effect mainly on the early phase of wound healing. Therefore, if they have to be given, they are given 7–10 days after operation.
- **Jaundice**: It is associated with delayed angiogenesis and reduced collagen synthesis. Even then in most of the cases the wound heals satisfactorily.
- **Renal failure**: It suppresses cell division, re-epithelialization, and formation of connective tissue.
- **Smoking**: Long-term smoking causes chronic hypoxia, vasoconstriction, and vascular disease. These factors combine to inhibit wound healing.
- **Other causes**: Obesity, immunodeficiency, cardiac failure, chronic respiratory disease, severe anemia, and hemorrhagic diathesis delay wound healing.

Types of Wound Healing

There are three types of wound healing.

Healing by primary intention

It occurs in a clean incised wound after it is closed by stitching within 6 hours of injury. The wound heals rapidly without granulation tissue formation with minimal scarring. It is the target of all modern operations.

Healing by secondary intention

It occurs in an infected wound when the wound is left open to heal by granulation tissue, contraction, and epithelialization. This type of healing takes a lot of time and produces a significant scar. The differences between two types of healing are given in Table 9.6.

Healing by tertiary intention

It follows delayed primary closure of a contaminated wound. It is a combination of the first two types of healing and is followed by lesser scarring than healing of secondary intention.

Table 9.6 Differences between healing by primary intention and secondary intention

Features	Healing by primary intention	Healing by secondary intention
Time taken in healing	Few days	Weeks and months
Rate of healing	Rapid	Slow
Pus formation	Does not occur	Significant
Granulation tissue formation	Hardly any	Significant
Scar	Minimal, linear, supple, and nontender	Significant, broad, firm, and may be tender

Scars of Wound Healing

The result of wound healing is a scar which is of five types.

Normal healthy scar

It is a scar of healing by primary intention. It is linear, thin, soft and supple, nontender, smooth, and nonadherant (Fig. 9.7).

Scar of healing by secondary intention

It is irregular and thin, may be a little depressed from the surface, and may be depigmented and firm.

Scar contracture

It is different from contraction of wound during healing. It is contraction of scar after healing resulting in deformity and functional deficiency. The scar contracture is often seen in the front of the neck and flexor surfaces of joints.

Hypertrophic scar

It is excessive fibrous tissue formation that is limited to the scar. It stops growing after some time (Fig. 9.8).

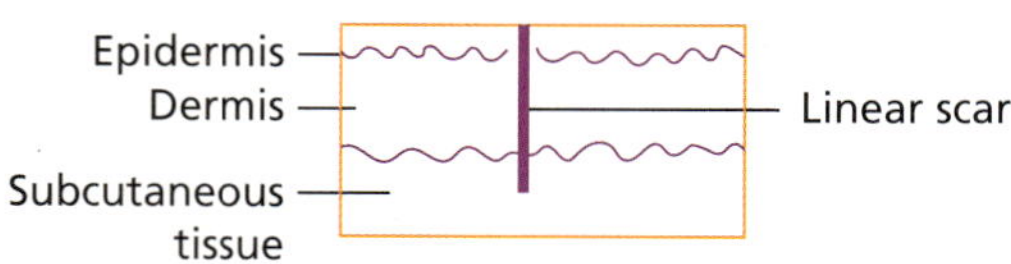

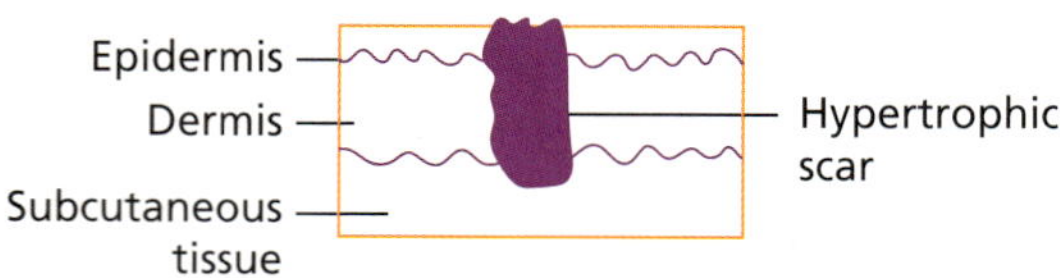

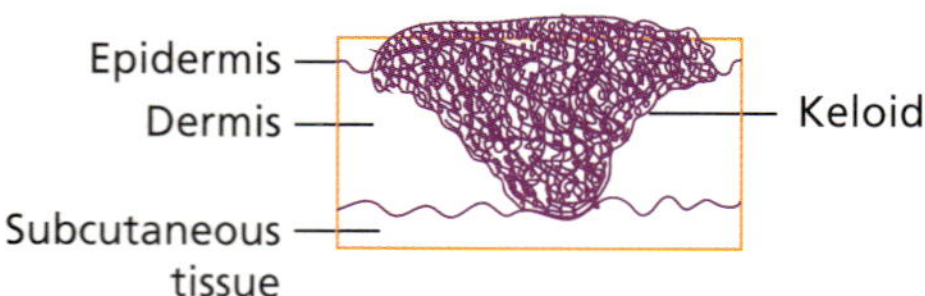

Figure 9.7 Three types of scars of healing.

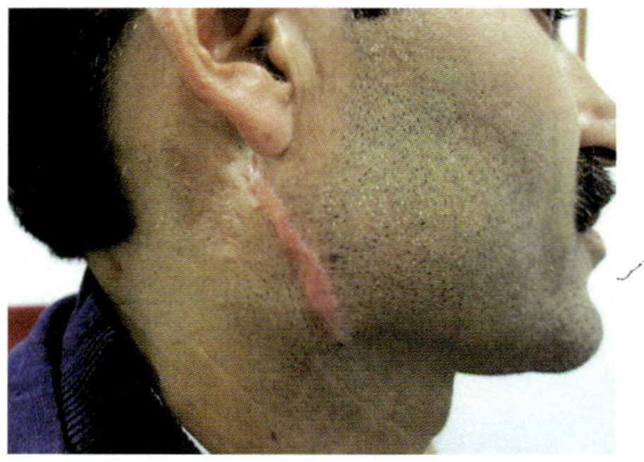

Figure 9.8 Hypertrophic scar near the angle of mandible. (Courtesy: Dr. A.C. Dwivedi)

Keloid

It is the excessive growth of fibrous tissue in a scar which extends into the surrounding normal tissue with claw-like processes (Fig. 9.9).

- **Pathogenesis**: The rate of collagen synthesis in keloid fibroblast culture is significantly greater than normal. The equilibrium is further disrupted by collagenase inhibitor alpha-2-macroglobulin which is abundant in a keloid. It also produces more cytokines.
- **Treatment**: Keloids are difficult to treat. Intralesional injection of triamcinolone 2 mL (40 mg/mL) every 6–8 weeks is the usual treatment. Local application of clobetasol propionate cream may improve the results. Newer methods of treatment include local injection of interferon, cryosurgery, laser, silicon elastomer locally, and use of pressure garments.

The differences between a hypertrophic scar and a keloid are given in Table 9.7.

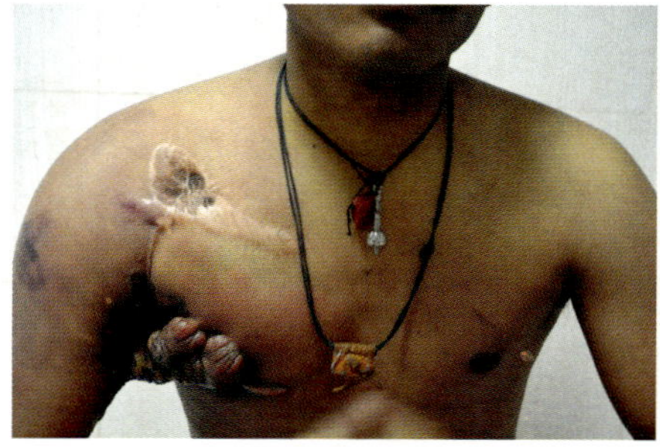

Figure 9.9 Keloids of right lower chest wall having claw-like processes on a scar of operation. (Courtesy: Professor Sandeep Tewari)

Table 9.7 Differences between a hypertrophic scar and a keloid

Features	Hypertrophic scar	Keloid
Predisposing factors	Prolonged inflammatory phase of healing, young age, scar crossing skin creases	Black race, heredity, tuberculous diathesis, puncture or incision of ear lobule or presternal skin
Clinical features		
Age	Common in children	Common at 10–30 years of age
Sex	Equal in both sexes	More in females
Itching	May be present	Prominent feature
Tenderness	Nontender	Tenderness at margins
Extent	Limited to scar	Extends into normal skin around scar
Appearance	Usually regular	May have claw-like processes
Vascularity	Normal	Appears red or erythematous due to increased vascularity
Natural history	Stops growing usually after 6 months and then starts regressing	Continues to grow for a few years
Complications	Usually no complications	Ulceration and infection
Recurrence	Very little chance of recurrence	Very much likely to recur

KEY POINTS

- Injury or trauma is the most primitive or natural disease of living beings and one of the commonest causes of death.
- The main effects of trauma/injury are production of a wound and bleeding. The other effects are secondary depending on the site, type, and severity of injury.
- Closed injury wounds include abrasion, contusion, and hematoma. Open injury wounds include incised wound, laceration, stab wound, and penetrating wound. Complicated wounds involve injury to deeper vital structures.
- Hematoma is due to tearing or rupture of blood vessels where the blood accumulates in tissues, tissue spaces, and body cavities. A small hematoma resolves by itself, but a large or compressing hematoma requires urgent evacuation.
- Incised wound is produced by horizontal movement of a sharp-edged weapon with pressure on the body surface. It tends to gape with protrusion of subcutaneous tissue. Its edges are clean cut and bleed freely. Treatment includes hemostasis and suturing.
- Stab or punctured wounds are caused by vertical movement of a knife or dagger on the body. Penetrating or perforating wounds are produced in a similar manner by a sharp-pointed weapon or a bullet penetrating or perforating a body cavity such as thorax or abdomen.
- Lacerated wounds are caused by blunt objects or weapons, road traffic accidents, shell fragments, and industrial accidents. The surface is broken and the tissues around are crushed and devascularized, and liable to subsequent infection. The wound is irregular and does not bleed freely. Treatment includes excision of damaged tissue followed by primary closure, delayed primary closure, no closure, or skin grafting.
- Bleeding is the second most common manifestation of trauma and priority must be given to arrest it. It can cause hypovolemic shock and compression of the vital organs in cavities in which they are contained, for example, cardiac tamponade due to hemopericardium.
- Respiratory difficulty is another important manifestation of trauma. Most of the traumatic injuries can cause obstruction of breathing or depression of respiratory center leading to death.
- Wound infection can be accidental or intraoperative. Accidental wounds are heavily contaminated that need prompt treatment. Operative wounds are classified as clean wounds, clean-contaminated wounds, contaminated wounds, and infected/dirty

(CONTD...)

KEY POINTS (...CONTD)

wounds depending on the extent of contamination and chances for infection.

- Emergency treatment is done according to the mnemonic ABCDEF which stands for airway, breathing, circulation, disability, exposure, and fluid resuscitation.
- The first step in wound care is achieving proper hemostasis. Tidy wounds are sutured and covered by polymeric films such as Opsite or Tegaderm which are adhesive transparent dressings or a stretchable adhesive dressing.
- If there is doubt regarding cleanliness of the wound, it may be kept covered by a sterile gauze for 3–4 days. If the wound remains clean, it is suture closed; if not, it is treated by excision and dressing, and suture closed when it becomes clean.
- Wounds can be closed using suture material, tapes, staples and adhesives, and coverage with split-thickness or full-thickness grafts or flaps.
- Large dermal wounds, for example, donor sites of split skin grafts, require epithelialization only. They are dressed with scarlet red which forms a scab under which the epithelium migrates. They may be dressed with alginate mesh.
- Wound healing is a natural process and occurs in three phases: inflammatory, proliferative, and maturation phases. Wound healing can be inhibited or delayed due to local and general factors.
- Wound healing by primary intention occurs in a clean incised wound with minimal scarring. This scar is linear, thin, soft and supple, nontender, smooth, and nonadherant.
- Wound healing by secondary intention occurs in an infected wound when the wound is left open to heal by granulation tissue, contraction, and epithelialization. This type of healing takes a lot of time and produces a significant scar which is irregular and thin, may be a little depressed from the surface, and may be depigmented and firm.
- Scar contracture may occur after healing, resulting in deformity and functional deficiency. It is often seen in the front of the neck and flexor surfaces of joints.
- Hypertrophic scar is excessive fibrous tissue formation that is limited to the scar. It stops growing after some time.
- Keloid is the excessive growth of fibrous tissue in a scar which itches and extends into the surrounding normal tissue with claw-like processes. It continues to grow for few years and may result in ulceration and infection.

SELF-ASSESSMENT

Long answer questions

1. What are the common causes of trauma? Describe the effects of trauma on the human body.
2. What are the types of wounds produced by trauma? Describe their features and treatment.

Short answer questions

1. Abrasion
2. Contusion
3. Incised wound
4. Lacerated wound
5. Healing of wounds
6. Keloids

Multiple choice questions

1. Which of the following is the commonest cause of death?
   (a) Tetanus
   (b) Gas gangrene
   (c) Major trauma
   (d) Fracture of both bones of forearm
2. A glass cut wound is bleeding freely and has sharp cut edges. What is the type of wound among the following?
   (a) Lacerated wound
   (b) Incised wound
   (c) Penetrating wound
   (d) Abrasion

(CONTD...)

SELF-ASSESSMENT *(...CONTD)*

3. Which of the following is the first step in the treatment of a wound?
   (a) Arrest of hemorrhage
   (b) Tetanus prophylaxis
   (c) Administration of antibiotics
   (d) Pain relief
4. An itchy scar of previous trauma in the front of chest has overgrown with claw-like processes going into neighboring skin. What is the diagnosis?
   (a) Hypertrophic scar
   (b) Keloid
   (c) Scar contracture
   (d) Marjolin's ulcer
5. The best dressing for a wound with skin loss is
   (a) Skin autograft
   (b) Eusol dressing
   (c) Scarlet red dressing
   (d) Prolene mesh

Answers

1. (c) 2. (b) 3. (a) 4. (b) 5. (a)

Thermal Injury (Burns) and Skin Grafting

10

Definitions

The body tissues can be injured by excessive heat [e.g., burns (Fig. 10.1) and scald] and excessive cold (e.g., frostbite and trench foot) resulting in coagulative necrosis of tissues.

- **Burns**: A burn is an injury of tissues produced by dry heat and characterized by coagulative necrosis of skin and other tissues.
- **Scalds**: It is a superficial burn caused by hot liquids or hot moist vapor and characterized usually by vesicles and bullae formation.

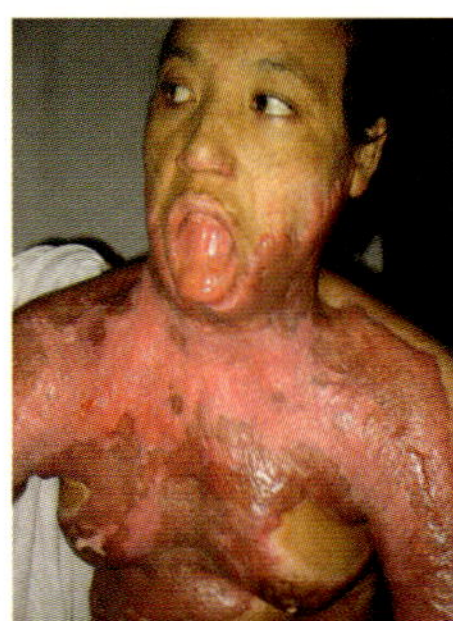

Figure 10.1 A case of extensive burn of neck, shoulders, and upper chest. (Courtesy: Professor Brijesh Mishra)

Pathophysiology

The burns damage the skin and the damaged skin may harm the body as described in the following (Fig. 10.2):

- Immediately following burn, the skin swells up due to inflammatory reaction characterized by vasodilatation and increased capillary permeability which causes loss of fluid into extravascular compartment and outside through the burnt skin surface. It causes hypovolemia and hypovolemic shock.
- Through the burn wound, all types of bacteria (resident and environmental) can enter the body, especially *Staphylococcus aureus* and *Pseudomonas aeruginosa*. The burn wound infection may produce bacteremia, septicemia, and septic shock (MODS, MSOF).
- Other effects of burns are loss of protein and electrolytes along with the fluid leading to hypoproteinemia and electrolyte imbalance.
- Severe burns can cause anemia (post-burn anemia due to burning of red blood cells and bone marrow depression.

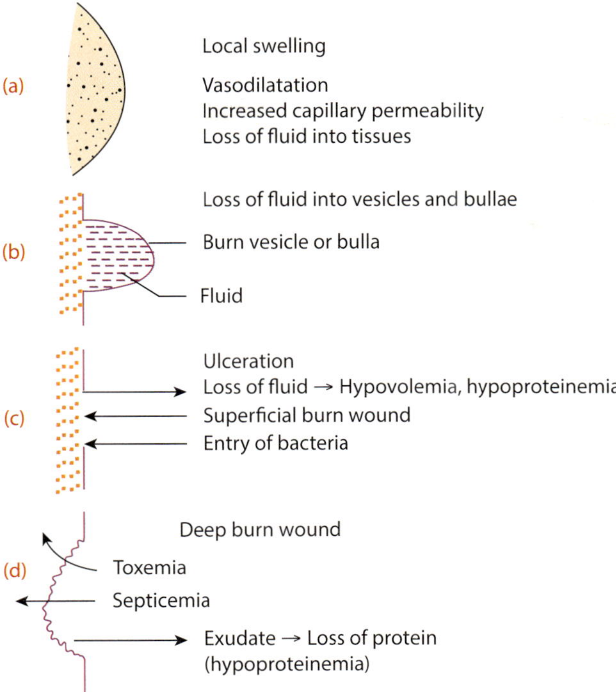

Figure 10.2 Pathophysiology of burns.

Etiology

- Thermal burns
  - Burns due to dry heat
    - Flame burns
    - Hot metal touch
    - Radiant heat, actinic rays
  - Burns due to moist heat—scald
    - Hot tea, coffee, or milk spillover
    - Steam exposure
- Chemical burns—strong acids, alkalies, and other chemicals
- Electrical and lightening burns
- Radiation burns

Assessment of burns

Depth of Burns

Partial-Thickness Burns Partial-thickness burns are characterized by damage to superficial layers of skin exposing the nerve endings of the skin leading to severe pain.

Full-Thickness Burns They are characterized by destruction of full thickness of skin destroying the nerve endings. Hence, the pain is less.

Degree of Burns

Another method of classification depending on the depth of burns is degree of burns (Table 10.1).

Extent of Burns

The extent of burn is assessed by Wallace's rule of nine where the burnt area is calculated by taking into account the extent of burn in various parts of body (Box 10.1).

Treatment of burns

To prevent further thermal injury, "stop, drop, and roll" is used by rescuer.

The airway must be patent. It may require endotracheal intubation or tracheostomy.

Table 10.1 Assessment of degree of burns

Degree of burns	Clinical features	Healing
First degree	Epidermal injury and severe pain with erythema and edema	Heal with supportive treatment within 3–5 days without scarring
Second degree	Involvement of dermis also with pain and blistering	Heal in 10–14 days with hypertrophic scarring
Third degree	Burning of full thickness of skin with less pain and eschar formation	• Require skin grafting for healing • Heal with significant scarring and deformity

Box 10.1 Wallace's rule of nine

- Head and neck: 9%
- Front of chest: 9%
- Back of chest: 9%
- Front of abdomen: 9% limb: 9%
- Back of abdomen: 9%
- Right upper limb: 9%
- Left upper limb: 9%
- Front of right lower limb: 9%
- Back of right lower limb: 9%
- Front of left lower
- Back of left lower limb: 9%
- External genitalia: 1%

Other measures include cold water bath maintaining the circulation, pain relief, broad-spectrum antibiotics, maintenance of nutrition, tetanus prophylaxis, and prevention of erosive gastritis by ranitidine or omeprazole.

Whatever is done by burns to the body has to be undone by treatment. The essentials of treatment are given in the next subsections.

Fluid Replacement

The fluid lost from the body is replaced by employing Muir–Barclay formula or Parkland formula (Box 10.2).

The fluids used for replacement are normal saline, Ringer's lactate, Hartmann solution, and plasma. Ringer's lactate is the fluid of choice.

Box 10.2 Calculation of fluid replacement

- **Muir–Barclay formula**

$$\text{One ration of fluid} = \frac{[\text{percentage of burn}] \times [\text{weight (kg)}]}{2}$$

Of this, three rations are given in the first 12 hours, two rations in the next 12 hours, and one in the next 12 hours

- **Parkland's formula**: A total of 4 mL/kg/% of burn fluid is given in the first 24 hours, half of which is given in the first 8 hours and half in the next 16 hours

Treatment of Burn Wound

Treatment of Superficial Burn Wound A superficial burn wound is cleaned and silver sulfadiazine cream or mafenide is applied locally and left open (exposure method), or covered with cotton and bandage (closed method).

Scald It is treated like a superficial burn wound. The skin of the vesicles or bullae may be excised or retained. It dries up and heals.

Treatment of Deep Burn Wound A deep burn is treated by tangential excision and skin grafting after 24–48 hours of injury. The skin can be obtained from unburnt areas or skin bank. It results in early healing and prevents wound infection and contractures.

Escharotomy In circumferential full-thickness burns of the torso and limbs the rigid dry eschar may produce a tourniquet effect and compartment syndrome. It is treated by escharotomy at bedside with electrocautery avoiding nerves and blood vessels and taking the incision beyond the eschar.

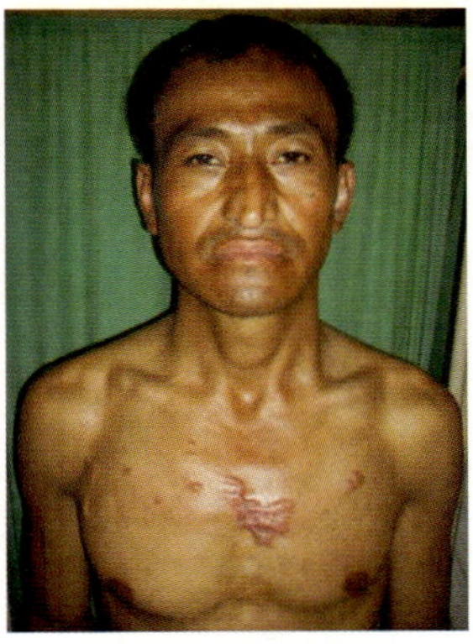

Figure 10.3 Postburn keloid in front of lower chest. (Courtesy: Professor Brijesh Mishra)

Complications of burns

- Shock
- Wound infection
- Septicemia
- Contractures
- Keloids (Fig. 10.3)
- Marjolin's ulcer (it is a squamous cell carcinoma which occurs on an old scar of a burn)
- Death (burns are a common cause of death which occurs due to hypovolemic shock, airway obstruction, and septic shock)

Skin grafting

Skin grafting is required to cover raw areas of the body surface and sometimes mucosal defects. Now skin grafts are also being used for reconstruction of some structures, for example, breast and urethra.

Contraindications of skin grafting include if the wound contains pus, dead tissue, β-hemolytic *Streptococcus*, and bacterial concentration more than 10^5 organisms per gram of tissue.

Definitions

The skin grafts are segments of epidermis and dermis that have been detached from their native blood supply to be transplanted at another area where the skin is missing.

Donor area is the place from where the skin grafts are taken. In adults they are taken from thighs, and from buttocks in children. Recipient site is the area which is raw and requires coverage by skin graft/grafts.

Types of Skin Grafts

Based on Source of Skin Graft

- **Autograft**: An autograft is one which is taken from the same person.
- **Allograft**: An allograft is taken from a genetically dissimilar individual of the same species, usually a cadaver.
- **Xenograft**: Xenograft is taken from a different species, usually pigs.
- **Cultured skin**: Cultured skin can be grown from human epidermal cells. It is most useful for extensively burned patients because more surface area can be covered, but this skin tends to be very thin.

Based on Thickness of the Skin Graft (Table 10.2)

- **Split-thickness skin grafts:** They are sometimes called Thiersch grafts and contain epidermis and a portion of dermis. They are further divided into thin (epidermis only), medium (epidermis and superficial dermis), and thick (epidermis and dermis) types based on the amount of dermis included in the graft (0.010–0.025 inch). The abdomen, buttocks, and thighs are the common donor sites.
- **Full-thickness skin grafts:** They contain epidermis and full thickness of dermis without subcutaneous fat. They are most useful for covering defects of face and hands which are not amenable to coverage with a skin flap. Postauricular and supraclavicular areas provide a good match of skin color. Periauricular grafts provide the best color match for the face.

Technique of Taking Skin Grafts

Split-thickness skin grafts can be taken with a handheld knife or powered skin knives (electrical dermatome). The knife is kept slightly oblique on the stretched skin and

Table 10.2 Differences between split-thickness and full-thickness skin grafts

Characteristics	Split-thickness skin graft	Full-thickness skin graft
Contents of the skin graft	Contains epidermis and a portion of dermis	Contains epidermis and full thickness of dermis without subcutaneous fat
Types	Thin, medium, and thick	Full thickness of skin
Indications	Temporary wound closure before better secondary correction is possible	For smaller areas where good elastic skin which will not contract is required, for example, eyelids, fingers, and facial parts
Donor sites	Abdomen, buttock, and thighs	Postauricular and supraclavicular areas, periauricular grafts
Advantages	• Large supply of donor areas • Ease of harvesting • Availability of the same donor site for reuse in 10–14 days • Coverage of large surface areas • Ability to store for later use	• Cosmetic superiority to split-thickness skin grafts • Decreased secondary contracture • Increased durability
Disadvantages	• Cosmetic inferiority to full-thickness skin grafts • Decreased durability • Hyperpigmentation • Increased secondary contracture	• Limited donor sites • Increased primary contracture

moved horizontally in a to-and-fro motion. The donor area is pressed with a warm moist sponge for hemostasis and dressed with scarlet red ointment or tulle gras.

Healing of Skin Grafts

Plasma Imbibition Survival of free grafts depends on imbibition of plasma during the first 48 hours. Fibrin is laid down to hold the graft in place.

Inosculation Plasma imbibition is followed by inosculation (vascular budding) when the graft is usually supported by true circulation by the fourth to seventh day when the graft begins to turn pink. Lymphatic connections develop by the fifth day. Contact of skin graft is essential for inosculation to take place. The factors which lead to loss of contact are given in Box 10.3.

Box 10.3 Factors causing loss of contact of skin graft

- Tension on the graft
- Fluid (blood, serum, or pus) under the graft
- Movements between the graft and its bed
- Infected wounds (they do not support skin grafts; the critical bacterial concentration appears to be 10^5 organisms per gram of tissue)

Composite grafts

These grafts consist of a unit of multiple tissues, for example, fingertip containing skin, subcutaneous tissue, fat and bone, or a segment of pinna containing skin and cartilage. They are free grafts; hence, they are small. They establish a blood supply in the recipient area. Hair transplant graft is another example of composite grafts.

Flaps

Definition

Flaps are segments of skin and subcutaneous tissue which are moved from one part of the body to another either retaining or transplanting their blood supply. Due to their intrinsic blood supply, the flaps are useful for healing and for covering defects that require padding.

Indications of Flap

- Wound closure in areas of poor vascularity (e.g., wounds overlying bare bone, cartilage, nerves or tendons, and radiation-injured tissues)
- Facial reconstruction (e.g., nose or lips)
- Areas over bone where padding is needed (e.g., ischial tuberosity in pressure sores)

The **contraindications** for a flap are:

- Local sepsis in a septicemic patient
- Tobacco smoker who continues to smoke
- Poor anatomical knowledge of local blood supply

Types of Flaps

The flaps are of many types:

- Skin flap
- Muscle flap
- Fasciocutaneous and musculocutaneous flaps
- Free flap
- Pedicled flap (it is a part of skin which is free from three sides and attached at one side with the donor area for its blood supply called pedicle)
- Microvascular flap (it is a free skin graft with its blood supply identified to be anastomosed to similar-sized cut vessels in the recipient area)

Skin Flaps

Based on the vascular supply, skin flaps are of two types (Table 10.3):

1. **Random flaps**: They receive their vascular supply from the dermal–subdermal plexus.
2. **Axial flaps**: They have a direct cutaneous artery and vein supplying their subdermal plexus.

Muscle Flaps and Musculocutaneous Flaps

They contain a muscle with a named artery which must be identified and preserved. These flaps increase the blood supply of that area where they are grafted. When the overlying skin and subcutaneous tissue and muscle are included in the grafts, they are called myocutaneous flaps. The commonly used muscle and musculocutaneous flaps include latissimus dorsi flap, pectoralis major flap, tensor fascia lata flap, rectus abdominis flap, and other flaps.

Indications

They are used to cover bare bone. They have been most useful in reconstruction of areas of poor vascularity and of radiation damage.

Fasciocutaneous Flaps

They involve the transfer of skin, subcutaneous tissue, and the underlying fascia with an anatomically distinct artery. As the underlying muscle is not mobilized, there is less functional debilitation. These flaps are cosmetically inferior to muscle flaps. The examples of fasciocutaneous flaps include those overlying gastrocnemius, quadriceps femoris, and rectus abdominis muscles.

Table 10.3 Differences between random and axial skin flaps

Features	Random flaps	Axial flaps
Vascular supply	Dermal–subdermal plexus	Direct cutaneous artery and vein supplying their subdermal plexus
Reliability of vascular supply	Not reliable. They lack an anatomically recognized arterial and venous system	Reliable. Hence, flaps of greater length may be obtained and can be used as microvascular free flap
Examples	Z-plasty, V-Y advancement flap, rotation flap, and transposition flap	Forehead flap, groin flap, and deltopectoral flap

Free Flaps (Free Tissue Transfer)

In these flaps the native blood supply is completely severed with transplantation of flaps to separate body areas with microvascular anastomosis. The operative requirements include an operating microscope with two viewing binocular lenses and swaged on a needle of 60–80 mm and 8-0, 9-0, and 10-0 sutures. They can be muscle, myocutaneous, fasciocutaneous, or axial flaps. They may be used to provide function, for example, free neurotized muscle transfer for correction of facial nerve palsy. A composite free flap, for example, fibular flap with its overlying skin, is the most useful face flap for reconstruction of mandible following excision of a tumor.

Assessment of Flap Viability

The vascular patency of the flap can be assessed by color, temperature, Doppler flowmetry, fluoroscanning, and color Doppler.

The complications of flap surgery include improper vascular anastomosis resulting in failure of flap to take up and wound infection.

KEY POINTS

- Burns are caused by dry heat and scalds by moist heat. They cause coagulative necrosis of tissues.
- Immediately following burn, the skin swells up due to inflammatory reaction and there is loss of fluid into extravascular compartment and outside through the burnt skin surface. This causes hypovolemia and hypovolemic shock.
- *Staphylococcus aureus and Pseudomonas aeruginosa* cause burn wound infection and can cause bacteremia, septicemia, and septic shock (MODS, MSOF).
- Burns cause loss of protein and electrolytes along with the fluid leading to hypoproteinemia and electrolyte imbalance. Severe burns can cause anemia (anemia of burns) due to burning of red blood cells and bone marrow depression.
- Partial-thickness burns are characterized by damage to superficial layers of skin exposing the nerve endings of the skin leading to severe pain. Full-thickness burns are characterized by destruction of full thickness of skin destroying the nerve endings. Hence, the pain is less.
- First-degree burns involve epidermis and heal with supportive treatment within 3–5 days without scarring. Second-degree burns involve dermis and heal in 10–14 days with hypertrophic scarring. Third-degree burns involve full thickness of skin with less pain and eschar formation and require skin grafting for healing.
- The extent of burn is assessed by Wallace's rule of nine where the burnt area is calculated by taking into account the extent of burn in various parts of body.
- Replacement of fluid loss in a burn patient is done using Muir–Barclay formula or Parkland formula. The fluids used for replacement are normal saline, Ringer's lactate, Hartmann solution, and plasma. Ringer's lactate is the fluid of choice.
- A superficial burn wound is cleaned and dressed with silver sulfadiazine cream and left open (exposure method), or covered with cotton and bandage (closed method).
- A deep burn is treated by tangential excision and skin grafting after 24–48 hours of injury.
- Complications of burns include shock, wound infection, septicemia, contractures, keloids, Marjolin's ulcer, and death.
- The skin grafts are segments of epidermis and dermis that have been detached from their native blood supply to be transplanted at another area.
- Split-thickness skin grafts contain epidermis and a portion of dermis. They are further divided into thin, medium, and thick types based on the amount of dermis included in the graft.
- Full-thickness skin grafts contain epidermis and full thickness of dermis without subcutaneous fat. They are most useful for covering small defects of face and hands which are not amenable to coverage with a skin flap.
- Skin grafts heal by plasma imbibition and inosculation.
- Flaps are segments of skin and subcutaneous tissue which are moved from one part of the body to another either retaining or transplanting their blood supply. Due to their intrinsic blood supply,

(CONTD...)

KEY POINTS (...CONTD)

the flaps are useful for healing and for covering defects that require padding.

- Random skin flaps receive their vascular supply from the dermal–subdermal plexus. Hence, their vascular supply is not reliable as they lack an anatomically recognized arterial and venous system.
- Axial skin flaps have a direct cutaneous artery and vein supplying their subdermal plexus. Their vascular supply is reliable and hence flaps of greater length may be obtained and can be used as microvascular free flap.
- Muscle flaps contain a muscle with a named artery which must be identified and preserved. When the overlying skin and subcutaneous tissue and muscle are included in the grafts, they are called myocutaneous flaps. They are used to cover bare bone. They have been most useful in reconstruction of areas of poor vascularity and of radiation damage.
- Fasciocutaneous flaps involve the transfer of skin, subcutaneous tissue, and the underlying fascia with an anatomically distinct artery. As the underlying muscle is not mobilized, there is less functional debilitation. These flaps are cosmetically inferior to muscle flaps.
- In free flaps the native blood supply is completely severed with transplantation of flaps to separate body areas with microvascular anastomosis.
- The vascular patency of the flap can be assessed by color of the graft, temperature, Doppler flowmetry, fluoroscanning, and color Doppler.

SELF-ASSESSMENT

Long answer question

1. What are the causes of burns? What are their ill effects on the body and how will you treat them?

Short answer questions

1. Scald
2. Rule of nine
3. Parkland's formula
4. Partial-thickness graft
5. Random flap
6. Axial flaps
7. Free flaps

Multiple choice questions

1. Scald is defined as
   (a) Burn due to acid exposure
   (b) Burn due to contact with live electric wire
   (c) Burn due to dry heat
   (d) Burn due to wet heat
2. All of the following are the immediate effects of accidental burns, except
   (a) Local burning pain
   (b) Burn wound
   (c) Loss of fluid from burnt skin
   (d) Keloids
3. The extent of burns is assessed by
   (a) Wallace's rule of nine
   (b) Muir–Barclay formula
   (c) Parkland formula
   (d) None of the above
4. The immediate important steps in the management of burns are all of the following, except
   (a) Relief of pain
   (b) Correction of fluid loss
   (c) Tetanus prophylaxis
   (d) Release of contractures
5. Exposed bone denuded of periosteum should be ideally covered with
   (a) Thin split-thickness graft
   (b) Thick split-thickness graft
   (c) Full-thickness grafts
   (d) Muscle flaps

Answers

1. (d) 2. (d) 3. (a) 4. (d) 5. (d)

Head Injury

11

Introduction

Head injury accounts for almost 50% of trauma-related deaths in young people. It includes injury to the scalp, skull, and brain; hence, the term craniocerebral trauma is more appropriate. Figure 11.1 shows an unconscious patient with head injury having a forehead wound, left black eye, and dried-up blood in left nostril and on lips and teeth.

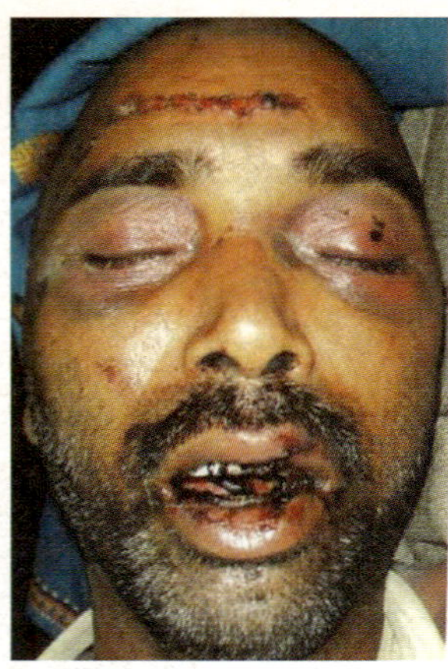

Figure 11.1 Patient with head injury. (Courtesy: Professor Sandeep Tewari)

Causes of head injury

The common causes of head injury include traffic accidents especially motor cycle accidents, fall from a height (roof or tree), homicidal attacks, industrial accidents, and fall in the bathroom.

Scalp injury

The scalp is the protective skin cover of skull. It is very hairy, thick, strong, and very vascular. Hence, it bleeds briskly and heals quickly after injury. Complications of scalp injuries include infection skin loss; wound infection may be with intracranial extension and bleeding. Common injuries of the scalp are described below.

Scalp Hematoma

Etiology It follows blunt trauma.

Clinical Features

- It feels hard at the periphery due to clotting of blood and soft in the center due to serum or liquid blood. Thus, it may give an impression of a depressed fracture.

- A lax hematoma in the temporal region may occur in fractures of squamous temporal and parietal bones and may be associated with extradural hematoma (middle meningeal hemorrhage).
- Sometimes an extensive hematoma may form in loose subaponeurotic space due to a linear fracture of skull.
- In a subpericranial hematoma the blood collects under the pericranium. Hence, it assumes the shape of the related skull bone.

Investigations They can be imaged by ultrasonography, CT scan, or MRI, but most of the time the diagnosis is clinical.

Complications The complications of hematoma include rupture with bleeding and secondary infection.

Treatment As a rule, these hematomas do not require treatment. A large hematoma may be aspirated or evacuated surgically.

Open Wounds of the Scalp

Lacerated Open Wound A lacerated wound follows blunt injury. It is irregular in shape and does not bleed freely. It is treated by excision and closure. The deficiency is made good by local adjustment or skin grafting.

Incised Open Wound An incised wound has sharp edges and bleeds freely. The bleeding can be stopped by pressing the edge of wound against the skull or by catching the edge of cut galea at various points by scalp hemostats and everting. It is closed by sutures.

Avulsion of Scalp

If the hair are caught in a rotating machine, the entire scalp may be avulsed. It usually hangs bleeding like a flap by the side of the head. It is washed clean and spread in the wound and sutured in position. It usually heals well as the scalp has a rich blood supply. If there is shortage of skin, grafting may be required. Large areas of skull may be covered by skin grafted with microvascular technique. The complications of avulsion of scalp include flap necrosis, wound infection, and bleeding.

Abrasions of the Scalp

Abrasions are common in the scalp. They are treated with local povidone–iodine paint or some antiseptic cream.

Skull injury (fractures of skull)

The injury of the skull is characterized by a fracture or fractures which usually follow blunt trauma. The common fractures of the skull are given in Box 11.1. The skull fractures can be compound when associated with scalp injuries. Figure 11.2 shows a patient with extensive injury of skull with avulsion of scalp and fracture of skull.

Box 11.1 Fractures of the skull

- Simple linear fracture
- Depressed fracture
- Anterior cranial fossa fracture
- Middle cranial fossa fracture
- Posterior cranial fossa fracture

(Anterior, middle and posterior cranial fossa fractures: Fractures of the base of skull)

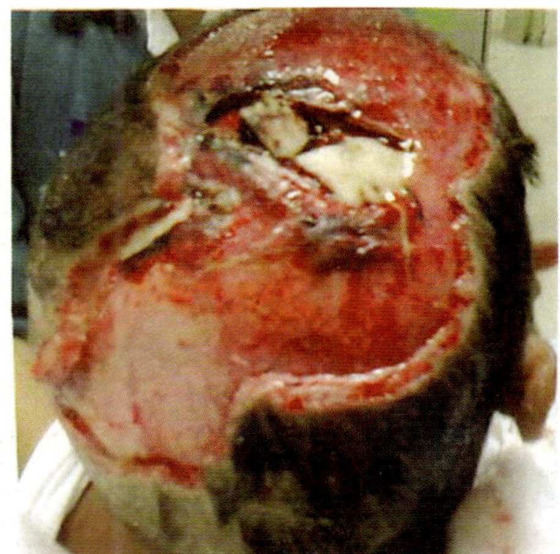

Figure 11.2 Extensive injury of head with avulsion of scalp and fracture of skull. (Courtesy: Dr. S.K. Vaish)

Simple Linear Fracture

- This fracture is characterized by an abnormal line on the skull in a radiograph.
- A linear fracture that crosses the middle meningeal artery groove may produce an extradural hematoma. It may be confused with a suture line in a radiograph. In such a case the patient is admitted for 24 hours for observation and a CT scan should be done, which will show the fracture and also the hematoma.
- As such a linear fracture does not require any treatment but with a hematoma an urgent operation is required.

Depressed Fracture

- It is caused by a localized impact or sharp trauma affecting the inner table more than the outer table. It can occur anywhere but the commonest site is frontal bone.
- The depressed fragment of the bone may lacerate the dura and brain when there is 15% risk of subsequent epilepsy.
- Pond fracture is a type of depressed fracture commonly seen in children characterized by a smooth concave depression similar to a dent in a ping-pong ball (ping-pong fracture).
- Investigations: CT scan of skull shows the fracture in which the injury to the inner table and the integrity of local dura is seen.
- Complications: The complications of a depressed fracture of skull are described in Box 11.2.
- Treatment: A depressed fracture is treated by debridement, irrigation, elevation of fracture, and duraplasty. If the bone fragments are heavily contaminated, they are removed, and a reconstructive acrylic cranioplasty should be considered at a later date.

Box 11.2 Complications of a depressed fracture of skull

- Intracranial hematoma, especially from injury to dural sinuses
- Local wound infection, osteomyelitis
- Cosmetic problem
- Epilepsy

Anterior Cranial Fossa Fracture

It is associated with subconjunctival hemorrhage without posterior limit, anosmia, epistaxis, nasal tip paresthesia, and CSF rhinorrhea.

Middle Cranial Fossa Fracture

It presents with CSF otorrhea, hemotympanum, ossicular disruption, Battle's sign, and seventh and eighth cranial nerve palsies.

Posterior Cranial Fossa Fracture

It may show ecchymosis over occipital region or even mastoids.

The clinical features of fractures of base of skull are described in Box 11.3.

Box 11.3 Clinical features of the fractures of the base of skull

Anterior cranial fossa fracture

- Anterior cranial fossa
- Subconjuntival hemorrhage without posterior limit
- Anosmia
- Epistaxis, CSF rhinorrhea
- Nasal tip anesthesia

Middle cranial fossa fracture

- CSF otorrhea, bleeding from ear, hemotympanum, ossicular disruption
- Hearing defect
- Battle's sign
- Seventh and eighth cranial nerve palsies

Posterior cranial fossa fracture

- Local tenderness, crepitus
- Ecchymosis over occiput and even mastoids may be present

Investigations

Radiography of skull reveals the fracture site and may also reveal pneumocranium or air-fluid level (aerocele). CT scan, or MRI especially for posterior fossa lesions, and cerebral angiography may be done if there is suspicion of intracranial injury including injury to cerebral circulation.

Complications

The bacteria may enter the intracranial compartments from the paranasal air sinuses causing meningitis. There is no evidence that prophylactic antibiotics protect against meningitis. Other complications include a variety of intracranial hematomas, aerocele, traumatic osteomyelitis of skull, and epilepsy.

Treatment of Fractures of Skull

- Uncomplicated fractures usually do not require any treatment except symptomatic.
- Depressed fractures are elevated. They may require open reduction and fixation.
- In fractures of the base, the patient should lie with head end of the bed elevated, should not blow the nose, and should wipe the leaking CSF with a sterile swab. With this treatment the CSF leak stops within 1–2 weeks.
- Persistent CSF leak should be investigated to find the site of leak so that it can be repaired by autologous vascularized graft and fibrin glue.

CSF rhinorrhea and CSF otorrhea

Clear watery discharge from the nose or ear after head injury is due to leakage of CSF (CSF rhinorrhea, CSF otorrhea). Rhinorrhea is more common than otorrhea which is due to fracture of cribriform plate. If it is a minor leak which is discolored with blood, it may be difficult to diagnose. Here the halo test may be helpful which is done by putting a drop of fluid on an absorbent surface such as fascial tissue. The drop will form a double ring with a darker central spot of blood.

It is treated by nursing the patient with head elevated, wiping the leak with a sterile swab and avoiding blowing the nose. A catheter may be placed in lumbar subarachnoid space to reduce normal CSF pressure. The antibiotics have hardly any role. Most of the CSF leaks heal with the treatment in a few days. If it persists, the leak is localized by isotope encephalography or CT cisternography, and repaired by duraplasty.

Brain injury

Brain injury is caused by transfer of energy of trauma to the brain. It is of two types: primary and secondary.

Etiopathogenesis

Primary brain injury

It occurs when the energy is being transferred to the brain as a ball striking the skull injures the brain (contusion of brain) at the site of impact. There are five mechanisms of primary brain injury.

Acceleration–Deceleration Acceleration or deceleration is the primary mode of injury in most closed or blunt head injuries where the injuring agent does not penetrate the skull and meninges. The brain dissipates the energy imparted to it by internal movements and gyrations, low-energy gyrations causing temporary disruption of function and high-energy gyrations causing disruption of neurons or even tearing of brain substance.

Direct Disruption in Open Head Injury Here the injuring agent penetrates the skull and meninges and injures the brain directly as a bullet causing injury to the brain.

Contusion It occurs when the brain strikes bony or dural structures during gyrations of its surface, or it may occur beneath the skull at the site of impact due to localized indenting of skull.

Contrecoup It is the injury of the brain at the point or pole opposite to where the blow was delivered. Contrecoup means opposite to blow. The injury of brain at the site of trauma is called coup.

Compression Compression of the head is an uncommon injury and occurs when the head is stamped upon by an assailant or trapped beneath a vehicle that falls off its jack.

Diffuse Axonal Injury It is due to rapid acceleration or deceleration and occurs when axons become sheared off at the junction between gray and white matter. It is characterized by depressed level of consciousness and further signs depend on whether there is intracerebral hemorrhage somewhere.

Penetrating Injury It is caused by a bullet or such other devices. It causes direct disruption of brain and direct transfer of energy which is directly proportional to the projectile mass and square of its velocity.

Secondary brain injury

The secondary brain injury does not occur at the time of trauma but later on (due to delay in treatment) and is caused by the intracranial lesions, for example, a hematoma produced by trauma (extradural, subdural, and intracerebral).

Other types of secondary brain injuries include traumatic cerebral edema, subdural hematoma (SDH), intracerebral hematoma, intraventricular bleeding, cerebral ischemia, coning and herniation, and entry of infection and air (aerocele) through fractures of base of skull.

The effects of brain injury are described in Box 11.4.

Box 11.4 Effects of brain injury

- Intracranial hematoma
- Traumatic cerebral edema
- Ischemia with infarction, cerebral necrosis
- Increased intracranial pressure
- Coning, herniation of contents of supratentorial compartment through the tentorial hiatus, and herniation of contents of infratentorial compartment through foramen magnum
- Hemiparesis, paralysis, cranial nerve palsies
- Convulsions
- Respiratory depression, failure

Assessment of Severity of Brain Injury

The patient is examined as a whole including the level of consciousness, reflexes, pulse, respiration, temperature, blood pressure, and other associated injuries, especially cervical spine.

Glasgow coma scale (GCS)

The severity of head injury is assessed by this clinical method of assessment as described in Box 11.5.

Box 11.5 Glasgow coma scale

Eye opening	Motor response	Verbal response
Spontaneous: 4	Obeys commands: 6	Oriented to place and time: 5
To speech: 3	Moves purposefully: 5	Confused conversation: 4
To pain: 2	Withdraws: 4	Inappropriate words: 3
No eye opening: 1	Abnormal flexion: 3	Incomprehensible sounds: 2
	Extension response: 2	No verbal response: 1
	No motor response: 1	

Maximum score is 15 which is normal

Minimum score is 3 which means very serious

The scores for various types of injuries are as follows:

- Mild head injury: 13–15
- Moderate head injury: 9–12
- Severe head injury: <8 (3–8)

Investigations

CT scan

The old method of investigation has been radiography of skull which detects the fractures of skull but gives hardly any information about the brain injury. The advent of CT scan has reduced the importance of X-ray of skull as even the skull can be assessed by CT using the bone windows. The indications for CT scan are described as follows:

- Persistently drowsy patient
- If the level of consciousness is going down
- Presence of lateralizing neurological signs
- Neurological deterioration
- Fracture of skull base

Cervical radiography

The cervical spine should be radiographed (C1–T1) in patients who have sustained significant head injury as it may also be injured along with head. In the absence of cervical fracture or cervical spinal cord deficit, flexion/extension views of cervical spine are required to rule out ligamentous injury.

Measuring intracranial pressure

A small hole is drilled in the skull and an intraparenchymal fiber-optic pressure transducer, called bolt, is placed in it. It allows intracranial pressure (ICP) monitoring.

Angiography

Transarterial catheter-based angiography is required to evaluate the vascular pathology of brain. For this both the carotid arteries and both the vertebral arteries may be injected as indicated and followed through arterial, capillary, and venous phases to obtain a complete cerebral angiogram.

Types of Brain Injuries

The clinical features, pathology, and treatment of various types of brain injury are given in Table 11.1.

Table 11.1 Management of various types of brain injuries

Type	Clinical features	Pathology	CT findings	Treatment
Concussion	Transient loss of consciousness with low heart rate and blood pressure, and respiratory arrest for a few seconds followed by retrograde amnesia for some time	Brain may be normal or may be contused at the site of impact (coup) or at the point just opposite the impact (contrecoup)	Diffuse cerebral edema	• ABCDE • Supportive treatment
Contusion or laceration	• Longer loss of consciousness • May cause death • May be severe residual neurological deficit	• Cerebral contusion, edema, hemorrhage, and necrosis • May be subarachnoid bleeding	Localized cerebral edema	• ABCDE • Reduction of intracranial pressure • Phenytoin if required
Extradural hematoma	• Two episodes of unconsciousness separated by a lucid interval • Headache, confusion, somnolence, seizures, and focal neurological deficit several hours after trauma that lead to coma, respiratory depression, and death	Rapid accumulation of blood in extradural space due to tear of middle meningeal artery	CT scan shows shadow of hematoma with convexity toward brain	• ABCDE • Surgical decompression in the "golden" hour

(CONTD...)

(...CONTD)

Table 11.1 Management of various types of brain injuries

Type	Clinical features	Pathology	CT findings	Treatment
Subdural hematoma	• Similar to extradural hematoma but the onset of symptoms is delayed	Slow accumulation of blood in the subdural space due to tear in veins from cortex to superior sagittal sinus	CT scan shows shadow of hematoma with concavity toward brain	• Surgical evacuation • Small hematomas may be managed conservatively
Cerebral hemorrhage	Occurs immediately after injury. Symptoms and signs like those of hypertensive hemorrhage	Accumulation of blood in cerebral parenchyma	• Cerebral edema • Shows small blood collections at multiple sites	• ABCDE • Supportive treatment • Sometimes evacuation of hematoma

Concussion

- It is the simple brain injury characterized by transient loss of consciousness with bradycardia, hypotension, and respiratory arrest for a few seconds.
- Grossly the brain may be normal or may be bruised at the site of impact (coup) or at a point just opposite the impact (contrecoup).
- It is followed by full recovery except for retrograde amnesia for some time.
- CT scan is normal or may show diffuse cerebral edema of the site of injury.

Contusion or laceration

- It is a more severe injury characterized by a longer loss of consciousness followed by some residual neurological deficit.
- The brain has some tissue injury characterized by edema, petechial hemorrhages, and necrosis.
- Subarachnoid bleeding may occur.

Extradural or epidural hematoma (EDH)

It is the accumulation of blood in the extradural space between dura and the skull.

- **Causes:** It is usually due to rupture of middle meningeal artery with fracture of temporal bone. Other vessels which may be involved include middle meningeal veins and anterior branch or posterior branch of middle meningeal artery.
- **Pathogenesis:** Box 11.6 explains the pathogenesis of extradural hematoma.

Box 11.6 **Pathogenesis of extradural hematoma**

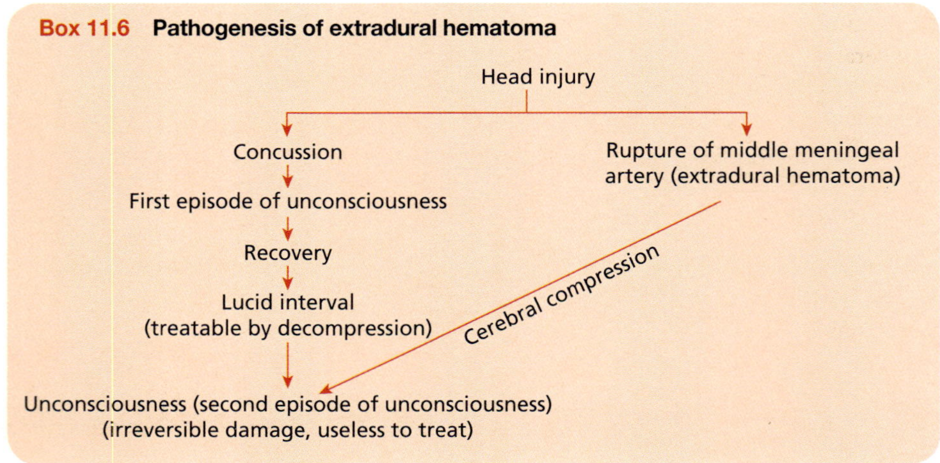

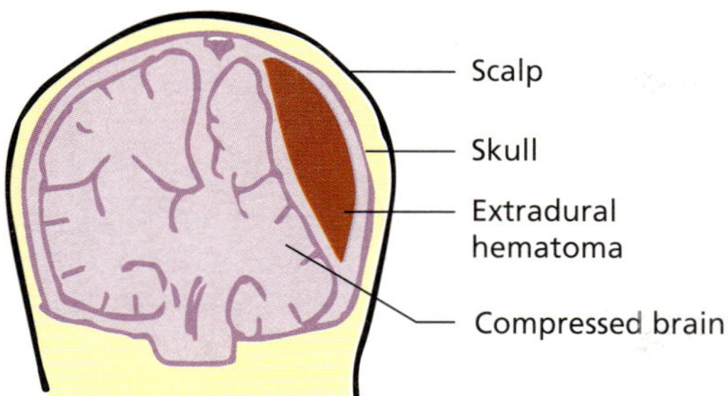

Figure 11.3 Head injury with extradural hematoma having biconvex shape (lenticular opacity).

- **Clinical features:**
  - It is characterized by two episodes of unconsciousness separated by a short interval (less than 1 hour) of clear consciousness called lucid interval. It varies from 6 to 12 hours; it may even be absent.
  - The second episode of unconsciousness is preceded by headache, confusion, somnolence, seizures, and focal deficit followed by coma, respiratory depression, and death.
  - The first unconsciousness is due to concussion which recovers after some time but by that time enough blood accumulates in the extradural space to cause symptoms of acute cerebral compression, that is, confusion, irritability, drowsiness, ipsilateral hemiparesis, and Hutchinson's pupils (papillary constriction followed by dilatation on the same side).
- **CT scan findings**: The hematoma is convex toward the brain (lenticular shadow) on CT scan (Fig. 11.3).
- **Complications**: Include third nerve palsy, contralateral hemiparesis, post-traumatic epilepsy, amnesia, and brain death.
- **Treatment**: It is treated immediately in the golden hour by making a 5-cm vertical incision and a burr hole in the temporal region, removing the blood and arresting bleeding.

A patient with clot volume <30 cm^3, maximum thickness <1.5 cm, and GCS score >8 may be managed conservatively.

Subdural hematoma

It is the collection of blood under the dura mater.

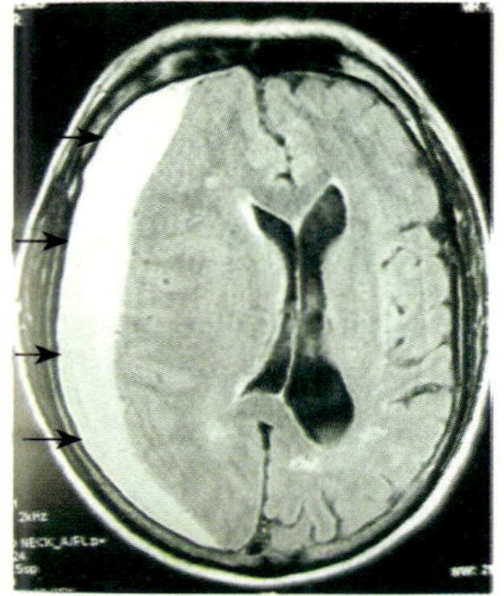

Figure 11.4 Axial CT scan of skull showing right-sided subdural hematoma with marked midline shift.

Cause It is usually due to the tear of veins from cortex to superior sagittal sinus or from cerebral laceration. It may be acute or chronic.

Clinical Features Acute hematoma is characterized by nearly the same symptoms and signs as those of extradural hematoma but the onset is slow and the duration is longer.

CT Scan Findings CT scan shows the hematoma of bright or mixed density with concavity toward the brain that conforms to the shape of brain surface and shows a marked midline shift (Fig. 11.4).

Chronic Subdural Hematoma It is seen in elderly, mostly in those on anticoagulants and having cerebral atrophy. It is usually 2–3 weeks old. There is slow-onset pressure symptoms of 2–3 weeks' duration. CT scan shows diffuse hypodense lesion with concavity toward brain.

Complications Include recurrence, wound infection, poor recovery, epilepsy, and a very high death rate.

Treatment A chronic SDH >1 cm or symptomatic SDH should by surgically evacuated.

An acute SDH is treated by conservative measures. If it has thickness more than 1 cm and midline shift more than 5 cm, it should be surgically evacuated.

Intracerebral hemorrhage

It is the bleeding in brain parenchyma and is of two types: diffuse and localized.

Diffuse bleeding is characterized by loss of consciousness and signs of raised ICP. It is treated by supportive treatment.

Localized intracranial bleeding is identified by focal signs depending on the site of bleeding. It is treated by operation if the clot volume is more than 50 cm^3 or is more than 20 cm^3 with referable neurological deterioration.

Arterial dissection

Head and neck trauma may be associated with traumatic dissection of arteries of brain, that is, carotid or vertebral arteries. It results in reduction of blood supply of brain, thromboembolism, and rupture of dissected arterial wall with bleeding.

The lesions are detected by four-vessel cerebral angiography. The findings include stenosis of lumen (string sign), visible intimal flaps, and contrast in the false lumen.

Surgical intervention is indicated in persisting embolic disease and vertebral dissection presenting with subarachnoid hemorrhage, and the treatment options include stenting and vessel occlusion (interventional radiology), or vessel legation or bypass grafting (open operation).

Cavernous sinus part of carotid artery may be injured with formation of a carotid–cavernous fistula damaging the contained cranial nerves (III, IV, and VI). It is treated by balloon occlusion (small fistula) or total occlusion of parent carotid artery.

Treatment of Brain Injuries

Observation and Supportive Therapy The treatment of most of the head injuries is careful observation of the patient for better or worse. There are hardly any drugs to treat this problem. Sedatives are not given; analgesics may be given. Anticonvulsants are required to treat convulsions and diuretics and corticosteroids are used to reduce cerebral edema.

Management of Increased Intracranial Pressure

- The most important effect of brain injury is increased ICP which should be brought down to maintain adequate cerebral perfusion pressure (above 50 mm Hg) to prevent irreversible ischemic injury.
- The first step is to monitor ICP by an intraventricular catheter or intraparenchymal monitor and then manage the ICP.
- The methods of reducing ICP include elevation of head end of the bed, hyperventilation, diuretics (mannitol, furosemide), barbiturates (sodium pentobarbital), and hypothermia.

Management of Post-Traumatic Epilepsy It is prevented by giving phenytoin.

Management of Concussion and Contusion These are treated by supportive measures. Intracranial hematomas require surgical decompression. There is hardly any other indication for surgery.

Surgery in Brain Injury It is mainly done to evacuate localized intracranial hematomas only. The site of hematoma is localized by signs and symptoms and imaging methods. A hole is made in the skull at the site of hematoma by perforator and burr (burr hole) and the hematoma is opened and evacuated.

Complications of head injury

The complications of head injury can be classified as early and late complications (Box 11.7).

Box 11.7 Complications of head injury

Early complications	Late complications
• Brainstem injury due to coning	• Post-traumatic hydrocephalus
• Compression of cerebellum and medulla	• Post-traumatic seizure disorder
• CSF rhinorrhea, otorrhea	• Post-traumatic headache
• Post-traumatic meningitis	• Post-traumatic amnesia
• Pituitary damage	• A variety of residual neurological deficits
• Aerocele	• Neuroendocrine and metabolic disorders, e.g., diabetes insipidus

KEY POINTS

- Head injury includes injury to the scalp, skull, and brain, hence called appropriately craniocerebral trauma.
- Scalp injuries include abrasion, contusion, cut, laceration, hematoma, and avulsion. Scalp wounds bleed profusely which can be stopped by pressure or catching the cut edge of galea and eversion. The avulsed skin is washed clean, spread over the raw area, and stitched.
- Skull may fracture and the fractures include a linear, depressed, and pond fracture, and fractures of base of skull. Linear fractures are of no consequence, but a fracture of temporoparietal region may result in an extradural hematoma which requires decompression in the "golden hour."
- Depressed skull fracture is caused by a localized impact or sharp trauma affecting the inner table more than the outer table. It may lacerate the dura and brain when there is 15% risk of subsequent epilepsy. Pond fracture is a type of depressed fracture similar to a dent in a ping-pong ball commonly seen in children.
- Anterior cranial fossa fracture is associated with subconjunctival hemorrhage without posterior limit, anosmia, epistaxis, nasal tip paresthesia, and CSF rhinorrhea.
- Middle cranial fossa fracture presents with CSF otorrhea, hemotympanum, ossicular disruption, Battle's sign, and seventh and eighth cranial nerve palsies.
- Posterior cranial fossa fracture presents with ecchymosis over occipital region or even mastoids.
- Acceleration or deceleration is the primary mode of injury in most closed or blunt head injuries where the injuring agent does not penetrate the skull and meninges.
- Direct disruption in open head injury involves penetration of the skull and meninges and injures the brain directly as a bullet causing injury to the brain.
- Contusion occurs when the brain strikes bony or dural structures during gyrations of its surface, or it may occur beneath the skull at the site of impact due to localized indenting of skull.
- Contrecoup is the injury of the brain at the point or pole opposite to where the blow was delivered.
- The severity of head injury is assessed by Glasgow Coma Scale (GCS). CT scan of the brain gives a definitive diagnosis about the nature of the brain injury. Cervical spine assessment should always be performed in patients with head injury.
- Extradural or epidural hematoma is the accumulation of blood in the extradural space between dura and the skull characterized by two episodes of unconsciousness separated by a short interval of clear consciousness called lucid interval. CT scan shows a lenticular shadow. It is treated by urgent evacuation.
- Subdural hematoma is the collection of blood under the dura mater. It is usually due to the tear of veins from cortex to superior sagittal sinus or from cerebral laceration. Onset of symptoms is slow and the duration is longer. It is seen in the elderly, mostly in those on anticoagulants and having cerebral atrophy. CT scan shows the collection with concavity toward the brain that conforms to the shape of brain surface and may show midline shift.
- Intracerebral hemorrhage is bleeding into the brain substance. It occurs immediately after injury and is characterized by symptoms and signs of site of involvement in the brain. A localized hematoma requires evacuation.

SELF-ASSESSMENT

Long answer questions

1. What are the common causes of head injury? Describe the various types of injuries of brain. How do you treat concussion?
2. What are the principles of treatment of injuries of brain?

Short answer questions

1. Avulsion of scalp
2. Cerebrospinal rhinorrhea
3. Extradural hematoma
4. Glasgow Coma Scale

(CONTD...)

SELF-ASSESSMENT (...CONTD)

Multiple choice questions

1. Bleeding from scalp wound is best controlled immediately by
   (a) Eversion of galea aponeurotica
   (b) Suturing
   (c) Digital pressure on the wound edge
   (d) Electrocoagulation of bleeding points
2. Cerebrospinal fluid rhinorrhea is due to
   (a) Fracture of middle cranial fossa
   (b) Fracture of posterior cranial fossa
   (c) Fracture of anterior cranial fossa
   (d) Fracture of mastoid process
3. A cricketer was injured by a ball striking the temporal region, followed by lucid interval. What is the most likely injury?
   (a) Intracerebral hemorrhage
   (b) Extradural hemorrhage
   (c) Cerebral concussion
   (d) Subdural hematoma
4. The most important investigation to diagnose intracranial injury is
   (a) Plain X-ray of skull
   (b) CT scan
   (c) Ultrasonography
   (d) Isotope scanning
5. What is the treatment of choice of extradural hemorrhage?
   (a) Hemostatics
   (b) Blood transfusion
   (c) Urgent decompression in the "golden hour"
   (d) Embolization of ipsilateral middle meningeal artery

Answers

1. (a) 2. (c) 3. (b) 4. (b) 5. (c)

Maxillofacial (Faciomaxillary) Injuries

12

Introduction

Faciomaxillary injuries are as common as head injuries. Face is an area of the body that has maximum cosmetic importance; the entry to air and food passages is situated on the face, also eyes and orbits on the front and ears on the sides. Hence, if not treated properly and in time, they can cause death and disfigurement. Figure 12.1 shows extensive avulsion injury of left half of the face, nose, and upper lip with loss of vision in left eye.

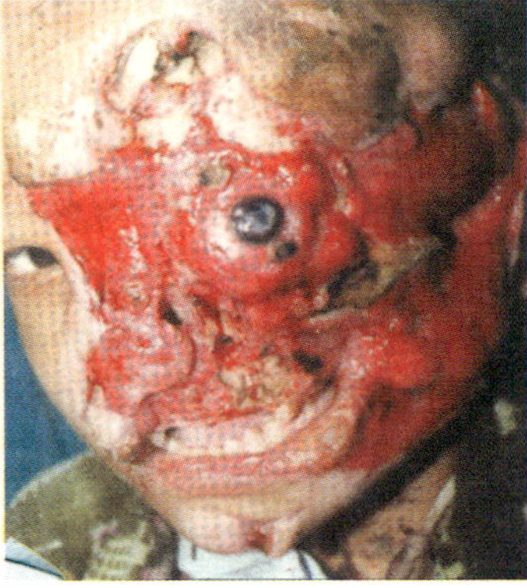

Figure 12.1 Extensive avulsion injury of left half of the face. (Courtesy: Dr. Sanjeev Bhatia)

Surgical anatomy of the face

The facial skin is very vascular. Hence, the wounds of the face heal very rapidly. Under the skin there is no deep fascia except in the parotid region (parotideomasseteric fascia) but there are many small muscles of facial expression which are supplied by five branches of facial nerve coming from stylomastoid foramen and through the parotid salivary gland situated in front of the external ear. Parotid gland is drained by Stensen's duct which runs forwards to open inside the cheek at the level of crown of second upper molar.

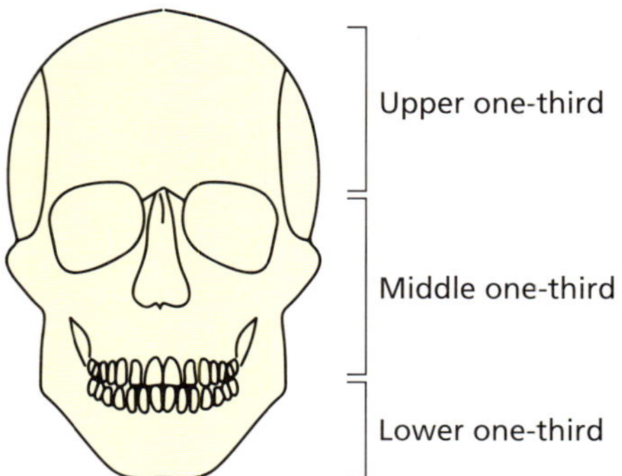

Figure 12.2 Diagram of the skull showing the three parts of skeleton of face.

All of these soft tissues are supported at the back by maxillofacial skeleton which can be divided into upper, middle, and lower thirds (Fig. 12.2):

- The upper third is constituted by frontal bone which has an air sinus of variable size in the central part.
- The middle third is mainly constituted by two maxillae and two zygomatic bones articulating with many small bones, that is, two nasal bones, two lacrimal bones, nasal septum, vomer, ethmoid, and pterygoid plates of ethmoid.
- The lower third of face is made up of mandible or lower jaw.

Etiology of maxillofacial injuries

The face is the most exposed and obvious part of the body, hence most likely to be injured in road traffic accidents, sporting activities (e.g., boxing), fall from a height, homicidal attacks, and wartime injuries. It may be injured by blunt trauma (e.g., traffic accidents) and by sharp cuts (e.g., glass cut injury) and firearm injury.

Types of maxillofacial injuries

The injuries of face may be soft-tissue injuries or injuries of maxillofacial skeleton (fracture and displacements).

Soft-Tissue Injuries The soft-tissue injuries include abrasions, contusions, cuts, and lacerations of facial skin; and injuries of facial nerve and Stensen's duct. They are mostly simple injuries and are not life-threatening, but may be disfiguring. They are the most common injuries of this region.

Hard-Tissue Injuries The injuries of maxillofacial skeleton include fractures and displacement of bones of face and jaws. They are more serious and sometimes complex injuries. The seriousness is further aggravated as they may be associated with (a) head injury (brain injury), (b) injury to cervical spine and spinal cord, and (c) injury to other organs of body, for example, splenic rupture. Hence, the patient must be carefully evaluated as a whole.

Clinicopathological effects

Apart from wound/wounds, disfigurement, and early onset of edema, there are two major effects or manifestations of these injuries which can kill the victim in a short time.

Bleeding As the facial structures are richly supplied with blood, these injuries are associated with severe or dramatic bleeding, at least initially, from facial wound, nose, mouth, or ears.

Respiratory Obstruction The nasal passage and mouth are the most prominent part of the face. Hence, maxillofacial injuries may cause immediate or delayed airway obstruction usually at the level of oropharynx. The causes of obstruction are enumerated in Box 12.1. Airway obstruction should be promptly diagnosed. It must be managed immediately before doing anything as it is an urgent threat to life. The symptoms and signs of airway obstruction are described in Box 12.2.

Clinical assessment

After injury, the patient may come himself/herself in case of a minor injury or may be brought to the hospital in case of a serious injury. The complaints

Box 12.1 Causes of airway obstruction in maxillofacial injuries

- Inhalation of teeth, pieces of denture, or a foreign body
- Accumulation of blood, oral secretions, vomitus, and cerebrospinal fluid (CSF) in oropharynx
- Falling back of tongue as occurs in a butterfly fracture of mandibular symphysis
- Rapid-onset edema (within 60–90 minutes) of tongue and facial and pharyngeal tissues (e.g., in Le Fort II and III fractures of maxilla). The edematous soft palate and tongue may come together to close the pharyngeal airway
- A large hematoma of floor of mouth
- Retroposition of maxilla in fractures of this bone with occlusion of oropharynx

Box 12.2 Symptoms and signs of airway obstruction

- Restlessness, apprehension, anxiety, tachypnea, tachycardia, and pallor
- Labored noisy breathing
- Rapid movement or fluttering of the alae of the nose
- Suprasternal indrawing and intercostal retraction
- Cyanosis (cyanosis is a late sign)

may be pain, bleeding, wound or wounds, swelling, and respiratory difficulty.

General Examination

Most often the injuries are complex and multiple involving other regions or parts of the body. Hence, the patient must be examined for other associated injuries (e.g. rupture of liver), which are less visible and may be more serious.

Local Examination

Ecchymosis, hematoma, and rapid onset of edema may make the local examination difficult. The examination is done in a systematic manner so as not to miss any injury.

Inspection of Face

- See for bleeding from nose, lips, mouth, and ear.
- See for cerebrospinal fluid (CSF) leak from nose (CSF rhinorrhea) or ear (CSF otorrhea).
- Examine the wound/wounds for site, size, edge, and depth.
- See for ecchymosis and hematomas, for example, subconjunctival hemorrhage in fractures of orbital margin (Fig. 12.3), and ecchymosis over the mastoid process in a fracture of middle cranial fossa (Battle's sign).
- See for any asymmetry, displacements and deformities, for example, open bite deformity in Le Fort II and Le Fort III fractures, depressed bridge of nose and telecanthus in fractures of nasoethmoidal complex, and loss of prominence of cheek in fractures of zygoma.

Palpation of Face The palpation of the injured part is done in a systematic manner from above downwards starting from forehead, supraorbital margin, nasal bridge, infraorbital margin, cheek, and zygomatic bone. The mandible is then examined starting at condyles by inserting the index finger in the ears, and then following the posterior and lower border into the symphysis.

- **Dental occlusion**: The patient is asked to open and close the mouth to see the dental occlusion. Normally the teeth of both the jaws "fit" into each other even if the grinding surfaces are naturally irregular. If they do not "fit," fracture of the jaw involving the dentoalveolar border is most likely present.

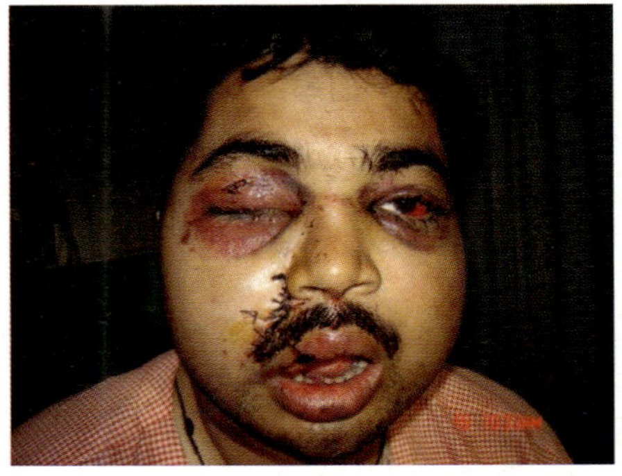

Figure 12.3 Faciomaxillary trauma with bilateral black eye and subconjunctival hemorrhage in left eye.

- **Gingivae**: A tear in the gingivae is a sign of fracture of jaw. It makes the fracture compound in the mouth.
- **Floor of mouth**: There may be hematoma in the floor of mouth which is a sign of fracture of lower jaw. It is called Coleman's sign.
- **Palpation of jaws**
  - The maxillary dental arch in the incisor region is grasped between the thumb, index finger, and middle finger of one hand and the forehead is stabilized with the other hand. Now gentle movements are made forwards and backwards and from side to side. Abnormal mobility is indicative of fracture.
  - The anterolateral surface of maxilla can be felt in the mouth above the maxillary teeth in labiogingival sulcus for any irregularity or crepitus. In zygomatic fracture the anterolateral wall above the upper molars may show irregularity.
  - The outer and inner surfaces of the mandible in the mouth are palpated for any irregularity or crepitus.
- **Palate**: The palate is inspected and palpated for any abnormality, for example, bruising and midpalatal split.

Examination of Cranial Nerves and Their Branches

- **Supraorbital nerve**: It may be injured in fractures of upper orbital margin. Hence, examine for anesthesia/paresthesia in its distribution.
- **Infraorbital nerve**: It may be injured in fractures of orbital floor. Hence, see for anesthesia/paresthesia in the cheek and upper lip.
- **Inferior dental nerve**: In fractures of body of mandible the lower lip may become numb due to injury to this nerve.
- **Facial nerve**: Facial cuts and lacerations and penetrating wounds of the parotid region may injure the facial nerve or its branches for which the patient must be examined.

Eyes If the eyes can be opened, they are examined for the level of globe, vision, movements, and diplopia. The pupils are also examined.

Nose The nose should be examined with a speculum and good light for epistaxis, CSF leak, tip and dorsal contour changes, intranasal laceration, septum deviation, and hematomas.

Classification of maxillofacial fractures

- **Depending on the bones involved**:
  - Fractures of upper third involving frontal bone and upper border of orbit
  - Fractures of middle third comprising maxilla, zygoma, nose, and orbit
  - Fractures of lower third comprising mandible
- **Depending on the involvement of dental occlusion**:
  - Fractures that do not involve dental occlusion, that is, fracture of zygoma, nose, and frontal bone
  - Fractures that involve the dental occlusion, that is, fracture of mandible and maxilla

Fractures of upper third of the face

These fractures are usually depressed fractures of the frontal bone involving either the anterior wall or both the walls of the frontal sinus. They usually result from direct impact leading to a depressed fracture involving the outer wall of the sinus. If the posterior wall of the sinus is fractured, the patient should be examined by a neurosurgeon also.

Fractures of middle third of the face

Le Fort Fractures

Rene Le Fort (1911) created fractures of middle third of the face in cadavers, employing different degrees of force, and classified the fractures thus produced into three groups (Fig. 12.4).

Le Fort I Fracture (Table 12.1) The fracture line runs horizontally above the alveolus and palate through the points of weakness from the pyriform

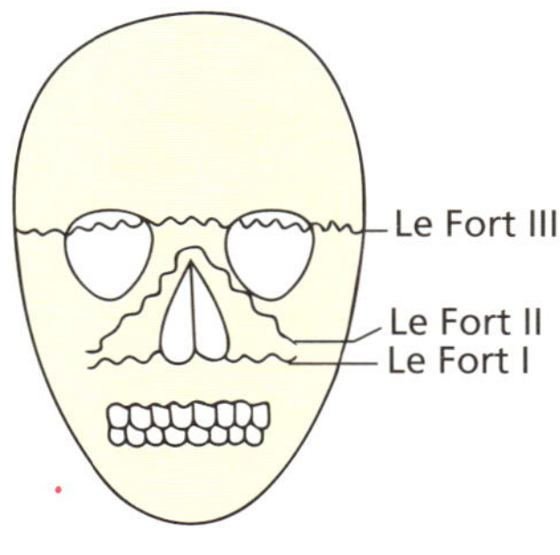

Figure 12.4 Le Fort fractures of midface.

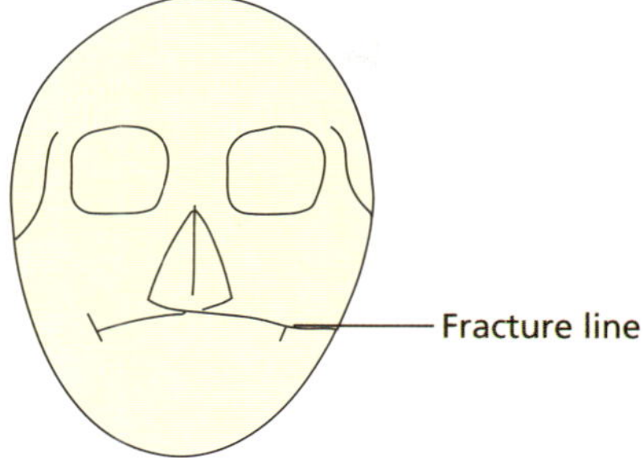

Figure 12.5 Le Fort I fracture of middle face.

Table 12.1 Features of Le Fort I fracture of middle third of face

Feature	Description
Shape	Horizontal (Fig. 12.5)
Level	Low level
Fracture line	Runs horizontally just above the floor of nasal cavity and separates alveolus and palate, lower third of nasal septum, and lower third of pterygoid plates from facial skeleton above
Essential anatomy	Most of the bones of middle third remain attached with skull
Symptoms and signs	• Slight swelling and edema of lower part of face including upper lip swelling • Ecchymosis of upper labial and buccal vestibule, laceration may be seen • Nasal bleeding • Mobile dentoalveolar portion of the maxilla (floating maxilla) • Occlusal derangement, posterior gagging of occlusion • Palatal ecchymosis (Guerin's sign)

aperture of the nose through the lateral and medial walls of maxillary antrum, running posteriorly to include the lower part of pterygoid plates.

Le Fort II Fracture or Subzygomatic Fracture (Table 12.2) The fracture line runs through the bridge of the nose and ethmoids continuing into

Table 12.2 Features of Le Fort II fracture of middle third of face

Feature	Description
Shape	Pyramidal (Fig. 12.6)
Level	Midlevel
Fracture line	Runs through the bridge of nose and ethmoids into the orbits on either side to the medial part of infraorbital rim and often through infraorbital foramen affecting the orbital floor. It then goes back through the lateral wall of maxillary antrum at a higher level into the pterygoid plates
Essential anatomy	Zygoma and lateral wall of orbit remain attached with skull
Symptoms and signs	• Gross edema of middle third of face (ballooning or moon face) • Circumorbital edema and ecchymosis (black eye/raccoon eye) • Subconjunctival hemorrhage confined to medial half of eye • Depressed nasal bridge (flat face), nasal disfigurement • Shortening of face if the fracture is impacted into cranial base with anterior open bite • Lengthening of face if there is downward and backward displacement of lower fragment with posterior gagging of occlusion and anterior open bite (dish-face deformity) • Nasal bleeding, may be CSF rhinorrhea • Tenderness and step deformity of infraorbital margin • Difficulty in mastication and speech • Anesthesia/paresthesia of cheek may be present

CSF, cerebrospinal fluid.

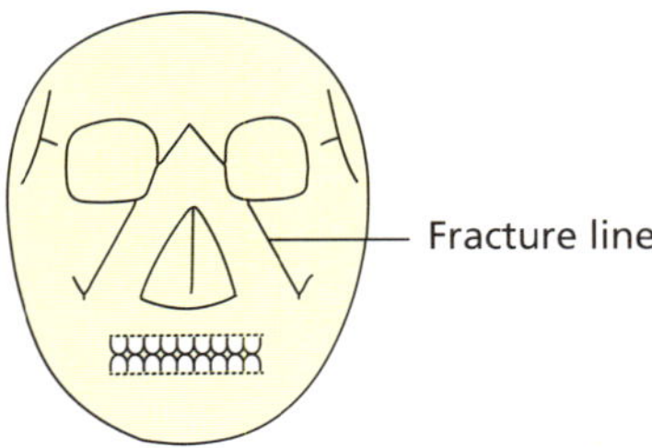

Figure 12.6 Le Fort II fracture of middle face.

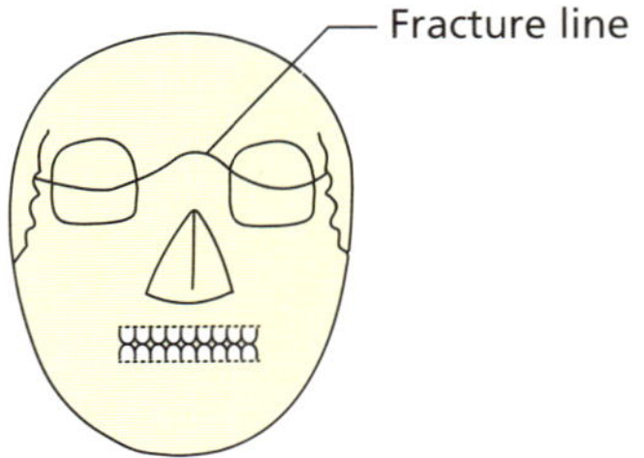

Figure 12.7 Le Fort III fracture of middle face.

the orbit to the medial part of infraorbital rim and often through the infraorbital foramen affecting the orbital floor. It then goes back through the lateral wall of maxillary antrum at a higher level than the Le Fort I, and into pterygoid plates.

Le Fort III Fracture or Craniofacial Dysjunction/Suprazygomatic Fracture (Table 12.3) The fracture line separates the middle third facial skeleton from the base of skull and runs through the nasal bridge, septum, and ethmoids and irregularly through the bones of orbit to the frontozygomatic suture, lateral wall of maxillary antrum, and the pterygoid plates at a higher level.

In Le Fort II and III fractures the cribriform plate of the frontal bone may be fractured leading to dural tear and CSF rhinorrhea. Another important feature of Le Fort fractures is midpalatal split. A natural line of weakness exists at the sutural interface between the two palatine bones of maxilla. It may split following a high-level impact.

Zygomatic Complex Fractures

They are the most common fractures after the fractures of nasal bones. Zygomatic complex fractures are caused by direct trauma. The fracture occurs through the points of weakness, that is, infraorbital margin, frontozygomatic suture, zygomatic arch, and the anterolateral wall of antrum. After fracture the bone may be displaced usually in the posterior direction which can be assessed by occipitomental radiography (Figs 12.8 and 12.9). The clinical features of zygomatic complex fractures are given in Box 12.3.

Blowout Fractures of Orbit

- A direct blow on the globe of eye may push it back fracturing weaker plates of bone, without necessarily fracturing the bones of orbital rim.
- The weakest plate of bone is orbital floor, the fracture of which results in herniation of orbital

Table 12.3 Features of Le Fort III fracture of middle third of face

Feature	Description
Shape	Horizontal or transverse (Fig. 12.7)
Level	High level
Fracture line	Fracture line runs parallel to the skull base, and passes through the nasal bone, lacrimal bones, ethmoids, optic foramina, inferior orbital fissures, pterygomaxillary fissure, and lateral orbital walls with frontozygomatic suture with zygomatic arch
Essential anatomy	Total separation of middle third bones from base of skull (craniofacial dysjunction)
Symptoms and signs	• Nasal bleeding, CSF rhinorrhea • Airway obstruction • Swelling of middle face (ballooning) • Circumorbital ecchymosis with edema (raccoon eye) • Subconjunctival hemorrhage with posterior limit not seen • Lengthening of middle face with lowering of ocular level • Enophthalmos, may be diplopia • Monoblock abnormal mobility of facial bones

CSF, cerebrospinal fluid.

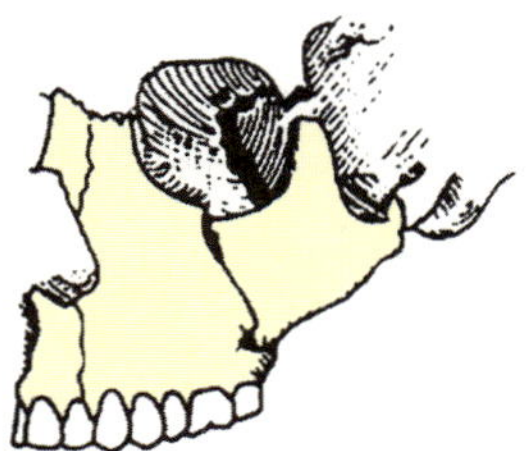

Figure 12.8 Fracture of left zygoma with downward and inward displacement.

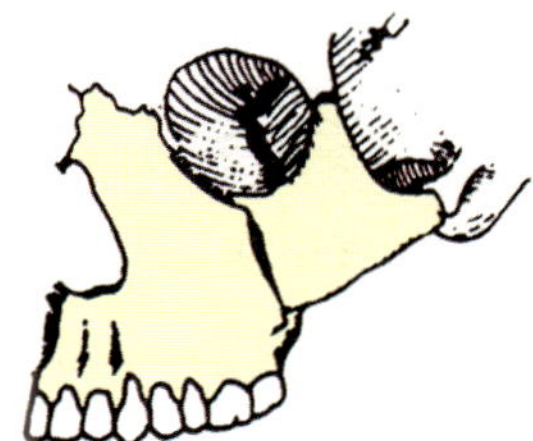

Figure 12.9 Fracture of left zygoma with backward and inward displacement.

> **Box 12.3 Clinical features of zygomatic complex fractures**
>
> - Flattening of prominence of cheek
> - Ecchymosis
> - Periorbital swelling and subconjunctival hemorrhage
> - Epistaxis
> - Numbness and paresthesia in the distribution of infraorbital nerve
> - Diplopia, enophthalmos, lowering of level of pupil
> - Tenderness and step deformity at frontozygomatic and infraorbital margins
> - Trismus and limitation of mandibular movement

contents down into the maxillary antrum. It results in dysfunction of eye muscles, especially inferior oblique and inferior rectus leading to failure of the eyeball to rotate upwards.

- When the periorbital swelling subsides, enophthalmos and diplopia become manifest.
- Classical finding of herniation of the orbital contents into the maxillary antrum can be seen in sagittal CT (Fig. 12.10) or in a radiograph occipitomental view.

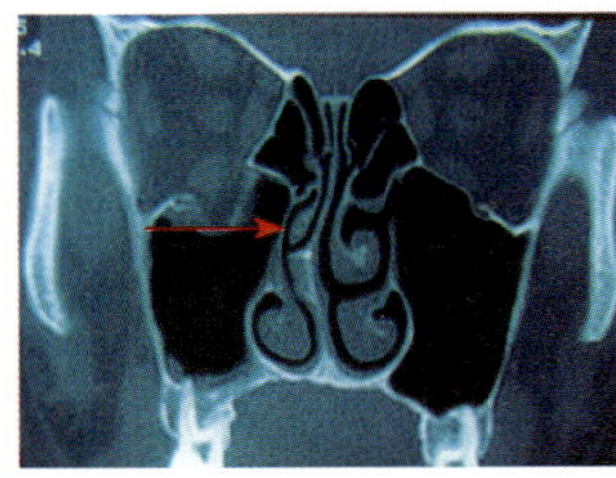

Figure 12.10 Sagittal CT scan showing fracture of right orbital floor with herniation of orbital contents into maxillary antrum. (Courtesy: Professor Surajit Bhattacharya)

Nasoethmoidal Complex Fractures

These fractures can be of two types:

1. Isolated nasal bone fracture with or without fracture of septum (Fig. 12.11) (nasal bone fractures are the most common fracture of the face)
2. Comminuted fractures involving nasal bones, frontal process, and the anterior wall of frontal sinus

These fractures can cause nasal bleeding, significant deformity, CSF rhinorrhea, traumatic telecanthus, subconjunctival bleeding, and crepitus over nasal bridge.

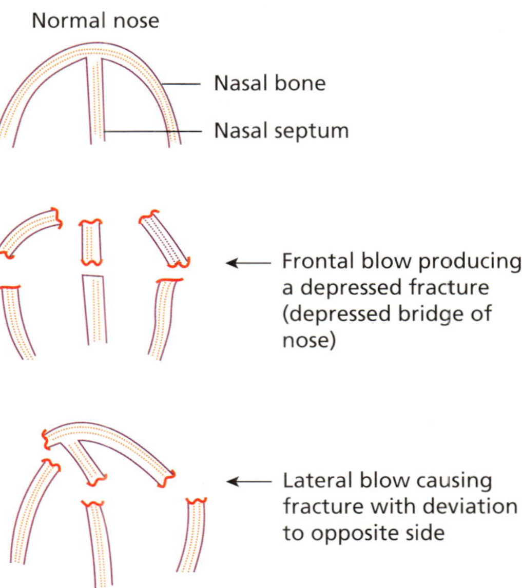

Figure 12.11 Fractures of nasal bones.

Fractures of lower third of the face

The fractures of mandible are included in this category. These fractures are quite common.

Classification of Mandibular Fractures Based on Site

- Common fractures (Fig. 12.12)
  - Condylar fracture (most common)
  - Angle of mandible through the last molar
  - Body of mandible in the region of canine
- Less common fractures
  - Fracture of coronoid
  - Fracture of ascending ramus
  - Symphyseal fracture
  - Dentoalveolar fracture

Out of these, condylar fracture, fracture of coronoid, and fracture of ascending ramus are usually simple fractures; rest are compound fractures in the mouth.

Etiology of Mandibular Fractures

Direct Injury The mandible may break at the point of impact (direct injury)

Indirect Injury The mandible may break at the point of weakness away from the site of impact due to transmission of force (indirect injury) as seen in a guardsman's fracture where a blow on the chin may cause a symphyseal or parasymphyseal fracture due to direct blow, and a unilateral or bilateral fracture of condylar neck due to transmitted force (indirect injury). Blows from below may thrust the mandible upwards fracturing the alveolus and teeth as they are pushed against maxillary teeth.

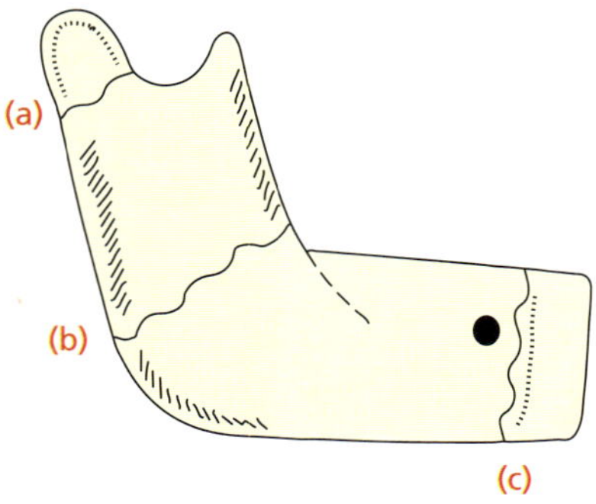

Figure 12.12 Common fractures of mandible: (a) condylar fracture, (b) angle of the mandible fracture, and (c) fracture of body of the mandible in the region of canine tooth.

Fracture of Condylar Neck

- It is the commonest fracture of the mandible as the neck of condyle is the weakest area. It is usually a simple fracture and may be unilateral or bilateral. The upper fragment may remain at its site or may be displaced.
- Clinical features: Following fracture there is local pain and may be bleeding from the ear, tenderness, and swelling. In unilateral fracture the jaw deviates to the affected side when the patient tries to open the mouth. In bilateral fracture there is anterior open bite.
- Cause of anterior open bite: The open bite occurs due to vertical pull of muscles of mastication, shortening the height of ramus. The posterior teeth come in contact earlier and the anterior teeth remain apart. Functionally and cosmetically, it is a very undesirable problem which is difficult or impossible to treat. Hence, it should be treated and corrected early at the time of injury.

Fracture of Angle of Mandible Through Last Molar

It follows direct trauma. It is characterized by local pain, tenderness, swelling, local ecchymosis in oral cavity, step deformity, and occlusal discrepancy.

Fracture of Body (Horizontal Ramus)

It is characterized by local tenderness and step deformity at the lower border of mandible at the site of fracture. The dental alignment is

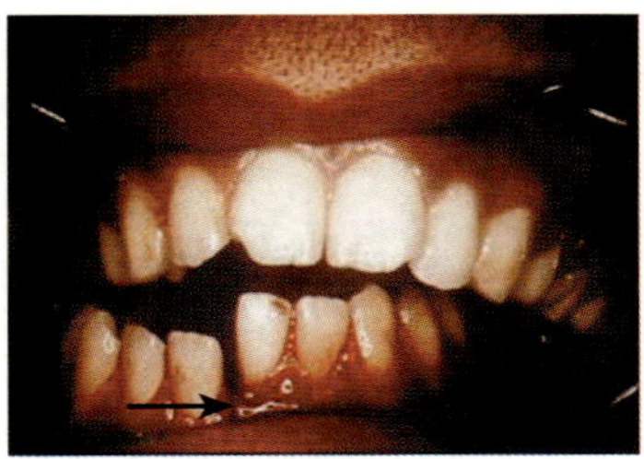

Figure 12.13 Complete fracture of lower jaw with superoinferior displacement between the right two incisors. (Courtesy: Professor Surajit Bhattacharya)

disturbed (Fig. 12.13) and there may be sublingual ecchymosis. The patient may not be able to close the mouth resulting in drooling of saliva.

Fracture at the Canine Region or Parasymphyseal Fractures

It is also called butterfly fracture as a butterfly-like segment of mandible is detached from the rest of mandible at both canine regions due to a direct blow on the chin from the front. This segment has insertion of lingual muscles at genial tubercles. Hence, the tongue may fall back to occlude the pharyngeal airway if the patient is kept in supine position.

Fracture of Ascending Ramus

It is characterized by local pain and tenderness, ecchymosis, and swelling.

Dentoalveolar Fracture

It is caused by direct trauma and characterized by local pain, mobile dentoalveolar segment, occlusal derangement, laceration of related gingiva and subluxation, avulsion, or horizontal/vertical split of tooth.

Symphyseal Fracture

It is characterized by inability to close the mouth, drooling of saliva, step deformity of lower border, sublingual ecchymosis, and discrepancy of occlusion.

Fracture of Edentulous Mandible

These fractures are seen in edentulous elderly people where the mandible is atrophic with thin atrophic periosteum and poor blood supply. Hence, there is considerable risk of ischemic necrosis of bone if open reduction is done.

Investigations in maxillofacial injuries

Laboratory Studies Hemoglobin, blood counts, blood sugar, urea, creatinine, serum calcium, and blood grouping are the usual investigations.

Radiography Properly done radiography diagnoses most of the fractures accurately. Boxes 12.4 and 12.5 enumerate the basic radiographs required for diagnosing the maxillofacial fractures. CT scan is a good investigation to see the details of fractures, especially the complex fractures of midface (Figs 12.14 and 12.15). Orthopantomography is the best investigation to see the lower jaw injuries and the injuries of both rows of the teeth (Fig. 12.16).

Box 12.4 Radiographs in maxillofacial fractures

Fractures of upper third	Fractures of middle third (Fig. 12.14)	Fractures of lower third (Figs 12.15 and 12.16)
• Lateral skull • Occipitofrontal radiographs	• Submentovertex view • Cranial posteroanterior view of skull • Lateral view of skull • PA view—Water's position • 15° and 30° occipitomental view	• Orthopantomogram (OPG) • PA view—Water's position • Right and left lateral oblique views • Towne's view for seeing the fractured condyles

Box 12.5 Radiographs for fracture of faciomaxillary bones

Injured bone	Radiographic views
Frontal bone	Lateral skull, occipitofrontal radiography
Maxilla	15° and 30° occipitomental view
Zygoma	15° and 30° occipitomental view, submentovertex view
Orbit	15° and 30° occipitomental view
Nasal bones	Lateral view of nasal bones, occipitofrontal view
Mandibular body and ramus	• Orthopantomogram • Lateral oblique • Lower occlusal • PA mandible
Mandibular condyles	• Orthopantomogram • PA mandible with mouth open • Toller transpharyngeal views

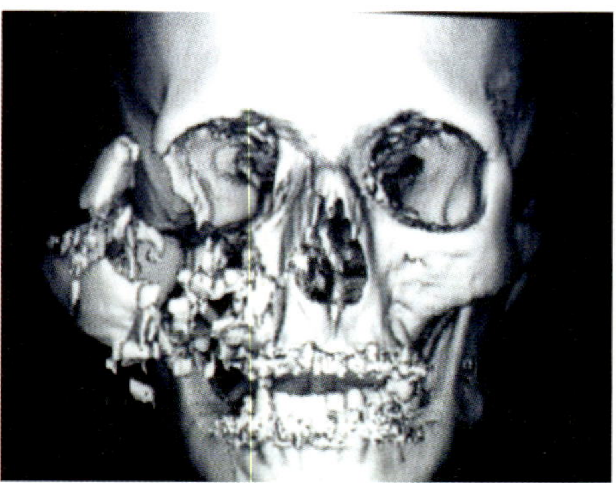

Figure 12.14 3D CT reconstruction of middle face showing extensive injury of right midface: maxilla, zygoma, nasal bone, nasal septum, and the alveolar borders. (Courtesy: Professor Surajit Bhattacharya)

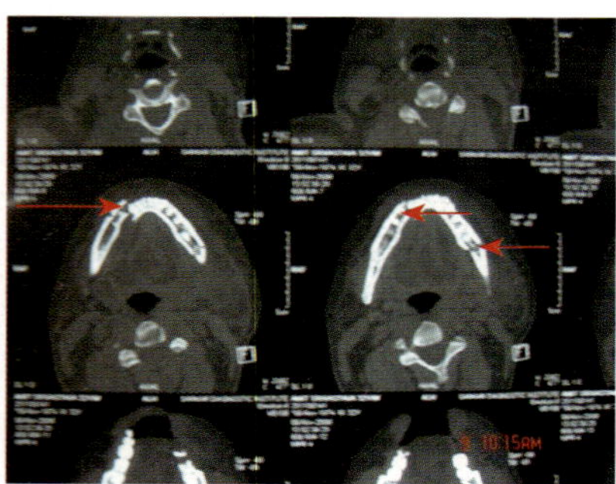

Figure 12.15 Axial CT scan of lower face showing fractures of mandible. (Courtesy: Professor Surajit Bhattacharya)

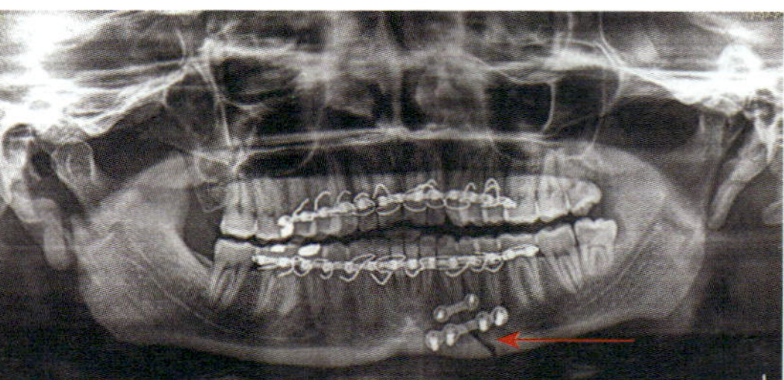

Figure 12.16 Orthopantomogram showing a treated case of fracture of mandible near symphysis with plates and screws. (Courtesy: Dr. S.S. Sarkar, Sarkar Diagnostics)

Treatment of maxillofacial fractures

The comprehensive management of maxillofacial injuries is given in Flowchart 12.1.

General Measures

Airway The airway must be kept clear and patent by the following measures:

- The oropharynx and trachea is cleared of blood clot, saliva, mucus, and foreign bodies by fingers, forceps, or suction (Fig. 12.17).
- The patient should be kept in semiprone position with head supported on one arm,

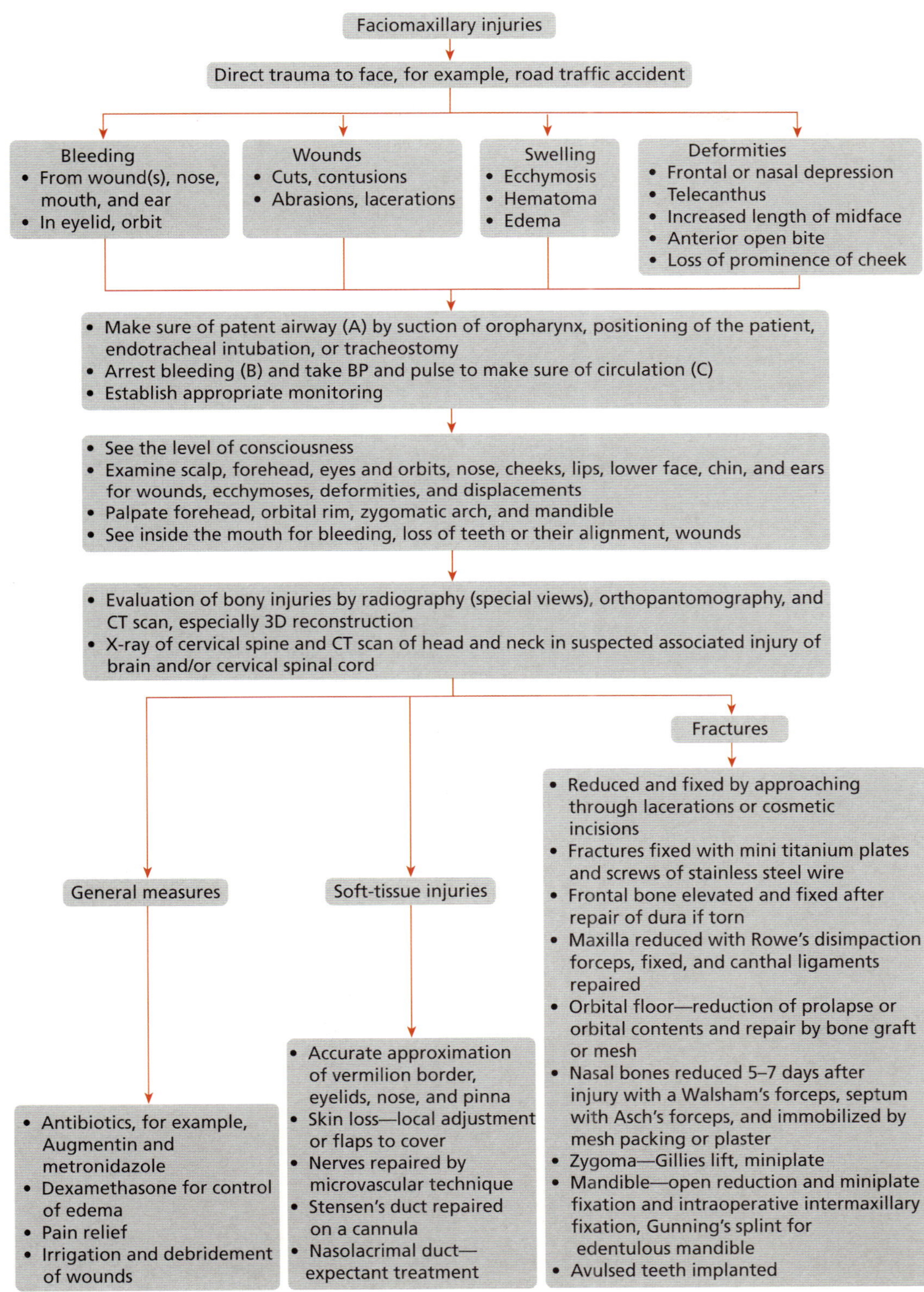

Flowchart 12.1 Management of maxillofacial injuries.

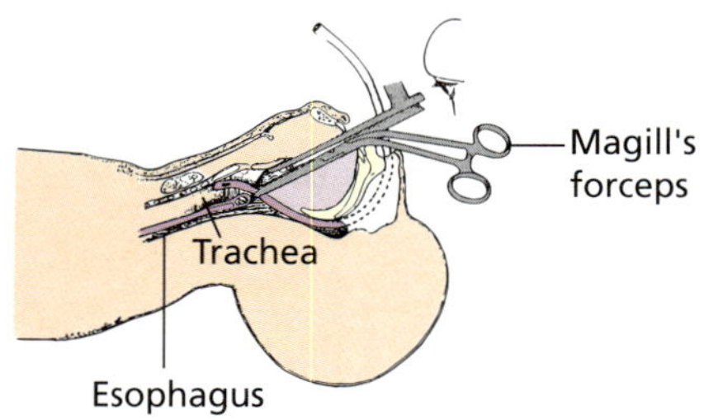

Figure 12.17 Method of guiding aspirating catheter into trachea under direct vision for removal of tracheal blood and mucus.

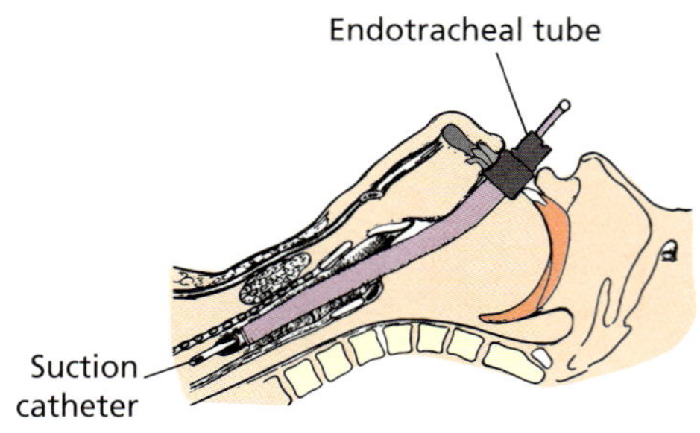

Figure 12.18 Method of removing mucus from the trachea through an endotracheal tube.

or prone with head down so that blood and secretions from the mouth come out. A protective collar is applied to the neck till an associated cervical spine injury is excluded by radiography.

- Endotracheal intubation or tracheostomy is often required in severe faciomaxillary injury for giving oxygen and keeping the airway clear of secretions by suction (Figs 12.18 and 12.19).
- In fractured and displaced maxilla the obstructed nasopharynx can be opened by putting index and middle fingers behind the soft palate and thumb on the upper incisor region and pulling it anteriorly and downwards. It is followed by passing one or two nasopharyngeal tubes.

Arrest of Bleeding Bleeding must be controlled quickly initially by digital compression or compression dressing as applicable. Subsequently injured vessels should be clamped and ligated or repaired. Soft-tissue wounds should be repaired. Deep wounds may be packed till definitive measures can be taken. Nasal bleeding is arrested by packing with ribbon gauze soaked in 1:1000 adrenaline.

Other Measures Most of the maxillofacial fractures are compound. Hence, antibiotic treatment is always indicated. The patient may be given penicillin, amoxicillin, cephalosporins, and gentamicin singly or in combination. Metronidazole may also be given to look after the anaerobes. Dexamethasone may be given to reduce traumatic edema.

Treatment of Soft-Tissue Injury

Skin Wounds The facial soft tissues have very good blood supply. Hence, they heal quickly.

- Contusions and abrasions are painted with Betadine.
- All open wounds are cleaned, explored, debrided, and suture closed. The edges of the wound should be accurately approximated, especially in areas of cosmetic importance, for

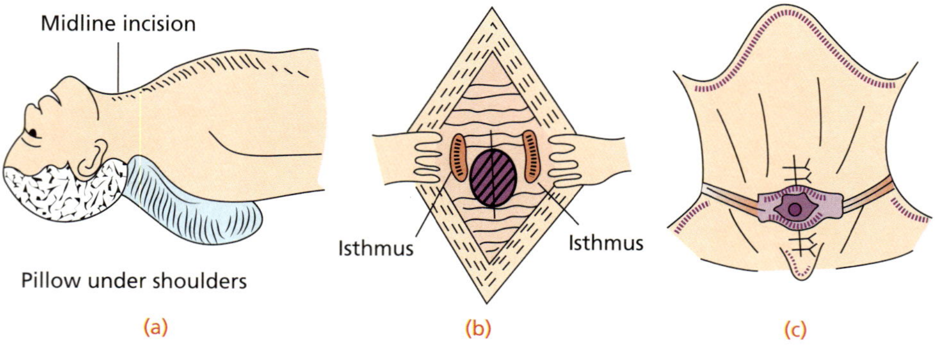

Figure 12.19 Essential steps of tracheostomy: (a) Position of the patient, (b) making a hole through third and forth rings of trachea, and (c) completed tracheostomy with tube tied in position.

example, vermilion border, eyelids, nose, and pinna.
- The muscles and subcutaneous tissues are stitched by absorbable fine sutures (Vicryl) and the skin is then closed by fine (5/0 or 6/0) monofilament unabsorbable sutures, for example, nylon or polypropylene.

Facial Nerve Injury The facial nerve is repaired using an operating microscope and fine nylon sutures.

Parotid Duct Facial wounds in the region of Stensen's duct may injure it. The severed ends are identified and repaired on a fine cannula which is passed from the ductal orifice in the oral cavity into the divided ends. The cannula is kept in position for a week.

Nasolacrimal Duct The nasolacrimal duct may be severed in the injuries of maxilla, but usually nothing can be done to repair it.

Treatment of Fractures

The two essential points in fracture management are reduction of fracture ends in correct position and retaining them in that position till healing occurs which is a natural process.

Treatment of upper third fractures

Incision and Exposure The fracture site may be approached through the laceration but for better and wider exposure, a bicoronal scalp flap has to be raised.

Fractures of Anterior Wall of Frontal Sinus The fractures of the anterior wall are treated by reduction and fixation using small titanium plates and screws. If there is bone tissue deficiency, it should be made good by bone grafting to avoid forehead depression.

Fracture of Posterior Wall of Frontal Sinus If the posterior wall of the frontal sinus is fractured, neurosurgical collaboration is required.

Treatment of middle third fractures

Four types of fractures are included under this group. Their treatment is described in the next subsections.

Maxillary fractures

The maxillary fractures are treated by open reduction and internal fixation.

Incision and Exposure The upper part of maxilla is approached by incisions in the lower eyelid (blepharoplasty incision), lower conjunctival sac, or infraorbital region to treat fractures of infraorbital rim, fractures of orbital floor, and orbital blowout fractures. The lower maxilla is approached through a gingival sulcus incision above the teeth extending up to the second molar.

Reduction of Maxilla The maxilla is reduced with Rowe's disimpaction forceps which holds the palate between the nasal and palatal mucosa to give a series of downward, forward, and sideway movements (Fig. 12.20).

Methods of Fixation
- **Direct fixation/internal fixation**: The fractures of lower maxilla are fixed by plates or wires. The dental arch is restored to normal. This can be checked by approximating the maxillary teeth with mandibular teeth. Dental arch bars or eyelet wires may have to be used. The plates used for fixation are made of stainless steel or titanium (more recent). Intermaxillary wiring is an old method of treatment of fractures of the jaws.
- **Indirect skeletal fixation/external fixation**: It is done using the pins, frames, and halos but they are rarely used now due to the advent of more sophisticated plating systems. In comminuted fractures when the restored maxilla remains unstable, external fixation is indicated. Here the mandible is fixed to the skull and the maxilla is "sandwiched" in between. The skull fixation is done with a halo frame or supraorbital pins and the mandible is fixed by pins inserted in its body on each side.

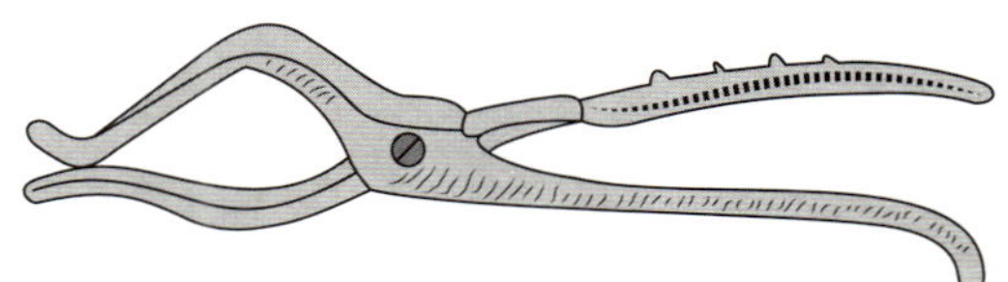

Figure 12.20 Rowe's maxillary disimpaction forceps.

Table 12.4 Management of maxillary fractures

Surgical technique	Description	
Incision and exposure	• Blepharoplasty incision • Subconjunctival incision • Infraorbital incision • Gingival sulcus incision	
Reduction of maxilla	Rowe's maxillary disimpaction forceps (downward, forward, and sideway movements)	
Fixation	Direct skeletal fixation	• Intermaxillary wiring (oldest method) • Eyelet wiring • Dental arch bars • Stainless steel plates and screws • Titanium plates and screws
	Indirect skeletal fixation (rarely used)	• Pins, for example, supraorbital pins • Halos and frames

Now all the pins are joined together by connecting bars secured by universal joints.

A brief outline of treatment of fractures of maxilla is described in Table 12.4.

Zygomatic complex fractures

- **Gillies temporal approach**: It is used to reduce most of the zygomatic fractures.
- **Incision**: A 1.5-cm-long incision is given in the hairline in the temporal fossa at 45° to vertical. It is deepened down to prepare a channel through the temporal fossa down to the body of zygoma and its arch.
- **Reduction**: A Bristow's or Rowe's zygoma elevator is inserted below the zygomatic body or arch depending on the site of fracture and the fracture is reduced by applying force in the direction opposite to the fracture displacement (Figs 12.21 and 12.22). The accuracy of reduction is confirmed by palpating the bony prominences of the zygomatic arch, and the lateral and inferior orbital margin.
- **Fixation**: The unstable fractures of zygoma are treated by open reduction and fixation by interosseous wires or titanium plates and screws.

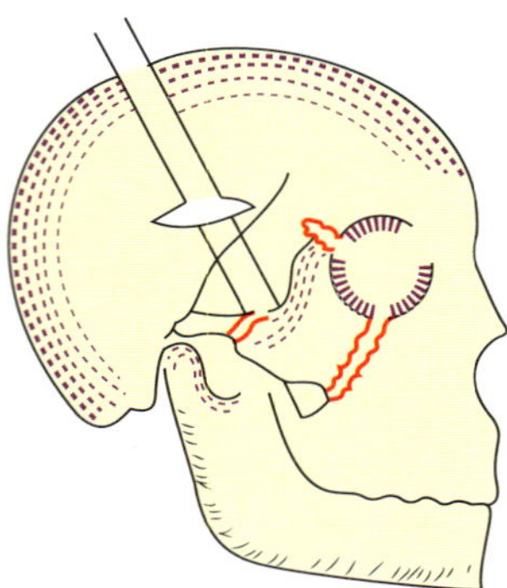

Figure 12.21 Technique of elevation of fractured zygoma by Bristow's elevator.

Blowout fractures of the orbit

- Involvement of orbital floor in the fracture is tested by forced duction test. If the floor seems to be involved, it should be explored and treated.
- They are treated by repair of orbital floor and correction of downward displacement of orbital contents.
- Incision: The orbital floor is explored through a blepharoplasty incision in the lower eyelid or through the inferior fornix.
- Fixation: The repair is done by bone grafts, titanium mesh, or alloplastic materials fixed in place by wires, screws, or plates (Fig. 12.23). If the defect is very large and the repair is unstable, packing of antrum via a Caldwell-Luc approach is indicated. The packing is done from above downwards by ribbon gauze soaked in Whitehead's varnish. Overpacking is avoided. The pack is removed after 3 weeks.

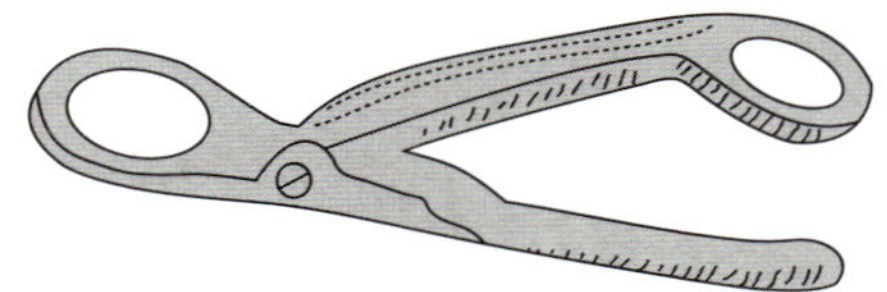

Figure 12.22 Rowe's zygoma elevator.

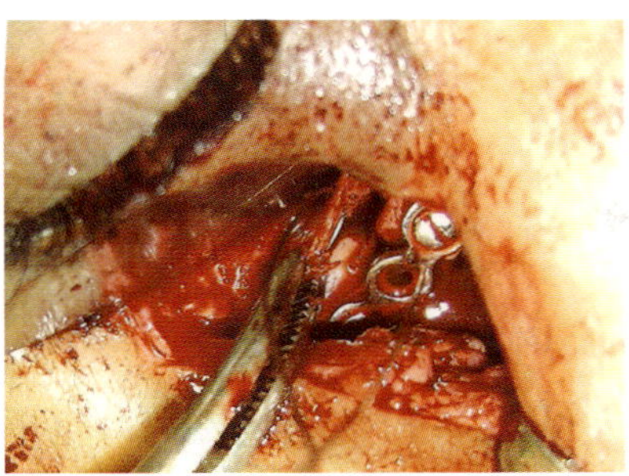

Figure 12.23 Fracture of lower orbital margin and floor is being treated with nails and plate, Prolene mesh, and wiring. (Courtesy: Professor Surajit Bhattacharya)

Nasoethmoidal complex fracture

- **Timing**: The fracture of nasal bones is reduced as soon as the edema subsides, but it should be done within a week of injury as subsequently it becomes difficult or impossible to reduce.
- **Reduction**
  - *Walsham's forceps*: The nasal bones are repositioned with the help of a Walsham's forceps, the external blade of which is covered with rubber tubing to avoid damage to nasal skin. The bones are pushed laterally to disimpact and then medially to reposition them correctly.
  - *Asch's forceps*: The nasal septum is grasped with Asch's forceps and manipulated to make it straight. It is then repositioned in the groove of nasal crest and vomer. If it cannot be adequately reduced, it will require septoplasty later on.
- **Fixation**: The nasoethmoidal fractures are treated by open reduction and fixation. The disrupted medial canthal attachments may require repair to correct telecanthus. It is followed by supporting the nasal bones by a pack behind the nasal bridge which is removed after 2–3 days. A protective nasal plaster may be applied for 5–7 days.
- Septal hematoma should be surgically evacuated. Septal perforation may be closed by insertion of a silastic biflanged prosthesis.

Lower third or mandibular fractures

The treatment of choice for most of the mandibular fractures is open reduction and fixation by plating system of stainless steel or titanium.

Treatment of Fractures of Dentate Mandible

- The fracture site is explored by intraoral or extraoral approach.
- To achieve a correct dental occlusion, intraoperative intermaxillary fixation (IMF) utilizing eyelet wires is advisable (Figs 12.24–12.26) which is removed after the rigid plate fixation is done.
- Sometimes in spite of rigid fixation with titanium miniplates, IMF is required in the postoperative phase. In such a case, the IMF done during operation is removed in the recovery room when the patient is recovering from anesthesia to avoid the risk of airway obstruction. IMF is done again as soon as the patient has fully recovered from anesthesia.

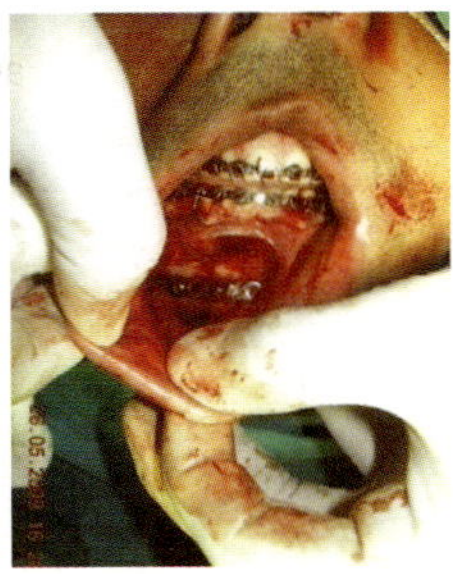

Figure 12.24 Fracture of mandible treated with open reduction and fixation with plate and screws by intraoral approach and interdental wiring. (Courtesy: Dr. R.K. Mishra, Sushrut Institute of Plastic Surgery Hospital, Lucknow)

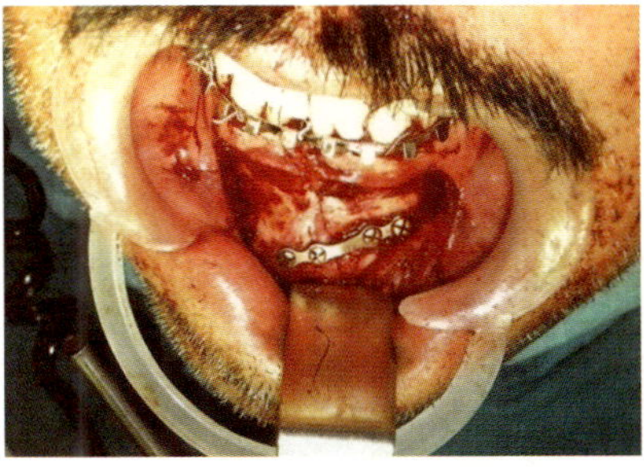

Figure 12.25 Fracture of symphysis menti of mandible treated with open reduction and internal fixation using plate and screws with interdental wiring. (Courtesy: Dr. R.K. Mishra, Sushrut Institute of Plastic Surgery Hospital, Lucknow)

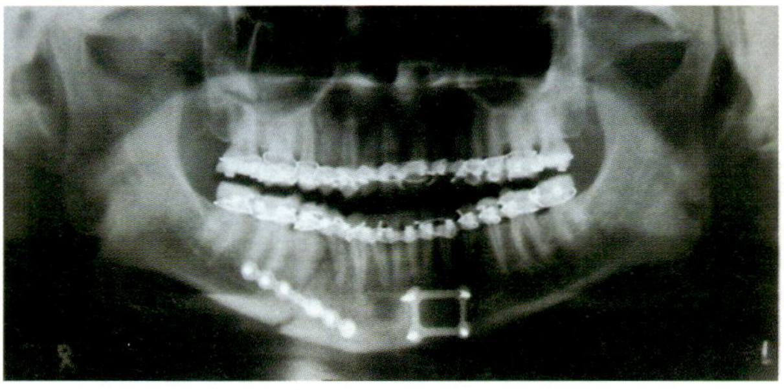

Figure 12.26 Orthopantomogram showing treatment of fracture of mandible by open reduction and fixation with plates and screws with interdental wiring. (Courtesy: Professor Divya Mehrotra)

- The results of treatment are usually good; rarely malunion may occur due to displacement of fractures (Fig. 12.27).

Treatment of Condylar Fractures

- **No treatment**: A condylar fracture with minimal displacement and minimal disturbance of occlusion usually requires no active treatment.
- **Open reduction and fixation**: A condylar fracture if displaced or bilateral with considerable occlusal disturbance is treated by open reduction and fixation with titanium plates to prevent an anterior open bite within 7–10 days of injury (Fig. 12.28).

Treatment of Fracture of Edentulous Mandible

- **Open reduction and fixation**: These fractures can be treated by open reduction and fixation provided minimal periosteal mobilization is done as it may compromise mandibular blood supply.
- **Gunning's splints**: When it is certain that the blood supply is likely to be seriously impaired by open reduction, Gunning's splints may be used for fixation. They consist of arc-like grooved upper and lower dentures having hooks in place of teeth. Each splint is wired to one jaw, the lower one to mandible by circummandibular wires and the other to maxilla to a stable point of middle third. The fracture is reduced and the splints are fixed to jaws by wires and the splints are tied to each other on the hooks.

Treatment of Avulsed Tooth

- If the tooth is preserved in saliva or milk, it can be implanted up to 6 hours of injury.

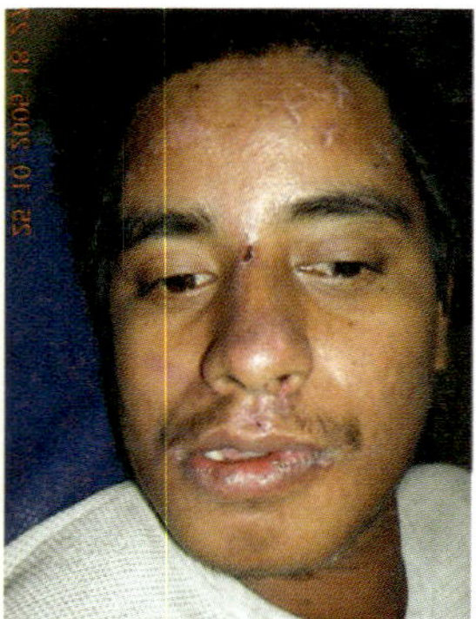

Figure 12.27 Treated case of fracture of mandible with the butterfly segment which was displaced down. (Courtesy: Dr. R.K. Mishra, Sushrut Institute of Plastic Surgery Hospital, Lucknow)

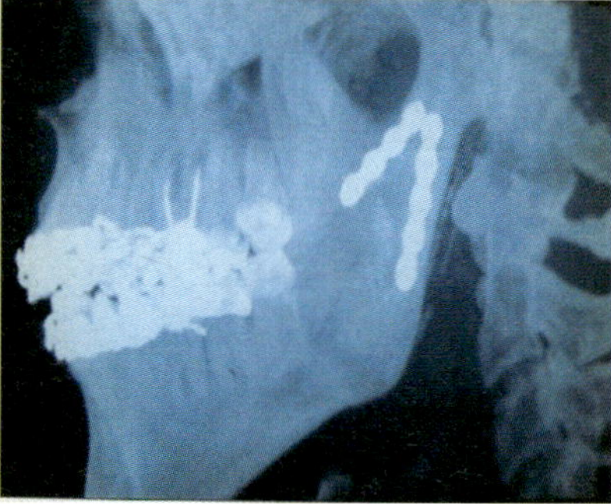

Figure 12.28 Left lateral view of lower facial skeleton showing fracture of condyle of mandible treated by open reduction and fixation with plates and screws. (Courtesy: Professor Divya Mehrotra)

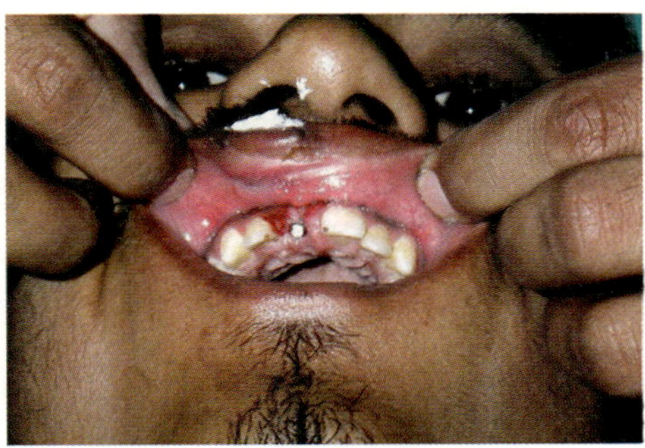

Figure 12.29 Titanium dental implant in situ for replacing a lost tooth. (Courtesy: Professor Divya Mehrotra)

- If the tooth is lost, titanium dental implantation can be done after the socket heals (Fig. 12.29).

Treatment of Less Common Fractures Fracture of coronoid process requires immobilization for 12 weeks if there is not much displacement. Significant displacement is treated by operative reduction and miniplate fixation.

Ascending ramus is well padded by muscles; hence, its fracture requires 6- to 8-week rest till it becomes painless.

Symphyseal fractures require open reduction and fixation. Dentoalveolar fracture is treated by interdental wiring.

Complications of maxillofacial injuries

The classification of maxillofacial fractures can be classified as immediate and delayed complications.

Immediate Complications

- Hemorrhage
- Airway obstruction
- Wound infection including traumatic osteomyelitis of the bones injured

Delayed Complications

- Malunion of fractured bones
- Nonunion (common causes of nonunion include loose or broken tooth coming in fracture line, infection, inadequate immobilization, and systemic factors)
- Deformities
  - Forehead depression in frontal fractures
  - Depressed or crooked nose in fracture of nasal bones
  - Flattening of midface, dish-face deformity, anterior open bite with gagging of molars, telecanthus, strabismus (squint), and enophthalmos in fractures of midface
  - Asymmetry of face and anterior open bite with gagging of molars in bilateral condylar fractures
  - Occlusal derangement
  - Ankylosis of temporomandibular joint due to intracapsular fracture, hemarthrosis, prolonged immobilization, and contracture of soft tissue around the joint
- Neurological deficits
  - Supraorbital and supratrochlear nerve injury: Anesthesia of skin of forehead
  - Olfactory nerve injury in fractures of cribriform plate: Anosmia
  - Infraorbital nerve injury: Anesthesia of lower eyelid, lateral part of nostril, upper lip, and anterior maxillary teeth
  - Superior orbital fissure syndrome in fractures of zygomatic complex leading to injury of oculomotor, trochlear, and abducent nerves resulting in ptosis, proptosis, paralysis of extrinsic eye muscles (ophthalmoplegia), and a fixed dilated pupil (mydriasis)
- Nasal obstruction due to nasal depression and deviation of nasal septum
- Epiphora (overflow of tears) due to nasolacrimal duct injury in fractures of midface
- Double vision in fractures of orbit

KEY POINTS

- Faciomaxillary injuries are as common as head injuries and include soft-tissue injuries of facial skin, facial nerve, Stensen's duct, and faciomaxillary skeleton.
- Bleeding and respiratory obstruction are two serious effects of these injuries that require urgent attention.
- Faciomaxillary skeleton is divided into upper, middle, and lower thirds—the upper constituted by frontal bone, middle by two maxillae and zygomatic bones articulating with many small bones, and lower by mandible or lower jaw.
- Fractures of the upper third are usually depressed fractures of the frontal bone involving either the anterior wall or both the walls of the frontal sinus. The first one is treated by open reduction and second one requires neurosurgical help.
- Fractures of middle third are classified as Le Fort fractures: The fracture line of Le Fort I runs horizontally just above the floor of nasal cavity; of Le Fort II through the bridge of nose and ethmoids into the orbits on either side to medial part of orbital rim and often through infraorbital foramen affecting orbital floor; and of Le Fort III runs parallel to the skull base and passes through nasal bones to lateral orbital walls with frontozygomatic suture with zygomatic arch.
- Zygomatic complex fractures are characterized by flattening of the prominence of the cheek, swelling, and subconjunctival hemorrhage.
- Blowout fractures of the orbit occur due to a direct blow on the globe of eye which may push it back fracturing weaker plate of bone, that is, orbital floor, resulting in herniation of orbital contents down into the maxillary antrum.
- Nasoethmoid complex fractures occur as isolated nasal bone fractures with or without fracture of septum (most common fracture of face) or as comminuted fractures involving nasal bones, frontal process, and the anterior wall of frontal sinus.
- Fractures of the lower third (mandible) involve neck of condyle (most common), angle, ramus, body, symphysis, and dentoalveolar segment.
- X-rays are used for diagnosis. Occipitomental view is useful to diagnose midface fracture. For mandibular fractures orthopantomogram is the radiograph of choice. CT scans are the most effective tool as they can assess fracture and its displacement three-dimensionally.
- The maxilla is reduced with Rowe's disimpaction forceps. Direct fixation is done through arch bars and eyelet wires with titanium plates and screws across the fracture site. Indirect skeletal fixation is done by "sandwiching" the maxilla between mandible and the skull using pins, and a halo frame.
- Gillies temporal approach is used for reducing fractures of the zygoma and zygomatic arch using Bristow's or Rowe's zygoma elevator.
- The orbital floor fracture is treated with bone grafts, titanium mesh, or alloplastic materials fixed in place by wires, screws, or plates.
- Nasal bone fractures must be treated within a week. They are reduced using Walsham's forceps. The nasal septum is reduced using Asch's forceps.
- Septal hematoma should be surgically evacuated. Septal perforation may be closed by insertion of a silastic biflanged prosthesis.
- In unilateral condylar fracture, the jaw deviates to the affected side when the patient tries to open the mouth. In bilateral condylar fracture, there is anterior open bite.
- Fractures of the body of mandible present with loss of dental alignment, local tenderness at the fracture site associated with step deformity, and sublingual ecchymosis.
- Fracture of the parasymphysis at both canine regions results in a butterfly fracture. This fracture can prove fatal as the tongue may fall back to occlude the pharyngeal airway if the patient is kept in supine position.
- A condylar fracture with minimal displacement requires no active treatment. But if displaced with considerable occlusal disturbance, it is treated by open reduction.
- Treatment of dentate mandibular fractures requires open reduction and internal fixation using miniplates and screws. Gunning's splints are used to treat edentulous mandible fractures because periosteal stripping in open reduction can compromise vascular supply.
- An avulsed tooth, if preserved in saliva or milk, can be reimplanted up to 6 hours after injury. If the tooth is lost, titanium dental implants are the choice of treatment.

SELF-ASSESSMENT

Long answer questions

1. Describe the etiology, clinical features, and treatment of fractures of mandible.
2. What are the types of fractures of maxilla? Discuss their management.

Short answer questions

1. Le Fort fracture II
2. Fracture of zygoma
3. Fracture of nasal bones
4. Fracture of mandibular condyle
5. Anterior open bite
6. Fracture of edentulous mandible
7. Gunning's splints

Multiple choice questions

1. All of the following statements are true about frontal bone, except
   (a) It is a bone of forehead
   (b) It is a single bone not paired like parietal or temporal bones
   (c) It is a solid bone
   (d) It fractures following direct impact resulting usually in a depressed fracture
2. All of the following statements are true about the frontal bone fracture, except
   (a) It usually fractures following a direct impact
   (b) Both the tables of bone are always fractured
   (c) It is treated by open reduction
   (d) For treating the fracture of inner table, the help of a neurosurgeon is required
3. All of the following statements are true about maxillofacial skeleton, except
   (a) The upper third is constituted by frontal bone
   (b) The middle third is constituted by two maxillae
   (c) The middle third is constituted by two maxillae and two zygomatic bones articulating with nasal bones, lacrimal bones, nasal septum, vomer, ethmoid, and pterygoid plates
   (d) The lower third is made up of mandible
4. Epistaxis is defined as
   (a) Bleeding from the ear
   (b) Bleeding from the nose
   (c) Bleeding from the eye
   (d) Bleeding from the mouth
5. Epistaxis usually occurs or can occur in all of the following fractures, except
   (a) Fracture of frontal bone
   (b) Fracture of maxilla
   (c) Fracture of nasal bones
   (d) Fracture of horizontal ramus of mandible
6. Match the injuries with nerve injuries

(a) Supraorbital nerve	(1) Wounds of parotid region
(b) Infraorbital nerve	(2) Fracture of upper orbital margin
(c) Facial nerve	(3) Fracture of horizontal ramus of mandible
(d) Inferior dental nerve	(4) Fracture of orbital floor

7. Le Fort I fracture is defined as
   (a) Fracture of upper orbital margin
   (b) Fracture of orbital floor
   (c) Horizontal fracture of maxillary alveolus and palate with fracture line running horizontally on either side from the pyriform aperture of nose
   (d) Fracture of horizontal ramus of mandible
8. All of the following are symptoms and signs of a fracture of zygomatic arch, except
   (a) Flattening of prominence of cheek
   (b) Numbness and paresthesia in infraorbital area
   (c) Normal eye and vision
   (d) Tenderness and step deformity at frontozygomatic and infraorbital margins
9. A fracture of zygoma is associated with all of the following clinical manifestations, except
   (a) Diplopia
   (b) Lowering of level of pupil
   (c) Subconjunctival hemorrhage
   (d) Proptosis
10. All of the following statements are true about CSF rhinorrhea, except
    (a) It is the leakage of CSF from the nose

(CONTD...)

SELF-ASSESSMENT *(...CONTD)*

(b) It is due to fracture of cribriform plate of frontal bone
(c) It is usually associated with normal sense of smell
(d) It may sometimes require duraplasty to control leakage

11. Which of the following is the first step in emergency management of faciomaxillary injuries?
(a) Arrest of bleeding
(b) To maintain a patent airway
(c) To give prophylactic antibiotics
(d) To relieve pain

Answers

1. (c) 2. (b) 3. (b) 4. (b) 5. (d) 6. (a)—(2), (b)—(4), (c)—(1), (d)—(3) 7. (c) 8. (c) 9. (d) 10. (c) 11. (b)

Hemorrhage and Blood Transfusion

13

Introduction

Hemorrhage or bleeding is a common effect or symptom of trauma or disease. Minor bleeding may not be significant but a major bleeding if not treated immediately may result in loss of life.

Etiology of hemorrhage

- Trauma
- Surgery
  - Intraoperative or primary
  - Postoperative—reactionary and secondary
- Spontaneous bleeding
  - Local causes
    - Infections and inflammations
      - Tuberculosis, for example, pulmonary tuberculosis
      - Others, for example, peptic ulcer, ulcerative colitis, reflux esophagitis
    - Tumors
      - Benign, for example, nasopharyngeal fibroma, papilloma of urinary bladder, rectal polyp
      - Malignant, for example, carcinoma of tongue, larynx, lung, kidney, and urinary bladder
    - Mechanical disorders, for example, varicose veins, hemorrhoids, esophageal varices, arteriovenous malformation, arterial aneurysm
  - General causes
    - Defect of blood vessels, for example, vascular purpura, telangiectasia, vasculitis
    - Disorders of platelets (bleeding time is elevated), for example, reduced number of platelets, abnormal platelet function
    - Deficiency of coagulation factors (coagulation time is elevated), for example, congenital coagulation disorders (hemophilia, Christmas disease), acquired coagulation disorders (hypovitaminosis K, anticoagulant drugs)

Trauma is the commonest cause of bleeding.

Table 13.1 Differences between arterial, venous, and capillary bleeding

Features	Arterial bleeding	Venous bleeding	Capillary bleeding
Color	Bright red	Dark red and the color darkens further due to oxygen desaturation when the blood loss is severe. Exception is pulmonary vein where the color is bright red due to presence of oxygenated blood	Bright red
Flow	Spurts as a jet with a pulse wave	Steady flow	Ooze or like "sweating" from many points
Complications	• Significant blood loss in a short time • Early hemorrhagic shock	Hemorrhagic shock of slow onset	• The bleeding may continue for several hours resulting in a significant blood loss • Disseminated intravascular coagulation (DIC)
Examples	Ruptured arterial aneurysm	Ruptured esophageal varices of portal hypertension, varicose veins of lower limb, neck veins during cervical lymph node dissection	Prolonged operation covering a wide area

Classification of hemorrhage

According to the Nature of the Bleeding Vessel Depending on the nature of bleeding vessel, hemorrhage can be classified as arterial hemorrhage, venous hemorrhage, and capillary hemorrhage (Table 13.1).

According to the Time of Hemorrhage Depending on the time of hemorrhage, hemorrhage can be classified as primary, reactionary, and secondary (Table 13.2).

According to the Visibility of Hemorrhage

- **Revealed or external bleeding**: It is visible external bleeding as occurs from an open wound.
- **Concealed or internal bleeding**: In this type the bleeding occurs in a body cavity, for example, pleural or pericardial cavity, or in tissues as occurs in a closed fracture of shaft of femur. Hence, the bleeding is not visible.
- **Initially concealed and later revealed**: An example of this bleeding is a bleeding peptic ulcer in upper gastrointestinal tract which reveals later as melena.

Hemostasis

Hemostasis is a complex process whose job is to limit blood loss from an injured vessel. This process is completed in four physiological events.

Vascular Constriction It consists of vascular constriction following injury which reduces the lumen of injured vessel. It is subsequently linked to platelet plug formation leading to production of thromboxane A2 via release of arachidonic acid from platelet membranes which is a potent constrictor of smooth muscle.

Platelet Plug Formation Platelets do not normally adhere to each other or vessel wall but can form a plug when vascular disruption occurs with injury to intima.

Fibrin Production Through a complex sequence of events and intrinsic and extrinsic pathways, the prothrombin is converted into thrombin which converts fibrinogen into fibrin that forms the clot which stops bleeding.

Fibrinolysis Finally during the process of wound healing with restoration of continuity of injured tissues, the clot undergoes clot lysis with the help of plasmin. It results in restoration of blood flow in the injured tissues.

Table 13.2 Differences between primary, reactionary, and secondary hemorrhage

Features	Primary hemorrhage	Reactionary hemorrhage	Secondary hemorrhage
Time of bleeding	Occurs at the time of injury/surgery	Occurs within 24 hours of trauma or operation, usually within 4–6 hours	Occurs 7–14 days after operation or trauma
Causes	Trauma due to injury or surgery	• Slipping of ligature • Dislodgement of clot • Rising blood pressure Most commonly arise from small blood vessels	• Wound infection which leads to sloughing of a part of wall of local vessels • Predisposed by pressure of a drainage tube or a fragment of bone
Examples	Mixed type of bleeding depending on type of vessel injured	In thyroid operations as coughing and vomiting causes acute engorgement of veins in the neck	• Tuberculous pulmonary cavity bleeding • Peptic ulcer bleeding • Hemorrhoidectomy • Bleeding following arterial surgery and amputation • Erosion of a vessel by cancer or its metastases, for example, from carotid artery in carcinoma of tongue

Clinical features of hemorrhage

Acute Hemorrhage

- The external bleeding is diagnosed by the visible loss of blood.
- The internal bleeding is diagnosed by pallor, progressive rise of pulse rate, cold and moist skin, rapid shallow breathing, and fall of blood pressure (hypovolemic shock).
- At the site of bleeding, there may be diffuse swelling due to hematoma, or signs of fluid accumulation if the bleeding has occurred in a closed cavity, for example, hemothorax and hemoperitoneum.

The acute hemorrhage can be of four grades depending on the volume of blood loss and other features as described in Table 13.3.

Chronic Blood Loss

- It can be obvious bleeding as occurs in piles.
- Chronic blood loss can be due to occult bleeding as occurs in gastrointestinal cancers when it presents as iron deficiency anemia.

Estimation of blood loss

Blood loss is estimated in relation to preexisting circulating blood volume (average 6 L in an adult) which is determined by the following formula:

- **In an infant**: 80–85 mL/kg
- **In an adult**: 65–75 mL/kg

The methods of assessing blood loss are described as follows:

- **Size of blood clot**: A clot equal to the size of clenched fist is equal to about 500 mL.
- **Degree of swelling in a closed fracture**: Moderate swelling in a closed fracture of tibia means 500–1500 mL blood loss and that in a closed fracture of shaft of femur equals 500–2000 mL blood loss.
- **Swab weighing**: During an operation the blood loss can be estimated by weighing all the swabs and sponges after use and subtracting their dry weight from it. To this must be added the blood in the suction or drainage bottle.
- **Hemoglobin and PCV estimation** is also a method of assessing blood loss.
- **Blood volume estimation**: This involves use of radioiodine technique or microhematocrit method.

Treatment of hemorrhage

The treatment of bleeding includes two major components: control of bleeding and restoration of blood volume.

1. **Control of bleeding**: The further blood loss is stopped by pressure, packing, use of local hemostatic agents (gelatin sponge, oxidized

Table 13.3 Grades of hemorrhage

Features	Grade I hemorrhage	Grade II hemorrhage	Grade III hemorrhage	Grade IV hemorrhage
Volume of lost blood	Up to 750 mL	750–1500 mL	1500–2000 mL	Above 2000 mL
Percent of total blood volume	Up to 15% of total blood volume	15–30% of total blood volume	30–40% of total blood volume	More than 40% of total blood volume
Pulse rate	Up to 100 beats/minute	100–120 beats/minute	120–140 beats/minute	More than 140 beats/minute
Blood pressure	Normal	Normal in recumbent position, falls on standing (orthostatic hypotension)	Hypotension even on lying	Marked hypotension
Effect on brain	Normal	Anxious	Confused	Obtunded
Urine output	Normal	Slightly reduced	Reduced	Markedly reduced
Treatment	• Arrest of bleeding • Intravenous fluids • Supportive treatment	• Arrest of bleeding • Intravenous fluids • May need blood transfusion	• Arrest of bleeding • Supportive treatment • Always needs blood transfusion	• Arrest of bleeding • Massive blood transfusion • Supportive treatment

cellulose, collagen sponge, thrombin, bone wax), ligation of a bleeding vessel, repair of an injured vessel, therapeutic embolization, and removal of a bleeding tumor. The methods of arrest of various types of bleeding are given in Table 13.4. The common bleeding encountered by a dentist is bleeding from an extracted tooth socket (Box 13.1).

2. **Restoration of blood volume**: Blood transfusion or infusion of 4.5% albumin, saline, Haemaccel (gelatin), dextran, and plasma is required when there is significant loss of blood altering the hemodynamics of cardiovascular system (≤15% of total blood volume).
3. **Other measures**: Elevation of foot end of bed, oxygen support, pain relief, urethral catheterization, monitoring, and ventilator support are used as required.

Table 13.4 Methods of arresting various types of bleeding

Type of bleeding	Methods of arrest of bleeding
Arterial bleeding	Ligation if not important; repair or reconstruction if large
Venous bleeding	Ligation of bleeder, clipping, banding, or excision
Capillary bleeding	Pressure, packing, use of local hemostatic agents, for example, gel foam, Oxycel, bone wax
Primary hemorrhage	• Ligation or repair of bleeding vessel
	• Coagulation of small vessels
	• Packing with hemostatic in diffuse bleeding
Reactionary hemorrhage	Same as primary hemorrhage
Secondary hemorrhage	• Antibiotics
	• Packing with a hemostatic after cleaning, for example, packing with a gauze soaked in eusol

Box 13.1 Arrest of bleeding from tooth socket after extraction

- In most of the cases the bleeding stops after pressure packing the socket for some time, maybe with some local hemostatic
- If bleeding continues, make sure there is no bleeding disorder
- If it is present, it should be treated. Sometimes local gum flaps are sutured over the socket

Blood transfusion

It was possible to do blood transfusion after the discovery of blood groups by Landsteiner in 1920. It is a great help in the management of bleeding which may be a manifestation of bleeding disorders, major trauma, and major operations.

Indications for Blood Transfusion

The indications of blood transfusion or restoration of blood volume are described in Box 13.2.

Box 13.2 Indications of blood transfusion

- Severe blood loss (≥15% of total blood volume) due to trauma or disease, for example, bleeding esophageal varices
- Major operations where a certain amount of blood loss is inevitable, for example, repair of aortic aneurysm
- Severe burns with associated hemolysis
- Chronic anemia (give packed red cells)
- For arresting hemorrhage in thrombocytopenia, hemophilia, and liver disease

Steps in Blood Transfusion

Blood grouping

The blood grouping of recipient and donor is the first step. It is based on two groups of antigens of red cells:

1. **Antigens of ABO blood group**: The red cells contain two antigens A and B and the serum contains antibodies, namely anti-A and anti-B. On this basis, there are four blood groups A, B, AB, and O.

   Blood grouping based on ABO and Rh is described in Table 13.5.

2. **Antigens of Rhesus blood group**: Rh(D) is strongly antigenic and is present in about 85% of population. Antibodies to this antigen are not naturally present in the serum of remaining 15% of people (Rh-negative), but they may be acquired by transfusion of Rh-positive blood in a Rh-negative recipient. It also occurs during pregnancy with a Rh-positive fetus in a Rh-negative mother.

Blood collection

- The donor must be fit without any infections such as HIV-1 and HIV-2, hepatitis B and C, and malaria. The weight of the donor should be more than 45 kg.
- The antecubital vein of the arm is punctured and the blood is collected in a sac containing 75 mL of citrate phosphate dextrose (CPD) solution.

Blood storage

Collected blood is stored in a special refrigerator at 4°C. CPD blood can be stored for 3 weeks. The

Table 13.5 Blood groups—ABO and Rh

Blood group	Antigen in red cells	Antibody in serum
A	Antigen A	Anti-B antibody
B	Antigen B	Anti-A antibody
AB	Antigens A and B	No AB antibody
O	No A and B antigens	Anti-A and anti-B antibodies
Rh-positive	Presence of D antigen	Absent
Rh-negative	Absence of D antigen	Absent but may be acquired later on

storage of blood results in rapid loss of platelets and WBCs and some loss of clotting factors, but RBCs remain alive till expiry of blood but their oxygen-releasing property is reduced gradually.

One unit of blood consists of 350 mL of blood and raises hemoglobin by 1 g/dL.

Cross-matching

Direct matching of recipient's serum with donor's red cells is done to confirm ABO compatibility and to find if Rh and any other blood group antibody is present in the serum of the recipient.

Blood transfusion protocols

- **Checking of donor blood**: Check donor blood, especially reference number, names ward/bed, blood group, and date of expiry before transfusion. The blood type compatibility chart is given in Table 13.6.
- **Selection and preparation of site**: Select and prepare site for transfusion and insertion of a suitable cannula, preferably a Teflon cannula, and starting transfusion of blood (Fig. 13.1).
- **Regulating the appropriate rate of transfusion**: Regulate the appropriate rate of transfusion, for example, 40 drops/minute allows 540 mL of blood to be transfused in 4 hours.
- **Filter**: A filter with absolute filtration rating of 40 μm filters off platelet aggregates and leukocyte membranes of stored blood.
- **Warming of blood**: It is required when rapid major blood transfusion is being done to prevent hypothermia and cardiac arrest.

With the modern technique of blood transfusion, the complications are rare; even then they can occur, especially with whole blood transfusion. Hence, these days there is more and more stress on the transfusion of blood fractions where the chances of reactions are even less. If there is a suspicion of reaction, the transfusion must be stopped and treatment is given depending on the nature of reaction. The common complications of blood transfusion are given in Box 13.3.

- **Simple allergic reaction:** It is controlled by giving an antihistaminic parenterally, for example, chlorpheniramine 10 mg intravenously.
- **Incompatibility**: It is a serious problem. The patient develops rigor, fever, and pain in the flanks, and may be markedly alarmed. The residual blood is sent for checking and a closed watch is kept on the pulse, blood pressure, and urine output. Furosemide 80–120 mg may be given if urine output is less than 30 mL/hour. Dialysis may be required.

Table 13.6 Blood type compatibility chart

Donor blood group	Recipient blood group
A	A, AB
B	B, AB
AB	AB (universal recipient) only
O	All blood groups (universal donor)

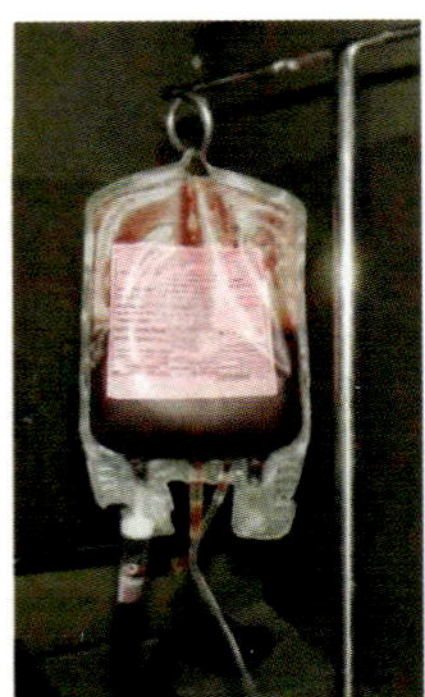

Figure 13.1 Blood transfusion with simultaneous intravenous fluid infusion from the same stand.

Box 13.3 Complications of blood transfusion

- Hemolytic reaction due to mismatched transfusion
- Transmission of infection, for example, AIDS, hepatitis B and C, syphilis, malaria, and brucellosis
- Allergic reactions such as urticaria, bronchospasm, and febrile reactions with shivering
- Congestive heart failure especially in elderly if too rapid infusion of large volumes of blood is done
- Thrombophlebitis at the site of venepuncture
- Air embolism
- Abnormal coagulation due to low platelet count, low fibrinogen level in serum, and an increase

Blood fractions

Blood is made up of many components and all the components (whole blood) are not required in all the patients. Hence, different fractions of the blood are identified and separated and they are now available for use in particular deficiencies. One unit of whole blood raises hemoglobin by 1 gm%.

Packed Red Cells

Packed red cells (blood minus two-third plasma) are given to correct anemia, especially in elderly and small children. They are obtained by centrifuging whole blood at 2000–3000 × g for 15–20 minutes. One unit of packed red blood cells (PRBCs) is expected to raise circulating hemoglobin by 1 g/dL.

Frozen Red Cells (Cryopreserved)

Cryopreservation extends the life of red cells almost indefinitely, but it is expensive. They are frozen with the help of glycerol. They are used in the treatment of anemia.

Washed Red Cells

They contain less than 5% of plasma and contain no white cells and platelets. They are useful in patients who react to platelets and white cell antigens. They are useful in patients who require transfusion over a long period of time, for example, renal transplantation.

Plasma

It is obtained by centrifugation of blood. It is used in burns and for treating hypoalbuminemia. It can be fractionalized into many constituents:

- **Human serum albumin**: It can be stored for several months at 4°C. Two strengths of albumin solution are available, that is, 5% and 20%. The first one is osmotically equivalent to plasma and used with crystalloid solution such as Ringer's as a plasma substitute in burns. A 20% solution (100 mL) is used to restore serum albumin in liver or renal disease.
- **Fresh frozen plasma (FFP)**: It is plasma removed from fresh blood and kept in a frozen state. If thawed and immediately used, it provides all the coagulation factors (except platelets). One unit of FFP increases the level of clotting factors by 3%.
- **Cryoprecipitate**: It is rich in factor VIII and fibrinogen. It is cryoglobulin fraction of plasma obtained by thawing a single donation of FFP at 4 ± 2°C. It is used to treat bleeding disorders.
- **Fibrinogen**: It is obtained by organic liquid fractionation of plasma. It is used for correction of severe depletion of fibrinogen in disseminated intravascular coagulation (DIC). Fibrinogen is given when its level falls below 80–10 mg/dL.
- **Factor VIII and factor IX concentrates**: They are available in freeze-dried forms and used in the treatment of hemophilia and von Willebrand disease.

Platelet-Rich Plasma

It is obtained by centrifugation of freshly donated blood for 15–20 minutes. It contains 5.5×10^9/L platelets in 50 mL plasma. It can be random-donor platelet-rich plasma or single-donor platelet-rich plasma. One unit of single-donor platelet-rich plasma is equal to 8 units of random-donor platelet-rich plasma. It is used in the treatment of thrombocytopenia, for example, hypersplenism.

Platelet Concentrate

It is obtained by centrifugation of platelet-rich plasma. It is used in thrombocytopenia and drug-induced hemorrhage. Its transfusion is required only if the platelet count is below 50,000. A single donor unit of platelets raises the platelet count by 50,000–60,000 platelets per mcL.

Prothrombin Complex Concentrate

It contains factors II, IX, and X, and is used in emergency reversal of warfarin therapy in uncontrolled hemorrhage.

Sodium Chloride, Adenine, Glucose–Mannitol Blood (SAG-M Blood)

In some blood donations the plasma is removed completely and is replaced by 100 mL of solution containing 877 mg sodium chloride, 16.9 mg adenine, 181 mg glucose (anhydrous), and 525 mg mannitol. It contains no protein. It allows good viability of cells. Hence, it is very useful in correcting anemia.

Artificial Blood

Perfluorocarbon (Fluosoleda) is a synthetic oxygen carrier having a half-life of 7 days. It is a RBC substitute. It is emulsified with albumin or lipids before infusion.

Bleeding disorders

Classification of Bleeding Disorders

- **Defects of blood vessel wall**: Vascular purpuras, telangiectasia, vasculitis
- **Disorders of platelets**: Thrombocytopenia, abnormal platelet function, antiplatelet drugs, for example, aspirin, clopidogrel
- **Deficiency of coagulation factors**
  - *Congenital coagulation disorders*: Hemophilia, Christmas disease, von Willebrand disease
  - *Acquired coagulation disorders*: Hypovitaminosis K, anticoagulant drugs

The investigations and treatment depend on the cause.

Hemophilia A (Classic Hemophilia)

It is an inherited bleeding disorder (X-linked recessive) due to deficiency of coagulation factor VIII. It is the most common bleeding disorder.

Grading of hemophilia

It is classified into three grades depending on the level of factor activity in the plasma as described in Table 13.7. The patients with more than 25% factor activity rarely fail to clot after major trauma or operation.

Clinical features of hemophilia A

- Females are asymptomatic carriers and males are the sufferers.
- The severe disease is generally noted at birth or in the first year of life; mild disease may not be recognized until young adulthood.
- Bleeding may occur anywhere in the body, the most common sites being joints (knees, ankles, elbows), muscles, and gastrointestinal tract. Spontaneous hemarthrosis (often repeated) is so characteristic that it is virtually diagnostic of this disease.
- If this condition is not known, the patient may have life-threatening bleeding even after dental extraction.

Diagnosis

- Low factor VIII levels
- Prolonged partial thromboplastin time (PTT)
- Normal platelet count, prothrombin time, and bleeding time

Treatment of hemophilia A

- These patients can be operated safely in hospital where adequate facilities are available. Aspirin should be avoided.

Table 13.7 Grading of hemophilia

Grade of hemophilia	Level of factor activity	Severity of bleeding
Severe hemophilia	Less than 1%	Bleeds spontaneously
Moderate hemophilia	1–5%	Bleeds with mild trauma or operation
Mild hemophilia	More than 5%	Bleeds after major trauma or surgery

- Plasma-derived factor VIII or recombinant factor concentrate is the mainstay of treatment in the dose of 50 units/kg body weight.
- In mild hemophilia it may be necessary to raise factor VIII level to 25% with one infusion. Mild hemophilia may respond to intravenous or intranasal treatment with DDAVP.
- In moderate disease the level is raised to 50% and maintained above 25% with repeated infusions for 2–3 days.
- For major surgery the level should be raised to 100% and then maintained above 50% continuously for 10–14 days.
- It requires 1000 units of concentrate to raise level to 25%. The half-life of factor VIII is 12 hours.

Hemophilia B (Christmas Disease)

It is identical to hemophilia A and is due to factor IX deficiency and inherited as X-linked autosomal recessive trait. It is treated by factor IX product and may be aminocaproic acid.

von Willebrand Disease

It is due to deficiency of the larger component (99%) of the factor VIII—vWF. It is an autosomal dominant disease with normal bleeding time and platelet count. Hemarthrosis is not common in this disease. It is of two types: 1 and 2 (ABMN). It is treated by DDAVP and vWF as required.

KEY POINTS

- Hemorrhage or bleeding is a common effect or symptom of trauma or disease, trauma being the most common cause. It is of three types: arterial blood is bright red in color and spurts as a jet; venous bleeding occurs as a steady flow and is dark red; and capillary blood is bright red in color and occurs as an ooze.
- Primary hemorrhage occurs at the time of injury/surgery, reactionary within 24 hours of trauma or operation, usually within 4–6 hours, and secondary hemorrhage 7–14 days after operation or trauma due to wound infection.
- Visible external bleeding occurs from an open wound. Concealed or internal bleeding occurs in a body cavity and hence is not visible.
- External bleeding is diagnosed by the visible loss of blood while internal bleeding is diagnosed by pallor, progressive rise of pulse rate, cold and moist skin, rapid shallow breathing, and fall of blood pressure (hypovolemic shock).
- It is of four grades depending on the volume of blood lost.
- Arrest of bleeding includes pressure, packing, use of local hemostatic agents (gelatin sponge, oxidized cellulose, collagen sponge, thrombin, bone wax), ligation of a bleeding vessel, repair of an injured vessel, therapeutic embolization, and removal of a bleeding tumor. Simultaneously restoration of blood volume is done by blood transfusion or infusion of 4.5% albumin, saline, Haemaccel (gelatin), dextran, and plasma.
- Indications of blood transfusion are severe blood loss (>15% of total blood volume), major surgeries, severe burns, and chronic anemia, and for arresting hemorrhage in thrombocytopenia, hemophilia, and liver disease.
- Complications of blood transfusion include hemolytic reaction due to mismatched transfusion, transmission of infection, allergic reactions and febrile reactions, congestive heart failure, thrombophlebitis at the site of venipuncture, air embolism, and abnormal coagulation.
- Blood fractions include packed red cells given to correct anemia, frozen red cells, washed red cells, platelet-rich plasma, platelet concentrate, fresh frozen plasma, and cryoprecipitate. One unit of fresh frozen plasma (FFP) increases the level of clotting factors by 3%. Fibrinogen is used for correction of severe depletion of fibrinogen in disseminated intravascular coagulation (DIC).
- Hemophilia A is due to deficiency of coagulation factor VIII. The patients with more than 25% factor activity rarely fail to clot after major trauma or operation. Hemophilia B is characterized by deficiency of factor IX. It is treated by replacement of deficient factors.
- von Willebrand disease is an autosomal dominant disease with deficiency of the larger component (99%) of the factor VIII—vWF. It has normal bleeding time and platelet count.

SELF-ASSESSMENT

Long answer questions

1. What are the causes and types of bleeding? Describe the treatment of bleeding, especially the treatment of a bleeding socket after dental extraction.
2. What are the indications of blood transfusion? Describe the technique and complications of blood transfusion.

Short answer questions

1. Blood groups
2. Rh factor
3. SAG-M blood
4. Hemophilia

Multiple choice questions

1. The primary hemorrhage is defined as
   (a) Bleeding occurring at the time of injury or operation
   (b) Bleeding occurring 4–6 hours after injury or operation
   (c) Bleeding occurring 7–14 days after injury or operation
   (d) None of the above
2. The secondary hemorrhage is defined as
   (a) Bleeding occurring at the time of injury or operation
   (b) Bleeding occurring 4–6 hours after injury or operation
   (c) Bleeding occurring 7–14 days after injury or operation
   (d) None of the above
3. Of the following causes of bleeding, the commonest cause is
   (a) Tuberculosis
   (b) Cancer
   (c) Trauma
   (d) Rupture of an arterial aneurysm
4. All of the following signs are the signs of severe internal bleeding, except
   (a) Pallor
   (b) Progressive fall of blood pressure
   (c) Rising pulse rate
   (d) Hot and dry skin
5. The average blood volume in an adult is
   (a) 4 L
   (b) 6 L
   (c) 8 L
   (d) 10 L
6. Which of the following blood groups is universal donor?
   (a) Group A
   (b) Group B
   (c) Group AB
   (d) Group O
7. Which of the following blood groups is universal recipient?
   (a) Group A
   (b) Group B
   (c) Group AB
   (d) Group O
8. Which of the following diseases is not transmitted by blood transfusion?
   (a) Syphilis
   (b) AIDS
   (c) Diabetes mellitus
   (d) Hepatitis B
9. Hemophilia A is due to deficiency of factor
   (a) VII
   (b) VIII
   (c) IX
   (d) XI
10. All of the following facts are true about SAG-M blood, except
    (a) The plasma is removed completely
    (b) The plasma is substituted by a solution containing sodium chloride, adenine, and glucose
    (c) It contains serum proteins
    (d) It can be used for top-up transfusion in anemia

Answers

1. (a) 2. (c) 3. (c) 4. (d) 5. (b) 6. (d) 7. (c) 8. (c) 9. (c) 10. (c)

Shock; Water, Acid–Base and Electrolyte Balance, and Nutrition

14

1. SHOCK

Definition

Shock is a state of poor perfusion of blood into the tissues and organs with impaired cellular metabolism manifesting with hypoxia and severe pathological abnormalities.

Types of shock

- Hypovolemic shock
  - Loss of blood
  - Loss of plasma, for example, extensive burns
  - Fluid loss due to severe diarrhea and vomiting
- Cardiogenic shock
  - Acute myocardial infarction
  - Acute pulmonary embolism
  - Cardiac tamponade
- Septic shock due to severe infection especially with Gram-negative organisms with release of toxins
- Neurogenic shock due to sudden severe anxiety and painful stimuli causing widespread splanchnic vasodilatation
- Anaphylactic shock due to type I hypersensitivity reaction

Pathophysiology of shock

At cellular level hypoxia causes changes in normal aerobic and anaerobic metabolism causing lactic acidosis. Lysosomes from cells get released into blood causing cell lysis. Intracellular potassium is released into circulation. Hypoxia and acidosis through complements release free

Box 14.1 Pathophysiology of shock

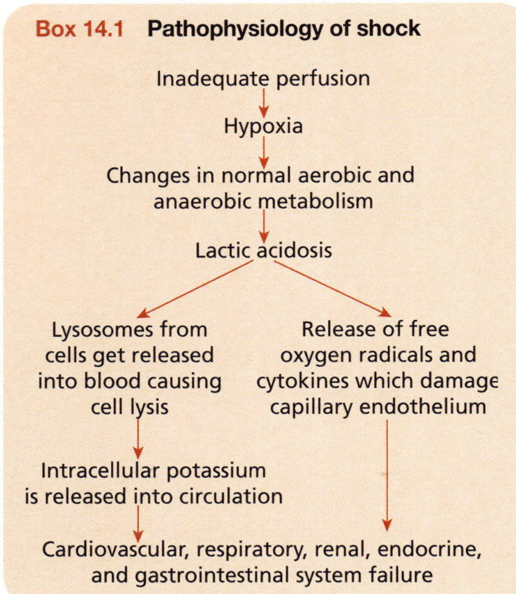

oxygen radicals and cytokines which damage capillary endothelium. Eventually cardiovascular, respiratory, renal, endocrine, and gastrointestinal systems will be affected presenting with systemic features (Box 14.1).

Consequences of unresuscitable shock

If hypotension and poor perfusion persists, it leads to irreversible shock which ultimately ends in damage to vital organs and death (Box 14.2).

Box 14.2 Consequences of unresuscitable shock

- Reperfusion injury
- End-organ damage
- Multiple organ failure
- Acute respiratory distress syndrome
- Renal failure
- Acute liver insufficiency
- Coagulopathy
- Cardiovascular failure

Clinical features of various types of shock

Hypovolemic Shock

- Initially the patient is thirsty, subcutaneous veins collapse, and the peripheries are cold, pale, and sweaty with poor capillary filling. It is followed by oliguria.
- Soon cardiovascular instability occurs which is manifested by tachycardia, thready pulse, and hypotension.
- Hypovolemia may also produce depressed sensorium, mental confusion, and restlessness and even coma.

Cardiogenic Shock

It is due to some cardiac disease, the symptoms and signs of which are obvious. In right-sided disease the neck veins may be prominent with hepatic enlargement and pedal edema. In left-sided disease there may be pulmonary rales and a third heart sound.

Septic Shock

It is initially a "warm shock" as the periphery is warm with full veins. The hypotension may be mild and the urine output may be normal. The patient has spikes of fever with rigor. The cause of septicemia is obvious.

As time passes, the hypotension increases with collapse of peripheral veins, oliguria, and cold and clammy skin.

Neurogenic Shock and Anaphylactic Shock

The neurogenic shock is of sudden onset and is caused by failure of autonomic nervous system and may follow regional or general anesthesia or spinal trauma. The patient is hypotensive with warm skin and flushing in the anesthetized and denervated areas.

The anaphylactic shock is a sudden fall of blood pressure following an unusual or exaggerated allergic reaction to a foreign protein (antigen–antibody reaction) with release of histamine, increased capillary permeability, and fatal consequences.

Monitoring of patient in shock

The patient is admitted to ICU and should be continuously monitored by recording of pulse, blood pressure, blood gases, central venous pressure (CVP), pulmonary capillary wedge pressure (PCWP) by passing a Swan-Ganz catheter, urine output, and serum electrolytes (Box 14.3).

Box 14.3 Monitoring a patient in shock

- **Essential parameters to be monitored**
  - Electrocardiography
  - Pulse oximetry
  - Blood pressure
  - Urinary output
- **Other parameters to be monitored**
  - Central venous pressure (CVP)
  - Invasive blood pressure
  - Cardiac output (CO)
  - Blood gas analysis

Investigations

Investigations depend on the cause and type of shock, for example, pus, urine, and blood culture in septic shock, and ultrasonography, echocardiography, CT scan, and others as required.

Treatment of shock

The general measures include maintenance of a patent airway, central venous catheterization, fluid resuscitation, treatment of the cause, and mechanism of shock.

Hypovolemic Shock

- The bleeding must be arrested by pressure, direct intervention, or operation, for example, excision of a bleeding tumor.
- The foot end of bed is elevated.
- The blood volume is restored by an appropriate fluid, for example, blood, plasma, plasma substitutes, or electrolyte solutions depending on the cause and the nature of fluid required, for example, blood for blood.
- The open wounds are cleaned, debrided, and repaired and fractures reduced and fixed.

Cardiogenic Shock

The cause is removed, for example, in cardiac tamponade the pericardial fluid is aspirated and myocardial infraction is treated with the help of a physician.

Septic Shock

- The focus of infection is controlled by appropriate combination of intravenous antibiotics including metronidazole, surgical drainage, and debridement.
- Fluid is replaced by Ringer's lactate or normal saline.
- Corticosteroids may be required.

Neurogenic Shock

Neurogenic shock is treated with relief of pain and anxiety and supportive treatment.

Anaphylactic Shock

It is managed with intravenous adrenaline 100 µg, corticosteroids, and supportive treatment. Vasopressors and bronchodilators may be required.

The etiology, clinical features, and treatment of various types of shock are described in Table 14.1.

Syncope

It is transient loss of consciousness due to generalized cerebral ischemia. It is usually accompanied by hypotension and bradycardia.

Table 14.1 Management of hypovolemic, cardiogenic, and septic shock

Features	Hypovolemic shock	Cardiogenic shock	Septic shock
Etiology	Reduction of blood volume due to massive bleeding or fluid loss due to extensive burns, severe diarrhea, and vomiting	Disturbed cardiac function, for example, acute myocardial infarction, cardiac tamponade	Severe infection, for example, peritonitis, urinary tract infection, diabetic cellulitis
Clinical features	• Cold and clammy skin • Tachycardia • Hypotension • Increased thirst • Collapsed subcutaneous veins	• Cold and clammy skin • Arrhythmias • Crepts at bases of lungs • Prominent neck veins • Hepatomegaly • Pedal edema	• Pink or cyanosed • Attacks of fever with rigor • May be jaundiced • Obvious septic focus
Central venous pressure	Low	High	Low or normal
Treatment	• Restore blood volume • Remove the cause	• Inotropic drugs • Cardiac support • Decompression of pericardial cavity	• Antibiotics • Drainage and debridement • Corticosteroids

Etiology

It may occur in response to emotional stress, postural hypotension, vigorous exercise in hot environment, obstructed venous return to heart, acute pain or its anticipation, fluid loss, and a sensitive carotid sinus.

Clinical Features

A prodroma of malaise, nausea, headache, diaphoresis, pallor, visual disturbance, loss of postural tone, sense of weakness, and impending loss of consciousness is followed by actual loss of consciousness. Although the patient is usually flaccid, some motor activity may be seen. Urinary incontinence (rarely fecal) may also occur as in a seizure.

Treatment

The patient should be made recumbent immediately which leads to rapid recovery. Medications associated with postural hypotension should be discontinued or reduced in dose.

Cardiac arrest

It is the cessation of activity of heart resulting in circulatory arrest due to any cause, for example, anoxia due to respiratory insufficiency or obstruction, prolonged and deep hypotension, and reaction to some drugs. It is important to recognize it immediately and start treatment to restore circulation within 3 minutes to prevent ischemic brain injury.

Diagnosis

It is diagnosed by absence of carotid pulse, heart sounds, and spontaneous breathing. If facilities are available, the patient is put on a cardiac monitor.

Treatment

- The first step in the treatment is to re-establish circulation by external cardiac massage given at the rate of 60–70/minute by pressing over the lower sternum just above xiphoid. Intracardiac or intravenous injection of calcium chloride and 1:10,000 adrenaline help to start cardiac function.
- The second step is to restore breathing initially by mouth-to-mouth breathing, and later on by an Ambu bag or a ventilator connected to the endotracheal tube passed into the trachea.
- The third step is to correct metabolic acidosis by giving sodium bicarbonate solution intravenously.

2. WATER BALANCE

Distribution of water in the body

Water comprises approximately 60% of the body mass in a young man due to more muscle mass. It is reduced to 54% in men older than 60 years. In young women it is 51% due to greater content of fat which is reduced to 46% in women older than 60 years. The water content is higher in infants and children.

Distribution of water in fluid compartments

The body water is distributed in three physiological compartments: intracellular (40%), extravascular (interstitial 55%), and intravascular (5%) (Fig. 14.1). These compartments are separated by semipermeable membranes.

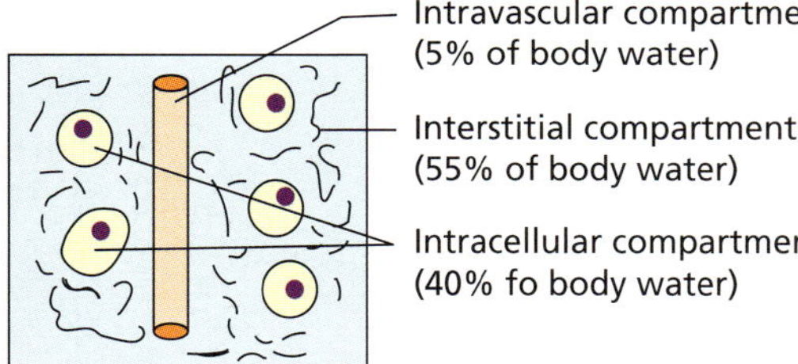

Figure 14.1 Fluid compartments.

Water intake and output

The body water contains a variety of solutes in a fixed concentration. The water acts as a vehicle for the transport of nutrients to the cells and tissues and for the elimination of end products of metabolism. In hot climate both intake and output of water increase to compensate for the loss of water due to excessive heat. A minimum output of urine is essential to excrete the end products of metabolism. It is about 400 mL/day and known as obligatory volume.

Daily water balance in a 70-kg adult is described in Table 14.2.

Regulation of water balance

The water balance inside the body is mainly regulated by thirst which regulates the water intake and the urinary excretion by the kidneys (Box 14.4). The thirst is under control of thirst center in the hypothalamus and the urinary volume is regulated by antidiuretic hormone (ADH) of posterior pituitary.

Water depletion (dehydration)

Cause It may be due to decreased water intake or excessive water loss. The decreased water intake

Table 14.2 Daily water balance in a 70-kg adult

Water intake/output	Sources	Quantity (mL)
Water intake	Drinking water and other fluids	1200
	Water in solid food	1000
	Endogenous production during oxidation of foods	300
	Total water intake	2500
Water output	Urine	1500
	Exhaled air	600
	Skin	300
	Stool	100
	Total water output	2500

Box 14.4 Regulation of water balance

- **Thirst center in hypothalamus**: Regulates volume of water ingested
- **Antidiuretic hormone (ADH) of pituitary**: Regulates volume of urine excreted
- **Plasma volumes, plasma osmolality, and angiotensin**: Regulates thirst center and plasma ADH

occurs when the patient is unable to take fluid due to painful conditions of mouth or pharynx or due to esophageal obstruction. Increased water loss may be renal (e.g., diabetes insipidus) or extrarenal (e.g., extensive burns).

Clinical Features The clinical features of water depletion are increased thirst, dryness of mucous membranes, for example, tongue, oliguria, and muscle weakness.

Diagnosis In severe water depletion the packed cell volume (PCV) rises above 50% with a serum osmolality more than 150 mEq/L. The water deficit can be calculated by the following equation:

$$\text{Water deficit} = \frac{(\text{normal body water volume}) - (\text{normal serum Na}) \times \text{normal body water volume}}{\text{Current serum Na}}$$

Treatment The pure water depletion is treated with water without electrolytes given orally or rectally. Isotonic solution of 5% glucose may be given parenterally. Half of water deficit is corrected in the first 24 hours and the other half in the next 24 hours.

Water excess or water intoxication (fluid overload)

Causes It is mostly a complication of fluid therapy (iatrogenic water excess), the examples of which include excessive infusion of 5% glucose, and excessive bowel or prostatic bed wash out with plain water.

Clinical Features The symptoms appear suddenly and include confusion, drowsiness, or convulsions with normal blood pressure and pulse rate.

Diagnosis The CVP may be elevated and the hematocrit is low. Serum electrolytes, especially sodium, and the serum osmolality are low.

Treatment It is better to prevent this problem. In an established problem, do not give fluids for 24 hours. In severe cases, 6 mL of 5% sodium chloride solution per kilogram body weight may be given to raise serum sodium. Intravenous furosemide may also be given with a mineralocorticoid to conserve sodium.

3. ACID–BASE BALANCE

Normal health is the result of a balanced chemical reaction. One component of this balance is acid–base balance of body fluids which is indicated by pH.

Concept of pH

It is the symbol relating the hydrogen ion (H^+) concentration or activity of a solution to that of a given standard solution. Numerically the pH is approximately equal to negative logarithm of H^+ concentration expressed in osmolality. pH 7 is neutral; above it the alkalinity increases and below it the acidity. The pH of pure water is 7, that is, 10^{-7} mol/L of H^+, the logarithm of which is 7. The normal pH of the body fluids is 7.36–7.44 and that of blood is 7.4 which is slightly alkaline.

Maintenance of Normal pH

The pH of body fluids is maintained within normal limits in spite of a large load of acids produced endogenously as a by-product of body metabolism. These acids are neutralized by the buffer systems of the body and then excreted by lungs as CO_2 and by kidneys as urea. Some important buffers are:

- Proteins and phosphate (HPO_4, H_2PO_4) buffers in intracellular pH
- Bicarbonate and carbonic anhydrase system in the extracellular fluids
- Hemoglobin

A buffer system consists of a weak acid or base and salts of that acid or base. The buffering effect is the result of the formation of an amount of weak acid or base equal to the strong acid or base added to the system. Hence, there is a compensatory mechanism in an attempt to maintain normal pH.

The standard bicarbonate level of blood is 22–25 mmol/L. The control of intracellular pH which is slightly lower than extracellular pH is essential to sustain the normal biochemical reactions in the cell.

With the help of **Henderson-Hasselbalch equation**, the pH of plasma or a solution can be found if the molar concentrations of the bicarbonate ion and dissolved carbon dioxide are known. It is given as follows:

$$pH = 6.1 + \log \frac{HCO_3^-}{CO_2}$$

Acid–base disorders

Acidosis is the process characterized by accumulation of H^+ ions due to increase in PCO_2 (respiratory acidosis) or due to decrease in HCO_3^- (metabolic acidosis). Acidemia is said to be present if pH is less than 7.36.

Alkalosis is the process that causes bases to accumulate due to decrease in PCO_2 (respiratory alkalosis) or due to increase in HCO_3^- (metabolic alkalosis). In alkalosis base accumulates in the body; alkalemia is said to be present if pH is more than 7.36.

The diagnosis of acid–base imbalance is made by doing blood gas analysis (increased PCO_2 in acidosis and decreased PCO_2 in alkalosis) and measuring the pH. The arterial pH normally ranges from 7.36 to 7.44 with an average of 7.4. The disorders of acid–base balance are described in brief in Table 14.3.

Table 14.3 Acid–base disorders

Disorder	Defect	Etiology	Compensation
Metabolic acidosis (pH lowered)	• Retention of fixed acid or loss of base (HCO_3^-) • PCO_2 lowered (compensatory)	Diabetic ketoacidosis, renal failure, severe diarrhea, small bowel fistula	• Increased rate and depth of respiration (hyperventilation) • Renal route is slow
Metabolic alkalosis (pH elevated)	• Loss of fixed acids and gain of base (HCO_3^-) • PCO_2 elevated (compensatory)	Persistent vomiting, nasogastric suction, excessive intake of alkalies, hyperaldosteronism	• Decreased rate and depth of ventilation • Renal route is slow
Respiratory acidosis (pH lowered)	• Accumulation of CO_2 with increased $PaCO_2$ • HCO_3^- elevated (compensatory)	Airway obstruction, failure of neuromuscular mechanism of respiration, pulmonary edema, chest injuries	Renal retention of bicarbonate (HCO_3^-)
Respiratory alkalosis (pH elevated)	• Excessive loss of CO_2 with decreased $PaCO_2$ • HCO_3^- lowered (compensatory)	Rapid respiration induced by psychoneurosis or overventilation on a ventilator	Increased renal excretion of bicarbonate (HCO_3^-)

Metabolic Acidosis

Causes It is the most common disorder seen in a hospital and occurs due to decrease in HCO_3^-, for example, diarrhea and small bowel fistula. It can occur due to overproduction of acids (H^+), for example, diabetic ketoacidosis and renal failure using HCO_3^- ions for buffering. The causes include diabetic ketoacidosis, renal failure, diarrhea, trauma, and small bowel fistula.

Clinical Features It is characterized by reduced cardiac output, pulmonary hypertension, arrhythmia, oliguria, respiratory difficulty, and hyperventilation. Kussmaul breathing is a late sign. Most of the patients of acidosis are treated early; hence, Kussmaul breathing is very rarely seen.

Diagnosis Anion gap (AG) is important in assessing the cause of metabolic acidosis. It may help in differentiating between metabolic acidosis caused due to excess of acid and due to loss of HCO_3^-:

$$AG = Na^+ - (Cl + HCO_3^-)$$

Normally it is less than 12. The highest normal value varies from institution to institution.

Treatment The cause is treated and if the pH is less than 7.2, sodium bicarbonate is given according to the following formula:

Bicarbonate requirement (mmol) = body weight (kg) × base deficit (mmol/L) × 0.3

Each milliliter of 8.4% $NaHCO_3$ solution contains 1 mmol of HCO_3^-.

Metabolic Alkalosis

Causes It is characterized by increased plasma levels of HCO_3^- and occurs due to loss of acid gastric juice in persistent vomiting and nasogastric suction. It also occurs following excessive intake of alkalies in the treatment of peptic ulcer and hyperaldosteronism.

Clinical Features These include excitable nervous system, hypokalemia, that is, paresthesias, tetany, and convulsions. Cheyne–Stokes respiration may be seen in terminal phase of alkalosis.

Treatment It is treated with administration of saline and potassium as required. Severe alkalosis (pH more than 7.6) is treated with 0.1% hydrochloric acid in 5% glucose at a rate less than 0.2 mmol/kg/L.

Respiratory Acidosis

Causes It occurs due to interference in exchange of gases across the alveolar membrane as may happen in airway obstruction, failure of neuromuscular mechanism of respiration, pulmonary edema, and chest injuries (flail chest). It results in accumulation of CO_2 in the blood which forms carbonic acid (H_2CO_3) and releases H^+ ions causing acidosis.

Clinical Features The clinical features of respiratory acidosis depend on the cause and include a varying combination of stridor, shallow rapid breathing, and may be cyanosis (late sign). It is mostly recognized by the presence of its cause.

Treatment It is treated by removal of cause, for example, removal of airway obstruction, diuretics in pulmonary edema, and ventilator support.

Respiratory Alkalosis

Causes It occurs due to primary decrease in $PaCO_2$ caused by rapid respiration induced by psychoneurosis or overventilation in patients on ventilator.

Clinical Features Acute hypocarbia can result in cerebral vasoconstriction and reduced cerebral blood flow leading to confusion, seizures, and tetany. It can cause tachycardia and ventricular arrhythmia.

Treatment It is treated by removal of cause. Insufflation of carbon dioxide may be used in patients having respiratory arrest.

4. ELECTROLYTE BALANCE

Water is present in all the cells, tissues, and spaces of body. Nowhere it exists in pure form. It contains a variety of solutes which normally have a fixed concentration that is expressed in milliequivalents per liter or millimoles per liter.

Measurements of electrolytes

Milliequivalents Per Liter

The equivalent weight of an ion or a molecule is its atomic or molecular weight in grams divided by its valency. A milliequivalent is one-thousandth of equivalent weight. Thus, 1 mEq of Na^+ is equal to 23 mg, and 1 mEq of Cl^- is equal to 35.5 mg. It is more appropriate to describe the concentration of particles of a solute in milliequivalents per liter rather than in milligrams, as it describes the number of charge on each particle.

Millimoles Per Liter

A mole is equal to the quantity of a chemical compound whose weight in grams is equal to its molecular weight. A millimole is one-thousandth of a mole. In case of sodium, potassium, chloride, and bicarbonate, the concentration in millimoles is the same as in milliequivalents.

Milliosmoles

When two solutions are separated by a semipermeable membrane, the nondiffusible ions and molecules exert an osmotic pressure which causes movement of water across the membrane to achieve osmotic equilibrium. When a molecule breaks into ions, each ion then exerts osmotic pressure independently.

One gram molecular weight of a nonionizable substance is 1 Osm. As the osmotic pressure is determined by the number of particles, if a chemical ionizes into two ions (as sodium chloride into Na^+ and Cl^-), then half of the gram molecular weight of such a chemical is 1 Osm. A milliosmole is one-thousandth of 1 Osm.

Osmolality

The tonicity of plasma is determined by the solutes, for example, sodium and corresponding anions, chlorides, and bicarbonates together with substances such as glucose, urea, and proteins. They are osmotically active; hence, the tonicity is described as milliosmole per liter. It is calculated by the following equation:

$$\text{Osmolality} = 2 \times Na^+ + \frac{\text{glucose (mg\%)}}{18} + \frac{\text{blood urea (mg\%)}}{6}$$

Hence, the level of sodium contributes most to the osmolality of plasma.

Osmolarity

Osmolarity is the osmolar concentration as osmoles per liter of water. In body fluids the two values are nearly the same.

Electrolyte composition of body fluids

Na^+ is the major cation of the extracellular fluid while the potassium is of the intracellular fluid. Cl^- and HCO_3^- are the major anions of the extracellular fluid and the HPO_4^+ is of the intracellular fluid. The total number of cations is equal to the total number of anions. The levels of various electrolytes in the body fluids (mEq/L) are described in Table 14.4.

Disorders of electrolytic balance

Sodium pump pumps Na^+ out of cell in exchange of K^+ which is driven into the cells. This

Table 14.4 Distribution of electrolytes in body fluids (mEq/L)

Ions	Electrolytes	Intracellular fluid (ICF)	Interstitial fluid (ISF)	Intravascular fluid (plasma)
Cations	Na^+	10	144	142
	K^+	150	4	4
	Ca^+	2	3	5
	Mg^+	40	2	3
Anions	Cl^-	10	114	103
	HCO_3^-	10	30	27
	PO_4^-, SO_4^-	150	3	3
	Proteins	40	1	16
	Organic acids	—	5	5

mechanism also ensures a higher concentration of ions within the cell, thus maintaining a potential difference across the cell membrane.

Sodium Abnormalities

The normal sodium level in blood is 135–145 mEq/L. It is unusual to have pure sodium loss or excess. It is always associated with some change in the volume of extracellular fluid.

Hyponatremia

It is said to occur when the sodium level is below 135 mEq/L, the critical level being less than 125 mEq/L.

Causes The causes of hyponatremia are given as follows:

- Inadequate intake, starvation
- Excessive loss
  - Gastrointestinal loss
    - Excessive diarrhea
    - Repeated vomiting
  - Renal loss
    - Chronic renal failure
    - Salt-losing nephropathy
    - Diuretic therapy
    - Hypoadrenalism
  - Internal loss into the body
    - Acute pancreatitis
    - Acute generalized peritonitis
  - Skin loss
    - Excessive sweating
    - Extensive burns
- Increased extracellular volume (dilutional hyponatremia)
  - Congestive heart failure
  - Compulsive water drinking
  - Excessive electrolyte-free infusion

Clinical Features A rapid loss of sodium with water produces hypovolemia and shock. A slow deficiency causes muscle weakness, fatigue, and muscular cramps.

Treatment The treatment is removal of cause. Hyponatremia with contracted volume is treated with isotonic sodium chloride given intravenously. Hyponatremia with expanded volume is treated with administration of sodium chloride, water restriction, and spironolactone.

Hypernatremia

It occurs when the blood sodium level goes above 145 mEq/L, the critical level being more than 155 mEq/L.

Causes The causes of hypernatremia are given as follows:

- Excessive intake of sodium
  - Oral ingestion of sodium chloride
  - Use of hypertonic saline for induction of abortion and injection sclerotherapy
  - Sodium bicarbonate administration after cardiac arrest
- Reduced sodium excretion (sodium retention)

  - Acute renal failure
  - Hyperaldosteronism
- Excessive water loss
  - Hot weather
  - Febrile states
  - Diabetes insipidus
  - Peritoneal dialysis
  - Mannitol administration
- Poor intake of water—coma
- Essential hypernatremia

Clinical Features The symptoms and signs of hypernatremia include lethargy, fatigue, hyperactive deep tendon reflexes, seizures, and coma. They are rare with sodium less than 150 mmol/L.

Treatment It results in cellular dehydration. It is treated with a loop diuretic if the renal function is normal and replacement of fluid by 5% dextrose.

Potassium Abnormalities

The normal potassium level in blood is 3.5–5.0 mEq/L. It may be reduced or increased in many disease states.

Hypokalemia

It is the presence of less than normal potassium in the blood; a level less than 3 mEq/L is dangerous.

Causes The causes of hypokalemia are given as follows:

- Deficient intake
  - Anorexia nervosa
  - Prolonged intravenous fluid therapy without potassium supplementation
  - Excessive water drinking
- Increased loss
  - Increased gastrointestinal loss
    - Persistent vomiting
    - Severe diarrhea
    - High-output small bowel fistula
  - Increased renal loss
    - Renal tubular acidosis
    - Mineralocorticoid excess, for example, hyperaldosteronism
    - Diuretics, for example, chlorothiazide, mercurial
- Shift of potassium into intracellular compartment
  - Alkalosis, may be alkali induced
  - High dose of insulin and/or glucose
  - Barium ingestion

Clinical Features It is usually associated with hyponatremia and water loss, and characterized by anorexia, nausea, vomiting, abdominal distension, muscle weakness, hypotonia, and ECG abnormalities.

Treatment It is treated by giving potassium orally in the form of fruit juice or potassium chloride, or parenterally under careful control.

Hyperkalemia

It is the presence of more than normal (5.0 mEq/L) potassium in the blood. It is dangerous to life if it becomes more than 6 mEq/L.

Causes The causes of hyperkalemia are given as follows:

- Excessive intake of potassium
  - Potassium chloride orally or parenterally
  - Fruit juice ingestion
  - Transfusion of stored blood
- Diminished excretion of potassium
  - Renal failure
  - Addison's disease
  - Hypoaldosteronism
  - Potassium-conserving drugs, for example, amiloride, triamterene
  - Renal transplant rejection
- Shift of potassium from intracellular compartment
  - Extensive soft tissue destruction, for example, crush injury, rhabdomyolysis
  - Acidosis

Clinical Features It is characterized by muscle weakness, flaccid paralysis, and ECG changes (tall, peaked T waves and reduced QT interval).

Treatment It is treated by removal of cause, and initially by administration of 25% glucose with 1 unit of plain insulin for every 5 g of glucose followed by 500 mL of 5% glucose intravenously. Calcium gluconate 10 mL of 10% solution is given intravenously at the rate of 2 mL/minute.

Administration of sodium bicarbonate also lowers potassium levels. Dialysis is required in patients with renal failure.

Calcium Abnormalities

The normal calcium level in the blood is 8.5–10.5 mg/dL and approximately half of this is nonionized and bound to plasma proteins.

Hypocalcemia

It is less than normal calcium in the blood. If it falls below 6.5 mg/dL, it is dangerous to life.

Causes The common causes of hypocalcemia are given as follows:

- Absence or deficiency of parathormone
  - Accidental removal or injury to parathyroids during thyroid surgery
  - Parathyroidectomy for hyperparathyroidism
  - Neoplastic infiltration
  - DiGeorge syndrome
- Ineffectiveness of parathormone
  - Chronic renal failure
  - Deficiency or ineffectiveness of active vitamin D
  - Pseudohypoparathyroidism
- Increased calcium utilization
  - Medullary carcinoma of thyroid
  - Carcinoma of prostate
  - Acute pancreatitis

Clinical Features These include paresthesias, hyperreflexia, cramps, tetany, and convulsions.

Treatment Apart from the treatment of cause, 10% calcium gluconate or calcium chloride is given intravenously in tetany followed by oral calcium therapy.

Hypercalcemia

If the blood calcium level goes above 10.5 mg/dL, it is called hypercalcemia. If it is more than 13.5 mg/dL, it is critical level.

Causes The causes of hypercalcemia are given as follows:

- Parathyroid-related (hyperparathyroidism)
  - Parathyroid adenoma
  - Parathyroid hyperplasia
  - Parathyroid carcinoma
- Cancer-related
  - Osteolytic metastases
  - Paraneoplastic syndrome in renal cell carcinoma and bronchogenic carcinoma
  - Multiple myeloma
- Other causes
  - Hypervitaminosis D
  - High bone turnover, that is, hyperthyroidism, prolonged immobilization, Paget's disease of bone
  - Poor renal excretion, for example, renal transplantation
  - Excessive intake of calcium salts

Clinical Features These include fatigue, weakness, anorexia, nausea, and vomiting followed by drowsiness, stupor, and coma.

Treatment It is treated by hydration, correction of fluid deficit, and use of chelating agents.

Magnesium Abnormalities

Hypomagnesemia occurs in malabsorption syndrome, loss of gastrointestinal secretions, and prolonged infusion with magnesium-free fluids. The clinical features resemble those of hypocalcemia. The symptomatic patients are treated with magnesium sulfate 50% given parenterally. Hypermagnesemia is rare.

5. NUTRITION IN SURGICAL PATIENTS

Food (nourishment) is required for growth, normal functioning, and maintenance of life. The components of food are proteins, carbohydrates, fats, vitamins, and minerals, and have to be supplied from outside as they cannot be synthesized by the body.

Energy requirements

An average person requires 30–35 kcal/kg body weight per day, that is, 2200–2500 kcal for a man and 1800–2000 kcal for a woman. Of these, at least 500 kcal must be provided by carbohydrates. The requirement of energy increases in sepsis and other hypercatabolic states, for example, thyrotoxicosis.

Macronutrients

They are the body-building (proteins) and energy-yielding (carbohydrates and fats) nutrients. They are the main constituents of the diet.

Proteins

Proteins are complex organic nitrogenous compounds which are the principal constituent of cell protoplasm (body builder). Normally 1 g of protein per kilogram of body weight is required daily. It yields 4 kcal/g.

Carbohydrates

Carbohydrates, apart from carbon, contain hydrogen and oxygen in proportion to form water (CH_2O). They are the main energy-yielding components of diet, 1 g of glucose yielding 4 kcal. The carbohydrate metabolic abnormalities manifest as hypoglycemia and hyperglycemia.

The normal blood sugar level is 60–110 mg/dL; less than 40 mg/dL and more than 500 mg/dL are the critical levels and dangerous.

Hypoglycemia

It is characterized by low blood sugar level less than 60 mg/dL. The causes of hypoglycemia are described in Box 14.5.

Hyperglycemia

A plasma glucose level above 126 mg/dL is hyperglycemia (7 mmol/L). It is the main finding in diabetes mellitus. The causes of hyperglycemia are described in Box 14.6.

Box 14.5 Causes of hypoglycemia

- **Underproduction of glucose**
  - Deficiency of counter-insulin glucose regulatory hormone
    - Hypopituitarism (growth hormone deficiency)
    - Addison's disease (cortisol deficiency)
    - Catechol deficiency
    - Hypothyroidism (thyroid hormone deficiency)
  - Specific defects or deficiencies of glycogenolytic or neoglucogenetic enzymes, for example, glucose-6-phosphatase, liver phosphorylase, pyruvate carboxylase
  - Substrate limitation or deficiency
    - Carbohydrate deficiency: Starvation, upper gastrointestinal obstruction, anorexia nervosa
    - Late pregnancy
    - Malabsorption: Sprue, chronic diarrhea
  - Defective hepatic gluconeogenesis
    - Chronic hepatitis
    - Cirrhosis of liver
  - Drugs and chemicals: Aminobenzoic acid, haloperidol, propranolol
- **Overutilization of glucose**
  - Hyperinsulinism
    - Insulinoma
    - Islet cell hyperplasia
    - Sulfonylurea
  - Hypoglycemia with appropriate or low plasma insulin
    - Solid extrapancreatic tumors of large size, for example, fibrosarcoma, hepatoma
    - Cachexia with fat depletion
  - Other causes
    - Hypercatabolic states, for example, exercise, fever
    - Pregnancy
    - Renal glycosuria
    - Drugs: Pentamidine, phenformin

Box 14.6 Causes of hyperglycemia

- **Insulin deficiency due to diseases of pancreas**
  - Chronic pancreatitis
  - Pancreatectomy
  - Congenital absence of pancreas
- **Excess anti-insulin hormones**
  - Cushing's disease (glucocorticoid excess)
  - Pheochromocytoma (catecholamine excess)
  - Acromegaly (growth hormone excess)
  - Hyperthyroidism (thyroid hormone excess)
- **Impaired insulin action**
  - Insulin receptor defects
  - Anti-insulin antibodies
- **Drugs and chemicals**, for example, ACTH, corticosteroids, alloxan

Fats

Fat is an ester of glycerol with fatty acids which forms soft pads between various organs of the body and furnishes a reserve supply of energy. One gram of fat yields 9 kcal.

Vitamins and Minerals

Vitamins and minerals are necessary for normal metabolic functions of the body in very small amounts (micronutrients).

Nutritional deficiency

Overall nutritional deficiency is very common in our country. The nutritional excess manifests mainly as obesity. The causes of nutritional deficiency (protein–calorie deficiency) are described in Box 14.7. Methods of assessing adequate nutrition are given in Box 14.8.

Starvation during surgery

Many surgical patients require special care to maintain the nourishment of body because the patient may stop taking food due to disease, or food may not be given due to anesthesia and

Box 14.7 Causes of nutritional deficiency

- **Inadequate food supply**
  - Poor food production
  - Inadequate food supply
  - Poverty and inability to afford
- **Impaired ingestion**
  - Conditions in which the patient does not eat
    - Anorexia due to any cause including anorexia nervosa
    - Voluntary fasting
  - Conditions in which the patient cannot eat
    - Dysphagia due to obstructed food passage
    - Other problems of mastication and swallowing, for example, odynophagia, xerostomia, edentulism
- **Nutritional deficiency due to rejection of nutrition**
  - Persistent or recurrent vomiting
  - Chronic diarrhea
- **Impaired digestion and/or absorption**
  - Massive small bowel resection
  - Pancreatic insufficiency
  - Intestinal short circuiting due to internal fistula
- **Impaired assimilation due to chronic liver disease**
- **Excessive demands**
  - Hyperthyroidism
  - Malignancy
- **Abnormal excretion or loss of nutrition**
  - Nephrotic syndrome
  - Chyluria
  - Septic draining wounds

Box 14.8 Methods of assessing adequate nutrition

- Body weight
- Mid-arm circumference
- Triceps skin fold thickness
- Serum albumin
- Lymphocyte count

operation. Hence, the patient needs careful nutritional management to prevent starvation which leads to gradual depletion of glycogen, amino acids, and fat. Simultaneously it results in breakdown of body proteins leading to reduced muscle mass and poor wound healing. The overall effect of lack of nutrition is loss of body weight which if exceeds more than 30% of initial weight may have fatal consequences.

Nutritional supplementation

All patients of nutritional deficiency, for example, trauma and operation, require nutritional support.

The nutritional support can be given by enteral and parenteral routes.

Enteral Alimentation

Here the nutrition is administered directly into the stomach, duodenum, or jejunum (enteral) through tubes. The feed must provide the calorie and protein needs of the patient. Adequate amounts of vitamins, minerals, and trace elements should be included. The nutrition has to be given in the form of liquid food, for example, milk and liquidized food in a blender.

Elemental Diets

They are commercially available for tube feeding containing amino acids, fats, carbohydrates, vitamins, and trace elements. They do not cause lactose diarrhea but are more expensive than milk-based or blenderized feeds. The details of an elemental diet are described in Table 14.5.

Indications The enteral alimentation is indicated when the gastrointestinal tract is healthy but the patient cannot ingest food and drinks due to dysphagia caused by oropharyngeal and esophageal carcinoma.

Types of Enteral Alimentation The enteral alimentation is through a nasogastric or nasoduodenal tube or through a gastrostomy or jejunostomy tube.

Advantages It is safer, physiological, and cheaper than parenteral feeding.

Complications They include diarrhea, abdominal distension, and problems connected with tube, and nutritional deficiencies.

Parenteral Nutrition

Intravenous route may be used to provide nutritional requirements. It is indicated when oral and enteral feeding is not possible. The parenteral nutrition started with 5% dextrose and normal saline (0.9% NaCl), but now nearly all the nutritional requirements can be met by parenteral route.

When parenteral alimentation is required for short periods and the needs are small, it is done through a peripheral vein using solutions containing amino acids with 5% glucose and solutions of lipids. These solutions are not thrombogenic.

Total parenteral nutrition (TPN)

In TPN all the calorie and nutritional requirements are met with intravenous route. Since these solutions are thrombogenic, they are given through a central venous catheter inserted into the subclavian vein with its tip in superior vena cava. The water-soluble vitamins are given daily by infusion. Folic acid and vitamins B_{12}, A, D, and K are given once a week.

Table 14.5 Elemental diet

Contents	Percentage	Weight (gm)	Kilocalories
Proteins	42	105	420
Fats	3.36	84	756
Carbohydrates	13.36	334	1336
Water		2500 mL	
Total			2512

Table 14.6 Parenteral nutrition solutions

Nutrient	Percentage	Volume (mL)	Total (g)	Energy (kcal)
Amino acids with 10% sorbitol*	10	1000	• Protein 100 • Sorbitol 100	• 400 • 400
Dextrose with electrolytes	25	1000	250	1000
Lipid†	10	500	50	450
Total	—	2500	—	2250

* Consists of 8 essential and 12 nonessential amino acids.
† Consists of fractionated soybean oil, for example, phospholipids, glycerol, and water. Not more than 2.5 g/kg/day of fat is given.

The details of parenteral nutrition solutions are described in Table 14.6.

The comparison of enteral and parenteral alimentation is described in Table 14.7.

Complications of total parenteral nutrition

- **Catheter-related complications:** These include pneumothorax, hematoma, and hemothorax during insertion of catheter and subsequently catheter sepsis.
- **Metabolic complications**: A series of metabolic problems, changes in fluid and electrolyte balance, and pH may occur if the procedure is not correctly monitored by daily blood sugar, urea, creatinine, electrolytes, fluid balance chart and urine and plasma osmolality, and weekly liver function tests, coagulation studies, and hemogram.

Table 14.7 Comparison of enteral and parenteral alimentation

Features	Enteral alimentation	Parenteral alimentation
Route of administration	Through a tube into the stomach, duodenum, or jejunum	Intravenous into a peripheral or central vein
Care and supervision required	Less	More
Gut flora	Utilized	Not utilized
Sepsis	Lesser chances	More chances
Insulin response	More	Less
Salt and water retention	Less	More
Complications	Less	More
Cost of therapy	Less	More

KEY POINTS

- Shock is a state of poor perfusion of blood into the tissues and organs with impaired cellular metabolism manifesting with hypoxia and severe pathological abnormalities. If it persists, it leads to irreversible shock which ends in damage to vital organs and death.
- Hypovolemic shock is due to loss of blood, plasma, and fluid and characterized by tachycardia, altered sensorium, hypotension, and oliguria which can lead to death if untreated. Treatment includes removal of cause, arrest of bleeding, and restoration of fluids.
- Cardiogenic shock is due to cardiac conditions, that is, acute myocardial infarction, acute pulmonary embolism, and cardiac tamponade. Its treatment includes removal of cause, for example, decompression of pericardium, use of inotropic drugs, and cardiac support.

(CONTD...)

KEY POINTS *(...CONTD)*

- Septic shock is due to release of toxins by Gram-negative organisms. It is treated by intravenous broad-spectrum antibiotics including metronidazole, surgical drainage and debridement, and supportive treatment.
- Neurogenic shock and anaphylactic shock are of sudden onset. Neurogenic shock is treated with relief of pain and anxiety. Anaphylactic shock is managed with intravenous adrenaline 100 μg and corticosteroids.
- Patients with shock must be continuously monitored by recording of pulse, blood pressure, blood gases, central venous pressure (CVP), pulmonary capillary wedge pressure (PCWP) by passing a Swan-Ganz catheter, urine output, and serum electrolytes.
- Syncope is transient loss of consciousness due to generalized cerebral ischemia. The patient should be made recumbent immediately which leads to rapid recovery.
- Cardiac arrest is the cessation of activity of heart resulting in circulatory arrest. It is important to recognize it immediately and start treatment to restore circulation within 3 minutes to prevent ischemic brain injury.
- Water comprises approximately 51–60% of the body mass. It is higher in infants and children. It is distributed in three physiological compartments: intracellular (40%), extravascular (interstitial 55%), and intravascular (5%).
- Total water intake is equal to total water output which is 2500 mL. A minimum output of urine is essential to excrete the end products of metabolism. It is about 400 mL/day and is known as obligatory volume.
- Water depletion or dehydration may be due to decreased water intake or excessive water loss. It is treated with water without electrolytes given orally or rectally. Isotonic solution of 5% glucose may be given parenterally.
- Water intoxication/excess/fluid overload is mostly a complication of fluid therapy characterized by elevated central venous pressure and low hematocrit. Treatment is not to give fluids for 24 hours and intravenous furosemide with mineralocorticoids.
- The normal pH of the body fluids is 7.36–7.44 and that of blood is 7.4 which is slightly alkaline.
- The important buffer systems which neutralize the endogenously produced acids are proteins and phosphate (HPO_4, H_2PO_4) buffers which help in maintaining intracellular pH and bicarbonate and carbonic anhydrase system in the extracellular fluids. The standard bicarbonate level of blood is 22–25 mmol/L.
- Acidemia is said to be present if pH is less than 7.36. In alkalosis base accumulates in the body; alkalemia is said to be present if pH is more than 7.4.
- Metabolic acidosis is the most common disorder seen in a hospital and occurs due to decrease in HCO_3^- or overproduction of acids (H^+).
- Metabolic alkalosis is characterized by increased plasma levels of HCO_3^-.
- Respiratory acidosis occurs due to interference in gaseous exchange which results in accumulation of CO_2 in the blood which forms carbonic acid (H_2CO_3) and releases H^+ ion.
- Respiratory alkalosis occurs due to primary decrease in $PaCO_2$ caused by rapid respiration.
- The equivalent weight of an ion or a molecule is its atomic or molecular weight in grams divided by its valency. A milliequivalent is one-thousandth of equivalent weight.
- A mole is equal to the quantity of a chemical compound whose weight in grams is equal to its molecular weight. A millimole is one-thousandth of a mole.
- One gram molecular weight of a nonionizable substance is 1 Osm. A milliosmole is one-thousandth of 1 Osm.
- The tonicity of plasma is determined by the solutes which are osmotically active and described as milliosmole per liter. Osmolarity is the osmolar concentration as osmoles per liter of water.
- Na^+ is the major cation of the extracellular fluid while the K^+ is of the intracellular fluid. Cl^- and HCO_3^- are the major anions of the extracellular fluid and the HPO_4^+ is of the intracellular fluid. The total number of cations is equal to the total number of anions.
- The normal sodium level in blood is 135–145 mEq/L. Hyponatremia occurs when the sodium level is below 135 mEq/L, the critical level being less than 125 mEq/L. Hypernatremia occurs when the blood sodium level goes above 145 mEq/L, the critical level being more than 155 mEq/L.
- The normal potassium level in blood is 3.5–5.0 mEq/L. Presence of less than normal potassium in the blood, a level less than 3 mEq/L, is called hypokalemia. Presence of more than normal, 5.0

(CONTD...)

KEY POINTS (...CONTD)

mEq/L, potassium in the blood is called hyperkalemia. Both are dangerous conditions.

- The normal calcium level in the blood is 8.5–10.5 mg/dL. If it falls below 8.5 mg/dL, it is called hypocalcemia and if the blood calcium level goes above 10.5 mg/dL, it is called hypercalcemia.
- Many surgical patients require special care to maintain the nourishment of body because the patient may stop taking food due to disease, or food may not be given due to anesthesia and operation.
- The overall effect of lack of nutrition is loss of body weight which if exceeds more than 30% of initial weight may have fatal consequences.
- Enteral alimentation is when nutrition is administered directly into the stomach, duodenum, or jejunum (enteral) through tubes such as a nasogastric or nasoduodenal tube or through a gastrostomy or jejunostomy tube.
- Complications of enteral alimentation include diarrhea, abdominal distension, and problems connected with tube and nutritional deficiencies.
- Parenteral alimentation is when intravenous route is used to provide nutritional requirements. It is indicated when oral and enteral feeding is not possible. The solutions used here are not thrombogenic.
- In total parenteral nutrition (TPN) all the calorie and nutritional requirements are met with intravenous route. Since these solutions are thrombogenic, they are given through a central venous catheter inserted into the subclavian vein with its tip in superior vena cava.
- The water-soluble vitamins are given daily by infusion. Folic acid and vitamins B_{12}, A, D, and K are given once a week.

SELF-ASSESSMENT

Long answer question

1. Define shock. What are the types, clinical features, and treatment of shock?

Short answer questions

1. Syncope
2. Cardiac arrest
3. pH
4. Acidosis
5. Alkalosis
6. Hypokalemia
7. Hypercalcemia
8. Enteral alimentation
9. Total parenteral nutrition

Multiple choice questions

1. Septic shock is caused by
   (a) Reduction of blood volume
   (b) Severe infection especially with Gram-negative organisms
   (c) Spinal trauma or anesthesia
   (d) Antigen–antibody reaction
2. All of the following facts are true about anaphylaxis, except
   (a) It is caused by antigen–antibody reaction
   (b) It is never fatal
   (c) There is release of histamine which causes peripheral vasodilatation
   (d) The capillary permeability is increased
3. All of the following features are true about hypovolemic shock, except
   (a) It is caused by loss of blood volume
   (b) The cardiac output is reduced
   (c) The central venous pressure is low
   (d) It is mainly treated by corticosteroids
4. All of the following features are correct about cardiogenic shock, except
   (a) It is caused by acute myocardial infarction or cardiac tamponade
   (b) The cardiac output is reduced
   (c) The central venous pressure is high
   (d) It is treated by blood transfusion

(CONTD...)

SELF-ASSESSMENT *(...CONTD)*

5. Vasovagal syncope is caused by
   (a) Inadequate cerebral blood flow
   (b) Inadequate cardiac blood supply
   (c) Pulmonary insufficiency
   (d) Liver dysfunction
6. What is the percentage of water in a normal young man?
   (a) 50% of body mass
   (b) 60% of body mass
   (c) 70% of body mass
   (d) 80% of body mass
7. What is the percentage of water in a normal young woman?
   (a) 51% of body mass
   (b) 61% of body mass
   (c) 71% of body mass
   (d) 81% of body mass
8. What is the percentage of water in the body of a healthy elderly male about 60 years of age?
   (a) 50% of body mass
   (b) 54% of body mass
   (c) 60% of body mass
   (d) 64% of body mass
9. What is the average daily intake of water including the endogenous production in an adult of 70 kg body weight?
   (a) 1500 mL
   (b) 2000 mL
   (c) 2500 mL
   (d) 3000 mL
10. How much water is endogenously produced by oxidation?
   (a) 200 mL
   (b) 300 mL
   (c) 400 mL
   (d) 500 mL
11. On an average how much water is excreted in the urine daily?
   (a) 1000 mL
   (b) 1500 mL
   (c) 2000 mL
   (d) 2500 mL
12. On an average how much water is excreted in the stool daily?
   (a) 100 mL
   (b) 150 mL
   (c) 200 mL
   (d) 250 mL
13. On an average how much water is lost in the exhaled air daily?
   (a) 400 mL
   (b) 500 mL
   (c) 600 mL
   (d) 7030 mL
14. What is the obligatory volume of urine?
   (a) 300 mL
   (b) 400 mL
   (c) 500 mL
   (d) 600 mL
15. What percentage of total body water is intracellular?
   (a) 40%
   (b) 50%
   (c) 60%
   (d) 70%
16. What percentage of total body water is extravascular (interstitial)?
   (a) 55%
   (b) 20%
   (c) 25%
   (d) 30%
17. What percentage of total body water is intravascular?
   (a) 5%
   (b) 10%
   (c) 15%
   (d) 20%
18. What is the normal pH of blood?
   (a) 7
   (b) 7.4
   (c) 8
   (d) 8.4
19. What is the normal pH of water?
   (a) 6
   (b) 6.5
   (c) 7
   (d) 7.5

(CONTD...)

SELF-ASSESSMENT *(...CONTD)*

20. What is the normal bicarbonate level of blood?
    (a) 15–18 mmol/L
    (b) 22–25 mmol/L
    (c) 25–28 mmol/L
    (d) 28–31 mmol/L
21. Acidosis is said to be present when the pH is
    (a) Less than 7
    (b) Less than 7.1
    (c) Less than 7.36
    (d) Less than 7.4
22. Alkalosis is said to be present when the pH is
    (a) Less than 7
    (b) More than 7.1
    (c) More than 7.36
    (d) More than 7.4
23. The major cation in the extracellular fluid is
    (a) Potassium
    (b) Sodium
    (c) Calcium
    (d) Magnesium
24. The major cation in the intracellular fluid is
    (a) Potassium
    (b) Sodium
    (c) Calcium
    (d) Magnesium
25. Hyponatremia is said to occur when serum sodium level is
    (a) Below 130 mmol/L
    (b) Below 135 mmol/L
    (c) Below 140 mAvmol/L
    (d) Below 145 mmol/L
26. Hypernatremia is said to occur when the serum sodium level is
    (a) More than 140 mmol/L
    (b) More than 145 mmol/L
    (c) More than 150 mmol/L
    (d) More than 155 mmol/L
27. What is the normal serum potassium level?
    (a) 3.5–5 mmol/L
    (b) 6–6.5 mmol/L
    (c) 6.5–7.5 mmol/L
    (d) 7.5–8.5 mmol/L
28. Hypokalemia is said to occur when the serum potassium level is
    (a) Less than 3.5 mmol/L
    (b) Less than 4.5 mmol/L
    (c) Less than 5.5 mmol/L
    (d) Less than 6.5 mmol/L
29. Hyperkalemia is said to occur when the serum potassium level is
    (a) More than 4.5 mmol/L
    (b) More than 5.0 mmol/L
    (c) More than 6.5 mmol/L
    (d) More than 7.5 mmol/L
30. The normal serum calcium level is
    (a) 7.5–8.0 mg/dL
    (b) 8.5–10.5 mg/dL
    (c) 10.5–11.5 mg/dL
    (d) 11.5–12.5 mg/dL

Answers

1. (b) 2. (b) 3. (d) 4. (d) 5. (a) 6. (b) 7. (a) 8. (b) 9. (c) 10. (b) 11. (b) 12. (a) 13. (c) 14. (b) 15. (a) 16. (a) 17. (c) 18. (b) 19. (c) 20. (b) 21. (c) 22. (c) 23. (b) 24. (a) 25. (b) 26. (b) 27. (a) 28. (a) 29. (b) 30. (b)

Diseases of Face

15

1. CONGENITAL AND DEVELOPMENTAL DISORDERS

Macrostoma

It is the lateral facial cleft due to failure of fusion of the mandibular and maxillary processes resulting in a large opening of the mouth. Macrostoma may be unilateral or bilateral and may extend up to the pinna. It may be associated with other congenital anomalies, for example, cleft lip, anomalies of ear, lower eyelid coloboma, and hypoplasia or absence of ramus or condyle of mandible or zygoma. The deformity can be corrected by plastic reconstruction.

Microstoma

It is an abnormally small opening of mouth which may be congenital or acquired. The congenital microstoma occurs in association with other congenital anomalies, for example, craniocarpotarsal dysplasia, acro-osteolysis, and Moebius syndrome. The acquired microstoma may occur following burns of face and dystrophic form of epidermolysis bullosa due to scarring. The opening of the mouth can be enlarged and made normal with a plastic procedure.

Labial pits

They are usually bilateral symmetrically placed depressions or papillae which occur at the junction of mucosa and vermilion border of lower lip. They are blind sinuses, 0.5–2.5 cm deep, descending through the muscle of lip to communicate with the underlying minor salivary glands. They probably arise from persistent lateral median grooves in the mandibular arch seen in 10- to 16-mm embryo. Approximately half of the patients of labial pits have an associated cleft lip or palate or both. The pits are excised by an elliptical incision which includes all mucous glands draining into pits.

Macrocheilia

It is the enlargement of lip, the causes of which include Melkersson–Rosenthal syndrome characterized by chronic swelling of lips, recurrent peripheral facial palsy and sometimes fissured tongue, cavernous hemangioma, and lymphangioma. Macrocheilia is treated by removal of the cause and debulking of the lip to restore the shape of the lip.

Oblique facial cleft

It is a very rare congenital anomaly that is almost always associated with a cleft lip or cleft palate. It is considered to be due to failure of fusion of medial nasal, lateral nasal, and maxillary processes. The cleft extends from the upper lip lateral to philtrum along the alar base to the inner canthus. The defect should be corrected by a reconstructive procedure.

Preauricular sinus or pit

It is a developmental defect characterized by the presence of a small opening or pit at the root of the helix or on the tragus.

Pathogenesis The pinna develops from fusion of six tubercles around the external auditory canal. Imperfect fusion of anterior tubercles results in the formation of one or more blind pits in preauricular region.

Clinical Features

- As such, the preauricular sinus is an asymptomatic condition and the patient does not know about it. It is only when the external end of this blind track is obstructed, usually by an epithelial plug, that it may lead to the formation of a cyst.
- It may get infected to form an abscess which may rupture leading to the formation of an ulcer which refuses to heal as the infection is maintained through the sinus.
- The patient presents with local pain, swelling (cyst or abscess), ulceration, and preauricular lymph node enlargement.

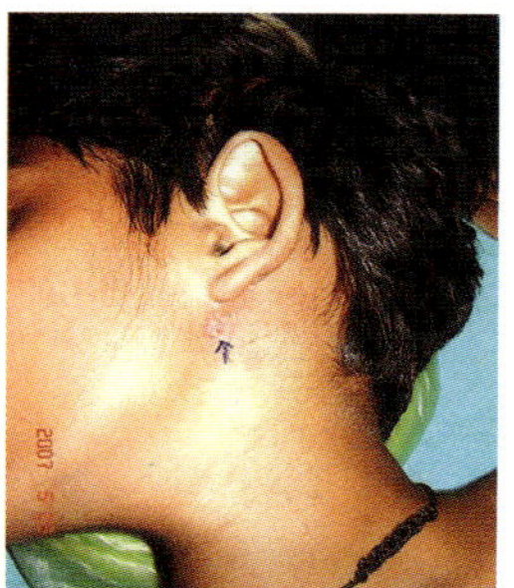

Figure 15.1 Preauricular sinus (left) just below the ear lobule. (Courtesy: Professor Surajit Bhattacharya)

- The opening of the sinus or pit is usually found at the root of the helix, on the tragus, or in the vicinity (Fig. 15.1).
- The track runs downwards and slightly forwards and ends blindly which can be confirmed by passing a nylon suture into the pit.

Treatment A symptomatic sinus is treated by complete excision which gives good results (Figs 15.2 and 15.3).

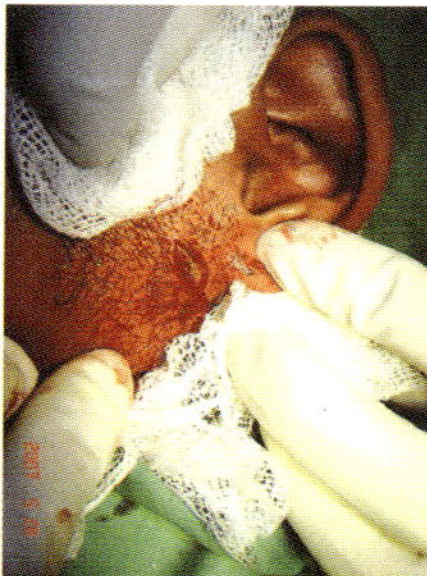

Figure 15.2 Preauricular sinus being excised by a perisinus incision. (Courtesy: Professor Surajit Bhattacharya)

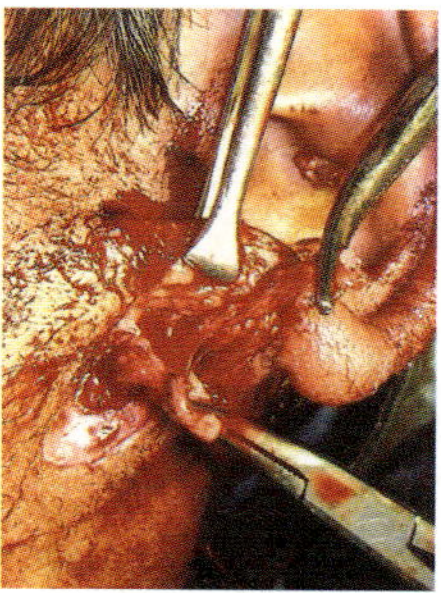

Figure 15.3 Preauricular sinus being mobilized for its excision. (Courtesy: Professor Surajit Bhattacharya)

2. INFLAMMATIONS AND INFECTIONS

Cheilosis

Causes This condition is characterized by moist crusting cracks at the angles of mouth. Angular cheilosis is the most common type of cheilosis, the causes of which are described in Box 15.1.

Box 15.1 Causes of angular cheilosis

It is infection of saliva-moist corners of mouth by *Candida* and staphylococci. The causes of persistent moist angles of mouth are:

- Repeated habitual licking of angles of mouth with tip of tongue (perleche)
- Sagging face and wrinkles of old age
- Deepening of the crease at the angles of mouth in an edentulous person, especially when the atrophy of ridges under the dentures leads to overclosure of mouth
- Sagging of angles of mouth due to loss of canine eminence

Clinical Features It usually occurs in middle-aged and elderly people but may occur in finger-sucking children. The patient presents with crusting cracks at the corners of mouth. There is usually local pain or burning sensation especially at the time of licking when the pale crusts separate with pain.

Treatment The patient is asked not to lick the corners of the mouth. A new denture is provided to elderly edentulous persons to prevent overclosure of jaws.

Local miconazole or clotrimazole cream controls the infection. Any atrophic candidiasis beneath the upper denture should be treated with systemic clotrimazole. With proper treatment, this condition heals without scarring.

Actinic cheilitis

It is chronic inflammation of lips that follows overexposure to sunlight. Actinic cheilitis is characterized by epithelial exfoliation of the lips, especially the lower lip. Small blisters recur at frequent intervals during summer months. Recurrent actinic cheilitis is a precursor of carcinoma of lip. Treatment includes prevention of sun exposure and the use of a sunscreen cream.

Syphilis

Rhagades

- They are multiple cracks at the corners of mouth seen in congenital syphilis.
- The cracks are deep and extend into the corners of mouth opposite to cracks of angular stomatitis which are superficial.
- They heal following antisyphilitic treatment, that is, benzathine penicillin G or tetracycline with local scarring.

Chancre of Upper Lip

- It is a clinical manifestation of primary syphilis which occurs due to transmission of infection (*Treponema pallidum*) by kissing.
- The patient presents with a painless ulcer with a dull red, clean base. It is hard and nontender. The submental and submandibular lymph nodes are significantly enlarged.
- The diagnosis is confirmed by dark-field microscopy of discharge which shows *Spirochaeta*.
- It is cured by antisyphilitic treatment, that is, benzathine penicillin or tetracycline.

Median mental sinus

It is caused by a periodontal abscess where the pus tracks down between two halves of lower jaw to the point of chin. The patient has a discharging sinus just below the chin in the midline. It does not heal following scraping. Radiography shows areas of rarefaction around the roots of lower incisors. It heals following extraction of affected lower incisors.

Carbuncle of face

It occurs commonly on the upper lip and adjacent area called "dangerous area of face" and is characterized by a swelling with pus discharge from multiple orifices.

- **Complications**: If it is pricked, squeezed, or tampered with, the infection may spread along the angular vein to the ophthalmic plexus and thence to cavernous sinus leading to its thrombophlebitis which is a dangerous complication.
- **Treatment:** The patient is given flucloxacillin, co-amoxiclav, or other broad-spectrum antibiotics till the infection comes under control. Hot applications of gauze soaked in a saturated solution of magnesium sulfate are recommended until the slough separates.

Pyogenic granuloma

- **Site**: It is a small inflammatory swelling occurring mostly on those parts of body which are likely to be injured frequently such as hands and face.
- **Pathology**: The recurrent or chronic infection in the wound stimulates the capillary loops to grow vigorously and form a protruding mass of granulation tissue which may be partly covered by epithelium. It may be confused with a hemangioma but the histology shows epidermal collarette.
- **Clinical features**: The patient presents with a small swelling which is bright red in color, bleeds readily on touch, and discharges serous or purulent fluid. It is moist, soft and slightly compressible, and nontender.
- **Treatment**: Following trauma it may break off from its base with slight bleeding but recurs in the next few days. Hence, it should be excised completely with electrocoagulation of its base.

Lupus vulgaris

It is a type of cutaneous tuberculosis of facial skin. Lupus vulgaris usually occurs between the ages 10 and 25.

- **Clinical features:** One or more small nodules appear on the face with congestion of surrounding skin. On applying pressure with a glass slide, the nodules are seen to be of the color of apple jelly (apple jelly granules). As the disease progresses, ulceration occurs which tends to heal in one area and extend in another. The regional lymph nodes are enlarged due to secondary and tuberculous infection.
- **Diagnosis:** The diagnosis can be confirmed by DNA–RNA amplification for tuberculosis in the discharge and biopsy.
- **Treatment:** It is treated by a full course of antituberculous drugs.

3. TUMORS OF FACE

Classification of tumors of face

Tumors are classified as benign and malignant tumors (Box 15.2).

Nevi

They are composed of modified melanocytes derived from neural crest. Nevi have excess melanin pigment; hence, they are tan brown or black in color. They are benign and are of many types.

Junctional Nevus

- **Site**: It is common in infants and located at dermoepidermal junction. It can occur anywhere in the body, but most nevi are seen on the palms, soles, and genitalia.
- **Clinical features**: It appears as a tan-brown to black macule. It is smooth, flat, and hairless. As it enlarges, it becomes slightly raised and

Box 15.2 Classification of tumors of face

Benign tumors
- Nevi
- Papilloma
- Lipoma
- Hemangioma
- Lymphangioma
- Neurofibroma
- Neurilemmoma (Schwannoma)
- Rhinophyma
- Keratoacanthoma

Malignant tumors
- Basal cell carcinoma
- Squamous cell carcinoma
- Malignant melanoma

may evolve into an intradermal or compound nevus. It has very little malignant potential.
- **Treatment**: It does not need any treatment, but if there is any change in the morphology, it should be excised.

Intradermal Nevus
- It can occur anywhere on the body and frequently contains hair.
- Intradermal nevus is typically dome-shaped, sometimes pedunculated, fleshy to a brown pigmented lesion seen in adults.
- Histologically it has melanocytes present in the dermis.
- It rarely turns malignant, hence requires no treatment.

Compound Nevus
- It has microscopic features of both junctional and intradermal nevi.
- Compound nevus is seen in adults, usually elevated, dome shaped, and light brown to dark brown in color.
- If there is no recent change in appearance, no treatment is needed.

Blue Nevus
- It appears in childhood as a slow-growing, well-defined nodule covered by a smooth intact epidermis.
- Blue nevus is a small, sharply defined, round, dark blue or grayish blue lesion that occurs most commonly on face, neck, hands, and arms.
- Histologically the melanocytes are limited to dermis intimately associated with fibroblasts. This together with extension of melanocytes deep into dermis may account for blue color.
- It does not need any treatment unless the patient wants its removal for cosmesis or for cancer phobia.

Giant Hairy Nevus
- It is a congenital lesion which can occur anywhere in the body and may be very large and may cover the entire trunk (bathing trunk nevus).
- Giant hairy nevus may turn into a malignant melanoma and may be associated with neurofibromas or melanocytic involvement of leptomeninges.
- Histologically it may have all the features of intradermal and compound nevi.
- Treatment is excision and skin grafting.

Papilloma

It is a benign tumor arising from skin or mucous membrane. Papilloma is etiologically related to human papillomavirus. It can occur in head and neck region, oral cavity, larynx, and other places. It is characterized by small finger-like projections having a central core of connective tissue, blood vessels, lymphatics, and nerve fibers, thus looks like a small tree. Treatment of a papilloma is excision.

Lipoma

It is a benign tumor of fatty tissue, the cause of which is not known.

Site It is a common tumor and can occur anywhere in the body where fat is found.

Types Depending on its site, it is of many types: subcutaneous, subfascial, subsynovial, intra-articular, intermuscular, parosteal, subserous, submucous, extradural, and intraglandular.

Clinical Features Subcutaneous lipoma is the commonest type. It is a painless, slow-growing swelling of insidious onset. It is smooth or lobulated and soft. It has a definite edge which slips under the finger. A subcutaneous lipoma may become pedunculated.

Diagnosis A subcutaneous lipoma can be easily diagnosed clinically. Other lipomas are diagnosed by imaging methods, that is, ultrasound, CT scan, or MRI.

Complications The complications of a lipoma include malignant transformation into a liposarcoma, myxomatous degeneration, and calcification. They are rare.

Treatment A symptomatic lipoma is excised surgically. It may be treated by liposuction, but then the chances of recurrence are more.

Hemangioma

It is a benign tumor of blood vessels which shows cellular endothelial hyperplasia with increased mast cells. Hemangioma is of two types: capillary hemangioma and cavernous hemangioma.

Capillary Hemangioma

It is of three types: salmon patch (stork bite), strawberry hemangioma, and port-wine stain (nevus flammeus).

Salmon Patch It presents at birth and occurs on nape of neck, scalp, and limbs. Salmon patch involves a wide area and occurs due to persistent fetal circulation. It usually disappears by itself completely in 1 year and usually does not require any treatment.

Strawberry Hemangioma

- It is the most common hemangioma and commonly occurs in head and neck region.
- Strawberry hemangioma may be present at birth or 1–3 weeks after birth and appears as a red mark which rapidly increases in size for 3 months. It is bluish, warm, and compressible. It begins to regress after 1 year of age and disappears completely in 7–8 years.
- It disappears spontaneously and usually does not require any treatment. The indications for surgery include uncontrolled growth, functional impairment of vision and hearing, and accidental hemorrhage.

Port-Wine Stain

- It is present at birth and persists throughout life. It is a smooth, flat, reddish blue/intensely purple area which is commonly seen in head, neck, and face in the maxillary and mandibular dermatomes of the fifth cranial nerve.
- A port-wine stain is difficult to treat. The treatment measures include laser (pulsed dye/diode), excision and grafting, and cosmetic coverage.

Cavernous Hemangioma

- It consists of large, thin-walled venous channels. It occurs in head, neck, face (Fig. 15.4), tongue, liver, and other regions.
- Cavernous hemangioma presents as a bluish red, smooth, soft, warm, compressible, nonpulsatile, and opaque swelling in the skin, subcutaneous tissue, and mucosa.
- It can be imaged by ultrasound, Doppler, and MRI (MR angiography).
- The main complications of a hemangioma are rupture and bleeding.
- The treatment methods include sclerotherapy with tetradecyl sulfate/hypertonic saline and

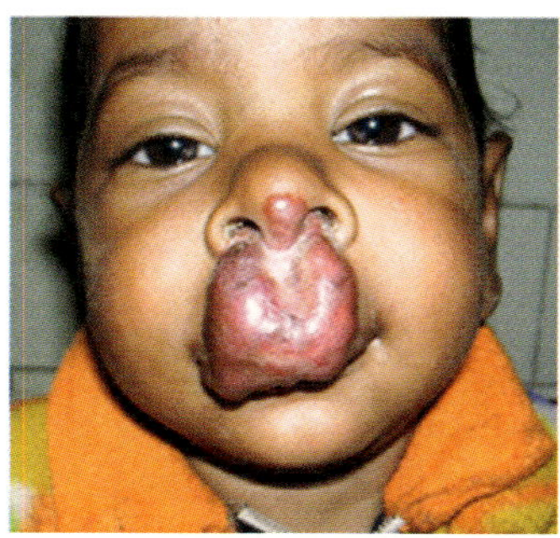

Figure 15.4 Hemangioma of upper lip and tip of nose. (Courtesy: Professor J.D. Rawat)

ligation of feeding artery followed by excision, therapeutic embolization, excision, and laser ablation.

Lymphangioma

It is a lymphatic malformation that is a benign, multilobular, multinodular cystic mass having multiple spaces lined by endothelial cells. Lymphangioma commonly affects face, lips (macrocheilia), and tongue (macroglossia). It is soft, nontender, and translucent. It may be excised to improve cosmesis and function.

Neurofibroma

It is a benign tumor of connective tissue of nerve sheath. It is of many types.

Solitary Neurofibroma It presents as a single, smooth, firm, and often tender swelling that can be moved across but not along the course of the nerve from which it is arising. There may be pain and hyperesthesia in the distribution of affected nerve.

Generalized Neurofibromatosis (von Recklinghausen's Disease) It is an inherited autosomal dominant disease characterized by multiple neurofibromas in the body associated with pigmented spots (café au lait). It may be associated with MEN type IIb syndrome.

Plexiform Neurofibromatosis It is characterized by thickening of skin which hangs down. It commonly occurs along the distribution of the fifth cranial nerve.

Pachydermatocele It is a variant of plexiform neurofibroma involving the neck and characterized by hanging thickened skin folds.

Elephantiasis Neurofibromatosa It is a congenital lesion of skin of limbs which is markedly thickened, dry, and coarse.

Treatment of Neurofibromas A localized symptomatic neurofibroma is excised which may be difficult and associated with some neurological deficit. The plexiform-type lesions are excised to improve cosmesis.

Neurilemmoma (schwannoma)

It is a benign tumor arising from Schwann cells. Neurilemmoma commonly affects the acoustic (eighth cranial) nerve but can arise from peripheral nerves. It is soft, lobulated, and well encapsulated, hence can be excised without damage to nerve fibers.

Keratoacanthoma (molluscum sebaceum)

It is a benign lesion but when fully developed may look like a carcinoma.

Etiology Its etiology is not known exactly but it may be caused by papillomavirus infecting a hair follicle during the anagen phase of the growth cycle. It has also been associated with smoking and chemical carcinogen exposure.

Clinical Features It is twice more common in men and usually occurs on the face of 50- to 70-year-olds. It commences as a tiny painless papule which grows rapidly to 1–3 cm size in about 6 weeks when it presents as a cup-shaped swelling that has symmetry about its middle. The central crater is filled with a plug of keratin (Fig. 15.5). After attaining full size, it resolves spontaneously within subsequent 6 months. Removal of central keratin plug may speed up resolution.

Treatment Although it resolves spontaneously, excision should be done as the differential diagnosis includes an anaplastic squamous cell carcinoma (SCC) and the scar of excision is better than the scar of spontaneous resolution.

Basal cell carcinoma (BCC)

It is a slow-growing locally invasive tumor of basal cell layer of skin and hair follicles, hence affects the pilosebaceous skin. It does not arise from mucosa.

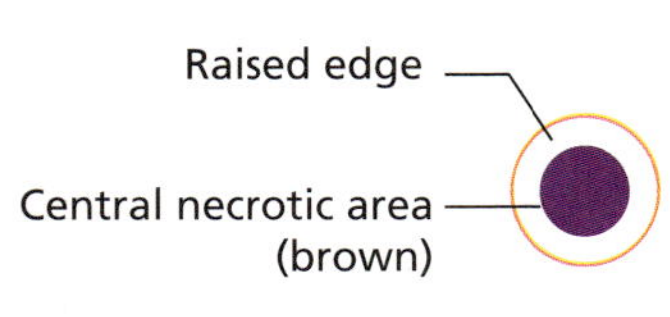

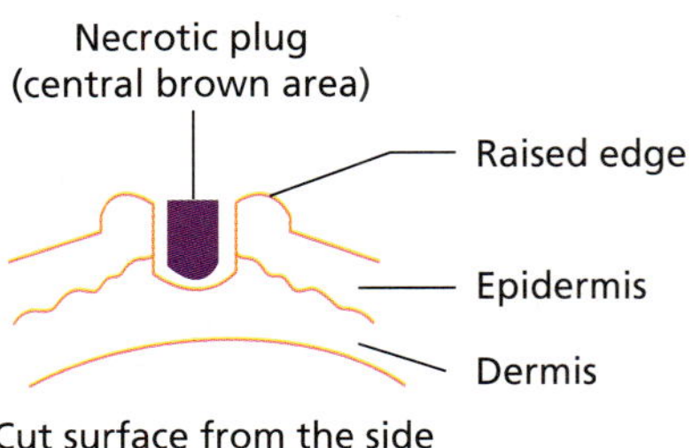

Figure 15.5 Keratoacanthoma.

Etiology

The etiology is not very clear. It is very common in certain parts of Australia where the sunlight is very bright, especially in fair-skinned people. Hence, etiologically it is related to actinic exposure. Other predisposing factors are exposure to arsenical compounds, coal tar, and aromatic hydrocarbons.

Clinical Features

The patient is usually a middle-aged or elderly person, more commonly a male who presents with this lesion on the face above the line joining the corner of mouth with the ear lobule (Fig. 15.6), in the area where the tears roll down ("tear cancer").

The signs of this cancer depend on its type.

Rodent Ulcer It is the most common presentation. The ulcer is characterized by a raised and beaded edge with induration. It bleeds on touch. It gradually destroys muscle, cartilage, and bone or whatever comes in its way (gnaws the tissues like a rodent, hence called rodent ulcer) and produces ghastly disfigurement. It does not metastasize.

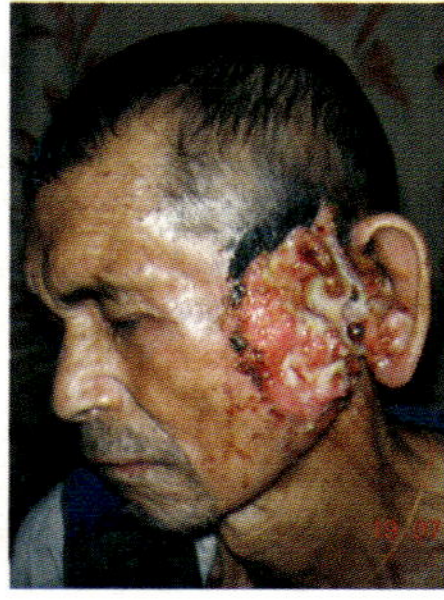

Figure 15.6 A large basal cell carcinoma—"field-fire" ulcer of left parotid region in an elderly male. (Courtesy: Professor Sandeep Kumar)

Nodulocystic Type It may present as a painless, firm, pearly nodule which is pigmented with fine vessels on its surface.

"Field-Fire" Ulcer It has an advancing active edge, with an inactive center which appears as if it is healing but not healing.

Diagnosis

Biopsy from the edge confirms the diagnosis. It is taken from the edge because of the following reasons:

- The edge is the growing part which has numerous cells.
- The center of the lesion has slough or scab which may not reveal malignancy.

Treatment

It is treated by a variety of methods.

Radiotherapy It is a radiosensitive tumor; hence, it can be treated by radiotherapy, the dose being 4000–6000 cGy. It is given if it is well away from eyes and not invading bone or cartilage.

Surgery The lesion is excised 1 cm beyond the margin of tumor as assessed and marked under loupe magnification and the excised tissue is sent for confirmation of cancer-clear margin. The resulting defect is closed by suturing, skin grafting, or rotation flaps.

Mohs Micrographic Surgery

- It is done by a dermatologist trained in the technique of cutaneous surgery and histopathology.
- In this method the tumor is excised under microscopic control to minimize recurrence

rates and maximize conservation of surrounding normal tissues. Hence, it is used to treat tumors close to eyes, nose, or ear. It is also used to treat SCC, dermatofibrosarcoma protuberans, and lentigo maligna.

- It is done under local anesthesia and involves an initial "saucerizing excision" of visible primary tumor which is then marked and oriented using different-colored stains in different quadrants.
- The complete excision of the tumor is confirmed in all directions histologically. Hence, further excision of residual tumor may be required from the mapped defect. In experienced hands, complete excision rates exceed 99%.

Treatment of Superficial Tumors Superficial tumors can be treated with topical 5-fluorouracil or imiquimod or cryotherapy.

Prognosis Out of all the three cancer of the face—BCC, SCC, and melanoma—it has the best prognosis (and melanoma has the worst).

Squamous cell carcinoma

It is the second most common skin cancer and four times less common than BCC. SCC is a malignant tumor of keratinizing cells of epidermis or its appendages. It also arises from stratum basale of skin. It expresses cytokeratins 1 and 10.

Etiology

It is strongly related to cumulative sun exposure. It frequently occurs in premalignant conditions of skin such as Bowen's disease, Paget's disease, leukoplakia, radiodermatitis, senile keratosis, chronic chemical irritation, chronic thermal irritation (kangri cancer) and xeroderma pigmentosa, chronic osteomyelitic sinus tract, preexisting scars, infection with HPV5 and HPV16, and immunosuppression.

Clinical Features

- It usually affects elderly people, more commonly a male.

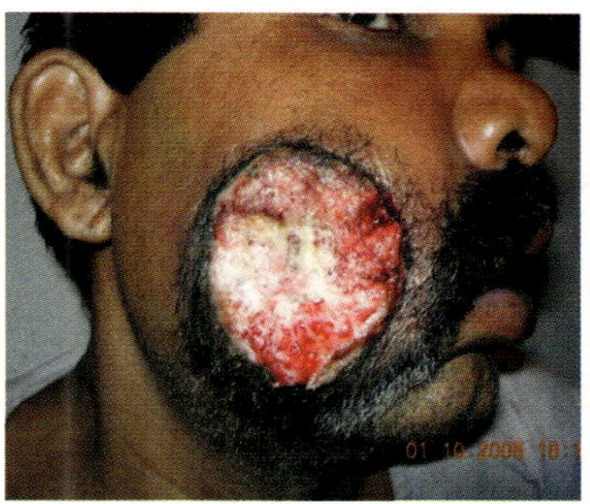

Figure 15.7 Squamous cell carcinoma of face. (Courtesy: Professor Sandeep Kumar)

- The common sites include dorsum of hand, limbs, face, and skin of abdominal wall. It can also affect external genitalia, mucocutaneous junctions, oral cavity, and anal canal.
- The early gross appearance of this tumor varies from a smooth nodular to verrucous, papillomatous, and ulcerating lesion, but all types eventually ulcerate and have an everted edge and are surrounded by inflamed indurated skin.
- The patient presents with a nonhealing ulcer or ulcerated swelling (Fig. 15.7). It is irregular in shape, and has an everted edge and indurated base. It may get fixed to the underlying structures as time passes.
- The regional lymph nodes are commonly involved and are hard and mobile or fixed.

Histopathology

Microscopically it shows whorls of squamous cells with epithelial or keratin pearls. Broder has described four grades of this tumor given in Box 15.3.

Box 15.3 Broder's histological grading

- **Grade I**: Well differentiated, 75% or more keratin pearls
- **Grade II**: Moderately differentiated, 50–75% keratin pearls
- **Grade III**: Poorly differentiated, 25–50% keratin pearls
- **Grade IV**: Undifferentiated/anaplastic, <25% keratin pearls

Diagnosis

- The diagnosis is confirmed by biopsy from the edge. During histopathological scrutiny, one should see the pathological pattern, cellular morphology, Broder's grade, depth of invasion, and perineural or vascular invasion.
- FNAC of palpable lymph nodes is done. Nonpalpable lymph nodes may be studied by sentinel node biopsy (SNB), if indicated.

Staging of SCC (Box 15.4)

The staging of the tumor is done to plan the treatment and to tell the prognosis.

Box 15.4 Staging of SCC

- **TNM staging**
  - *T1*: <2 cm
  - *T2*: 2–5 cm
  - *T3*: >5 cm
  - *T4*: Muscle or bony invasion
  - *N0*: No lymph node metastasis
  - *N1*: Positive regional lymph nodes
  - *M0*: No distant metastasis
  - *M1*: Distant metastasis present
- **Clinical staging**
  - *Stage I*: $T_1N_0M_0$
  - *Stage II*: $T_{2-3}N_0M_0$
  - *Stage III*: $T_4N_0M_0$, any TN_1M_0
  - *Stage IV*: Any TN_1M_1
- **Histological grading**
  - *G1*: Low grade
  - *G2*: Moderately differentiated
  - *G3*: High grade or highly anaplastic

Treatment

Surgery Wide excision is the treatment of choice. The margin of excision should be assessed by loupe magnification. A 4-mm clearance margin should be achieved if the lesion measures <2 cm across and a 1-cm clearance margin if it measures >2 cm.

Radiotherapy This tumor is radiosensitive and is treated by a variety of techniques, for example, needles, wire, or molds. A dose of 6000 cGy units over 6 weeks (5 days a week) is given. Radiorecurrent tumors are excised.

Chemotherapy Chemotherapy as such is not curative, but methotrexate, vincristine, and bleomycin can be used with other methods of treatment with advantage.

Neck Dissection Mobile involved lymph nodes are treated with block dissection.

Palliative Treatment Advanced disease with fixed lymph nodes is treated with palliative external beam radiotherapy.

Prognosis

Ninety-five percent of recurrences occur within 5 years of treatment; hence, follow-up beyond this period is not required. Poor prognostic factors of SCC are described in Box 15.5.

Box 15.5 Poor prognostic factors in SCC

- Tumor >2 cm
- Ill-defined border
- Associated immunosuppression
- Poor differentiation
- Perineural invasion
- Deeper invasion >6 mm
- Carcinoma of ear

Variants of Squamous Cell Carcinoma

Verrucous Carcinoma It is a type of SCC characterized by dry, exophytic, and warty growth. Verrucous carcinoma does not spread. It is treated by wide excision. Radiotherapy should not be given. One example of this tumor is Buschke–Lowenstein tumor of external genitalia.

Marjolin's Ulcer It is a SCC which occurs in old scars of burns or on a venous ulcer. Marjolin's ulcer does not spread till it is limited within the scar as the scar does not have lymphatics. As it grows beyond the scar, it may spread to regional lymph nodes. It is treated by wide excision. A large ulcer of a limb may require amputation. Radiotherapy should never be given to this lesion as it may turn it into a poorly differentiated SCC.

Carcinoma of lip

It is an epithelial malignant tumor of lips of unknown etiology characterized by an irregular ulcer or ulcerated mass. It is one of the common head and neck cancers.

Etiology

It is etiologically related to tobacco chewing, smoking, and actinic exposure. Many patients have a hyperkeratotic or leukoplakic patch on the lips.

Pathology

Histologically it is a SCC in 90% of patients, but in the upper lip the most common cancer is BCC. Most of the SCCs are well differentiated.

Clinical Features

- **Age**: Majority of patients are middle-aged and elderly (50–80 years) men.
- **Site**: Most of the cancers occur on the lower lip near the vermilion border (90–95%) and less often on the upper lip (2–7%) and commissures (1%).
- **Clinical presentation**: It may be an ulcerative or proliferative lesion, ulcer being the most common presentation. The ulcer initially may have repeated crusting or scabbing followed by necrosis. It is irregular and indurated, and has an everted edge (Figs 15.8 and 15.9). The submental lymph nodes may be enlarged. In lesions near the angle, the preauricular and submandibular lymph nodes may be enlarged.

Diagnosis

The diagnosis is confirmed by (incisional) biopsy. FNAC of enlarged lymph nodes may be done to find their involvement.

Treatment

Surgical Excision/Radiotherapy Early lesions (T_1) are treated by surgical excision or radiotherapy with equal success. The excision requires at least 3 mm of cancer-free margin.

Management of Lymph Node Involvement Supraomohyoid neck dissection is performed for tumors with clinically negative necks but with deeper primary invasion or size larger than 3 cm. In clinically evident nodal involvement, neck dissection with postoperative radiotherapy is the treatment of choice.

Reconstruction of Lips The lip needs reconstruction after surgery.

- The aims of reconstruction include reinstitution of oral competence, cosmesis, and maintenance of dynamic function while allowing adequate access for oral hygiene.

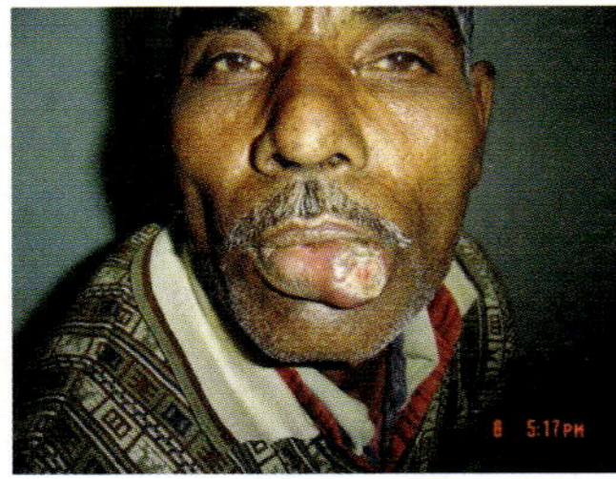

Figure 15.8 Carcinoma of lower lip in an elderly male. (Courtesy: Professor Surajit Bhattacharya)

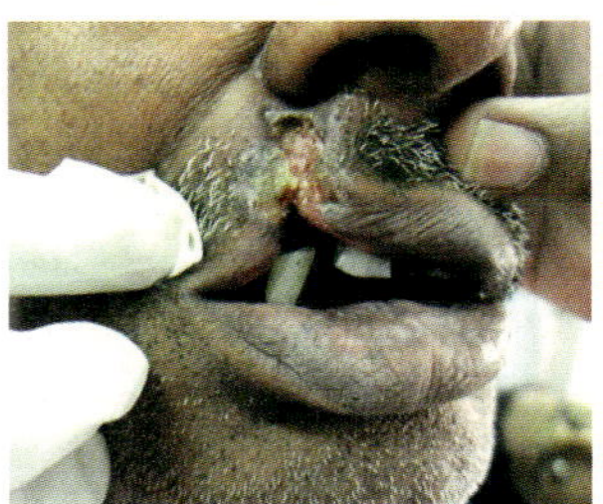

Figure 15.9 Carcinoma of upper lip with a fissure-type lesion. (Courtesy: Dr. A.C. Dwivedi)

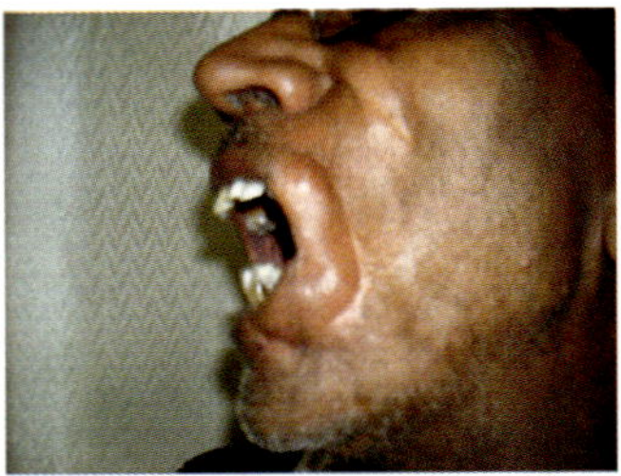

Figure 15.10 Carcinoma of lower lip after excision and repair with a flap. (Courtesy: Professor Surajit Bhattacharya)

- Half of the lip can be removed and then can be closed primarily, especially the lower lip which has excessive tissue than the upper lip. Care is taken to achieve accurate approximation of white line on either side of the defect at the vermilion border.
- Larger defects, more than half of lip, require reconstruction with Abbe-Estlander rotation flap located at the angle based on labial artery (Fig. 15.10). Reconstruction can be done with a free flap using microvascular technique.

Prognosis

The overall 5-year cure rate of 90% drops to 50% if the cervical nodes are involved.

Malignant melanoma

It is a malignant tumor of melanocytes that usually arises in the skin, but it can occur at other places where melanocytes exist, for example, bowel mucosa, retina, and leptomeninges.

Etiology

Exposure to sunlight (ultraviolet rays) is the main etiological factor especially in white-skinned races that are not suited to sun exposure. The risk factors include xeroderma pigmentosum, albinism, junctional nevus, dysplastic nevi, immunosuppression, and history of melanoma. Macroscopic features that suggest malignant change in a preexisting nevus are described in Box 15.6.

Box 15.6 Macroscopic features suggestive of malignant change in a preexisting nevus

- Change in size, shape, color, surface (nodularity or ulceration)
- Appearance of satellite lesions
- Tingling/itching/serosanguinous discharge
- Doppler-positive (blood supply) pigmented lesion

Methods of Spread

- **Lymphatic spread** occurs to regional lymph nodes by either permeation or embolism. In-transit satellite nodules are seen in the skin between the primary tumor and the regional lymph node region. It is due to **retrograde spread** into dermal lymphatics.
- **Hematogenous spread** occurs to lungs, liver, brain, skin, and bones. The metastases are typically black. The secondaries in liver produce a huge liver with excretion of melanin in urine (melanuria).

Clinical Features

It may start as a preexisting nevus (50–60%) or de novo cancer in normal skin (40–50%). It is unknown before puberty. The patient presents with ulceration, pigmentation, and bleeding. The lesion is irregular in surface and outline but has no induration. There are many types of malignant melanoma which have their own clinical features.

Types of Malignant Melanoma

Superficial Spreading Melanoma It is the most common type (64–70%) and most likely to arise in a preexisting nevus with a variegated irregular look. Superficial spreading melanoma has more radial growth and better prognosis. Nodularity in this lesion heralds the onset of vertical growth phase.

Nodular Melanoma It usually arises de novo, more commonly in men than in women, often in middle ages, and usually on the trunk, head, or

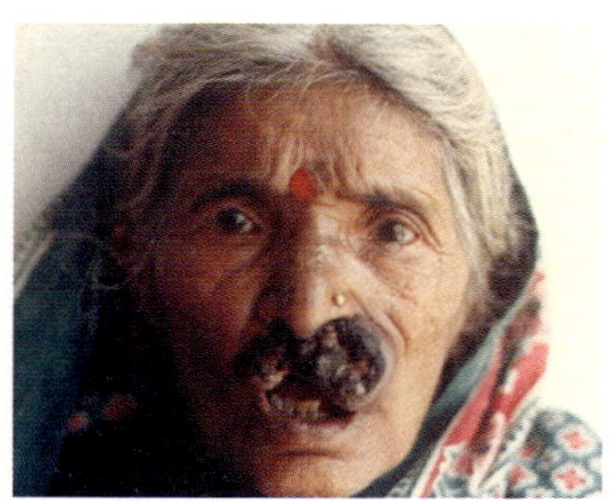

Figure 15.11 Malignant melanoma of the upper lip. (Courtesy: Professor Surajit Bhattacharya)

neck. Nodular melanoma appears as blue-black papules 1–2 cm in diameter. It lacks horizontal growth phase; hence, it is sharply demarcated.

Lentigo Maligna Melanoma It presents as a slow-growing, variegated brown macule (a lentigo) on the face, neck, or hands of elderly patients, more commonly women (Fig. 15.11). Lentigo maligna melanoma is related to prolonged intense sun exposure. It accounts for 5–10% of malignant melanomas. This tumor takes a longer period to enter in vertical growth phase when its metastatic potential is the same as other types of melanoma.

Acral Lentiginous Melanoma It affects the soles of feet and palms of hands and presents as a flat, irregular macule in later life. It is rare in whites but common in Asian people. Twenty-five percent of these lesions are amelanotic and may look like fungal infection or a pyogenic granuloma.

Subungual Melanoma It is usually a superficial spreading melanoma rather than an acral lentiginous melanoma. The classical sign of this lesion is Hutchinson's sign, that is, nail-fold pigmentation that widens progressively to produce a triangular pigmented macule with associated nail dystrophy. To confirm the diagnosis, it is important to biopsy the nail matrix rather than just the pigment on the nail plate.

Amelanotic Melanoma It is not pigmented, hence may be difficult to diagnose clinically.

Desmoplastic Melanoma It is also amelanotic, mostly occurs in head and neck region, and has a propensity for perineural invasion and local recurrence.

Histopathology

The malignant change is characterized by atypical melanocytes in the basal epidermis. In an in situ melanoma the atypical melanocytes remain at dermoepidermal junction without dermal involvement. Further growth of the lesion occurs in two phases.

Horizontal Growth Phase The cells spread along the dermoepidermal junction. They may breach the dermis but their migration is predominantly radial.

Vertical Growth Phase The dermis is invaded as the cells spread into the depth. The greater the depth of invasion, the greater is the metastatic potential of the tumor.

Investigations

Biopsy For confirming the diagnosis an excision biopsy with a 2-mm margin of skin and a cuff of subdermal fat is done. In a large lesion of face, however, an incisional biopsy can be done.

- **Breslow's depth:** The Breslow's thickness of the lesion can be measured by optical micrometer to nearest 0.1 mm from granular layer to the base of the tumor as described in Box 15.7. It is the most important prognostic variable.
- **Clark's level of anatomic invasion**: Clark has described five levels of invasion of melanoma in the skin as described in Box 15.8. The higher levels have worsening prognostic implications.

Box 15.7 Breslow's depth in malignant melanoma—prognostic indicator

- **I**: Less than 0.75 mm
- **II**: Between 0.76 and 1.50 mm
- **III**: Between 1.51 and 4.00 mm
- **IV**: More than 4.00 mm

- **Other investigations**: They include FNAC of palpable lymph nodes, SNB of impalpable nodes, ultrasound of the abdomen to find liver metastases, and X-ray of chest for pulmonary metastases.

Box 15.8 Clark's levels of invasion in melanoma

- **Level 1**: Tumor is confined to epidermis limited by basement membrane
- **Level 2**: Tumor extends into papillary dermis
- **Level 3**: Tumor reaches the interface between papillary dermis and reticular dermis
- **Level 4**: Tumor extends into reticular dermis
- **Level 5**: Tumor extends into subcutaneous fat

TNM Staging of Melanoma

TNM staging of malignant melanoma is described in Box 15.9.

Treatment

Surgery Surgical excision is the main method of treatment.

- Lentigo maligna (melanoma in situ) is excised with a 5-mm margin to prevent its entry into vertical growth phase when it will become lentigo maligna melanoma.
- Other melanomas: A tumor <1 mm deep is excised with a 1-cm margin. For deeper tumors a 2-cm margin is adequate as a margin wider than this is of no benefit.
- In tumors of extremities, if the primary area is wide, it is better to do amputation one joint above the lesion. In tumors of fingers and toes, disarticulation is required.

Treatment of Regional Lymph Nodes Clinically evident metastases are treated by block excision of lymph nodes. If the lymph nodes are not palpable, their involvement is found by SNB which is based on the hypothesis that the lymphatic metastases proceed as orderly processes which can be predicted by mapping the lymphatic drainage from the primary tumor to the first or sentinel node in the regional lymph nodes. There is hardly any benefit in doing SNB if the primary tumor is less than 1 mm because if it is <1.25 mm, only 4% of SNBs are likely to be positive.

Adjuvant Therapy Interferon alpha-2b is given intravenously in the maximally tolerated dose for 1 month followed by 11 months of subcutaneous injections three times weekly. The adverse effects include flu-like symptoms, fatigue, malaise, anorexia, neuropsychiatric side effects, and potential hepatotoxicity. It may prolong the time of recurrence but is unlikely to cure.

Box 15.9 TNM staging of melanoma

T: Tumor size

- **T1:** ≤1.0 mm
  - *T1a*: Without ulceration and mitosis <1/mm^2
  - *T1b*: With ulceration or mitoses ≥1 mm^2
- **T2:** 1.01–2.0 mm
  - *T2a*: Without ulceration
  - *T2b*: With ulceration
- **T3:** 2.01–4.0 mm
  - *T3a*: Without ulceration
  - *T3b*: With ulceration
- **T4:** >4.00 mm
  - *T4a*: Without ulceration
  - *T4b*: With ulceration

N: Node involvement

- **N1:** One node
  - *N1a*: Micrometastasis (after SNB)
  - *N1b*: Macrometastasis
- **N2**: Two or three nodes
  - *N2a*: Micrometastasis
  - *N2b*: Macrometastasis
  - *N2c*: In-transit metastasis(s)/satellite(s) without metastatic nodes
- **N3**: Four or more metastatic nodes or matted nodes, or in-transit metastasis/satellite(s) with metastatic node(s)

M: Metastasis

- **M1a**: Distant skin, subcutaneous, or nodal metastasis, LDH normal
- **M1b:** Lung metastasis, LDH normal
- **M1c:**
  - All other visceral metastasis, LDH normal
  - Any distant metastasis, LDH elevated

LDH, lactate dehydrogenase; *SNB*, sentinel node biopsy.

Radiation Therapy Melanoma is generally considered as relatively radioresistant. Hence, it is not irradiated routinely. It may be given in high-risk head and neck melanomas.

Prognosis

It is the worst tumor out of the three cancers of the face. The prognosis depends mainly on its vertical growth; the more the depth, the worse is the prognosis (Table 15.1).

Table 15.1 Five-year survival rates of malignant melanoma

Tumor depth (mm)	Five-year survivals (%)
<1.0	95–100
1.1–2.0	80–90
2.1–4.0	60–75
>4.0	50

The differences between the three malignant tumors of skin are described in Table 15.2.

Table 15.2 Differences between squamous cell carcinoma, basal cell carcinoma, and malignant melanoma

Features	Squamous cell carcinoma	Basal cell carcinoma	Malignant melanoma
Origin	Prickle cell layer of skin	Basal cell layer of skin	Pigment-forming cells (melanoblasts derived from neural crest)
Incidence	Common, 20–30%	Most common, 60–70%	10–20%
Etiology	Chronic irritation, ultraviolet light	Ultraviolet exposure, fair skin	Ultraviolet exposure, fair skin, preexisting mole
Sites of occurrence	Dorsum of hand, limbs, face, abdomen, oral cavity, penis	Part of the face above the line joining the lobule of ear with angle of mouth	Head and neck, face, digits, palm, and sole
Gross types	• Ulcerative or proliferative (cauliflower type) • Marjolin's ulcer	Nodular or ulcerative	Nodular or ulcerative
Edge	Everted	Raised and beaded	Irregular
Induration	Maximum	Moderate	Minimum
Scabbing	Never occurs	Occurs	Never occurs
Pigmentatum	Absent	Absent	Present in 90% of patients
Spread	• Mainly by lymphatics • Local invasion • Hematogenous spread is rare	• Spreads locally • Does not spread by lymphatics • Hematogenous spread is very rare	Mainly by lymphatics, also by bloodstream
Treatment	• Surgery is the most effective method of treatment • Radiotherapy is equally effective	Surgery and radiotherapy are equally effective	Surgery is the main modality of treatment

4. CYSTS

Labial retention cyst (mucocele)

It is a small cyst containing thick mucoid material. Labial retention cyst usually occurs in the lower lip and presents as a small, hemispherical, and translucent swelling (Fig. 15.12). It is usually caused by biting lips between anterior teeth resulting in damage to the duct of minor salivary glands of lips. It should be excised.

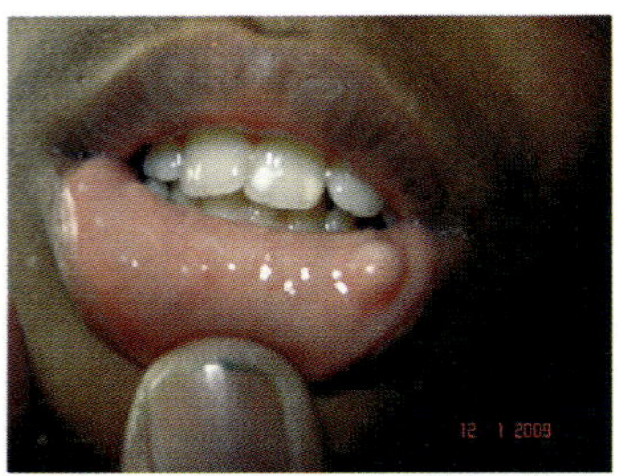

Figure 15.12 Mucus retention cyst of lower lip.

Periauricular dermoid cyst

It usually develops from inclusion of epithelium during fusion of two contiguous aural tubercles. The patient presents with a cystic swelling behind the pinna which is ovoid, soft, and nontender, and may be indented by a finger. Treatment is excision.

Periorbital cystic swellings

Sebaceous Cyst

It can occur anywhere on the face as a painless slow-growing hemispherical swelling. It usually has a small black dot on the top in the center (punctum). It is soft, nontender, and opaque. It is treated by excision (Fig. 15.13).

Lateral Angular Dermoid

It is one of the commonest types of dermoid cyst of head and neck region. The patient presents with a painless, slow-growing swelling at the lateral part of eyebrow. Lateral angular dermoid is smooth, soft, cystic, and not fixed to overlying skin. It may be indented by digital pressure. It is situated in a saucer-shaped depression of bone. It may have an intracranial extension which can be found by CT scan. It is excised.

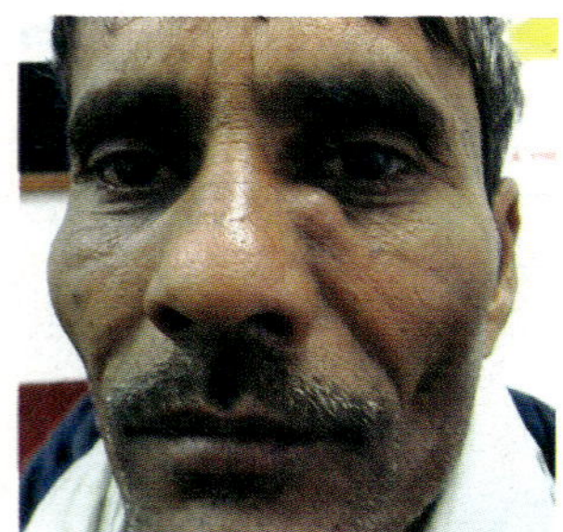

Figure 15.13 Sebaceous cyst of face in a middle-aged male.

Meibomian Cyst (Chalazion)

It is a retention cyst of Meibomian gland. It occurs in the upper eyelid and presents as a small swelling firm to hard in consistency, nontender, and slightly away from lid margin. Meibomian cyst is evacuated by a small incision on the lesion on the conjunctival surface.

Hordeolum Externum (Stye)

It is a small swelling of the eyelid due to infection of an eyelash follicle (Zeis gland). Hordeolum externum presents as a red, hard, and tender swelling of lid margin associated with marked edema. It is drained by pulling out the related hair.

Mucocele of Lacrimal Sac

The patient presents with a cystic swelling near the medial canthus of the eye. It is smooth, soft, and cystic and when pressed mucoid discharge fills up the medial canthus and the swelling becomes flat. It is treated by probing and syringing the lower lacrimal canaliculus so that the obstruction is relieved.

Cysts of root of nose

Dermoid Cyst

The patient presents with a painless, slow-growing swelling at the root of nose in midline. The swelling is cystic, nontender, and opaque, and does not empty on pressure. It is treated by excision.

Meningocele (Frontonasal)

The patient is a neonate or a child who presents with a transilluminant swelling at the root of the nose in midline. It may reduce slightly on pressure. It becomes tense when the child cries (Fig. 15.14).

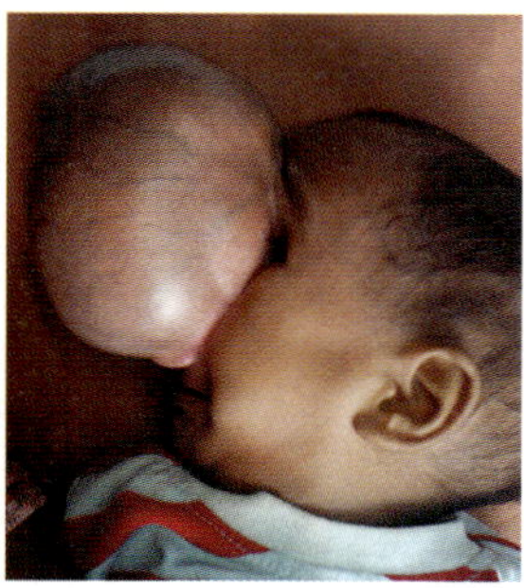

Figure 15.14 Frontonasal meningocele. (Courtesy: Professor J.D. Rawat)

Mucocele of Frontal Sinus or Ethmoid Cells

The patient has a soft, nontender, and translucent swelling at the root of nose above the medial part of the eye. X-ray may reveal clouding of the sinus with loss of scalloping outline which is so typical of frontal sinus. The ethmoidal sinuses can be imaged by CT scan. It is not strictly in midline. It is treated by frontoethmoidectomy with drainage of sinus into middle meatus of nose.

KEY POINTS

- The congenital and developmental defects of the face include macrostoma (large opening of mouth), microstoma (small opening of mouth), macrocheilia (large lip), labial pits, oblique facial cleft, and preauricular sinus. They usually require surgical treatment.
- A labial retention cyst (mucocele) is usually caused due to trauma to minor salivary glands in the lower lip and contains thick mucoid material.
- Angular cheilosis is characterized by moist crusting cracks at the angles of mouth which are infected by *Candida* and staphylococci.
- Actinic cheilitis is chronic inflammation of lips that follows overexposure to sunlight. Recurrent actinic cheilitis is a precursor of carcinoma of lip.
- Rhagades are multiple cracks at the corners of mouth seen in congenital syphilis. Chancre of upper lip is a clinical manifestation of primary syphilis which occurs due to transmission of infection *(Treponema pallidum)* by kissing.
- Squamous cell carcinoma (SCC) of lips is etiologically related to smoking and actinic exposure. It is characterized by an irregular ulcer. The treatment includes surgical excision, neck dissection in the presence of nodal involvement, and reconstruction with flap such as Abbe-Estlander flap.
- A dermoid cyst on face can occur at lateral angle of eye, behind the pinna, and at the roof of the nose.
- Medial mental sinus is caused by a periodontal abscess where the pus tracks down between two halves of lower jaw to the point of chin.
- Carbuncle of face commonly occurs on the upper lip and adjacent area called "dangerous area of face." If it is pricked or squeezed, it may result in cavernous sinus thrombophlebitis which is a dangerous complication.
- Lupus vulgaris is a type of cutaneous tuberculosis of face with superficial ulceration having nodules which if pressed with a glass slide appear like apple jelly granules.
- Nevi are benign tumors composed of modified melanocytes derived from neural crest. They have excess melanin pigment; hence, they are tan brown or black in color. They include junction nevus, intradermal nevus, compound nevus, blue nevus, and giant hairy nevus.
- Papilloma is a benign tumor arising from skin or mucous membrane. It is etiologically related to human papillomavirus.
- Cavernous hemangioma consists of large thin-walled venous channels. It occurs in head, neck, face, tongue, liver, and other regions. It is treated by sclerotherapy with tetradecyl sulfate/hypertonic saline and ligation of feeding vessel followed by excision, therapeutic embolization, excision, and laser ablation.
- Neurofibroma is a benign tumor of connective tissue of nerve sheath. It is of many types: solitary, generalized, plexiform, and elephantiasis neurofibromatosa.
- Keratoacanthoma (molluscum contagiosum) is a benign lesion but when fully developed may look like a carcinoma.
- Basal cell carcinoma (BCC) is a slow-growing locally invasive tumor which occurs on the face above the line joining the corner of mouth with the ear lobule. It is of three types: rodent ulcer,

(CONTD...)

KEY POINTS (...CONTD)

nodulocystic, and "field fire." It is treated by wide excision, radiotherapy, or Mohs technique.

- SCC is a malignant tumor of keratinizing cells of epidermis or its appendages. It presents as an irregular ulcer with everted edge. It is treated with wide excision with adjacent radiotherapy.
- Malignant melanoma is a malignant tumor of melanocytes that can occur on the face. It is of many types: superficial spreading, nodular, lentigo maligna, acral lentiginous melanoma, and amelanotic melanoma. Its treatment is excision, the extent of which depends on the depth of the lesion.
- Meibomian cyst (chalazion) and hordeolum externum (stye) are two small cysts of eyelids.
- Mucocele of lacrimal sac presents with a cystic swelling near the medial canthus of the eye. It empties on pressure and the contents fill the medial part of eye.
- Meningocele is a transilluminant swelling at the root of the nose in the midline seen in a newborn. Similarly a mucocele of frontal sinus or ethmoid cells present at the root of the nose by the side of midline.

SELF-ASSESSMENT

Long answer questions

1. Describe etiology, pathology, clinical features, investigations, and treatment of squamous cell carcinoma.
2. Discuss the etiology, pathology, clinical features, types, and treatment of basal cell carcinoma.

Short answer questions

1. Macrostoma
2. Cheilosis
3. Rhagades
4. Chancre of lip
5. Median mental sinus
6. Pyogenic granuloma
7. Lupus vulgaris
8. Lipoma
9. Rodent ulcer
10. Thickness of a melanoma

Multiple choice questions

1. Macrostoma is characterized by
   (a) Smaller opening of mouth
   (b) Larger opening of mouth
   (c) Enlarged lower lip
   (d) Enlarged tongue
2. Microstoma is characterized by
   (a) Smaller opening of mouth
   (b) Enlarged lower lip
   (c) Enlargement of both lips
   (d) Larger opening of mouth
3. All of the following facts are true about rhagades, except
   (a) They are caused by diabetes mellitus
   (b) They are a manifestation of syphilis
   (c) They are characterized by cracks at angles of mouth
   (d) They heal following antisyphilitic therapy
4. All of the following are false about chancre of lip, except
   (a) It is a type of carcinoma
   (b) It is caused by actinic exposure
   (c) It has an everted edge
   (d) It is a manifestation of primary syphilis
5. All of the following features are true about preauricular sinus, except
   (a) It is a congenital anomaly
   (b) It is a manifestation of tuberculosis of parotid salivary gland
   (c) It becomes symptomatic due to obstruction and infection
   (d) It is treated by complete excision of sinus tract

(CONTD...)

SELF-ASSESSMENT (...CONTD)

6. Pyogenic granuloma has all of the following features, except
   (a) It is a bright red swelling slightly compressible
   (b) It is often confused with a hemangioma
   (c) It is caused by tuberculous infection
   (d) Histology shows epidermal collarette

7. Lupus vulgaris is
   (a) A type of skin cancer
   (b) A type of cutaneous tuberculosis
   (c) A manifestation of syphilis
   (d) Ulceration of a sebaceous cyst

8. Which of the following is the most common cancer of skin of face?
   (a) Adenocarcinoma
   (b) Squamous cell carcinoma
   (c) Basal cell carcinoma
   (d) Malignant melanoma

9. Which of following lesions exhibits telangiectasis on its surface?
   (a) Nodular type of basal cell carcinoma
   (b) Squamous cell carcinoma
   (c) Malignant melanoma
   (d) Adenocarcinoma

10. Apple jelly granules are a feature of
    (a) Rodent ulcer
    (b) Lupus vulgaris
    (c) Keratoacanthoma
    (d) Malignant melanoma

11. Which of the following lesions of face is etiologically related to actinic exposure?
    (a) Cock's peculiar tumor
    (b) Lupus vulgaris
    (c) Basal cell carcinoma
    (d) Adenocarcinoma

12. The dermoid cyst of face can occur at all of the following sites, except
    (a) Behind pinna
    (b) At tip of nose
    (c) At the root of nose in midline
    (d) At the external angle of eyebrow

13. Which of the following statements is false about carcinoma of lip?
    (a) Lower lip is the commonest site of occurrence
    (b) It usually spreads to the lungs by bloodstream
    (c) It is etiologically related to smoking
    (d) Histologically it is squamous cell carcinoma

14. Which of the following is the commonest initial site of metastasis from squamous cell carcinoma of lip?
    (a) Submental nodes
    (b) Lungs
    (c) Supraclavicular lymph nodes
    (d) Liver

15. Carcinoma of the lip is treated by
    (a) Surgery
    (b) Radiotherapy
    (c) Both surgery and radiotherapy
    (d) Chemotherapy

Answers

1. (b) 2. (a) 3. (a) 4. (d) 5. (b) 6. (c) 7. (b) 8. (c)
9. (a) 10. (b) 11. (c) 12. (b) 13. (b) 14. (a) 15. (c)

Diseases of Nose and Paranasal Sinuses

16

Surgical anatomy

External Nose

It is a pyramidal hollow structure with its apex up and base downwards, situated in the central face. External nose has an osteocartilaginous framework with few small muscles (Fig. 16.1).

Internal Nose

It is divided into right and left nasal cavities by nasal septum. Each nasal cavity communicates with the exterior through a nostril, and with the nasopharynx behind through a posterior nasal aperture or choana. Each nasal cavity has a small skin-lined part in the front called vestibule and a mucosa-lined part, the nasal cavity proper. The boundaries of nasal cavity are given in the following text.

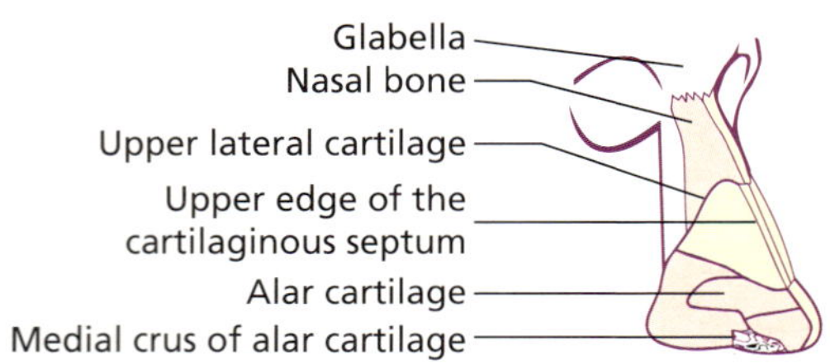

Figure 16.1 External nose.

Lateral Wall The lateral wall of the nose is marked by three scroll-like projections called turbinates or conchae. Below and lateral to each turbinate is the corresponding meatus of the nose.

Superior Wall The superior wall or roof is formed by nasal bones anteriorly, cribriform plate of ethmoid in the middle, and the body of sphenoid posteriorly. It contains the olfactory nerve fibers entering through cribriform plate.

Floor The anterior three-fourth part of floor of nose is formed by palatine process of maxilla and the posterior one-fourth is made by horizontal part of palatine bones.

Medial Wall (Nasal Septum) It consists of four parts: bony (perpendicular plate of ethmoid and vomer below and behind), cartilaginous, columellar, and membranous.

Little's Area It is a vascular area at the antero-inferior part of cartilaginous septum above the

Table 16.1 Paranasal sinuses and their drainage

Location	Paranasal sinuses	Drainage
Anterior sinuses	• Maxillary sinus • Frontal sinus • Anterior ethmoidal sinus	Middle meatus
Posterior sinuses	• Posterior ethmoidal sinus • Sphenoidal sinus	• Superior meatus • Sphenoethmoidal recess

Box 16.1 Functions of nose and paranasal sinuses

- Provide airway for breathing
- Air conditioning and filtration of inspired air
- Olfaction
- Resonance to voice
- Reduction of the number of bacteria, virus, and dust particles in the inspired air
- Nasal reflex function

vestibule. Little's area is the main site of bleeding (epistaxis) because of anastomosis of anterior ethmoidal artery, sphenopalatine artery, greater palatine artery, and septal branches of superior labial arteries and their accompanying veins (Kiesselbach's plexus).

Paranasal Air Sinuses

The paranasal sinuses are air-containing cavities in some bones around the nose lined by ciliated columnar epithelium. There are five sinuses on each side (Table 16.1). The functions of nose and paranasal sinuses are enumerated in Box 16.1.

Congenital disorder: choanal atresia

Etiology It is a developmental defect characterized by persistence of bucconasal membrane.

Types It may be unilateral or bilateral, complete or incomplete, and bony (90%) or membranous.

Clinical Features Unilateral atresia is more common and may remain undiagnosed till adulthood. The bilateral atresia presents with respiratory obstruction as the newborn has not learnt to breathe from the mouth.

Diagnosis This abnormality is diagnosed by the presence of mucoid discharge in the nose, absence of air bubble in discharge, and inability to pass a catheter in the nasopharynx. The obstruction can be confirmed by methylene blue studies and lateral radiography after instilling a radio-opaque contrast. CT scan may be done.

Treatment Bilateral atresia is an emergency. The neonate can be made to breathe by putting a feeding nipple with a large hole in the mouth between the lips (McGovern's method). Later the obstruction is removed by transnasal or transpalatal operation.

1. INFECTIONS AND INFLAMMATIONS

Rhinitis

Rhinitis is the inflammation of lining of nasal cavity. It is of many types as described in Box 16.2.

Acute Viral Rhinitis

It is a viral infection of nasal mucosa which is usually associated with involvement of lining of paranasal sinuses (rhinosinusitis).

Types of acute viral rhinitis

Etiologically it is of three types:

1. **Coryza or common cold**: It is caused by many viruses, that is, adenovirus, picornavirus, and its subgroups such as rhinovirus, coxsackievirus, and enteric cytopathic human orphan. The infection occurs by inhalation of airborne droplets. The incubation period is 1–4 days.

Box 16.2 Types of rhinitis

- Infective rhinitis
  - Acute viral rhinitis
  - Acute bacterial rhinitis
- Allergic rhinitis
  - Seasonal
  - Perennial
- Intrinsic or vasomotor rhinitis
- Unusual types
  - Atrophic rhinitis
  - Rhinitis medicamentosa
  - Hormonal rhinitis
  - Sarcoidosis
- Wegener's granulomatosis

2. **Influenza rhinitis**: It is caused by influenza virus A, B, or C.

3. **Rhinitis associated with exanthemas**: Rhinitis precedes exanthemas by 2–3 days. The examples include measles, rubella, and chickenpox.

Clinical features

- Nasal stuffiness, rhinorrhea, sneezing, and hyposmia are the main symptoms.
- Associated symptoms include malaise, chill, body ache, low-grade fever, and cough.
- Initially the discharge is watery and profuse. Later it may become mucopurulent due to secondary infection caused by *Streptococcus haemolyticus, Pneumococcus, Staphylococcus, Haemophilus influenzae, Klebsiella pneumoniae,* and *Moraxella catarrhalis.*

Complications

It is usually a self-limiting disease and resolves spontaneously within 2–3 weeks. However, the complications of this problem include sinusitis, pharyngitis, tonsillitis, bronchitis, pneumonia, and otitis media.

Treatment

There is no effective antiviral drug to prevent or treat this disease.

- Buffered hypertonic saline (3–5%) nasal irrigation relieves symptoms.
- Pseudoephedrine 30–60 mg orally every 4–6 hours or 120 mg twice daily may give relief in rhinorrhea and nasal obstruction.
- Oxymetazoline or phenylephrine sprays are rapidly effective but should not be used for more than a few days to prevent rebound congestion.
- Antibiotics have no role but may be prescribed if secondary infection has occurred.

Acute Bacterial Rhinitis

It is acute bacterial infection of nasal mucosa usually associated with involvement of paranasal sinuses (acute bacterial rhinosinusitis). It is less common as compared to viral rhinitis.

Causative bacteria

These include *Streptococcus pneumoniae*, other streptococci, *H. influenzae*, and less commonly *Staphylococcus aureus* and *M. catarrhalis.*

Clinical features

- The major symptoms include purulent nasal discharge, nasal obstruction or congestion, facial pain/pressure, altered smell, cough, and fever.
- The minor symptoms include headache, otalgia, halitosis, dental pain, and fatigue.
- It is distinguished from viral rhinitis by persistence of symptoms more than 10 days after onset or worsening of symptoms within 10 days.
- Intranasal examination may reveal a grayish white tenacious membrane in the nose on the inferior turbinate and nasal floor, attempted removal of which causes bleeding.

Complications

The complications of acute bacterial rhinosinusitis include orbital cellulitis and abscess, osteomyelitis, intracranial extension, and cavernous sinus thrombophlebitis.

Treatment

- The patient is given nonsteroidal anti-inflammatory drugs (NSAIDs) with oral or nasal decongestants, for example, oral pseudoephedrine 30–120 mg per dose up to 240 mg daily, nasal oxymetazoline 0.05%, or xylometazoline 0.05–0.1% one or two sprays in each nostril every 6–8 hours for up to 3 days.
- Most of the patients (80%) improve with this treatment within 2 weeks without antibiotic therapy.
- Antibiotics may be given if the symptoms last more than 10–14 days or are severe. The drugs of choice include amoxicillin, trimethoprim–sulfamethoxazole, doxycycline, and amoxicillin–clavulanate for 7–10 days.

Acute nasal diphtheria

Acute nasal diphtheria is a type of bacterial rhinitis which may be primary or secondary to pharyngeal diphtheria and may occur in acute or chronic form (Box 16.3).

Box 16.3 Acute nasal diphtheria

- **Causative organism**: Corynebacterium diphtheriae
- **Clinical features**
  - *Early stage:* There is often a transient rhinitis without membrane
  - *Later stages:* A thin grayish membrane is formed over the inferior turbinate due to exfoliation, necrosis, and fibrin deposition. Removal of membrane leads to bleeding
- **Diagnosis**: Culture of nasal swab
- **Treatment**
  - Diphtheria antitoxin 20,000–1,00,000 units depending on the severity
  - Penicillin 250 mg orally four times daily for 14 days. Erythromycin, azithromycin, and clarithromycin being other effective antibiotics

Allergic Rhinitis

Allergic rhinitis is an IgE-mediated immunological response of nasal mucosa to inhaled allergens and is characterized by sneezing, watery rhinorrhea, and itchy nose.

Types of allergic rhinitis

It is of two types: seasonal and perennial.

- **Seasonal allergic rhinitis**: It becomes symptomatic in a particular season when pollens of a certain plant to which the patient is allergic are present in the air.
- **Perennial allergic rhinitis**: It is symptomatic throughout the year.

Etiology

Two factors are mainly responsible in its etiology:

1. **Allergens**: Flowering shrubs and tree pollens are most common in the spring, flowering plants and grasses in the summer, and ragweed and molds in the fall. They produce seasonal rhinitis. Dust, household mites, air pollution, and pet dander are available all the time and produce perennial rhinitis.
2. **Genetic factors**: Chances of children developing allergy are 29%, and 47% if one or both parents suffer from allergy.

Pathogenesis

The pathogenesis of allergic rhinitis is described in Box 16.4.

Clinical features

- It can occur at any age and in both the sexes, 12–18 years of age being most vulnerable.
- Seasonal rhinitis is characterized by paroxysmal sneezing with 10–12 sneezes at a time, watery rhinorrhea, and nasal itching. The nasal symptoms are often accompanied by eye irritation, pruritus, conjunctival erythema, and excessive tearing. Many patients will have a strong family history of atopy or allergy.

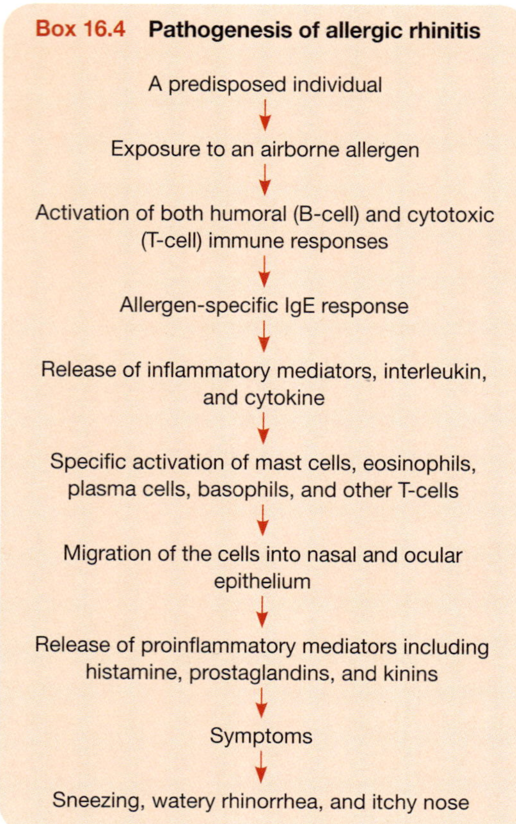

Box 16.4 Pathogenesis of allergic rhinitis

- Perennial rhinitis is characterized by milder symptoms, that is, frequent colds, persistent stuffy nose, loss of smell, postnasal drip, chronic cough, and hearing impairment.
- The nasal mucosa is pale, violaceous, and edematous. The turbinates are swollen and have a watery or mucoid discharge. It is in contrast with erythema of viral and bacterial rhinitis.

Differential diagnosis

Allergic rhinitis should be differentiated from vasomotor rhinitis which is caused by increased sensitivity of vidian nerve and is characterized by clear rhinorrhea in the elderly.

Investigations

The investigations include nasal smear which shows eosinophils, blood counts which show eosinophilia, and estimation of IgE which is elevated. Radioallergosorbent test (RAST) confirms the diagnosis.

Complications

The complications of allergic rhinitis include recurrent sinusitis, nasal polyps, serous otitis media, orthodontic problems, and bronchial asthma.

Treatment

Intranasal Corticosteroids They have revolutionized the treatment as they are more effective and frequently less expensive, but there may be delay in onset of relief for 2 or more weeks. They shrink hypertrophic nasal mucosa and nasal polyps providing improved nasal airway and osteomeatal complex drainage. The available sprays are listed in Table 16.2. The side effects are minimal but the most annoying is epistaxis which may be due to incorrect delivery of drug to nasal septum.

Antihistamines They offer immediate relief in most of the symptoms (Table 16.2). In some patients, the allergy symptoms return after several months of use.

Adjuvant Therapy Antileukotriene medications such as montelukast, cromolyn sodium, and sodium nedocromil work by stabilizing mast cells and preventing proinflammatory mediator release. Intranasal anticholinergic agents such as ipratropium bromide may be helpful adjuvants to control rhinorrhea, but they are not as effective as intranasal corticosteroids (Table 16.2). Saline irrigations may be used to flush the allergens out of nose.

Avoidance or reduction of exposure to airborne allergens may be very difficult and can be done by covering pillows and beds with plastic covers, substituting animal products, for example, wool with synthetic materials such as foam mattresses, and removing dust-collecting household fixtures, for example, carpets. Air purifiers and dust filters may be used.

Vasomotor Rhinitis

It is a nonallergic rhinitis that simulates allergic rhinitis with symptoms of nasal obstruction, rhinorrhea, and sneezing.

Table 16.2 Treatment of allergic rhinitis

Intranasal corticosteroids	Antihistamines	Adjuvant therapy
• Beclomethasone (42 µg/spray twice daily per nostril) • Flunisolide (25 µg/spray twice daily per nostril) • Mometasone furoate (200 µg once daily per nostril) • Budesonide (100 µg twice daily per nostril) • Fluticasone propionate (200 µg once daily per nostril)	**Nonsedating** • Loratadine (10 mg orally twice daily) • Fexofenadine (60 mg twice daily or 120 mg once daily) **Minimally sedating** • Cetirizine (10 mg orally) once daily **Sedating** • Brompheniramine (4 mg orally every 6–8 hours) • Chlorpheniramine (8–12 mg every 8–12 hours or a sustained-release tablet) • Clemastine (1.34–2.68 mg orally twice daily) • Desloratadine (5 mg twice daily) • H_1-receptor antagonist: Azelastine (1–2 sprays per nostril daily)	**Antileukotriene** • Montelukast (10 mg daily orally) alone or with cetirizine • Cromolyn sodium • Sodium nedocromil **Intranasal anticholinergic agents** • Ipratropium bromide 0.03% or 0.06% sprays (42–84 µg per nostril three times daily) • Intranasal saline irrigation to flush allergens out of nose • Avoidance or reduction of exposure to airborne allergens

Etiology

It is due to overactivity of parasympathetic system (vidian nerve) which causes excessive secretion of nasal glands. The nasal mucosa is hyper-reactive and hyper-responsive to several nonspecific stimuli, that is, changes in temperature, humidity, blasts of air, etc.

Clinical features

- The patient presents with bouts of sneezing just after getting out of bed in the morning, profuse watery rhinorrhea, and obstruction.
- The nose may drip when the patient leans forwards. The nasal obstruction alternates from side to side, more marked at night with blockage of the dependent side.
- On examination, the nasal mucosa of the turbinates is pale or bluish, congested, and hypertrophic.

Diagnosis

It is present throughout the year and tests of nasal allergy are negative.

Treatment

- The initiating factors, for example, sudden change in temperature and humidity, must be avoided.
- Antihistamines and nasal decongestants are given for symptomatic relief.
- Topical corticosteroid spray or aerosol may help when the above-mentioned measures do not help. Systemic steroids may be given for a short period in severe disease.
- Nasal obstruction may sometimes require reduction of size of turbinates by partial inferior turbinectomy, cauterization, cryosurgery, or laser.
- Excessive rhinorrhea may sometimes require division of parasympathetic secretomotor fibers to the nose (vidian neurectomy).

Atrophic Rhinitis (Ozaena)

It is a chronic inflammation of nose characterized by progressive atrophy of nasal mucosa and the underlying bone of the turbinates. There is a continuous discharge of viscid secretion which dries up to form foul-smelling crusts. The nasal passage increases in size. It is of two types: primary and secondary.

Primary atrophic rhinitis

Etiology

Its cause is not known. It may be related to heredity and racial factors (more common in white and yellow races), socioeconomic status (females of low social order), nutritional status (deficiency of vitamins A and D, iron, and proteins), infection (*Coccobacillus*, *Bacillus mucosus*, *Coccobacillus foetidus ozaenae*, and *Klebsiella ozaenae*), and autoimmunity.

Histology

The ciliated columnar epithelium of the nose is substituted by stratified squamous epithelium. There is atrophy of seromucous glands, venous blood sinusoids, and nerve elements. The bones of turbinates undergo resorption.

Clinical features

- It commonly occurs in females around puberty.
- There is foul smell from the nose (ozaena) which causes social problem. The patient is not aware of the smell due to anosmia (merciful anosmia).
- There may be nasal obstruction due to large crusts filling the nasal cavity.
- On examination, the nose is full with greenish or grayish black dry crusts on the turbinates and septum. An attempt to remove the crusts may cause bleeding (epistaxis). The posterior wall of nasopharynx may be easily visible due to atrophy of turbinates.
- It may be associated with pharyngitis sicca and atrophic laryngitis.

Investigations

Blood for hemoglobin and counts, X-ray of paranasal sinuses (Water's view), culture and sensitivity of nasal discharge, and serological tests for syphilis are the usual investigations.

Treatment

So far no curative treatment is available. The treatment includes:

- Maintenance of nasal hygiene
- Prevention of further crust formation by irrigation with lukewarm saline or alkaline solution (280 mL water + one teaspoonful of one part of sodium bicarbonate, one part of sodium biborate, and two parts of sodium chloride)
- Local instillation of 25% glucose in glycerine, estradiol in arachis oil 1000 units/mL local spray, and human placentrex injections submucosally and systemically

Surgical treatment may be required in some patients. It includes:

- Closing the nostrils by raising flaps from vestibule for 6 months or more (Young's operation)
- Closing the nostrils partially leaving 3- to 5-mm openings in the center
- Narrowing the nasal cavities by putting acrylic nasal implants in floor and lateral wall
- Injection of Teflon paste, insertion of cartilage, fat, or bone pieces in floor and lateral wall
- Displacement of lateral walls medially

Secondary atrophic rhinitis

The nasal mucosa may undergo atrophy in syphilis, lupus, leprosy, and many other diseases. The treatment of this type of atrophic rhinitis is removal of the cause.

Rhinitis Medicamentosa

Etiology It is because of long-term or excessive use of topical decongestants which cause intense ischemia during which some products of metabolism accumulate and cause rebound vasodilatation and congestion.

Clinical Features The nasal mucosa is chronically inflamed and swollen due to edema. The turbinates may undergo hypertrophy.

Treatment The causative nasal drops are stopped and a short course of corticosteroids is given. Surgical reduction of turbinates may be required.

Hormonal Rhinitis

Hypothyroidism inhibits sympathetic nervous system and promotes parasympathetic nervous system causing nasal stuffiness and symptoms of "common cold." It is cured by thyroid hormone supplementation.

Sarcoidosis

It is a granulomatous disease of unknown etiology resembling tuberculosis without caseation.

- **Site**: It involves lungs, skin, eyes, peripheral nerves, lymph nodes, and other tissues.
- **Clinical features**: In the nose, it presents with submucosal nodules involving septum or inferior turbinate with nasal obstruction, nasal pain, and sometimes epistaxis. Nodules may also form in the nasal vestibule or skin of face.
- **Diagnosis**: Biopsy of the nodule confirms the diagnosis.
- **Treatment**: It is treated with corticosteroids, that is, prednisone 0.5–1.0 mg/kg daily over months or years. For nasal symptoms, steroids can be given as nasal spray.

Wegener's Granulomatosis (Granulomatosis with Polyangiitis)

It is a systemic disease of unknown etiology having classic triad of upper and lower respiratory tract involvement and glomerulonephritis.

Clinical features

- In the early stage, the nasal symptoms include clear or blood-stained discharge which later becomes purulent. The patient often presents with persisting cold, or "sinus trouble" apart from manifestation of involvement of other organs and tissues.
- The nasal examination reveals crusting, granulations, septal perforation, and a saddle nose.
- Eyes, orbits, palate, oral cavity, pharynx, and middle ear may show destruction.
- The general symptoms include anemia, fatigue, night sweats, migratory arthralgia, cough, and hemoptysis. The renal involvement may end up in renal failure.

Diagnosis

The erythrocyte sedimentation rate (ESR) is elevated and antineutrophil cytoplasmic antibodies (ANCAs) usually directed against proteinase-3 are present in 90% of patients. Biopsy confirms the diagnosis.

Complications

The complications of Wegener's granulomatosis include bleeding from nose, nasal destruction, and renal failure.

Treatment

It is treated with cyclophosphamide plus corticosteroids or rituximab plus corticosteroids.

Nasal maggots (nasal myiasis)

It is the presence of maggots in the nose. The maggots are the larvae of house fly (Fig. 16.2).

Etiopathogenesis

The house flies (*Chrysomya*) are attracted by foul-smelling discharge of atrophic rhinitis, leprosy, syphilis, or any other infection of the nose, and then they lay eggs in the nose, about 200 at a time. They hatch into larvae within 24 hours.

Clinical Features

- They may infest the nose, nasopharynx, and paranasal sinuses.
- Initially for 3–4 days, there is intense irritation, sneezing, lacrimation and headache associated with blood-streaked discharge, and puffy eyelids and lips. Third to fourth day

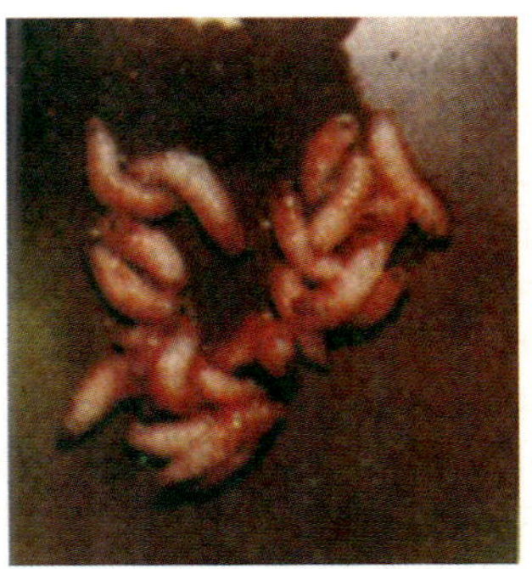

Figure 16.2 Maggots (larvae of house fly). (Courtesy: Professor R.M. Mathur)

onwards, the maggots crawl out of the nose. There is offensive smell around the patient.

- The maggots cause extensive destruction of the nose and tissues around may produce a fistula. Ultimately the patient may die of meningitis.

Treatment

- All visible maggots are removed with a forceps.
- Instillation of chloroform water with turpentine kills them. Then nasal douche with warm saline is used to remove slough and dead maggots.
- Further contact with flies should be avoided.

Syphilis of nose

Congenital Syphilis

- It may manifest in the first 3 months of life or around puberty.
- In infants, it presents as constant snuffles with an obstinate nasal discharge which dries up to form crusts. It leads to chronic irritation and then fissures of anterior nares.
- Around puberty, gummatous ulceration occurs which destroys the local tissues resulting in depressed bridge of nose. There is fetid crusting within the nose.
- Other congenital stigmata of syphilis may be present.

Acquired Syphilis

- Primary syphilis of the nose is rare but a syphilitic chancre can occur in the vestibule of nose.
- Late syphilis may manifest as mucous patches with rhinitis, crusting, and fissuring in nasal vestibule which manifests as a gumma of the septum of nose. It leads to ulceration and destruction of septum with fetid discharge and crusting leading to perforation. Finally, the bridge of the nose collapses causing a saddle-nose deformity.
- The serological tests of syphilis, for example, VDRL, TPHA, and FTA-ABS, are invariably positive.
- It is treated with benzathine penicillin 2.4 million units by intramuscular injection every week for 3 weeks. The nasal cavity is kept clean by irrigation with saline or alkaline solution and crust removal. Later on, surgical correction of nasal deformity is required.

Leprosy (Hansen disease) of the nose

Etiology It is a chronic infective disease caused by an acid-fast rod, *Mycobacterium leprae*. The lepromatous (multibacillary leprosy) commonly affects the nose. It has an insidious onset.

Site It is characterized by involvement of cooler body tissues, for example, skin, superficial nerves, nose, pharynx, larynx, eyes, and testicles.

Skin Lesions They include pale, anesthetic macules, 1–10 cm in diameter; discrete erythematous infiltrated nodules 1–5 cm in diameter; or diffuse skin infiltration.

Nasal Manifestations In lepromatous leprosy, there is bulbous thickening of nasal vestibule, obstruction of nasal cavity, extensive crusting, fetid purulent nasal discharge, ulceration, septal perforation, liquefaction of nasal framework, saddle nose, thick and deformed nasal ala, and leonine facies.

Diagnosis The diagnosis is confirmed by Ziehl–Neelsen staining of nasal smear to find the causative organism, and biopsy.

Treatment

- Lepromatous leprosy is treated with a triple-drug regimen consisting of rifampin 600 mg once a month, dapsone 100 mg daily, and clofazimine 300 mg once a month and then 50 mg daily for 12 months.
- Tuberculoid leprosy is treated with rifampin 600 mg once a month and dapsone 100 mg daily for 6 months. Two reactions—erythema nodosum leprosum and reversal reactions—may occur.

- Later on, deformities of nose and face are corrected by plastic surgical procedures.

Nasal polyps

They are non-neoplastic masses of edematous nasal or sinus mucosa caused by repeated attacks of allergic or vasomotor rhinitis combined with infection. Repeated blowing of the nose increases the size of polyp by pulling the polyp out.

Pathology

The polyp consists of hypertrophy of submucosa with increased intercellular serous fluid spaced in a fibrillar stroma. It is infiltrated with eosinophils, degranulated mast cells, and round cells. Initially it is covered with normal ciliated columnar epithelium; later on, it undergoes metaplastic changes to transitional and squamous type.

Types of Nasal Polyps

- Ethmoidal polyps
- Antrochoanal polyps

Ethmoidal Polyps

Clinical features

- **Sites**: The common sites of these polyps are uncinate process, bulla ethmoidalis, ostia of sinuses, and medial surface and edge of middle turbinate. They never arise from septum or floor of the nose.
- **Age**: They can occur at any age but are mostly seen in adults.
- **Symptoms**: The patient presents with total nasal obstruction with partial or complete loss of sense of smell. There may be repeated sneezing and watery nasal discharge and may be a mass protruding from the nostril. The nose may be broadened with increased intercanthal distance.

Diagnosis

- **Anterior rhinoscopy** shows smooth, glistening, sessile or pedunculated, grape-like masses, insensitive to probing and not bleeding on touch. They may be bilateral. The nasal cavity may have purulent discharge. If there is a solitary polyp, it must be probed to differentiate it from hypertrophy of turbinate or cystic middle turbinate.
- **X-ray of nose and paranasal sinuses** is usually normal.
- **CT scan** is required if there is suspicion of malignancy especially in patients above 40 years of age. It will show bone destruction while in a polyp the local bones are normal (Fig. 16.3).
- Biopsy is done if there is suspicion of a tumor.

Treatment

- In early stages, antihistamines do provide relief but occasionally recourse has to be taken to corticosteroids.
- If there are one or two pedunculated polyps, they are removed by snare.
- Multiple sessile polyps require a special forceps for uncapping of ethmoidal air cells by intranasal route.
- Recurrent polyps after intranasal procedures are treated by ethmoidectomy (external, intranasal, and transantral). They may be managed by endoscopic sinus surgery.

Antrochoanal Polyp

It arises from mucosa of maxillary antrum near the accessory ostium, comes out of it, and develops in choanae and nose. Thus, it has three parts: an

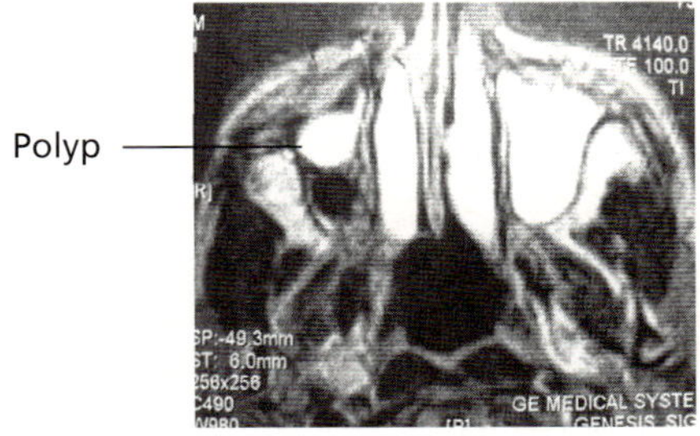

Figure 16.3 Axial MRI T2 image showing a small polyp in right maxillary antrum, fluid in left maxillary antrum, and edema of nasal mucosa. (Courtesy: Dr. S.S. Sarkar, Sarkar Diagnostics)

antral part which has a thin stalk, a choanal part which is round and globular, and a nasal part which is flat from side to side.

Clinical features

The patient is usually a child or young adult who usually has a single and unilateral polyp. It presents as unilateral nasal obstruction and mucoid discharge as it grows into nasopharynx. It may obstruct the opposite choana also.

Diagnosis

- **Anterior rhinoscopy** may show a large, smooth, soft, grayish mass which can be moved up or down by probe. It may be missed by anterior rhinoscopy.
- **Posterior rhinoscopy** may show a globular mass filling the choana or nasopharynx.
- **X-ray** may show opacified antrum and a soft tissue mass in the nose.

Differential diagnosis

A polyp has to be differentiated from a blob of mucus, hypertrophied middle turbinate, angiofibroma, and other tumors of nasopharynx. There may be underlying malignancy in a polyp; hence, every excised specimen must be sent for histopathology. A polyp in a child must be differentiated from an encephalocele or meningoencephalocele.

Complications

The complications include nasal obstruction with or without secondary infection.

Treatment

It is removed by avulsion through the nasal route. Recurrence is rare. A recurrent polyp requires a Caldwell-Luc approach or endoscopic sinus approach.

Acute paranasal sinusitis

It is the acute inflammation of paranasal sinus mucosa. Acute paranasal sinusitis may involve any sinus, but the maxillary sinus is the most commonly involved. Very often more than one sinus is inflamed.

Etiology

Causative organisms

Acute sinusitis usually starts as acute upper respiratory tract viral infection followed by secondary bacterial invasion. The common invading bacteria are *S. pneumoniae*, *H. influenzae*, *Branhamella catarrhalis*, *Streptococcus pyogenes*, and *K. pneumoniae*. The infection spreading into the sinus from the roots of upper lateral teeth is often caused by anaerobes.

Predisposing and Aggravating Factors

- **Infection from adjacent areas**: The sinus mucosa is continuous with nasal mucosa; thus, the organisms of the nose may infect the sinuses. The maxillary sinus may also be infected from the roots of upper molar and premolar teeth.
- **Swimming and diving**: These may cause entry of infected or chlorinated water into the sinuses through their ostia.
- **Obstruction to sinus ventilation and drainage**: It predisposes to infection. The causes of obstruction are deviated nasal septum, hypertrophied turbinates, edema of sinus ostia, nasal polyps, tumors, and nasal packing to control epistaxis.
- **Climate**: Sinusitis is common in cold and wet climate.

Pathology

The infection causes acute inflammation of the sinus mucosa which may take either catarrhal or purulent form. Failure of ostium to drain results in empyema of that sinus which is a severe form of inflammation characterized by accumulation of pus. The commonest site of empyema is maxillary sinus.

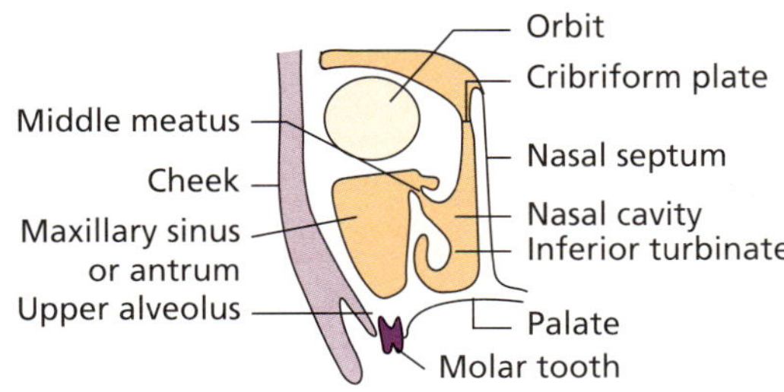

Figure 16.4 Anatomy of maxillary sinus or antrum.

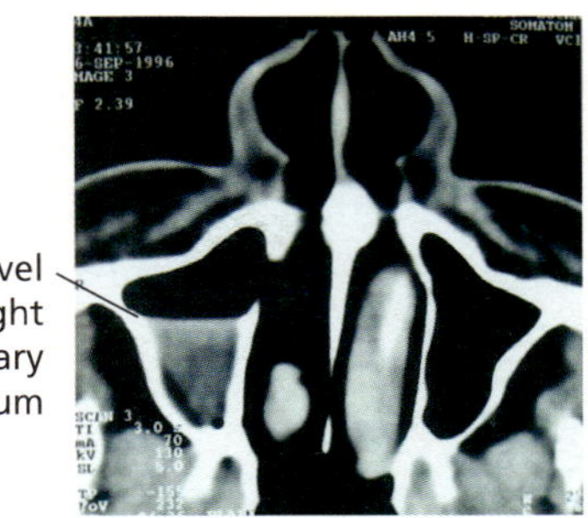

Figure 16.5 Axial CT scan of midface showing fluid collection with fluid level in right maxillary antrum.

Acute Maxillary Sinusitis

It is acute inflammation of the lining of maxillary sinus.

Surgical anatomy of maxillary sinus

It is the largest pyramidal-shaped cavity in the maxilla with base toward the lateral nasal wall and apex directed laterally toward the zygomatic arch. It opens in the middle meatus of nose. It has a capacity of about 15 mL in adults (Fig. 16.4).

Clinical Features It is characterized by fever, malaise, headache confined to forehead, and local pain over the maxilla aggravated by stooping, coughing, or chewing. There may be referred upper toothache due to irritation of superior alveolar nerve. On examination, pressure or tapping over the anterior wall of antrum produces pain. In children, the overlying cheek skin is red and edematous including lower eyelids.

Investigations

- **Anterior rhinoscopy** shows pus or mucopus in the middle meatus with inflamed local mucosa. If no pus is found, a pledget of cotton wool soaked in a vasoconstrictor is put locally and the patient is made to sit with the affected side turned up. The patient is examined again after 10–15 minutes for pus (postural test). About 10% of infections of maxillary antrum are due to dental sepsis caused by anaerobic organisms. In these patients, the nasal discharge has a foul smell. Transillumination shows an opaque sinus.
- **Radiography of maxilla (Water's view) including CT scan** shows either an opaque antrum or a fluid level (Fig. 16.5).
- Antral puncture can be done to obtain samples of pus for examination including culture and sensitivity.

Complications The complications of acute maxillary sinusitis include frontal sinusitis, osteitis or osteomyelitis of maxilla, orbital cellulitis, and empyema of maxillary antrum.

Treatment

- Fever and pain require symptomatic treatment.
- Nasal decongestants, for example, 1% ephedrine drops, may be used to decongest ostium and improve drainage.
- Steam inhalation provides symptomatic relief and improved sinus drainage.
- Local fomentation helps in resolution of inflammation.
- Antimicrobial drugs, for example, amoxicillin, erythromycin, doxycycline, cotrimoxazole, cefuroxime, or sparfloxacin, may be given as required. On receiving the culture report, appropriate changes are made in the treatment.

Chronic Maxillary Sinusitis

Etiopathogenesis If the acute sinus infection fails to resolve, the sinusitis becomes chronic and more difficult to treat. The acute infection destroys normal ciliated epithelium impairing sinus drainage. It is the most important causative factor for chronicity. Microscopically the mucosa and submucosa of sinus show chronic inflammation.

Clinical Features The symptoms and signs are often vague and are similar to those of acute sinusitis but of mild type. Pus discharge from the nose is the commonest symptom. Local pain and heaviness may be present.

Investigations

- Radiography shows opaque sinus.
- CT scan or MRI shows thickened mucosa (Fig. 16.6).
- Nasal endoscopy may reveal osteomeatal unit blockage, polypoidal mucosa, and purulent discharge from sinus ostium.
- Antroscopy may be done to see the antrum from inside and take biopsy if indicated.

Complications The complications include orbital cellulitis, abscess, extradural abscess, and cavernous sinus thrombosis.

Treatment The patient is given symptomatic treatment as described for acute sinusitis. It may give relief but more often some form of surgery is required:

- Antral puncture and irrigation helps in removal of pus and exudate from the sinus.
- Intranasal antrostomy: If irrigation fails, a window is created in the inferior meatus to provide free drainage and aeration of sinus.
- Caldwell-Luc operation: The antrum is entered through its anterior wall by a sublabial incision. A window is created between the antrum and upper sublabial sulcus to provide for free drainage. All this work is now being done by intranasal endoscopic techniques. The antrum can be entered through the antrostomy using a combination of 30° and 70° rigid endoscopes.

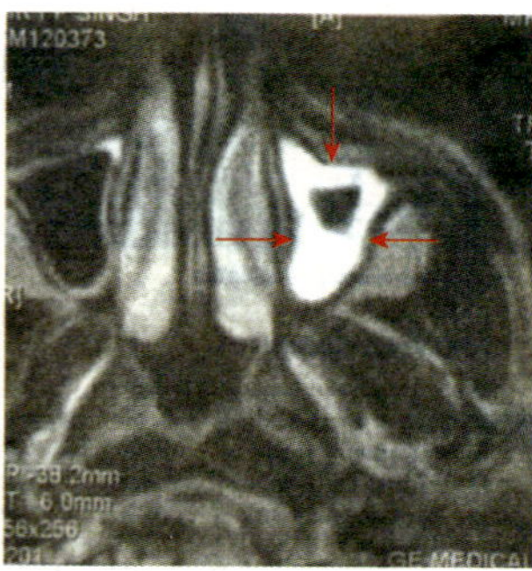

Figure 16.6 Axial MRI of face showing mucosal thickening of left maxillary antrum suggestive of chronic sinusitis. (Courtesy: Dr. S.S. Sarkar, Sarkar Diagnostics)

Frontal Sinusitis

Clinical Features It is commonly associated with ethmoid sinusitis wherein the patient presents with frontal headache with periodicity, that is, the pain appears on waking up in the morning, gradually increases and reaches its peak about mid-day, and then starts subsiding ("office headache"). It is aggravated by forward bending of head as when doing writing work. On examination, there is edema of upper eyelid and tenderness over the floor of frontal sinus just above the medial canthus.

Investigations

- Anterior rhinoscopy shows inflamed nasal mucosa in the middle meatus and a vertical streak of mucopus high up in the anterior part of middle meatus.
- Radiography shows opaque sinus or a fluid level in the sinus. Further details can be seen by a CT scan.

Treatment Treatment is done on the same principles as described for maxillary sinusitis. The obstructed frontal sinus is trephined and the chronic disease may require external frontoethmoidectomy (Howarth or Lynch operation) or osteoplastic flap operation.

Ethmoid Sinusitis (Ethmoiditis)

Clinical Features Acute ethmoiditis is often associated with infection of other sinuses. It is common in infants and children. It is characterized by pain which is localized over the bridge of the nose, medial canthus, and deep in the eye. It is aggravated by the movements of the eyeball, and associated with edema of both eyelids and excessive lacrimation.

Investigations Anterior rhinoscopy may reveal pus in middle or superior meatus depending on the involvement of anterior or posterior group of ethmoid sinuses. The middle turbinate is swollen.

Complications These include orbital cellulitis, abscess, blindness, cavernous sinus thrombosis, extradural abscess, meningitis, and brain abscess.

Treatment It is treated on the same lines as described for acute maxillary sinusitis. Visual deterioration and exophthalmos indicate a posterior orbital abscess. It is drained into the nose by endoscopic method. Chronic ethmoiditis is treated with ethmoidectomy by transantral approach or intranasal endoscopic method.

Sphenoiditis

It is characterized by pain localized to occiput or vertex and postnasal drip. Chronic disease may require surgery when sphenoid can be approached with trans-septal approach or endoscopy.

2. TRAUMA OF THE NOSE AND PARANASAL SINUSES

Deviated nasal septum

Deviated nasal septum is a very common problem and one of the important causes of nasal obstruction.

Etiology

- **Trauma**
  - A lateral blow on the nose may cause displacement of nasal cartilage to the opposite side.
  - A blow from the front may cause buckling, twisting, fracture, and duplication of nasal septum with telescoping of its fragments. The injuries to the nasal septum are common during childhood and even during delivery when they are often overlooked.
- **Developmental defect**
  - Unequal growth of face between palate and base of skull resulting in buckling of septum
  - Mouth breathing with high-arched palate
  - Cleft lip and palate
  - Dental abnormalities

Types of Deviated Septum

- **Columellar deviation or anterior dislocation**: The septal cartilage is deviated to one side due to dislocation of anterior inferior border from sulcus to one side. It can be seen by looking into the nose with the patient's head tilted backward.
- **C-shaped deformity**: The septum is deviated to one side in a C-like curve with obstruction on the side of convexity and a wide nasal chamber on the side of concavity.
- **S-shaped deformity**: The septum is S-shaped in vertical or anteroposterior plane. Hence, it may cause bilateral nasal obstruction.
- **Spur**: It is a shelf-like projection of bone from the junction of vomer and cartilage of septum. It may press on the lateral wall.
- **Thickened septum**: It is due to organized septal hematoma or over-riding of dislocated septal fragments.

Clinical Features

- It can occur at any age. It is more common in males than in females and presents with unilateral or bilateral nasal obstruction, headache, sinusitis, epistaxis, hyposmia or anosmia, nasal deformity, and epiphora.
- The high septal deviation causes more obstruction, particularly in inspiration, while low deviation causes less obstruction.
- Headache is due to pressure of bony spurs on the lateral nasal wall.
- Sinusitis is caused by blockage of osteomeatal unit caused by deviated septum.
- Epistaxis occurs from the mucosa over sharp bony spur or from dried and ulcerated mucosa.

- Hyposmia and anosmia are due to prevention of flow of air current through the olfactory area.

Diagnosis

The diagnosis can be confirmed by radiography and/or CT scan (Fig. 16.7).

Complications

The complications include sinus infection and bleeding and septal necrosis.

Treatment

Minor deviation does not require any treatment. Major or symptomatic deviation requires surgical help but the septal surgery is usually advised after the age of 17 years so as not to affect the nasal and facial bony development.

- **Septoplasty**: In this procedure, cartilage is preserved as much as possible; only the most deviated part is removed, and the rest of the framework is corrected and repositioned.
- **Submucous resection (SMR)**: It can be done under general or local anesthesia. The deviated part of bony and cartilaginous septum is excised subperiosteally and subperichondrially and the mucosal flaps are repaired. A 5- to 8-mm strip of cartilage on the dorsum is left for support to prevent possible saddle-nose deformity.

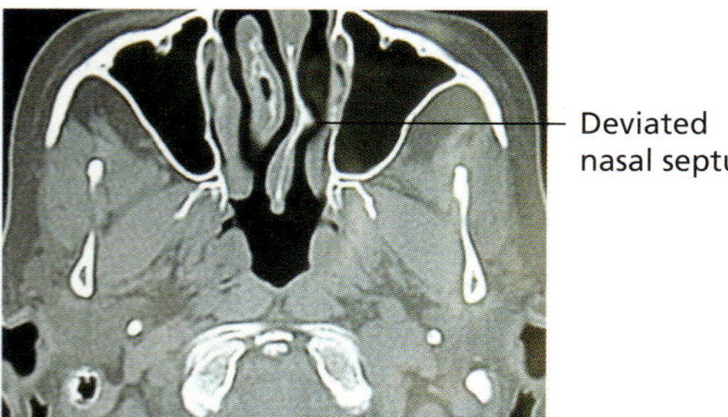

Figure 16.7 Axial CT scan of midface showing deviated nasal septum to left side. (Courtesy: Dr. Satyavan)

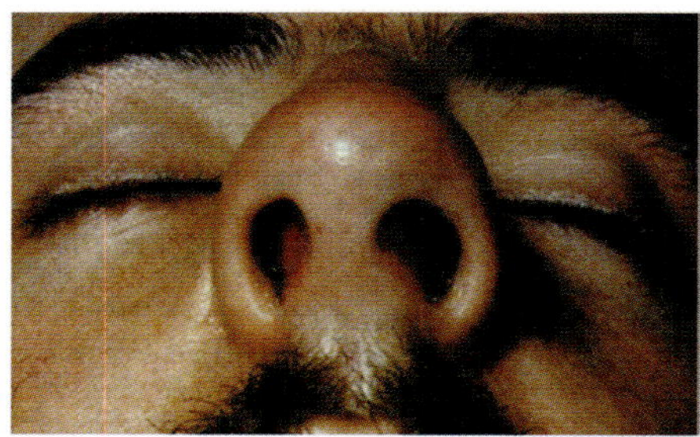

Figure 16.8 Photography of the midface with extended neck showing nasal septal hematoma. (Courtesy: Professor Surajit Bhattacharya)

Septal hematoma

It is the collection of blood under the perichondrium or the periosteum of nasal septum.

Etiology It occurs following local trauma and septal operations and may occur in bleeding disorders.

Clinical Features The patient presents with bilateral nasal obstruction which may be associated with frontal headache and a sense of pressure over the nasal bridge. There is a soft, smooth, rounded, and fluctuant swelling on both sides of nasal septum. It may be tender (Fig. 16.8).

Complications These include thickening of septum and septal abscess due to secondary infection.

Treatment A small hematoma is treated by aspiration with a large-bore needle. A large hematoma is evacuated by an anteroposterior incision parallel to nasal floor. Removal of a small piece of mucosa from the edge of the wound helps in better drainage. Antibiotics are given to prevent secondary infection.

Septal abscess

Etiology It usually follows secondary infection of a septal hematoma. Septal abscess may follow a furuncle of nose or upper lip. It may be a complication of systemic infections, for example, typhoid and measles.

Clinical Features The patient presents with severe bilateral nasal obstruction and pain, and may be associated with fever with chills and frontal headache. The skin over the nose may be red and swollen. Both sides of nasal septum are swollen and red. Fluctuation may be present. The submental and submandibular lymph nodes may be enlarged and tender.

Treatment The pus is drained with an incision on the most dependent part of abscess. A part of mucosa of the wound edge is excised. Even then it may require to be reopened after 2–3 days. Broad-spectrum antibiotics are usually given.

Perforation of nasal septum

The causes of perforation of nasal septum are described in Box 16.5.

Clinical Features It may be asymptomatic. A small perforation may cause whistling during breathing. Crusting may occur around perforation and a large crust may obstruct the nose. It may cause epistaxis when efforts are made to remove it.

Box 16.5 Causes of perforation of nasal septum

- **Traumatic perforation**
  - Injury to flaps during submucosal resection of septum
  - Cauterization of septum with chemical or electrocautery
  - Deliberate puncture to wear a nose ring ("nath")
  - Frequent nose-picking
  - Cocaine sniffing
- **Spontaneous perforation**
  - Septal abscess
  - Nasal myiasis
  - Rhinolith or retained foreign body causing pressure necrosis
  - Chronic granulomatous infections—tuberculosis and leprosy destroying cartilaginous septum, syphilis destroying the bony part
  - Wegener's granulomatosis
- **Idiopathic**

Diagnosis The cause of perforation is identified by the history, physical signs, and biopsy from the edge of perforation or granulations.

Treatment The nose is kept crust-free by alkaline nasal douches and application of a bland ointment and the cause is treated. A small perforation may be closed by a local flap. A large perforation may be difficult to close. It may be closed by a silicon button.

Foreign bodies in nose

Foreign bodies in the nose are very common and are mostly seen in children (also in those with some mental problem).

Etiology The common foreign bodies include buttons, seeds, pebbles, pieces of paper, hairpin, etc. A cotton swab or gauze piece may be left in the nose during nasal surgery. Most of the foreign bodies enter the nose through the nostrils. Large pieces of food may enter the nose through the posterior nares during vomiting.

Clinical Features The patient is usually brought with a positive history. If it is not reported immediately, the child presents with unilateral nasal discharge which may be foul smelling or blood-stained. Hence, if a child is brought with such a history, a foreign body in the nose must be ruled out. A radio-opaque foreign body can be imaged by radiography of nose.

Complications The complications of nasal foreign body include nasal infection, epistaxis, sinusitis, rhinolithiasis, and inhalation into tracheobronchial tree.

Treatment Pieces of paper, gauze piece, or a cotton swab can be removed with a forceps. Rounded objects can be hooked by passing a blunt hook past the foreign body and bringing it out along the floor. Noncooperative children may require general anesthesia.

Nasal trauma

Nasal injuries are quite common. They may vary from cut nose (Fig. 16.9) to fracture of nasal

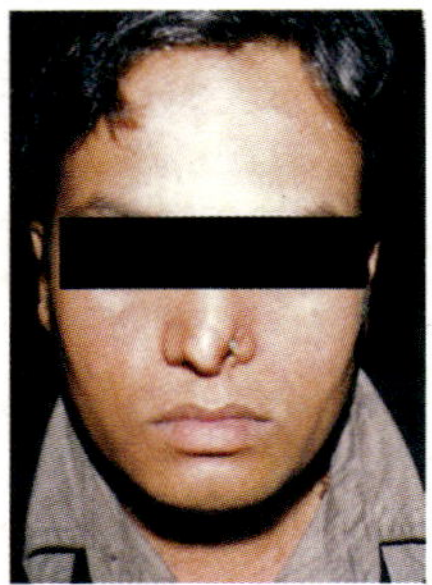

Figure 16.9 Partial cut nose involving left ala. (Courtesy: Professor S.P. Agarwal)

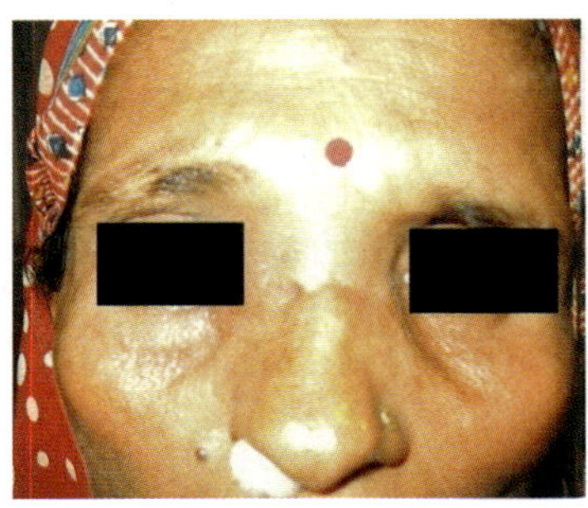

Figure 16.10 Depressed scar of old nasal injury. (Courtesy: Professor S.P. Agarwal)

bones. If not treated properly and in time, they may result in nasal deformity and disfigurement (Figs 16.9 and 16.10).

Fracture of Nasal Bones

Fractures of the nasal bones are an important component of maxillofacial trauma. They occur due to direct trauma and are characterized by nasal obstruction, bleeding, and nasal deformity. For further details, refer to Chapter 12, *Maxillofacial (Faciomaxillary) Injuries.*

Nasal Septal Injury

Etiology It follows direct trauma to the nose—from the front, the side, or below.

Clinical Features The septum may buckle on itself, fracture vertically or horizontally, or be crushed into pieces. The broken pieces may overlap each other or project into the nasal cavity through mucosal tears. The septal cartilage may get dislocated from its vomerine groove. The patient may present with profuse epistaxis or a septal hematoma if mucosa is intact.

Complications If these injuries are not treated properly, they may result in the deviation of cartilaginous nose and asymmetry of nasal tip, columella, or the nostril.

Treatment The dislocated and broken fragments should be repositioned and supported between mucoperiosteal flaps with mattress sutures and nasal packing.

3. TUMORS OF NOSE AND PARANASAL SINUSES

Rhinophyma (potato nose)

It is a disease of sebaceous follicles of nasal skin, especially of its distal part, causing immense thickening of the skin. It is commonly seen in middle-aged males.

Clinical Features The distal nose is covered by many overlapping irregular bosses on which the openings of sebaceous follicles are prominently visible (Fig. 16.11). It has dilated capillaries on its top imparting a bluish red color to it.

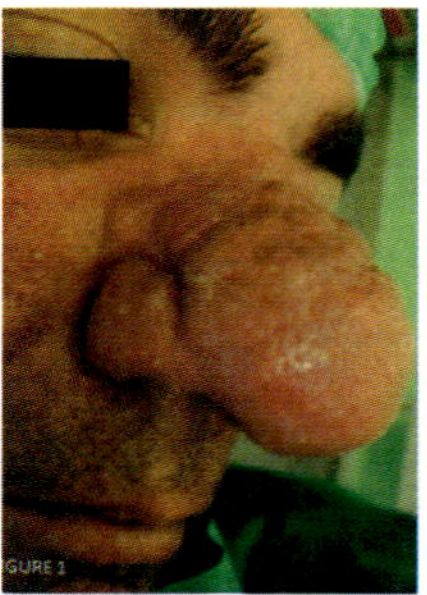

Figure 16.11 Rhinophyma of external nose showing swollen bluish distal nose with bosselated surface and shallow pits. (Courtesy: Dr. Surajit Bhattacharya)

Histology Histologically it is an aggregation of sebaceous adenomata. In 3% of patients, it may have an occult basal cell carcinoma in it.

Treatment

- **Surgery:** Paring away the protruding masses till the normal-appearing nose is visible is the treatment. Injury to the nasal cartilage must be avoided. There occurs brisk hemorrhage which is controlled by hot compresses. It is followed by dressing with the tulle gras. Skin grafting is usually not required.
- It can be treated by dermabrasion or laser resurfacing.

Polymorphic reticulosis (lethal midline granuloma, midline malignant reticulosis)

- The nature of this lesion is not well understood but it appears to be a nasal T-cell or NK-cell lymphoma.
- Contrary to granulomatosis with polyangiitis, the involvement is limited to midface with extensive bone destruction.
- It resembles non-Hodgkin lymphoma of either NK-cell or T-cell origin. Hence, immunophenotyping, especially for CD56 expression, is essential for histological evaluation.
- The complications include bleeding, disfigurement, and destruction of central face and meningitis.
- It is treated with radiotherapy followed by debridement and a nasal prosthesis. Recent treatment trends include cyclophosphamide and prednisone.

Benign and malignant tumors

A large number of tumors can occur in the nose and paranasal sinuses. They can occur in any of these structures but the commonest site is maxillary antrum. The classification of tumors of nose and paranasal sinuses is given in Box 16.6.

- A tumor of nose may present with unilateral nasal obstruction, unilateral persistent rhinorrhea, postnasal drip, and epistaxis, but these symptoms are nonspecific. Hence, too often the diagnosis is delayed.
- A tumor of paranasal sinuses presents with facial pain, swelling, proptosis, diplopia, and epiphora. Some of these signs are indicative of orbital involvement. Nerve involvement is heralded by numbness in the distribution of infraorbital nerve.

Box 16.6 Classification of the tumors of nose and paranasal sinuses

- **Benign tumors**
  - *Soft-tissue tumors*
    - Squamous papilloma
    - Transitional cell papilloma (inverted papilloma, Ringertz tumor)
    - Pleomorphic adenoma
    - Schwannoma
    - Meningioma
    - Cavernous hemangioma
    - Angiofibroma
    - Glioma
  - *Bone tumors*
    - Osteoma
    - Chondroma
- **Malignant tumors**
  - *Soft-tissue tumors*
    - Carcinoma
    - Malignant melanoma
    - Olfactory neuroblastoma
    - Hemangiopericytoma
    - Lymphoma
    - Plasmacytoma
    - Sarcoma
  - *Bone tumors*
    - Osteosarcoma
    - Chondrosarcoma

Papilloma

A papilloma is classified into three types.

Septal Papilloma (50%)

- **Site**: It arises from nasal vestibule and lower part of nasal septum.
- **Clinical features**: It may be single or multiple, exophytic and pedunculated, or sessile. It does not undergo malignant change.
- **Treatment**: It is treated by excision and cauterization of base. It can be treated with cryosurgery or laser.

Inverted Papilloma (47%)

- It is so named because the neoplastic (hyperplastic) epithelium is seen to grow toward underlying stroma rather than on the surface. It is covered by transitional epithelium.
- **Site:** This tumor occurs in the nose (lateral wall) and paranasal sinuses.
- **Clinical features:** The patient is usually 40–70 years of age, mostly a male, and presents with a unilateral tumor. Inverted papilloma presents as red or gray, firm, and vascular mass which may be translucent like a nasal polyp. When large or extensive, it can erode the lateral nasal wall and infiltrate the antrum or ethmoid. It may show calcification within and sclerosis at the margins of growth. It can undergo malignant change.
- **Investigation:** CT scan is required to see the extent of lesion.
- **Treatment:** It is treated by wide excision by lateral rhinotomy or medial maxillectomy and en bloc ethmoidectomy.

Cylindrical Cell Papilloma (3%)

- **Site**: It arises on the lateral nasal wall or from the paranasal sinuses.
- **Clinical features**: It causes nasal obstruction. It is associated with malignant transformation in 10–15% of patients into a squamous cell carcinoma.
- **Treatment**: It is excised widely.

Pleomorphic Adenoma

It is a rare tumor arising from nasal septum. It is treated by wide excision to avoid recurrence.

Schwannoma and Meningioma

They are uncommon tumors of nose and removed through a lateral rhinotomy.

Cavernous Hemangioma

It presents as an intranasal soft swelling arising from turbinates and lateral nasal wall. Cavernous hemangioma is bluish red in color and compressible. It is excised with preliminary cryotherapy.

Angiofibroma

It is a tumor of nasopharynx but mentioned here as it arises from the posterior part of cavity near the sphenopalatine foramen.

Glioma

Of all the gliomas (a tumor of glial tissue of brain), 30% are intranasal. They usually occur in infants and children and present as a firm polyp-like swelling protruding at anterior nares.

Osteoma

It is not an uncommon tumor and usually detected on a radiograph as an incidental finding. Osteoma is mostly seen in frontal or ethmoidal sinuses. It may cause headache and recurrent sinusitis. Radiography shows a calcified and well-demarcated lesion.

Chondroma

It is a painless, slow-growing swelling arising from ethmoid, nasal cavity, or septum. Chondroma is smooth or lobulated and firm. It may be a pure cartilage tumor or may be mixed type containing fibrous, osteoid, and angiomatous tissue apart from cartilaginous tissue.

- Intracranial lesions, for example, encephaloceles and meningoceles, may extend into nasal cavity and look like nasal lesions. Hence, biopsy must never be done before excluding such a possibility by CT scan or MRI.

- Chondromas are treated by excision. A large recurrent tumor should be widely excised due to the possibility of malignant transformation.

Carcinoma

Primary carcinoma of the nose is rare. It may be an extension of maxillary or ethmoid carcinoma. It is squamous cell carcinoma in 80% of cases; rest are adenocarcinomas and adenoid cystic carcinomas.

Squamous cell carcinoma

- **Clinical features**: Squamous cell carcinoma may arise from vestibule, anterior part of nasal septum, or lateral wall. The patients are mostly men above 50 years of age. The vestibular carcinoma may extend into the columella, nasal floor, and upper lip with metastasis to preauricular nodes. Septal carcinoma arises from mucocutaneous junction and causes burning and soreness. It is often called nose-picker's cancer. It is usually a tumor of low-grade malignancy. Lateral wall is the most common site of involvement. It extends into ethmoid or maxillary sinus easily. The patient presents with a polypoidal mass arising from the lateral wall.
- **Treatment**: It is treated with wide excision with postoperative radiation or chemoradiation. Low-grade tumors limited to lateral nasal wall, ethmoid sinuses, or septum can be treated by endoscopic techniques. Advanced disease is treated by a combination of chemotherapy, radiotherapy, and surgery.

Adenocarcinoma

Adenocarcinoma arises from glands of mucous membrane and is related etiologically to exposure to hard wood dust in furniture industry. It is treated by wide excision with cancer-clear margin.

Adenoid cystic carcinoma

Adenoid cystic carcinoma arises from ectopic minor salivary glands of the nose. This tumor may spread along with local nerves into the cranium which may require craniofacial resection.

Carcinoma of maxillary antrum

Carcinoma can arise from the epithelial lining of maxillary antrum. Its cause is not known but it is etiologically related to exposure to nickel. Its clinical presentation depends on the site of its origin as described in Table 16.3.

- **Treatment**: It is treated by wide excision which may amount to total maxillectomy. The cervical lymph nodes are treated by radiotherapy or radical node dissection.

Malignant Melanoma

- It affects the anterior part of nasal septum followed by middle and inferior turbinates. It spreads to cervical lymph nodes by lymphatics and anywhere in the body by bloodstream.

Table 16.3 Clinical features of carcinoma of maxillary antrum

Site of tumor	Clinical manifestation
Tumor of floor	Palatal bulge, may be pain in the teeth which may become loose
Tumor of medial wall	Unilateral nasal obstruction, epiphora, may be bleeding from obstructed nostril
Tumor of anterolateral wall	Asymmetrical swelling of face, pain, anesthesia of cheek including upper lip
Tumor of roof or orbital wall	Elevated inferior orbital margin, proptosis, diplopia
Tumor of posterior wall	Difficult to detect till late; trismus, paresthesia over cheek, gums, lower lip, postnasal discharge, swelling of the temporal region
Tumor without local signs (confined to antrum)	Metastatic enlargement of upper cervical lymph nodes, that is, submandibular and upper jugulodigastric

- The patient is usually around 50 years of age and presents with a slate gray or bluish black polypoid mass in the nose.
- It is treated by wide excision with a 5-year survival rate of 30%.

Olfactory Neuroblastoma

- It can occur at any age in any sex. There is a cherry-red polypoidal mass in the upper third of nasal cavity. It bleeds freely if an attempt is made to do biopsy. Lymphatic and systemic metastases can occur.
- It is treated by excision and postoperative radiotherapy. Craniofacial excision may be required for tumors of cribriform palate.

Hemangiopericytoma

- It is a rare tumor from the pericytes of capillaries. The patient is usually 60–70 years of age and presents with epistaxis.
- Biopsy confirms the diagnosis but results in brisk bleeding.
- It is treated with wide excision. Radiotherapy is indicated in inoperable and recurrent tumors.

Lymphoma

Sometimes a non-Hodgkin lymphoma occurs in the septum of the nose. It is treated by a combination of chemotherapy and radiotherapy.

Plasmacytoma

Solitary plasmacytoma can occur in the nose. It usually occurs in males over 40 years of age. After confirming the diagnosis by biopsy, it is treated by radiotherapy followed 3 months later by surgery, if total regression does not occur. As it may later result in a multiple myeloma, long-term follow-up is required.

Sarcoma

All types of sarcoma—osteosarcoma, chondrosarcoma, rhabdomyosarcoma, and angiosarcoma—and malignant histiocytoma can occur in the nose. The diagnosis is confirmed by radiography CT scan, and biopsy. The treatment depends on the nature of tumor.

4. OTHER DISEASES OF NOSE AND PARANASAL SINUSES

Rhinolithiasis

Etiology Rhinolithiasis is formation of a stone in the nasal cavity which usually forms around a foreign body, blood clot, or inspissated secretion by gradual deposition of calcium and magnesium salts. Over a period of time, it grows into a large irregular mass that fills the nasal cavity. It may cause pressure necrosis of septum and lateral wall of nose.

Clinical Features The patient is usually an adult who presents with unilateral nasal obstruction with foul-smelling discharge which may be blood-stained. When ulceration occurs, frank epistaxis and neuralgic pain may occur.

Diagnosis Anterior rhinoscopy shows a gray, brown, or greenish black mass which is irregular, hard, and brittle, present between the nasal septum and turbinates. It may be surrounded by granulations.

Treatment It is removed under general anesthesia. It may have to be broken into pieces for removal. Some very large and hard stones may require lateral rhinotomy.

Mucocele of paranasal sinuses

Pathology It is cystic lesion of a paranasal sinus containing thick mucus and lined by pseudostratified or low columnar epithelium.

Pathogenesis It can affect any sinus but the frontal sinus is affected most frequently. As time passes, the cyst grows in size and the increasing intracystic pressure converts its bony sinus wall into fibrous and the cyst grows into the direction of least resistance, that is, into the orbit.

Clinical Features The patient presents with a painless, slow-growing swelling in the orbit over a period of months or years. It may cause diplopia. There is smooth, globular, and tender swelling at upper medial half of the orbit or medial canthus area. The eyeball is usually pushed inferolaterally with proptosis.

Investigation The lesion is best imaged by CT scan.

Treatment It is treated with drainage by an open operation or endoscopically.

Epistaxis (rhinorrhagia)

It is the bleeding from the nose which may be venous or arterial. In about 90% of patients, it is from the venous Kiesselbach's plexus of Little's area.

Etiology

The most frequent causes of epistaxis are nose-picking, hypertension, and anticoagulant drugs. The causes are listed in Box 16.7.

Box 16.7 Etiology of epistaxis

- **Trauma**
  - Nose-picking
  - Fractures of nasal bones, maxilla, and anterior cranial fossa
  - Foreign body in nose
  - Barotrauma—high altitudes, caisson disease
  - Extremes of heat and cold
- **Spontaneous**
  - Infections and inflammations of nose—atrophic rhinitis, rhinitis sicca, nasal myiasis
  - Tumors of nose and nasopharynx, for example, angiofibroma, carcinoma, hemangioma, midline granuloma
  - Venous epistaxis due to sudden rise of venous pressure in retrocolumellar veins
  - Nose blowing, sneezing
  - Straining, violent coughing
  - Arterial epistaxis of old age—arteriosclerosis with or without arterial hypertension
  - Systemic causes—bleeding disorders, hereditary hemorrhagic telangiectasia
- **Iatrogenic**
  - Operations on nose, nasal intubation

Treatment of Epistaxis

Depending on the site of bleeding, it may be anterior bleeding or posterior bleeding. The commonest cause of anterior bleeding is nose-picking and the commonest cause of posterior bleeding is arterial hypertension. The anterior bleeding is easy to treat, while the treatment of posterior bleeding is difficult.

General measures

The patient is made to sit up in the bed, blood is cleaned, and the nose is pinched for 10 minutes. Cold fomentations may be helpful. If the bleeding point is visible, it can be cauterized by 50% trichloroacetic acid or electrocautery. If the bleeding is significant and not controlled by the above-mentioned measures, the patient is admitted to the hospital. The cause of bleeding if known is treated, for example, trauma and tumors.

Treatment of anterior nasal bleeding

Anterior nasal bleeding is treated by anterior nasal packing with either Vaseline-impregnated ribbon gauze or absorbable sponge. An alternative to anterior nasal packing is the use of an inflatable epistaxis balloon catheter.

Treatment of posterior nasal bleeding

Posterior nasal packing may be required which is done under general anesthesia. Sometimes arterial embolization or ligation of bleeding vessel is required to control bleeding.

Nasal obstruction

Etiology

- **In the lumen**: Foreign body, mucus plug, nasal snuff, rhinolith
- **In the wall**
  - Congenital—choanal atresia
  - Infections
    - Infective rhinitis
    - Sinusitis
    - Granulomatous infections, for example, tuberculosis, syphilis
    - Septal abscess
  - Trauma
    - Fracture of nasal bones
    - Fractures of maxilla
    - Hematoma of nasal septum
  - Allergy
    - Allergic rhinitis
    - Vasomotor rhinitis
    - Rhinitis medicamentosa
  - Tumors
    - Angiofibroma
    - Carcinoma
    - Others—sarcoma, lymphoma
  - Other causes
    - Deviated nasal septum
    - Nasal polyp
    - Adenoid hypertrophy
- **Outside the wall**
  - Maxillary sinusitis
  - Tumors of paranasal sinuses, for example, carcinoma, sarcoma, lymphoma
- **General causes**
  - Hypotensive drugs
  - Hypothyroidism
  - Smoking, alcoholism
  - Exposure to cold air, chill

The investigations and treatment of epistaxis depend on the cause.

KEY POINTS

- Choanal atresia is a developmental defect characterized by persistence of bucconasal membrane detected by the presence of mucoid discharge in the nose, absence of air bubble in discharge, and inability to pass a catheter in the nasopharynx. Bilateral atresia is an emergency.
- Rhinitis is inflammation of the lining of the nose which may be infective due to viruses and bacteria, allergic due to inhaled allergens, vasomotor due to overactivity of parasympathetic system, atrophic due to atrophy of nasal mucosa, and medicamentosa due to use of topical drugs.
- Rhinitis is characterized by varying combination of rhinorrhea, sneezing, loss of sense of smell, and nasal obstruction. They are treated by removal of cause and symptomatic treatment.
- Wegener's granulomatosis is a systemic disease of unknown etiology having classic triad of upper and lower respiratory tract involvement and glomerulonephritis.
- In nasal myiasis, maggots (larvae of flies) are found in nose, nasopharynx, and paranasal sinuses. They cause extensive destruction of the nose and tissues around and may produce a fistula. Ultimately the patient may die of meningitis.
- Congenital syphilis of nose presents as snuffles with an obstinate nasal discharge and as a gummatous ulcer which destroys the local tissues resulting in depressed bridge of nose.
- Lepromatous leprosy presents with bulbous thickening of nasal vestibule, obstruction of nasal cavity, extensive crusting, fetid purulent nasal discharge, ulceration, septal perforation, liquefaction of nasal framework, saddle nose, thick and deformed nasal ala, and leonine facies.
- Nasal polyps are non-neoplastic masses of edematous nasal or sinus mucosa caused by repeated attacks of allergic or vasomotor rhinitis combined with infection.
- Maxillary sinus is most commonly involved in acute inflammation of paranasal sinuses. It impairs the sinus drainage. Surgical treatment of sinus infection includes antral puncture and irrigation, intranasal antrostomy, and Caldwell-Luc operation.
- Frontal sinusitis is commonly associated with ethmoid sinusitis. The patient presents with frontal headache with periodicity, that is, the pain appears on waking up in the morning, gradually

(CONTD...)

KEY POINTS (...CONTD)

increases and reaches its peak about mid-day, and then starts subsiding ("office headache").

- Deviated nasal is an important cause of nasal obstruction. Septoplasty and submucous resection are the surgical procedures for major septal deviation.
- Septal perforation may be due to trauma, infections, and idiopathic. A small perforation may cause whistling during breathing. It is treated by repair or blocked by a prosthesis.
- Foreign bodies in the nose are very common and are mostly seen in children. Most of the foreign bodies enter the nose through the nostrils. They are removed by manipulation.
- Trauma to nose causes fracture and nasal septal injury. Severe trauma to the nose may result in fracture of frontal and ethmoidal sinuses extending into anterior cranial fossa with dural tear with cerebrospinal fluid rhinorrhea.
- Rhinophyma (potato nose) causes immense thickening of distal nose characterized by swollen bluish nose with bosselated surface and shallow pits.
- Lethal midline granuloma resembles non-Hodgkin lymphoma of either NK-cell or T-cell origin. In contrast to granulomatosis with polyangiitis, the involvement is limited to mid face with extensive bone destruction
- A tumor of nose may present with unilateral nasal obstruction, unilateral persistent rhinorrhea, postnasal drip, and epistaxis, but these symptoms are nonspecific. Hence, too often the diagnosis is delayed.
- A tumor of paranasal sinuses presents with facial pain, swelling, proptosis, diplopia, and epiphora. Some of these signs are indicative of orbital involvement. Nerve involvement is heralded by numbness in the distribution of infraorbital nerve.
- Carcinoma and sarcoma are the two important malignant tumors of maxilla/antrum. Both of them present with swelling and bleeding. They are treated by a combination of surgery, radiotherapy, and chemotherapy.
- Mucocele is common in frontal sinus. As time passes, the cyst grows in size and the increasing intracystic pressure converts its bony sinus wall into fibrous and the cyst grows into the direction of least resistance, that is, into the orbit.
- Epistaxis is bleeding from the nose which may be venous or arterial. In about 90% of patients, it is from the Kiesselbach's plexus of Little's area. The most frequent causes of epistaxis are nose-picking, hypertension, and anticoagulant drugs. It requires emergency treatment.

SELF-ASSESSMENT

Long answer question

1. What is rhinitis? What are its types? Describe the etiology, clinical features, and treatment of allergic rhinitis.

Short answer questions

1. Atrophic rhinitis
2. Wegener's granulomatosis
3. Midline granuloma
4. Deviated nasal septum
5. Rhinophyma
6. Nasal polyp
7. Chronic maxillary sinusitis
8. Inverted papilloma

Multiple choice questions

1. All of the following statements are true about allergic rhinitis, except
   (a) Epistaxis is a common symptom of this disease
   (b) It may be seasonal or perennial
   (c) It is IgE mediated
   (d) It is characterized by sneezing and watery rhinorrhea
2. Vasomotor rhinitis is due to
   (a) Nasal allergy
   (b) Overactivity of parasympathetic system
   (c) Viral infection
   (d) Long-term use of antihypertensive drugs

(CONTD...)

SELF-ASSESSMENT *(...CONTD)*

3. All of the following points are true about primary atrophic rhinitis, except
   (a) Its cause is not known
   (b) It is characterized by atrophy of nasal mucosa
   (c) There is foul smell from the nose
   (d) It is a curable disease
4. All of the following statements are true about nasal myiasis, except
   (a) It is a fungal infection of nose
   (b) It is the presence of maggots in the nose
   (c) It is due to laying of eggs in the nose by houseflies
   (d) It can cause death by meningitis
5. All of the following statements are true about a nasal polyp, except
   (a) It is a neoplastic disease
   (b) It is related to allergy
   (c) The polyps are of two types—ethmoidal and antrochoanal
   (d) An antrochoanal polyp arises in maxillary antrum
6. Sinusitis most commonly affects
   (a) Frontal sinus
   (b) Ethmoidal sinus
   (c) Sphenoidal sinus
   (d) Maxillary sinus
7. The most common site of empyema is
   (a) Sphenoidal sinus
   (b) Ethmoidal sinus
   (c) Maxillary sinus
   (d) Frontal sinus
8. All of the following are features of empyema of maxillary antrum, except
   (a) There is collection of pus in the maxillary antrum
   (b) The nasal discharge may have foul smell
   (c) X-ray of antrum is normal
   (d) Transillumination shows an opaque sinus
9. Which one of the following paranasal sinuses is the most common site of tumorigenesis?
   (a) Ethmoidal sinus
   (b) Sphenoidal sinus
   (c) Maxillary sinus
   (d) Frontal sinus
10. Deviated nasal septum can cause all of the following problems, except
    (a) Nasal obstruction
    (b) Nasal malignancy
    (c) Sinusitis
    (d) Nasal deformity
11. Rhinophyma is a
    (a) Viral infection
    (b) Bacterial infection
    (c) Fungal infection
    (d) Neoplastic process
12. Which one of the following is the most common type of carcinoma of maxillary antrum?
    (a) Adenocarcinoma
    (b) Transitional cell carcinoma
    (c) Mucoepidermoid carcinoma
    (d) Squamous cell carcinoma
13. Exposure of which one of the following metals is a risk factor for the development of maxillary carcinoma?
    (a) Nickel
    (b) Arsenic
    (c) Cobalt
    (d) Cadmium
14. Epistaxis is defined as
    (a) Bleeding from the ear
    (b) Bleeding from the nose
    (c) Bleeding from the larynx
    (d) Bleeding from trachea
15. The commonest site of bleeding in epistaxis is
    (a) Roof of nose
    (b) Lateral wall of the nose
    (c) Little's area
    (d) Floor of the nose

Answers

1. (a) 2. (b) 3. (d) 4. (a) 5. (a) 6. (d) 7. (c) 8. (c)
9. (c) 10. (b) 11. (d) 12. (d) 13. (a) 14. (b) 15. (c)

Diseases of Oral Cavity

17

Anatomy of oral cavity

The oral cavity extends from the lips to the oropharyngeal isthmus. It has the following parts: lips, cheeks, gums (gingivae), retromolar trigone, palate, anterior two-thirds of tongue (oral tongue), and floor of mouth.

Types of oral mucosa

Oral mucosa is of two types.

Masticatory Mucosa It is the mucous membrane which covers the alveolar process, retromolar trigone, and hard palate. It is keratinized and firmly attached to underlying periosteum and bone, hence called mucoperiosteum. It is relatively resistant to injury.

Papillated Mucosa It is the mucosa of dorsum of tongue. It is also keratinized, and is tough and firmly attached to the underlying muscles of tongue. Some diseases of oral cavity have a definite relationship with different types of oral mucosa.

Bacteriology of oral cavity

Many types of bacteria are present in the oral cavity. In the normal circumstances, most of them are harmless to the individual. The number (and virulence) of these bacteria is controlled by the following factors:

- Regular desquamation and replacement of surface cells
- Continuous washing of oral cavity by saliva
- Mild antibacterial activity contained in saliva
- The health and integrity of lining epithelium

Some oral commensals are facultative pathogens and take advantage of any weakness in the defenses of oral mucosa to produce an infective lesion in the mouth. Certain other microorganisms produce specific infective lesions and are true pathogens.

The cultivable organisms in the adult oral cavity (gingival crevice, dental plaque, tongue, and saliva) are described in Box 17.1.

Box 17.1 Bacteria in oral cavity

- Gram-positive facultative cocci, for example, streptococci, *Streptococcus salivarius*, enterococci, and staphylococci
- Gram-positive anaerobic cocci
- Gram-negative facultative cocci
- Gram-negative anaerobic cocci
- Gram-positive facultative rods
- Gram-positive anaerobic rods
- Gram-negative facultative rods
- Gram-negative anaerobic rods, for example, *Fusobacterium*, *Bacteroides melaninogenicus*, *Vibrio sputorum*, and other *Bacteroides*
- Spirochaetes

1. INFLAMMATION AND INFECTIONS

Aphthous ulcer (canker sores, aphthous stomatitis)

Aphthous ulcers are the most commonly reported oral ulcers occurring in approximately one-fourth of population.

Etiology The cause of these ulcers is uncertain, although an association with human herpes virus 6 has been suggested.

Clinical Features

- Site: They occur on nonkeratinized mucosa (buccal and labial) and not on gingivae or palate.
- They present as single or multiple, round or oval, discrete erythematous macules 2–30 mm in diameter that rapidly indurate and ulcerate but do not vesiculate like herpetic lesions. They have yellow-gray fibrinoid centers surrounded by red halos (Fig. 17.1).

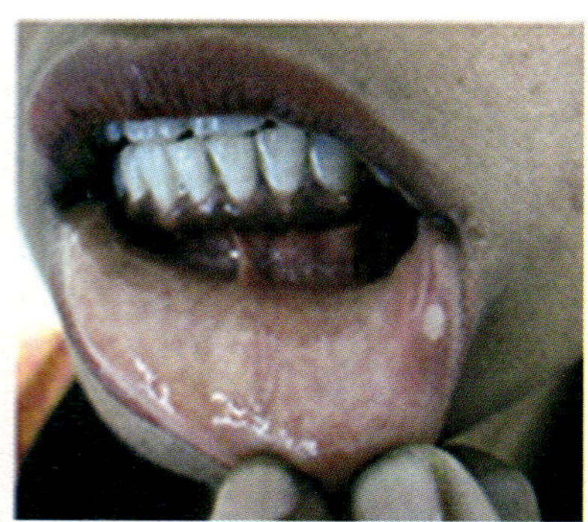

Figure 17.1 Aphthous ulcer of lower lip.

- They are quite painful as they interfere with mastication and speaking. The painful stage lasts for 7–10 days and the healing of ulcers is completed in 1–3 weeks without scarring.

Treatment

- Triamcinolone acetonide 0.1% or fluocinonide ointment 0.05% in an adhesive base is applied locally.
- Other topical therapies include diclofenac 3% in hyaluronan, 2.5% doxymycine-cyanoacrylate mouthwashes containing the enzymes amyloglucosidase and glucose oxidase, and amlexanox 5% oral paste.
- One-week tapering course of prednisone 40–60 mg/day has also been used successfully.
- In recurrent ulcers, cimetidine maintenance therapy may be helpful. Thalidomide can be given to HIV-positive patients with recurrent aphthous ulcers.

Herpetic stomatitis

Etiology It is caused by human herpes virus type 1 (HHV-1).

Types It is of three clinicopathological types:

1. Primary gingivostomatitis
2. Herpes labialis
3. Intraoral herpes

Clinical Features

- It presents as multiple small vesicles that rupture soon resulting in small yellow-white superficial ulcers surrounded by a red halo, located on the attached gingivae and mucocutaneous junctions of the lips, but can also form on the tongue, buccal mucosa, and soft palate.

- In severe disease, the gingivae are edematous and bleed readily. The primary type is accompanied by fever, pain, malaise, and cervical lymphadenopathy. Although this lesion is self-limiting, the virus may be reactivated by physical trauma and endogenous stress.
- The recurrent HHV-1 disease must be differentiated from recurrent aphthous ulcers. In contrast to recurrent aphthous ulcers, recurrent HHV-1 lesions are limited to attached gingivae and hard palate.

Treatment The treatment measures include the following:

- Topical anesthetic is used in solution or troche form.
- Disseminated infection or disease in an immunocompromised host is treated with systemic acyclovir 200–800 mg five times daily for 7–14 days. Newer antiviral agents, for example, valacyclovir and famciclovir, may be used.
- Topical acyclovir has limited usefulness, but penciclovir cream is reported to be effective.

Acute necrotizing ulcerative gingivitis (Vincent's gingivitis)

Etiology Gingivitis frequently occurs as a result of poor oral hygiene, heavy smoking, and lowered body resistance. Acute necrotizing ulcerative gingivitis is common in young adults under stress and occurs due to overgrowth of normal oral bacterial symbionts (spirochaetes, fusiform bacilli).

Clinical Features It is characterized by painful hemorrhagic gums, halitosis, ulceration, fever, cervical lymphadenopathy, and a yellowish-gray gingival pseudomembrane.

Treatment The treatment includes warm half-strength H_2O_2 rinses, maintenance of oral hygiene, removal of plaque and tartar of the tooth margins, and oral penicillin 250 mg three times daily for 10 days or clindamycin in penicillin-resistant cases.

Cancrum oris (noma)

Etiology It is an infective gangrene of oral cavity which is a severe form of Vincent's acute ulcerative gingivitis and stomatitis (noma means to devour or consume destructively). It is due to *Borrelia vincentii* and *fusiformis* infection.

Clinical Features The patient is usually a poorly nourished and ill child. Cancrum oris starts as a gingival ulcer with inflammation and rapidly progressive necrosis of tissues of gums, lips, cheek, jaw bones, and soft tissues in the vicinity with extensive tissue loss with severe toxemia and fetid odor. It may occur after an attack of measles, gastroenteritis, typhoid, or bronchopneumonia. This condition is associated with high morbidity and mortality.

Treatment The treatment includes intravenous antibiotics (penicillin/metronidazole), nasogastric tube feeding or total parenteral nutrition (TPN), and irrigation and excision of gangrenous tissue. Later on, the tissue defect/deformity requires reconstructive surgery.

Nutritional stomatitis

Many types of nutritional deficiencies produce some changes in the oral cavity called nutritional stomatitis (Table 17.1).

Table 17.1 Oral manifestations of nutritional deficiency

Nutritional deficiency	Oral manifestations
Riboflavin (B_2)	Cheilosis, angular stomatitis, and glossitis
Nicotinic acid	Soreness of mouth, stomatitis, and glossitis (pellagra)
Vitamin C	Bleeding gums and loosening of teeth (scurvy)
Iron	Atrophy of papillae, smooth tongue, and superficial glossitis

2. CYSTS OF MOUTH

Mucocele

It is a mucous-containing cyst of lips. It probably occurs due to trauma to the ducts of minor salivary glands of the lips resulting in extravasation of mucus in the tissues. It is described in detail in Chapter 15, *Diseases of Face*.

Ranula

It is a cyst of floor of mouth which resembles the belly of a small frog (rana means a small frog), hence this name (Fig. 17.2). It is smooth, bluish, and transilluminant, and may have a cervical extension. It is excised per orally along with sublingual salivary gland, and the plunging ranula with excision of submandibular salivary gland also.

Sublingual supramylohyoid dermoid

It is a sequestration dermoid that occurs in the floor of mouth either in the anterior midline below the tongue (median sublingual dermoid) or in the lateral side (lateral sublingual dermoid). It is smooth, soft, and opaque (Fig. 17.3). The treatment is excision.

Thyroglossal Cyst

It is a tubulodermoid which develops from thyroglossal tract which extends from foramen cecum of tongue to the isthmus of thyroid. It is usually present in the neck in midline in the vicinity of hyoid bone. Rarely it may occur in the floor of mouth or substance of the tongue.

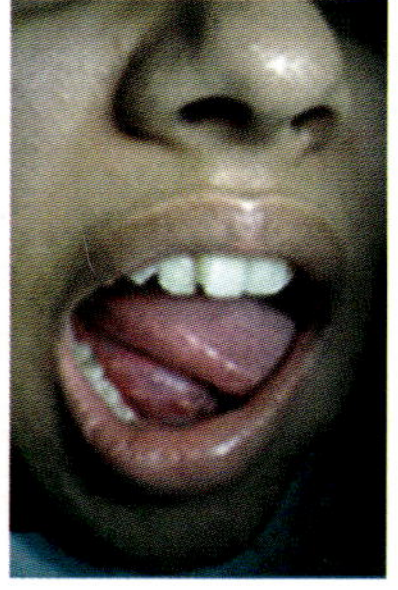

Figure 17.2 Ranula of floor of mouth. (Courtesy: Professor Surajit Bhattacharya)

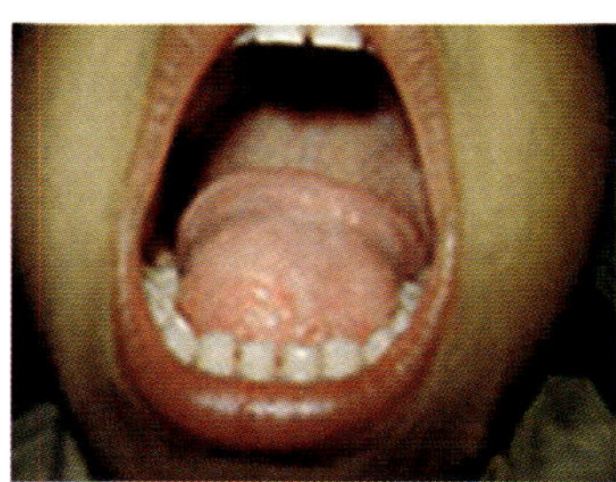

Figure 17.3 Sublingual supramylohyoid dermoid (median supramylohyoid type). (Courtesy: Professor Surajit Bhattacharya)

3. TUMORS OF ORAL CAVITY

A tumor can occur in the oral cavity. Their classification is described in Box 17.2.

Squamous cell papilloma

As the name suggests, it is a papilloma like that of skin lined by squamous cells. It can occur anywhere in the oral cavity, but usually arises from the epithelium of palate, fauces, and gingivae in children and young adults. Squamous cell papilloma has small, whitish, finger-like processes. It may have a pink cauliflower-like appearance, if its keratin is lost. It may be sessile (Fig. 17.4) or pedunculated. It should be excised with base electrocoagulated.

Box 17.2 Tumors of the oral cavity

Benign tumors

- Squamous cell papilloma
- Lipoma
- Hemangioma
- Granular cell myoblastoma
- Neural tumors
- Pleomorphic adenoma

Malignant tumors

- Squamous cell carcinoma
- Salivary carcinoma, for example, adenoid cystic carcinoma, mucoepidermoid carcinoma
- Malignant melanoma
- Lymphoma, leukemia
- Metastatic tumors

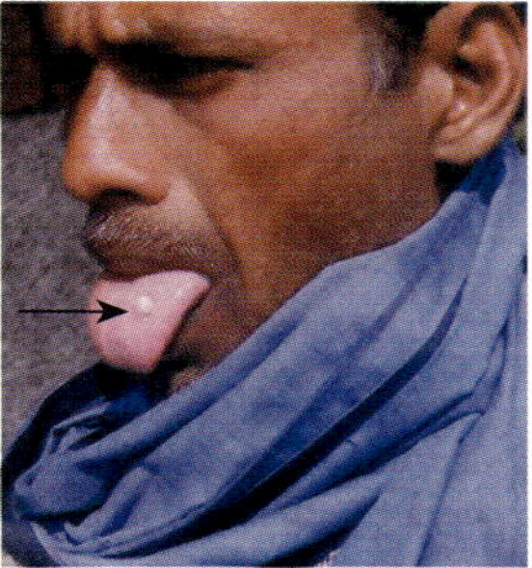

Figure 17.4 Papilloma of tongue.

Lipoma

It is a benign tumor of fatty tissue. Lipoma is a rare tumor of oral cavity but may occur in the floor of mouth or cheeks as a painless, slow-growing, pale, soft and smooth, or lobulated swelling of insidious onset. Treatment is excision.

Hemangioma

Hemangioma is a benign tumor comprising dilated thin-walled blood vessels. It may be localized (hemangioma) (Fig. 17.5) or diffuse (vascular malformation).

Localized Hemangioma The localized type varies from small multiple telangiectasia or spider nevi as seen in hereditary hemorrhagic telangiectasia to disfiguring port-wine stain. It is treated by excision, cryosurgery, or laser beam.

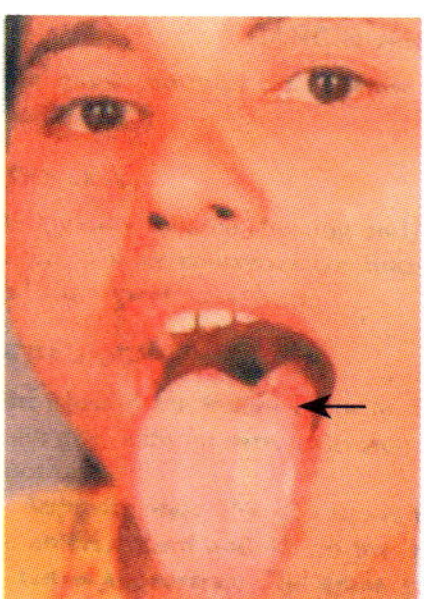

Figure 17.5 Hemangioma of tongue of posterior third, left side. (Courtesy: Professor Rajiv Agarwal)

Diffuse Hemangioma The diffuse type varies from cavernous venous malformation to cirsoid aneurysm. It is often extensive and involves large areas of gingivae, alveolar bone, and tongue. It needs to be treated if there are repeated episodes of bleeding, if a tooth is to be extracted, or for cosmetic reasons. The full extent of the lesion is assessed by CT scan, venography, intralesional contrast, and carotid arteriography. It may sometimes be possible to excise the lesion after ligation of external carotid artery and/or its branches. It is often combined with preoperative injection of sclerosant solutions or percutaneous embolization.

Granular cell myoblastoma

It is an uncommon tumor of tongue that occurs in middle-aged people and presents as a small rounded swelling in the substance of tongue or beneath the surface mucosa. Microscopically it consists of eosinophilic large granular cells frequently in continuity with muscle fibers. Hence, it was once considered to arise from striated muscle, but is now considered to be of neural origin. Pseudoepitheliomatous hyperplasia of the overlying epithelium often occurs when it may be mistaken for carcinoma. It is treated by complete excision; otherwise, it will recur.

Neural tumors

Neural tumors sometimes occur in the oral cavity as small painless nodules of insidious onset. A central neurilemmoma (schwannoma) may occur from the inferior dental nerve in the mandible expanding it. In von Recklinghausen's neurofibromatosis, the face and mouth may be affected extensively with multiple soft pedunculated swellings of oral mucosa or gingivae. They may involve the underlying bone causing deformity and interference in eruption of teeth. They may be associated with café au lait spots. The symptomatic tumors are excised.

Pleomorphic adenoma

All types of salivary tumors can occur in the oral cavity from sublingual salivary gland and minor salivary glands which are present all over the oral cavity but mostly in the palate. Pleomorphic adenoma is the commonest salivary tumor.

It occurs typically at the junction of hard and soft palate. It is a painless, slow-growing, rubbery hard swelling of insidious onset covered by normal mucosa. The tumor is excised completely together with overlying mucosa. The resultant wound is left to granulate and epithelize which occurs quite rapidly.

Squamous cell carcinoma of oral cavity

It is an epithelial malignant tumor of oral mucosa especially related to tobacco and alcohol habit and characterized by an irregular nonhealing ulcer. It is very common in our country.

Etiology

This cancer is etiologically related to tobacco habit (chewing and smoking) and heavy drinking. Furthermore, it is etiologically related to many lesions of oral mucosa which are associated with an increased risk of oral carcinoma. The premalignant lesions and conditions of oral mucosa are enumerated in Box 17.3.

Box 17.3 Premalignant lesions or conditions of oral mucosa

- **Premalignant lesions: Conditions having a definitive risk of cancer**
  - Oral leukoplakia
  - Erythroplakia
  - Speckled leukoplakia
  - Speckled erythroplakia
  - Chronic hyperplastic candidiasis
- **Premalignant lesions: Conditions associated with a higher than normal risk of cancer**
  - Oral submucous fibrosis
  - Syphilitic glossitis
  - Sideropenic dysphagia (Plummer–Vinson syndrome)

Pathology

It can occur anywhere in the oral cavity, the most common sites being labiogingival sulcus, cheeks, and gingivae (alveolus) (Fig. 17.6). It may produce an ulcerative or a proliferative lesion, the former being more common. Microscopically, it is a squamous cell carcinoma. It spreads mainly by local infiltration, and by lymphatics to locoregional lymph nodes. It usually does not spread by bloodstream.

Clinical Features

- This disease commonly occurs in middle-aged or elderly people, more commonly in males.
- It may remain asymptomatic in the beginning of the disease. As the disease advances, it

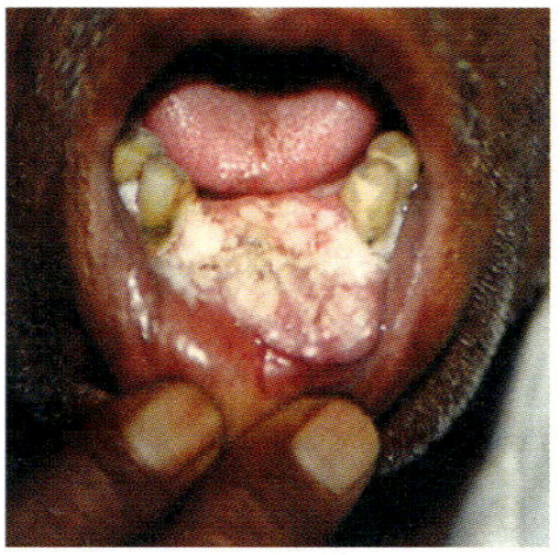

Figure 17.6 Carcinoma of lower central alveolus.

becomes symptomatic, the symptoms being a nonhealing ulcer, odynophagia (painful swallowing), otalgia (pain in the ear) in a posterior lesion, trismus, halitosis, toothache, and cervical lymphadenopathy.

- Irregular indurated ulcer in the oral cavity that bleeds on touch is the commonest presentation of carcinoma of oral cavity.
- Some other site-specific manifestations include slurring of speech (carcinoma of tongue), tooth extraction socket that fails to heal (carcinoma of alveolus), and gingival inflammation on which the dentures do not fit.
- The cervical lymph nodes are enlarged, hard, and mobile or fixed in 50–58% of cases. Occult microscopic metastases are present in 12–30% of cases with nonpalpable nodes.

TNM Staging

The TNM staging of the tumor is described in Box 17.4. The stage grouping based on the TNM classification helps in determining the line of treatment and prognosis of this disease. The stage grouping is described in Table 17.2.

Box 17.4 TNM staging of squamous cell carcinoma

- **T: Tumor size**
  - *T1*: Up to 2 cm in its greatest dimension
  - *T2*: 2–4 cm in size
  - *T3*: More than 4 cm
  - *T4*: Tumor of any size invading adjacent structures, for example, muscles, mandible, maxilla
- **N: Nodal involvement and size**
  - *N1*: Ipsilateral single lymph node up to 3 cm
  - *N2a*: Ipsilateral single lymph node 3–6 cm in size
  - *N2b*: Ipsilateral multiple nodes 3–6 cm in size
  - *N3*: Lymph node more than 6 cm in size
- **M: Metastasis**
  - *M0*: No distant metastasis
  - *M1*: Presence of distant metastases which are very rare in this cancer

Table 17.2 Stage grouping of squamous cell carcinoma with prognosis

Stage	TNM grouping	Prognosis
Stage I	T1N0M0	Very good
Stage II	T2N0M0	Good
Stage III	T3N0M0, T1–3N1M0	Bad
Stage IV	T4N0M0, T1N2–3M0, T any N any M1	Very poor

Investigations

Laboratory Studies The blood is sent for hemoglobin, counts, ESR, sugar, urea, creatinine, and others as required.

Radiography

- Orthopantomography of the jaws is done to see for bony involvement, that is, erosion or destruction.
- CT scan and/or MRI are sometimes required to find the extent of disease. MRI is better to study the soft-tissue spread of the disease.

Biopsy It is taken from the edge of the lesion from two sides under local anesthesia. It should not be taken from center as it often contains necrotic tissue. The histological features of this tumor are malignant squamous cells with epithelial pearls (keratin pearls).

FNAC FNAC is done from lymph nodes of neck to find their involvement.

Treatment

The treatment modalities of squamous cell carcinoma of the oral cavity are described in Table 17.3.

Surgery

The surgery involves en bloc resection of tumor combined with radical neck dissection of lymph nodes. If the tumor is attached to the mandible without eroding into it, partial-thickness removal of mandible is done with the tumor retaining the mandibular arch. If the tumor is eroding into the bone, a full-thickness portion of the involved bone is removed (Fig. 17.7) and the defect is

Table 17.3 Treatment modalities for squamous cell carcinoma of oral cavity

Stage	Treatment
T1N0M0 (stage I) tumors	Either radiotherapy or wide surgical excision (with microscopic confirmation of cancer clearance) with equal results
T2 and larger tumors (but excisable)	Combined surgery and radiotherapy
Stages II and III (tumor cannot be excised)	• Stage II: Wide excision followed by radiotherapy (RT) • Stage III: Downgrading by RT or CT followed by wide excision
Stage IV (T4 tumor)	Combination of radiotherapy and chemotherapy

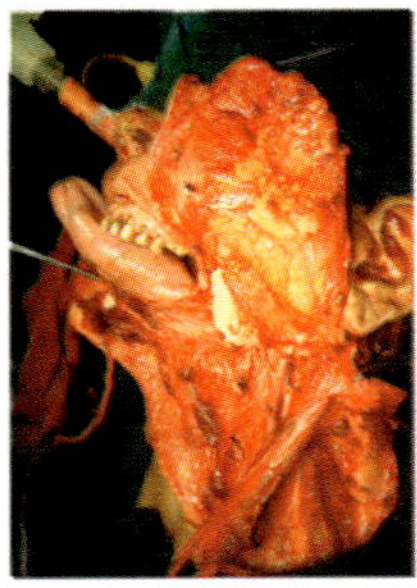

Figure 17.7 Appearance after radical excision of carcinoma of left alveolus with cervical lymph node dissection. (Courtesy: Professor Surajit Bhattacharya)

bridged by a bone graft obtained from iliac crest or fibula. The soft-tissue anatomical defects left after excision are reconstructed with the use of various flaps. Microvascular surgical techniques may be employed in reconstruction.

Neck dissection

The level of lymph node involvement is important in deciding the extent of lymph node dissection. The five levels of cervical lymph nodes are given in Table 17.4. Most of the oral cancers spread up to level III. Levels IV and V may be involved in advanced disease.

Table 17.4 Levels of lymph node involvement

Level	Lymph node involvement
Level I	Submental and submandibular
Level II	Upper jugular chain
Level III	Middle jugular chain
Level IV	Lower jugular chain
Level V	Lymph nodes of posterior triangle of neck along the spinal accessory nerve

Types of neck dissection

Classic Radical Neck Dissection It is resection of lymph nodes of levels I–IV, fat, fascia, sternomastoid, omohyoid, internal jugular vein, external jugular vein, accessory nerve, submandibular salivary gland, lower part of parotid, and prevertebral fascia en bloc (Crile's operation).

Modified Radical Neck Dissection (MRND) It is done in well-differentiated and less aggressive tumors. It is just like radical neck dissection with preservation of three important neck structures (N-nerve; M-muscle; V-vein); hence, it is of three types:

1. **MRND type I, N preserved**: Spinal accessory nerve preserved
2. **MRND type II, NM preserved**: Spinal accessory nerve and sternomastoid muscle preserved
3. **MRND type III, NMV preserved**: Spinal accessory nerve, sternomastoid muscle, and internal jugular vein preserved

Bilateral Neck Dissection Sometimes bilateral neck dissection is required in which the internal jugular vein of one side is preserved to prevent cerebral congestion and edema (dangerous). The side of which the vein is to be preserved is operated first.

Radiotherapy

Radiotherapy techniques include external beam radiotherapy and Co-60, and brachytherapy using cesium-137 needles or iridium-192 wires. If the tumor is in intimate contact with the bone, radiotherapy is not given for fear of radio-osteonecrosis.

Chemotherapy

The drugs used are cisplatin, methotrexate, and bleomycin. The chemotherapy may downstage the tumor when it can be excised.

Prognosis

The overall survival for all cancers of oral cavity is about 65%. In carcinoma of lip, the 5-year survivals are as high as 90%. The prognosis is worse in carcinoma of tongue. The overall 5-year survivals in the anterior lesions are more than 65% and less than 40% in a posterior lesion.

Carcinoma of Floor of Mouth

- It is a rare cancer in India but second common oral cancer in Western countries.
- It presents as an infiltrative ulcerative lesion that invades hyoglossus, mylohyoid, genioglossus, and anterior parts of mandible early.
- It is treated with wide excision including resection of mandibular rim through visor anterior approach. The mandibular defect is reconstructed with a bone graft and plates.
- Postoperative radiotherapy and later chemotherapy may be used to improve results. The prognosis is poor.

Carcinoma of Alveolus

It is a common oral cancer in India which arises from the gums (carcinomatous epulis). It involves the jaw bone early. Bilateral nodal involvement is common. It is treated with wide excision including the part of the bone involved and bilateral cervical node dissection.

4. OTHER DISEASES OF THE ORAL CAVITY

Abnormal labial frenum

Abnormalities of Labial Frenum

- Enlargement which is a congenital abnormality
- Scarring from injury or inflammation when occur repeatedly

Clinical Features

- It is mostly the upper labial frenum that is affected. It tends to become short, tethering the lip to the alveolar mucosa. It may restrict the mobility of lip, especially when smiling. In severe disease, the frenum extends from the central incisors to the palatine papilla causing a central diastema and reduction of the depth of the buccal sulcus. It may result in poor oral hygiene and periodontal disease. The frenal attachment to the crest of the edentulous alveolar ridge causes difficulty in retention of artificial denture.

Treatment The fibrous band within the frenum is excised and the mucosa is sutured to reconstitute the depth of the sulcus.

White patches in the oral cavity

White patches in the oral cavity are quite common. They show three main histological features: abnormal keratinization, hyperplasia or hypoplasia of epithelium, and disordered maturation (dysplasia). Dysplasia is a sign of possible malignant change. The important causes of white patches in the oral cavity are mentioned in the subsequent text.

Transient White Patches These patches appear and disappear after some time. They are seen in oral candidiasis and due to mucosal reaction to aspirin which is sometimes kept in the mouth to relieve toothache.

Fordyce Spots They are soft creamy white spots which are distributed symmetrically. They are a normal feature of oral mucosa. These spots are due to sebaceous glands which may appear in the mucous membrane of cheeks and sometimes the lips of elderly.

White Sponge Nevus It is a soft and uneven thickening of superficial layers of mucosa, sometimes involving extensive areas in the oral cavity. It is a familial disorder inherited as a simple dominant.

Tertiary Syphilis It usually causes chronic superficial glossitis. Microscopically it is a syphilitic granulomatous lesion with endarteritis of small arteries and one or more foci of malignant change. The serological tests for syphilis are positive. It is treated with penicillin and excision of the lesion.

Smoker's Keratosis

- This lesion is seen on the palate of heavy smokers.
- Clinical features: The thickened mucosa looks pale white with multiple small swellings of mucous glands surmounted with a red central orifice. These changes are especially seen in persons who indulge in reverse smoking. White patches may be seen on the floor of mouth in cheroot smokers.
- Treatment: The patient is advised to give up smoking which results in disappearance of lesions in most of the patients. Persistent patches are excised.

Frictional Keratosis It occurs due to chronic or recurrent irritation of mucosa by sharp teeth or ill-fitting denture and cheek biting. The lesion is recognized by its site and the cause. Removal of the cause results in its cure.

Chronic Candidiasis It is a common cause of white patches in the oral cavity. It is a common problem in infants and children and immunocompromised people. Chronic candidal infection causes epithelial proliferation and plaque formation which is not clinically distinguishable from leukoplakia.

Lichen Planus

It is a chronic inflammatory autoimmune disorder that affects 0.5–2% of population. Lichen planus is the most common cause of persistent white patches in the oral cavity which commonly affects the cheek mucosa (Fig. 17.8). This problem is commonly associated with anxiety or stress.

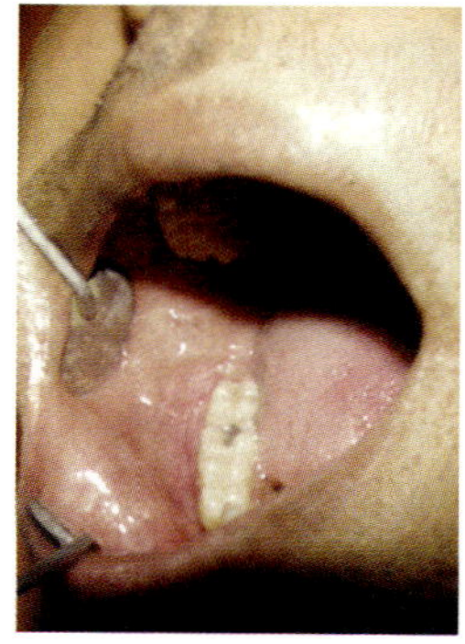

Figure 17.8 Lichen planus of right cheek. (Courtesy: Professor Divya Mehrotra)

Clinical Features The lesion is usually striated forming a lace-like pattern. It can be papular or confluent, especially on the tongue. It may be erosive and painful.

Diagnosis Exfoliative cytology or a small incisional or excisional biopsy is indicated, especially to rule out malignancy.

Treatment Treatment aims at relieving pain and discomfort. The cause is removed and corticosteroids are used locally and systemically. Cyclosporin and retinoids have also been used.

Oral Candidiasis

Oral candidiasis or thrush is a type of infection of the oral cavity caused by *Candida albicans* and is characterized by a white pseudomembranous lesion closely adherent to oral mucosa. It should always be remembered that candidiasis may be the first manifestation of HIV infection.

Etiology

C. albicans is a part of normal oral biology. It may become pathogenic due to systemic and local factors (Box 17.5).

Clinical features

This condition is usually painful and looks like creamy white curd-like patches sticking on erythematous mucosa. If this white area is rubbed off by a tongue depressor, the underlying

Box 17.5 Predisposing factors of oral candidiasis

Systemic factors

- Long-term administration of antibiotics
- Use of anticancer drugs
- Immune deficiency
- Corticosteroid therapy
- Diabetes mellitus
- Anemia
- AIDS (it causes oral candidiasis along with hairy leukoplakia caused by Epstein—Barr virus)

Local factors

- Radiotherapy given to oral cavity and pharynx
- Xerostomia
- Smoking
- Smokeless tobacco
- Mechanical changes in the oral environment such as dentures
- Poor oral hygiene

irregular erythema is seen. It produces four types of lesions:

1. Pseudomembranous lesion, being the most common (when it sloughs, it ulcerates and bleeds)
2. Hyperplastic form, characterized by superficial fungal invasion of epithelium and leukoplakia
3. Erythematous or atrophic form
4. Angular cheilitis

Investigations

- When the curd-like lesions are seen under high power (400×) using 10% potassium hydroxide, spores and nonseptate mycelia can be seen.
- Culture can be done.
- Biopsy will reveal intraepithelial pseudomycelia of *C. albicans*.
- It should always be remembered that candidiasis may be the first manifestation of HIV infection.

Treatment

- The cause must be treated.
- Antifungal drugs, for example, fluconazole 100 mg orally daily for 7 days, ketoconazole 200–400 mg orally with breakfast for 7–14 days, clotrimazole troches (10 mg dissolved orally five times daily), or nystatin mouth rinses (5,00,000 units; 5 mL of 1,00,000 units/mL) held in mouth before swallowing three times daily, are administered.
- Resistant cases to the above-mentioned drugs may need newer drugs, for example, voriconazole. Chlorhexidine 0.12% or half-strength hydrogen peroxide mouth rinses may provide local relief.
- Nystatin powder (1,00,000 units/g) applied to dentures three or four times daily for several weeks may be helpful in denture wearers.

Oral Leukoplakia

It is a persistent white patch on the oral mucosa which does not disappear on rubbing. It is a premalignant condition and likely to turn into malignancy in 2–4% of patients. It increases with age, duration of paan–tobacco chewing, and smoking.

Etiology

It is due to chronic persistent or recurrent irritation of oral mucosa in susceptible persons. The causes of irritation include drying and chemical effects of smoking, ill-fitting oral prosthesis, chewing tobacco and paan masala, and cheek biting. Its incidence is 20% in those who smoke or chew paan–tobacco, and 1% in those who do not smoke or chew paan–tobacco. The susceptibility to leukoplakia may be augmented by syphilis and alcoholism.

Pathology

The lesions vary from simple thickening to early carcinoma. Microscopically, it is of two types:

1. **Leukoplakia without cellular atypia**: It shows varying combinations of hyperkeratosis, parakeratosis, and acanthosis (simple leukoplakia).
2. **Leukoplakia with cellular atypia**: Apart from features of leukoplakia, described above, it shows varying degrees of dyskeratosis or atypia which may be minimal, moderate, or severe. Severe atypia is difficult to distinguish from carcinoma in situ.

Clinical features

- It can occur at any age but most of the patients are middle-aged or elderly, more commonly a male. The patient has a white patch/patches in the oral cavity (Figs 17.9 and 17.10) which varies from an isolated white patch to diffuse widespread mucosal involvement. There may be considerable variation in color and surface texture.

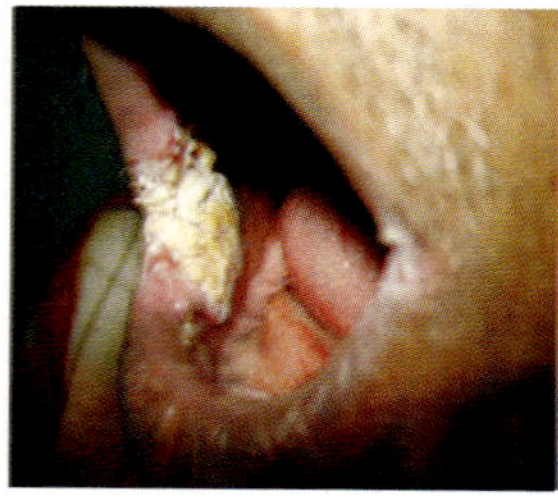

Figure 17.9 Leukoplakia of right commissure of lips, undergoing malignant change. The left angle also shows some changes. (Courtesy: Professor Surajit Bhattacharya)

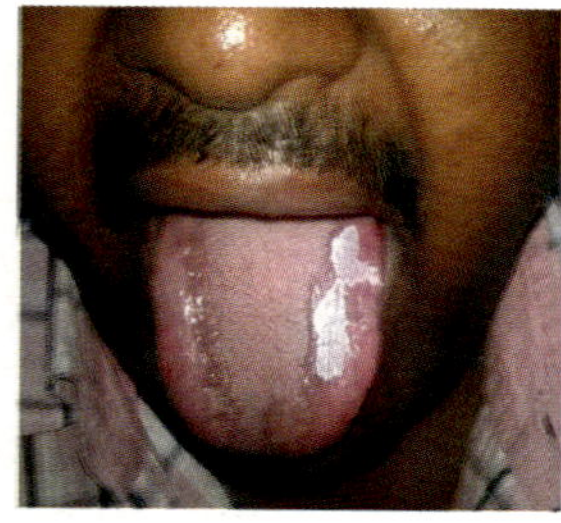

Figure 17.10 Leukoplakia of tongue. (Courtesy: Professor Surajit Bhattacharya)

- Site: It may occur anywhere in the oral cavity with the largest number of lesions developing on the mandibular alveolar ridge, gingivae, and mucogingival fold. In order of frequency the other common sites include buccal mucosa, palate, maxillary ridge, floor of mouth, lower lip, and tongue.
- The color may be white, grayish, or even light yellow. It may be stained to brownish hue in tobacco chewers. The surface texture may be smooth or deeply fissured and wrinkled.
- Speckled leukoplakia is a white leukoplakia interspersed with red areas. It is a more serious form of leukoplakia.

Diagnosis

The diagnosis is confirmed by biopsy taken from the area that displays the greatest surface irregularities such as cracks and fissures.

Treatment

- The simple leukoplakia is treated by removal of the cause, maintenance of oral hygiene, and periodic examination of the oral cavity. If the lesion does not disappear within 3–4 weeks, it is excised.
- The dyskeratotic leukoplakia is treated by excision or ablation (electrofulguration or cryosurgery) of the lesion. For example, a lip lesion is treated by lip stripping or lip shave.
- The use of beta-carotene, cyclooxygenase inhibitors (COX-2 inhibitors), vitamin E, and retinoids may be helpful in causing regression of the lesion.

Hairy leukoplakia

It occurs on the lateral border of tongue and is a common finding in patients with HIV infection. It usually develops rapidly and presents as a slightly raised leukoplakic area with corrugated or "hairy" surface. It usually responds to zidovudine or acyclovir.

Erythroplakia

It is a bright red velvety mucosal patch in the oral cavity of unknown etiology. Erythroplakia is a precancerous lesion. It is associated with epithelial dysplasia, carcinoma in situ, or carcinoma. Mashberg (1978) described two types of lesions:

1. A granular red velvet-like lesion having either speckled or patchy areas of white keratin on or peripheral to the lesion
2. A smooth red nongranular lesion with very little or no keratin, the red color being due to decreased keratin

Clinical Features It is common in lower alveolar mucosa, gingivobuccal sulcus, and floor of mouth. In both lesions, the mucosal surface appears inflamed. The limit of these lesions is often poorly defined, blending the inflamed with noninflamed mucosa. In many patients of cancer, erythroplakia appears long before ulceration, bleeding, induration, pain, or lymphadenopathy. It is 17–20 times more potentially malignant than leukoplakia.

Treatment It is treated by wide excision followed by microscopic scrutiny and appropriate long-term follow-up.

Oral submucous fibrosis

It is a chronic progressive disease characterized by the formation of fibrous bands beneath the oral mucosa.

Etiology It is not exactly known. It may occur due to hypersensitivity to chilies, betel nut, and tobacco. Vitamin deficiencies (vitamin A and riboflavin) may play a part. The betel quid or paan masala contains some alkaloids and collagenases that may be responsible for connective tissue changes leading to epithelial atrophy and malignant change.

Pathogenesis The arecoline of betel nut stimulates collagen synthesis and proliferation of buccal mucosal fibroblasts. The tannins of betel nut stabilize the collagen fibrils and render them resistant to degradation by collagenase. The newly formed fibrous bands progressively contract, limiting the ability to open the mouth. The fibrosis under the tongue mucosa restricts the movements of the tongue.

Pathology There occurs juxtaepithelial fibrosis with atrophy or hyperplasia of overlying epithelium, which has foci of epithelial dysplasia also.

Clinical Features

- It is a common problem in India which affects 5 people among 1000 persons. It is common in middle-aged and affects both sexes equally.
- The patient presents with severe limitation of the ability to open the mouth (extra-articular ankylosis of temporomandibular joint). The movements of the tongue are also restricted (ankyloglossia).
- The mucosa of the cheek, gingivae, palate, and tongue is thin and atrophic and shows a mottled/marbled pallor. The cheek loses its suppleness, elasticity, and stretchability. It feels hard like leather. These patients are more likely to develop oropharyngeal carcinoma.

Treatment

- The cause of this problem must be eliminated. The fibrosis is treated by intralesional injections of corticosteroids (triamcinolone).
- Excision of abnormal fibrous tissue with skin grafting may be required. Instead of skin, the raw area can be covered by a collagen sheet.

5. DISEASES OF TONGUE

Congenital and developmental disorders

Aglossia (Absent Tongue)

The tongue may be absent since birth due to defective growth of tuberculum impar often associated with maldevelopment of mandible.

Bifid Tongue

It is a congenital defect of tongue in which the tongue is divided into two parts by a longitudinal fissure. It is due to failure of fusion of two parts of tuberculum impar. It may be associated with inferior cleft lip and sometimes with cleft palate.

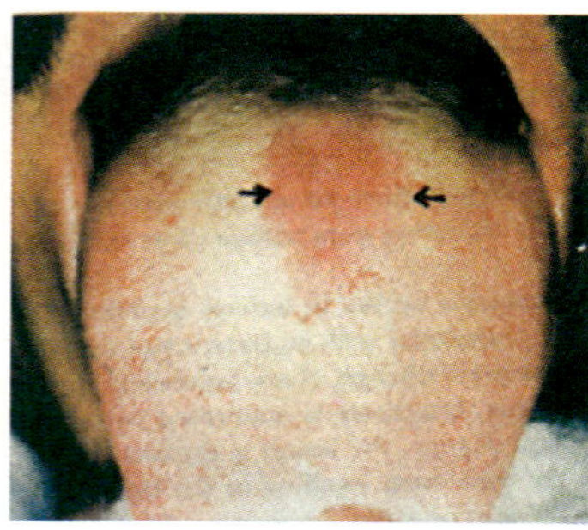

Figure 17.11 Median rhomboid glossitis. (Courtesy: Professor R.M. Mathur)

Infections and inflammations

Median Rhomboid Glossitis

It is a chronic disease of tongue characterized by rhomboidal redness with loss of papillae in the middle of the tongue with long axis anteroposterior with limit at the circumvallate papillae line (Fig. 17.11). It is a self-limiting problem that does not require any treatment. *Candida* infection can occur in it.

Syphilis of Tongue

The causative organism, *Treponema pallidum*, is transferred by licking or kissing, and rarely by passage of drinking cups, pipes, or spoons from one individual to another.

Clinical features of syphilis of tongue

Primary Syphilis Primary chancre on the tip of tongue or just behind is 1–3 cm in diameter, not indurated and associated with local edema. The submental and submandibular lymph nodes are enlarged sometimes considerably in size.

Secondary Syphilis

- **Mucous patches**: They are due to swelling of the papillae of tongue on which a grayish white film of dead epithelium appears. They may also be present inside the cheeks or faucial pillars.
- **Snail-track ulcers**: They are longitudinal shallow ulcers on the dorsum of tongue with sloping edges. They may also be present on the palate, tonsillar region, and the sides and undersurface of tongue.
- **Hutchinson's wart**: It is a condyloma of tongue which is strictly a median wart.

Tertiary Syphilis

- **Syphilitic leukoplakia**: It is a white patch of thickened epithelium in the middle of dorsum of tongue.
- **Gumma**: It is a painless hard swelling on the dorsum of tongue in the midline. It is of the size of a pea when superficial and the size of a walnut when deep. Gumma may rupture on the surface of the tongue to produce a gummatous ulcer.
- **Gummatous ulcer**: It is a chronic ulcer of midline of dorsum of tongue which has a punched-out edge, serpentine outline, and wash-leather slough. It is hard and nontender. It tends to heal in one part while spreading in other.
- **Diffuse gummatous inflammation**: Here the whole tongue is enlarged, hard, and nontender. Eventually it contracts due to fibrosis.

Management

The diagnosis is confirmed by serological tests for syphilis and sometimes biopsy. Benzyl penicillin injection 2.4 million units is the antibiotic of choice, once in primary syphilis and once weekly for 3 weeks in tertiary syphilis.

Tuberculosis of Tongue

The infection (caused by *Mycobacterium tuberculosis*) may involve the tongue by autoinoculation from infected tuberculous sputum, or by hematogenous and lymphatic spread from a distant focus.

Clinical manifestations

Tuberculous Ulcer

- It is the commonest tuberculous lesion. It may develop as a tiny tubercle which later ulcerates.

- Most of the patients are young, more commonly males, and have an ulcer close to the tip of tongue extending backwards on one side. It is painful, shallow, yellowish, and soft, and has unhealthy granulation tissue on the floor. The edge is sloping rather than undermined and the ulcer is deeper than it appears.
- There may be symptoms and signs of laryngeal or pulmonary tuberculosis.
- The discharge from the surface of ulcer may show tubercle bacilli. Biopsy may be required.

Tuberculoma It rarely occurs in the tongue. It presents as a nodule or a swelling as large as a walnut. It looks like syphilitic gumma and can be differentiated only by investigations. It ulcerates relatively early, resulting in a tuberculous ulcer. A tuberculoma may require excision.

Cold Abscess It is very rare in the tongue. It may be the result of softening of a tuberculoma. It presents as a painless soft swelling in the substance of the tongue. A cold abscess is either aspirated or surgically evacuated. The diagnosis can be confirmed by examination of aspirate for tuberculous infection.

Treatment

The patient is given four or five antituberculous drugs. In resistant cases, second-line drugs are administered.

Ulcers of Tongue

In the oral cavity, tongue is the most ulcer-prone. The mobility of tongue, infected environment of oral cavity, and its intimate relationship with teeth are etiologically related with the ulcers of tongue. The classification of the ulcers of the tongue is described in Box 17.6.

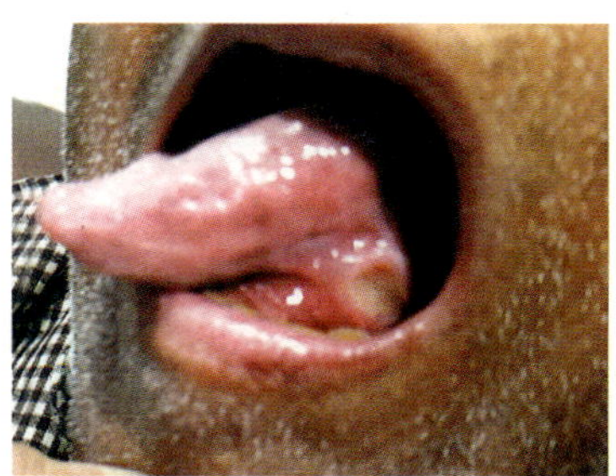

Figure 17.12 Dental ulcer of left side of floor of mouth adjacent to lateral border of tongue with sloping edge. (Courtesy: Professor Sandeep Kumar)

Clinical features of various ulcers of the tongue

Dental Ulcer

- It is caused by repeated trauma to the tongue by a decayed or broken sharp-edged or pointed tooth (usually the lower ones) or an ill-fitting denture. Hence, it is always situated at the borders of the tongue or just below.
- It is usually a painful, small elongated ulcer with sloping edge (Fig. 17.12). It is slightly indurated. It may become malignant if not treated in time. The treatment consists of removal of the cause, for example, rounding the sharp edge or point. The ulcer heals rapidly following removal of the etiological factor.

Aphthous Ulcer (Dyspeptic Ulcer) It is a small, rounded, painful erosion. It has a pale white center with a zone of hyperemia around. It often occurs near the tip of tongue. The other sites are lateral border and undersurface.

Post-Tussive Ulcer It is a small superficial ulcer that occurs on the frenum linguae in small children suffering with whooping cough. It is caused by trauma to the frenum during whoop by lower central incisors. Treatment is removal of

Box 17.6 Classification of ulcer of tongue

Nonspecific ulcers	Infective ulcers	Malignant ulcer
• Dental ulcer	• Syphilitic ulcers	• Carcinomatous ulcer
• Aphthous ulcer	• Tuberculous ulcer	
• Post-tussive ulcer (all of these are traumatic ulcers)	• Herpetic ulcer	

cause, that is, treatment of whooping cough with erythromycin.

Syphilitic Ulcers

- **Primary chancre**: The patient is an adult who presents with a painless ulcer usually on the tip of tongue. It is oval or round, raised, and superficial. The submental and submandibular lymph nodes are enlarged sometimes to a significant size.
- **Snail-track ulcers**: They are multiple superficial linear ulcers on the dorsum of tongue. Other features of secondary syphilis, that is, fever, rash, generalized lymphadenopathy, etc., are present.
- **Gummatous ulcer**: It is a solitary oval or round ulcer in the midline of dorsum of tongue. It has punched-out edge and wash-leather slough in the floor.

Tuberculous Ulcer The patient is usually young and may be suffering from pulmonary or laryngeal tuberculosis who is coughing and bringing out a lot of sputum. This ulcer is very painful and occurs near the tip. It is superficial, single or multiple, and soft, and has a sloping edge. It has watery granulation tissue in the floor.

Carcinomatous Ulcer The patient is usually a middle-aged or elderly person, more commonly a male who presents with a painless, nonhealing ulcer of the tongue of recent onset (but more than 3 weeks' duration). It can occur anywhere (Fig. 17.13) but is most commonly seen on the lateral border of tongue. It has an everted edge and indurated base. The submandibular lymph nodes may be enlarged, hard, and mobile or fixed.

Investigations

Biopsy It is the most important diagnostic investigation in a chronic nonhealing ulcer (of more than 3 weeks' duration). It is taken from the ulcer including a part of edge under local anesthesia. It is an absolute requirement for the diagnosis of a carcinomatous ulcer.

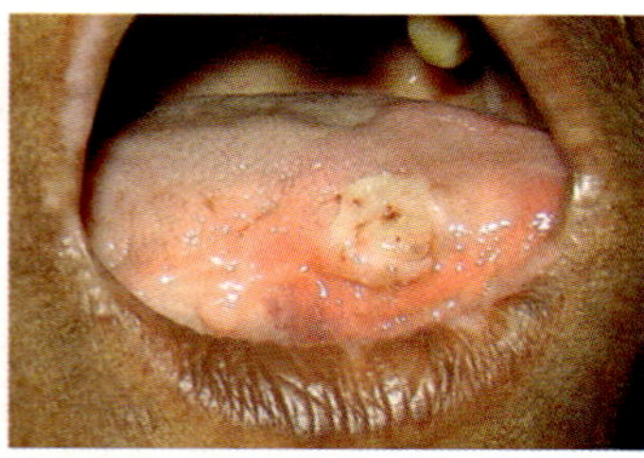

Figure 17.13 Carcinoma of tip of tongue.

Examination of the Discharge It is done by dark-field microscopy which may reveal *T. pallidum* in a syphilitic chancre. In a tuberculous ulcer, the patient is usually having productive cough and the examination of sputum may be positive for acid-fast bacilli. In a post-tussive ulcer, the sputum may have the causative organisms of whooping cough.

Other Investigations In a tuberculous ulcer, radiography of chest may show pulmonary tuberculosis, or laryngoscopy may reveal laryngeal tuberculosis. In snail-track ulcers and gummatous ulcers, serological tests of syphilis are usually positive.

Treatment

Treatment is the removal of the cause and maintenance of oral hygiene. Most of the ulcers heal after the cause is removed, except the carcinomatous ulcer, the treatment of which is described in the section "Carcinoma of Tongue."

Injuries of the tongue

The tongue may suffer with mechanical, thermal, or chemical injuries.

Mechanical Injury

Causes The causes of mechanical injury of tongue include:

- Tongue biting by an unconscious patient during anesthesia, epileptic fit, and coma
- Blow or fall while the victim is smoking a pipe which breaks and is driven into the substance of the tongue
- Accidental injury during operation in and around the oral cavity

Clinical Features Since the tongue is a very vascular organ, the injuries of the tongue bleed very briskly which may be aspirated into the airway. The tongue may be crushed, punctured, or lacerated. Sometimes a hematoma may form in the tongue which may spread into the floor of mouth and cause respiratory obstruction needing urgent tracheostomy.

Treatment

- The bleeding from the posterior part of tongue can be arrested by passing a finger as far back as possible and hooking the tongue forward on the jaw, thus applying pressure on the lingual artery.
- Subsequently under general anesthesia with endotracheal intubation, the bleeders are ligated and the wounds of the tongue are sutured. Even a loosely hanging segment should be sutured as these wounds heal rapidly with segments often remaining viable.
- Postoperatively the oral hygiene is maintained by frequent mouth washes.

Thermal Injury

The tongue may be burnt by accidental swallowing of very hot tea or coffee especially in those who are not used to taking very hot drinks. It usually causes a superficial burn. It is very painful and heals on its own in 2–3 days during which the oral hygiene is maintained by frequent mouth washes.

Chemical Injury

The accidental or intentional swallowing of corrosives may burn the tongue. The tip and dorsum of tongue are most affected. Repeated mouth washes are helpful.

Insect Bite

A wasp may bite the tongue. Classically it occurs when a holiday maker drinks from a beer bottle which has been left open. The tongue swells markedly immediately and may produce respiratory obstruction. It is treated by intravenous hydrocortisone and maintaining a patent airway.

Box 17.7 Classification of tumors of tongue

Benign tumors

- Papilloma
- Hemangioma
- Lymphangioma
- Neurofibroma
- Lipoma
- Osteoma
- Lingual thyroid

Malignant tumors

- Carcinoma—it is the commonest tumor of tongue
- Sarcoma
- Malignant melanoma

Tumors of tongue

A variety of tumors can affect the tongue. Their classification is described in Box 17.7.

Papilloma

It is the commonest benign tumor of tongue. Papilloma may be sessile or pedunculated and may have finger-like processes. It has a core of connective tissue covered by squamous epithelium. It should be excised with its base electrocauterized.

Hemangioma

It is a benign tumor or vascular malformation which consists of a bunch of thin-walled dilated vessels. It may be localized or diffuse. The tongue is having a localized or generalized swelling which is bluish, soft, and compressible (Fig. 17.14). It may be injured by teeth resulting in significant bleeding. A localized lesion is excised and a diffuse type is treated by injection of sclerosants or embolization.

Lymphangioma

It consists of a mass of dilated lymphatics. It causes diffuse and soft enlargement of tongue (macroglossia). It is treated by excision or glossoplasty.

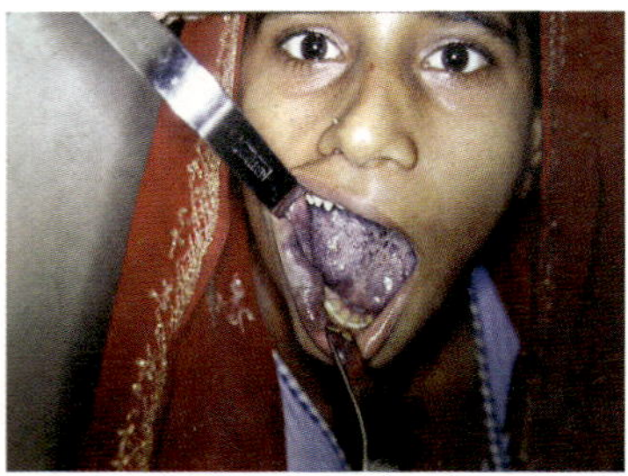

Figure 17.14 Hemangioma of tongue. (Courtesy: Professor Surajit Bhattacharya)

Neurofibroma

It may be localized or plexiform. The first one presents as a firm nodule while the second type causes macroglossia. It should be excised.

Lipoma

It is a rare tumor of tongue which presents as a small swelling of the size of a coffee bean. It is treated by excision.

Osteoma

It is a very rare tumor. The patient presents with a hard swelling in the posterior third of tongue, usually below foramen cecum. The bony tissue is derived from branchial arch remnants. It should be excised.

Lingual Thyroid

Sometimes ectopic thyroid tissue may be present in the tongue beneath foramen cecum which may enlarge due to some disease of thyroid. It may cause obstruction of oropharynx and disturbance of speech. It can be imaged by radio-iodine and CT scan/MRI. Neck should also be imaged for normal thyroid tissue. If it is causing symptoms, it has to be excised, and if it is the only thyroid tissue in the body, the patient has to be given thyroid hormone replacement.

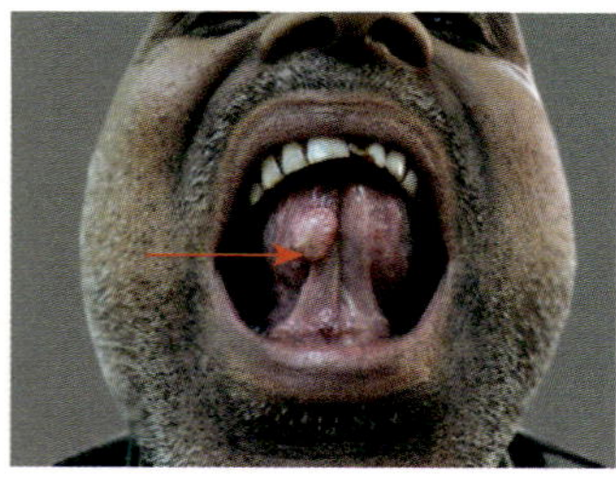

Figure 17.15 A small carcinoma of the undersurface of tongue. (Courtesy: Professor Surajit Bhattacharya)

Carcinoma of Tongue

It is an epithelial malignant tumor of the tongue etiologically related to tobacco and alcohol habit, characterized by an irregular ulcer or ulcerated swelling and poor prognosis. It is the commonest malignant tumor of tongue, and more common than all the benign tumors of tongue put together.

Clinical features

Commonly the patient is a middle-aged or elderly man. In the early stage of disease, there are no symptoms but an observant patient may notice the lesion, an ulcer, or a nodule in the tongue and come to the hospital (Figs 17.15 and 17.16). Most of the patients come when the disease is symptomatic and in advanced stage with the following clinical features:

- There is pain in the tongue (glossodynia) which may be referred to the ear of the same side.
- Excessive salivation occurs and the saliva may be blood-stained.
- The affected side of the tongue cannot be protruded out (ipsilateral ankyloglossia) due to infiltration of muscles. Hence, it deviates to the affected side.

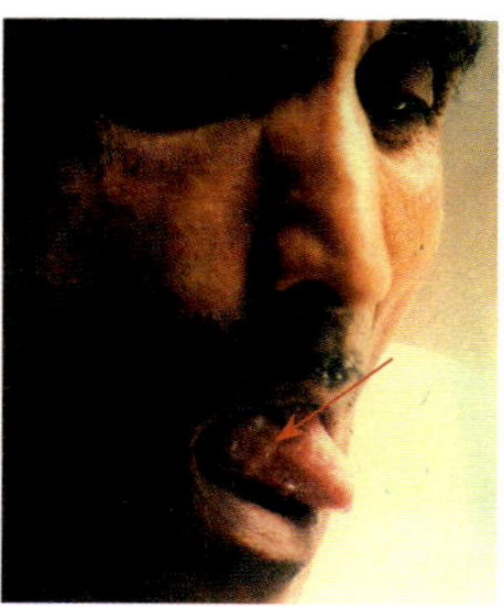

Figure 17.16 Carcinoma of right border of tongue.

- Dysphagia is a common symptom of cancer of posterior one-third of tongue; otherwise, it is due to fixation of tongue.
- There is inability to articulate clearly.
- Halitosis occurs due to local infection and necrosis of tumor.
- Palpable cervical lymph nodes—the cervical lymph nodes are palpable in 50% of patients. They are hard, nontender, mobile, or fixed. In 12% of patients, a lump in the neck may be the only presentation.

The lesion in the tongue is irregular, hard, and granular with a heaped-up or everted edge that bleeds on touch. It may cross the midline and may extend into floor of mouth and mandible. The lesions of posterior one-third are usually not visible but they can be palpated by a finger and can be seen with a pharyngeal mirror.

Treatment

The treatment of carcinoma tongue involves surgical excision, radiotherapy, and chemotherapy (Table 17.5).

Surgical Treatment

T1 Tumor

- A tumor less than 1 cm in size is excised with 1 cm clearance all around (Fig. 17.17). Laser (CO_2/diode) can be used.
- A tumor 1–2 cm in size is excised with 2 cm clearance all around (partial glossectomy) (Fig. 17.18) with removal of one-third of anterior two-third of tongue. This tumor can be treated by radiotherapy (brachytherapy using iridium-192 wires or cesium-137). It has the advantage of preserving the tongue.

Table 17.5 Treatment of carcinoma of tongue

Tumor	Treatment
T1 tumor <1 cm	• Excision with 1 cm clearance all around • Laser (CO_2/diode)
T1 tumor 1–2 cm	• Excision with 2 cm clearance all around (partial glossectomy) with removal of one-third of anterior two-third of tongue • Radiotherapy (brachytherapy using iridium-192 wires or cesium-137) preserves the tongue
T2 tumor	Hemiglossectomy with removal of diseased half of anterior two-third of tongue up to sulcus terminalis
T3, T4 tumors	Preoperative radiotherapy to downstage the disease and then resection
Posterior third of tongue tumor	• Radiotherapy • Wide excision after lip split and mandibulotomy
Cervical lymph nodes	• Neck dissection
Advanced unresectable tumor	• Palliative radiotherapy • Chemotherapy

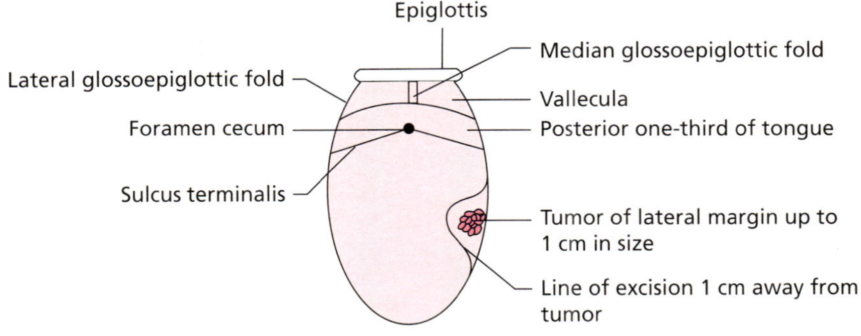

Figure 17.17 Surgical treatment—wide excision of a tumor up to 1 cm in size.

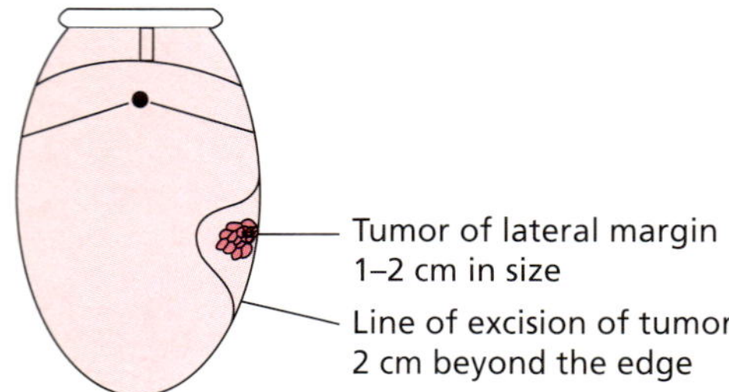

Figure 17.18 Partial glossectomy for a tumor of lateral border up to 2 cm in size.

T2 Tumor

- T2 tumor is treated with hemiglossectomy with removal of diseased half of anterior two-third of tongue up to sulcus terminalis (Fig. 17.19).
- The raw area of tongue in all the excisional procedures may be left as such to granulate and epithelize. If the area is small, it may be closed by primary suturing. A wide raw area is covered by pectoralis major myocutaneous flap or quilted split-skin graft.

Large Primary Tumors (T3, T4) They may be given preoperative radiotherapy to downstage the disease and then the resection is done. They may require major resection via a lip split and mandibulotomy.

Posterior Third Growth It is better treated with radiotherapy, although it can also be removed by lip split and mandibulotomy, but it carries a significant morbidity and mortality.

Preservation of Hypoglossal Nerve In these procedures, if possible, preserve one hypoglossal nerve as then the patient can relearn to speak and to swallow.

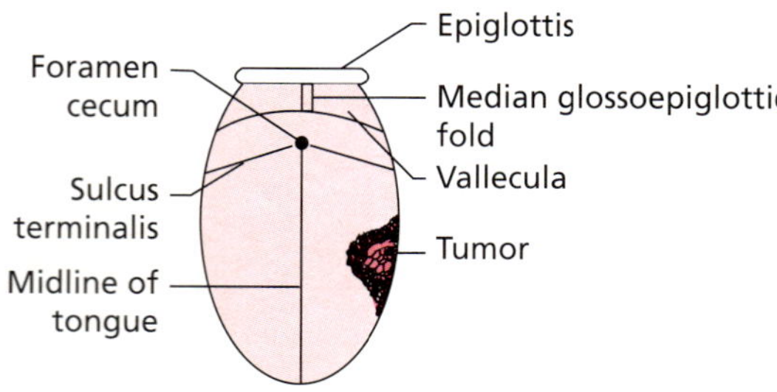

Figure 17.19 Hemiglossectomy for a tumor of margin of larger than 2 cm.

Commando Operation If the mandible is involved, the part involved is also removed which may amount to hemimandibulectomy. The full procedure involving wide excision or hemiglossectomy, hemimandibulectomy, and radical neck dissection is called commando operation.

Reconstruction The lost tongue may be reconstructed by deltopectoral flap, forehead flap, and pectoralis major flap.

Treatment of cervical lymph nodes

- The involved mobile cervical lymph nodes are excised by radical lymph node dissection which includes removal of internal jugular vein of the same side.
- In bilateral cervical disease, bilateral lymph node dissection is done preserving internal jugular vein of opposite side to maintain cerebral venous drainage. The latter type of lymph node dissection is known as functional lymph node dissection.
- Diseased neck nodes can be treated by radiotherapy (40 Gy) which is a good alternative to surgery and carries lesser morbidity than surgery.

Treatment of advanced unresectable tumor

- It is treated by palliative radiotherapy. It may reduce the tumor to make it excisable when it should be excised.
- Chemotherapy can be used to improve the results of treatment and also for palliation. The drugs include methotrexate, vincristine, Adriamycin, bleomycin, and mercaptopurine (Price-Hill regimen). They are given postoperatively. They may be given preoperatively to downstage the disease.

Treatment of carcinoma of posterior one-third of tongue

Radiotherapy is the preferred method of treatment. It can be excised by lip and mandibular split with bilateral neck node dissection with postoperative radiotherapy.

Prognosis

This cancer has a poor prognosis with 5-year survival of 50% in females and of 25% in males.

The differences between the carcinoma of anterior two-third and posterior one-third of tongue are described in Table 17.6. The overall prognosis of carcinoma of the tongue is poor with 5-year survival rates in females (50%) and in males (25%). It depends on the site of the lesion, the anterior lesions are better than the posterior lesions which are worse.

Other diseases of the tongue

Tongue-Tie (Inferior Ankyloglossia)

- In this congenital abnormality, the frenum linguae is short, restricting the mobility of tongue. The tip of tongue is doubled back on

Table 17.6 Differences between the carcinoma of anterior two-third and posterior one-third of tongue

Features	Carcinoma of anterior two-third of tongue	Carcinoma of posterior one-third of tongue
Incidence	More common	Less common
Symptoms	Remain asymptomatic for a short time	Remain asymptomatic for a long time
Presentation	As a nonhealing ulcer	As sore throat or throat discomfort
Referred pain to the ear of same side and blood-stained saliva	Early feature	Late feature
Clinical diagnosis	Cannot be easily missed	Can be missed easily
	Can be made by inspection	Can be made by palpation of posterior tongue by induration
Pathological feature of poor differentiation	Less common	More common
Lymphoepithelioma and transitional cell carcinoma	Do not occur in this part	Can rarely occur in this part
Local infiltration	Occurs in lower jaw, floor of mouth, and other half of tongue	Occurs in epiglottis, pre-epiglottic space, tonsillar pillars, and hypopharynx
Lymphatic spread	Less common, 50%	More common because of abundant lymphatics, 70%
	Bilateral spread less common	Bilateral spread more common because of cross-communication of lymphatics
Hematogenous spread	Rare	Can occur
CT scan/MRI	Not always needed to see the lesion and its extent	Always needed to see the lesion and its extent to plan therapy
Treatment	Wide excision is the preferred treatment	Radiotherapy is the preferred treatment
	Surgical treatment is relatively easy	Can be excised but needs mandibulotomy to do total glossectomy. Bilateral neck node dissection is required
	Postsurgical radiotherapy not always required	Postsurgical radiotherapy is usually required, especially if it is poorly differentiated and of the nodal status more than N1
Laryngectomy	Not required	Required in a T4 lesion
Prognosis	Better	Worse

itself and bent down to the floor of mouth. It may cause speech defect.

- Treatment: The tongue is lifted with the guard of a grooved director and the frenum is snipped near the floor of mouth to avoid injury to the frenal artery. Indiscriminate division should be avoided as it may lead to over mobile tongue which may result in speech defect and swallowing of tongue, blocking the pharyngeal airway.

Macroglossia

Etiology It is a chronic painless enlargement of tongue. Its causes include lymphangioma, muscular hypertrophy as seen in cretinism and some types of idiocy, neurofibromatosis, primary mesodermal amyloidosis, arteriovenous fistula (lingual gigantism), and edema due to carcinoma of posterior one-third of tongue.

Clinical Features It often causes difficulty in closing the mouth, speech, and mastication. It may cause proclination of lower incisors due to constant push from behind.

Treatment Treatment is removal of the cause. The hemangiomas are usually treated with cryosurgery or injection of sclerosants. Glossoplasty is required in other types. It is usually done by a V-shaped lateral incision. Care is taken not to injure the lingual arteries and nerves.

Geographical Tongue (Erythema Migrans)

- This lesion commonly occurs in unhealthy young children. Its cause is not known.

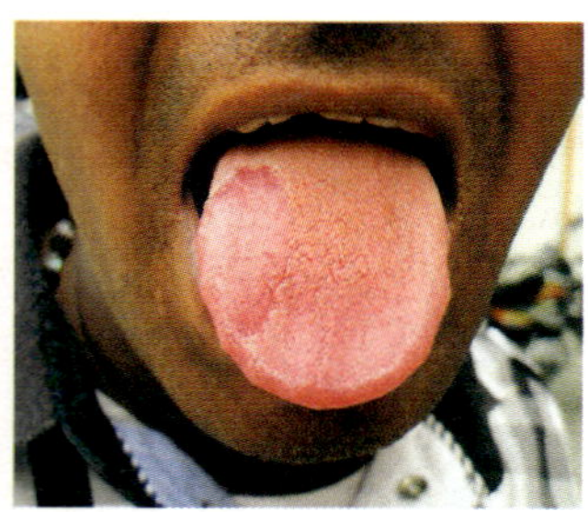

Figure 17.20 Geographical tongue.

- Clinical features: It is characterized by small, red, circular or oval patches on the anterior two-third of the tongue (Fig. 17.20). They gradually enlarge and appear as smooth denuded areas with a slightly elevated yellowish border and a peculiar irregular shape rather like the outline of a country on the map. That is why it is called geographical tongue. The filiform papillae disappear but the fungiform are present.
- When a patch reaches the border of tongue, it may creep around on the undersurface. When one spreading edge meets another edge, one often recedes while the other continues to spread. Each patch has a life of about 7 days.
- Treatment: This condition does not require any treatment except improvement of general health.

Black Hairy Tongue (Melanoglossia)

In this lesion, the tongue has a blackish patch on the dorsum of which the filiform papillae are elongated and thickened and appear like bristly hair (Fig. 17.21). It is due probably to one or other pigment producing molds which include *Aspergillus niger*. It may occur in people who suck on antibiotic lozenges for a substantial period. As such, it does not require any treatment except removal of the cause and maintenance of oral hygiene.

Fissuring of Tongue

Congenital Fissuring The congenital fissures of tongue are always transverse (Fig. 17.22a). They may be quite deep and may not be present at the

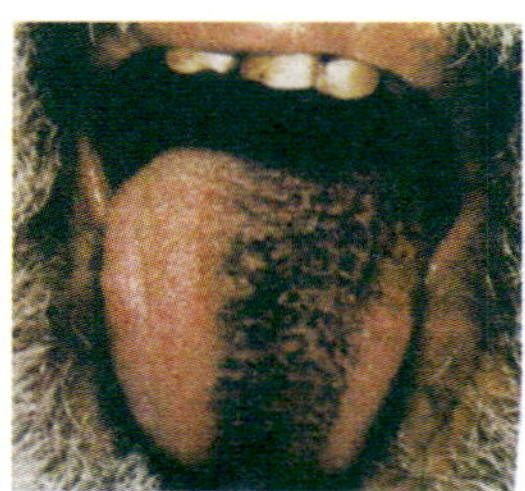

Figure 17.21 Black hairy tongue. (Courtesy: Professor R.M. Mathur)

time of birth, but may appear in early childhood. *Candida* infection can affect this tongue.

Syphilitic Fissuring The syphilitic fissures tend to be longitudinal (Fig. 17.22b). This tongue is usually bald and the fissures are deep.

Tuberculous Fissuring Tuberculosis rarely produces a single short and deep fissure in the tongue.

Treatment Treatment is removal of cause and maintenance of oral hygiene as the food residue in the fissures may cause infection.

Hemiatrophy of Tongue

Hemiatrophy of tongue is the result of injury of the ipsilateral hypoglossal nerve which causes paralysis of muscles of tongue of the same side. The paralyzed muscles gradually undergo atrophy. The affected half of tongue gets shriveled and cannot be protruded. Hence, the protruded tongue deviates to the side of the lesion.

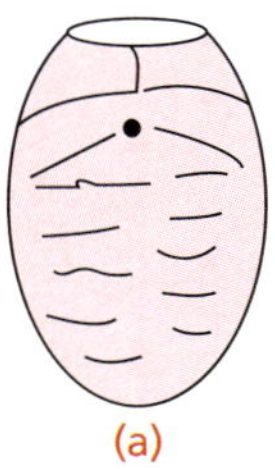

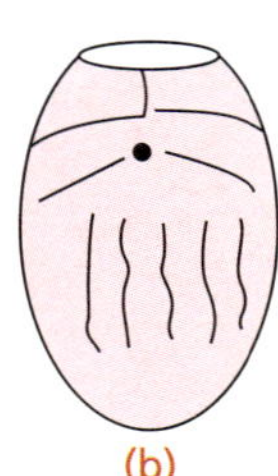

Figure 17.22 Fissuring of tongue. (a) Transverse fissures (congenital); (b) longitudinal fissures (syphilis).

The patient presents with some thickening of speech and difficulty in mastication and swallowing. There is no treatment of this problem but after a few months the patient learns to adjust to the lingual weakness.

Lingual Neuralgia

It is characterized by attacks of severe pain in one half of the tongue. Lingual neuralgia may be due to involvement of lingual nerve in scar tissue or neoplastic infiltration. It may follow lingual herpes. In a large number of cases, its etiology is not clear.

It is treated initially by carbamazepine which relieves a majority of patients. Other drugs which can be used include phenytoin and gabapentin. If the drug treatment does not help, the chorda tympani is divided in its canal close to the posterior border of tympanic membrane.

6. DISEASES OF PALATE

Inflammation and ulceration can occur in the palate as they can occur anywhere else in the oral cavity. Two problems need separate mention here and they include swellings and perforation of palate.

Swellings of palate

The classification of swellings of palate is described in Box 17.8.

Box 17.8 Classification of swellings of palate

Midline swellings

- Cyst of papilla or of incisive canal (nasopalatine cyst)
- Torus palatinus
- Epstein's pearls
- Syphilitic gumma

Lateral swellings

- Apical abscess or cyst
- Periodontal abscess or cyst from an upper molar
- Neurofibroma of greater palatine nerve
- Cancer of maxillary antrum extending downwards

Anywhere in the palate

- Ectopic salivary tumor
- Primary squamous cell carcinoma of palate
- Abscess

Clinical Features of Various Swellings of Palate

Cysts of Papilla or of Incisive Canal (Nasopalatine Cyst) The patient presents with a small swelling of long duration beneath the incisive papilla in the anterior palate. It is smooth and nontender. Radiography shows a well-defined, small, rounded, oval or heart-shaped radiolucency in the midline above or between the roots of upper central incisors.

Torus Palatinus It is a developmental defect characterized by nonpathological, localized, bony, hard, nontender protuberance in the center of hard palate. It is smooth, rounded, and symmetrical (in the mandible torus it presents on the mandibular lingual aspect, often bilateral in the canine–premolar area). It is excised if it interferes in fitting of dentures.

Epstein's Pearls The patient is an infant who has a diamond-shaped group of miniature white cysts at the junction of hard and soft palate in midline.

Syphilitic Gumma The patient is usually a child who has signs of congenital syphilis. There is a smooth, hard, and nontender swelling in the center of palate. Radiography shows an area of bone destruction and the serological tests for syphilis are positive.

Apical Abscess or Cyst The patient has a small swelling on the lingual aspect of upper lateral incisor. The abscess is of short duration and tender, while the cyst is of long duration and nontender. Radiography shows a localized area of radiolucency.

Periodontal Abscess or Cyst From an Upper Molar Like the apical abscess or cyst described above, this swelling arises from an upper molar. Hence, it is situated by its side. The abscess is of short duration and tender, while the cyst is of long duration and nontender. The swelling is round or oval and situated medial to tuberosity of maxilla and extending backwards toward the soft palate.

Neurofibroma of Greater Palatine Nerve It is a rare swelling of palate which cannot be clinically differentiated from ectopic salivary tissue. It occurs at the site of greater palatine nerve (on the sides of palate).

Carcinoma of Maxillary Antrum Extending Downwards The patient is usually an elderly person who displays signs of carcinoma of maxillary antrum, that is, nasal discharge, nasal bleeding, nasal obstruction, and epiphora. The palatal swelling usually presents in the region of tuberosity. Similarly a sarcoma of maxilla may bulge the palate down. The diagnosis can be confirmed by CT scan and/or MRI and FNAC.

Ectopic Salivary Tumor Small islands of ectopic salivary tissue can be present anywhere in the oral mucosa which can give origin to an ectopic salivary tumor. The forepart of the hard palate is the commonest site (Fig. 17.23). The swelling is smooth, firm or hard, and mobile. The diagnosis is confirmed by FNAC.

Primary Squamous Cell Carcinoma of Palate The patient is usually a middle-aged or elderly person, maybe a reverse smoker who presents with an ulcerated swelling or papillomatous lesion of the palate (Fig. 17.24). It

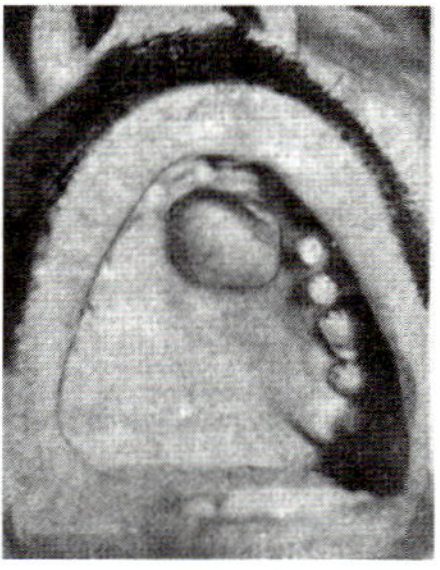

Figure 17.23 Pleomorphic adenoma of hard palate (ectopic salivary tumor).

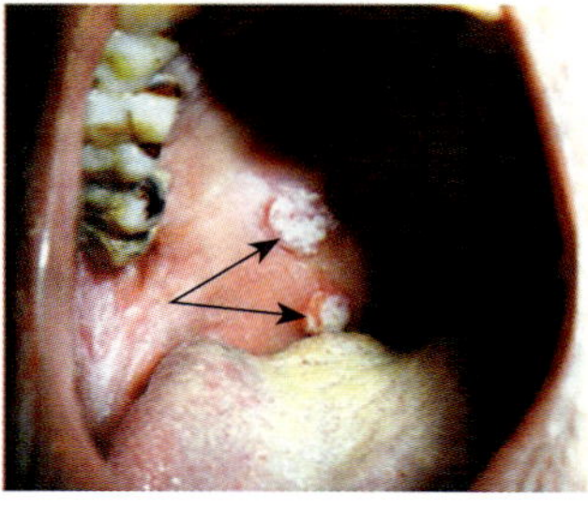

Figure 17.24 Papillomatous lesions (carcinoma) of palate. (Courtesy: Professor Sameer Gupta)

can occur anywhere in the palate but usually on the soft palate. It is hard and irregular and may bleed on touch.

Abscess It is a small painful swelling of short duration which can occur in the palate anywhere but commonly near the row of upper teeth. It is red, hot, and tender. The diagnosis can be confirmed by needle aspiration.

Treatment of Swellings of Palate

Treatment is removal of the cause.

- An abscess is treated by removal of pus and appropriate antibiotics.
- Cysts are either excised or deroofed, that is, a nasopalatine cyst can be easily enucleated by palatine approach.
- Torus palatinus is excised if it is interfering with fitting a denture plate.
- Epstein's pearls usually disappear spontaneously.
- Gumma is treated with antisyphilitic antibiotic, for example, penicillin.
- Ectopic salivary tumor is excised widely.
- Neurofibroma of greater palatine nerve is excised.
- The carcinoma of maxillary antrum and of palate is treated by wide excision (Fig. 17.25) and radiotherapy.

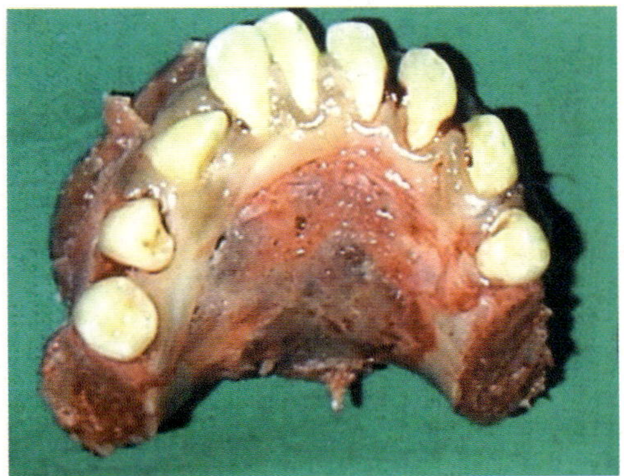

Figure 17.25 Excised palate in a patient of carcinoma of palate. (Courtesy: Professor Surajit Bhattacharya)

Box 17.9 Etiology of palatal perforation

Midline perforation

- Congenital, for example, cleft palate
- Spontaneous—rupture of gumma of palate
- Postoperative—failed cleft palate repair

Anywhere

- Trauma

Lateral perforation

- Erosion or destruction of palate by a malignant tumor of antrum or upper alveolus
- Extraction of upper lateral teeth
- Through the socket of palatally misplaced tooth

Perforation of palate

Etiology

The etiology of palatal perforation is described in Box 17.9.

Clinical Features

The patient presents with nasal voice and nasal regurgitation of food and drinks. A perforation is visible by inspection of palate. If there is suspicion of tumor, biopsy should be taken. The perforation and its pathology can be imaged by CT scan.

Treatment

The cause must be treated.

- If it is due to rupture of a gumma, a full course of antisyphilitic treatment is given.
- Perforation due to cancer is managed by a combination of wide excision and radiotherapy.
- For immediate relief, the perforation may be closed by an obturator or covered by a denture plate.
- For permanent solution of the problem, the defect is repaired by flaps based on one or both palatine arteries.

7. OTHER PROBLEMS OF MOUTH

Halitosis

It is a symptom characterized by offensive or bad breath. It is a common symptom. The bad smell may come from the nose or mouth during talking or mouth breathing.

Etiology

- **Nondisease states**
  - Diet—consumption of some smelly food, for example, garlic, onion
  - Poor oral hygiene
  - Mouth breathing
  - Smoking
  - Fear/anxiety halitosis
- **Diseases states**
  - *Diseases of oral cavity*
    - Infections and inflammations, for example, acute ulcerative gingivitis, dental caries, infected tooth socket, chronic periodontitis, pericoronitis, stomatitis including gangrenous stomatitis
    - Fungating malignant tumors, for example, carcinoma, sarcoma, and melanoma
  - *Disease of pharynx and esophagus*
    - Infections—septic tonsillitis, peritonsillar abscess (quinsy)
    - Pharyngeal diverticulum
    - Achalasia cardia
    - Carcinoma
  - *Diseases of nose and paranasal sinuses*
    - Atrophic rhinitis
    - Paranasal sinus infection
    - Foreign body in the nose
    - Nasal myiasis (maggots)
    - Fungating tumors, for example, carcinoma, sarcoma, Burkitt's tumor
  - *Diseases of bronchial tree and lungs*
    - Bronchiectasis
    - Lung abscess, gangrene of lung
    - Bronchial foreign body
  - *General diseases*
    - Acute infections, for example, enteric fever, acute appendicitis, acute peritonitis
    - Gangrene of bowel
    - Toxemia, septicemia
    - Gastrocolic fistula

The investigations and treatment depend on the cause, for example, biopsy and wide excision or radiotherapy in carcinoma of tongue. Maintenance of oral hygiene is most important.

Ptyalism

It is excessive secretion of saliva (polysialia).

Etiology

- **Excessive production of saliva**
  - *Diseases of oral cavity*
    - Stomatitis, for example, aphthous stomatitis, ulcerative stomatitis
    - Jagged carious tooth or teeth
    - Ill-fitting denture
    - Alveolar abscess
    - Salivary calculus disease
  - *Other diseases*
    - Spicy foods
    - Trigeminal neuralgia
    - Chronic duodenal ulcer
    - Nausea due to any cause
- **Difficulty in disposal of normally produced saliva**
  - Bulbar palsy
  - Myasthenia gravis
  - Parkinsonism
  - Botulism
  - Mental deficiency
  - Cretinism
- **Combination of both the factors**
  - Peritonsillar abscess
  - Carcinoma of tongue, palate, pharynx, and esophagus
  - Retropharyngeal abscess
  - Functional ptyalorrhea

The investigations and treatment depend on the cause, for example, the diagnosis of dental problems is confirmed by orthopantomography and treatment given according to the finding, for example, alveolar abscess is treated with antibiotics and removal of pus.

KEY POINTS

- Aphthous ulcers are the most commonly reported oral ulcers that occur on nonkeratinized mucosa (buccal and labial). They are quite painful and last for 7–10 days. They heal spontaneously within 1–3 weeks without scarring.
- Herpetic stomatitis is caused by human herpes virus (HHV) and presents as painful multiple small vesicles in gingiva and palate. The lesion is self-limiting.
- Vincent's gingivitis is caused by spirochaetes and fusiform bacilli and occurs as a result of poor oral hygiene, heavy smoking, and lowered body resistance. It is characterized by yellowish-gray gingival pseudomembrane.
- Cancrum oris is an infective gangrene of oral cavity which is a severe form of Vincent's gingivitis with rapid progressive necrosis of tissues of gums, lips, cheek, jaw bones, and soft tissues in the vicinity with severe toxemia and fetid odor. It is associated with a high morbidity and mortality.
- Nutritional deficiencies produce some changes in the oral cavity called nutritional stomatitis. Vitamin B_2 deficiency causes cheilosis, angular stomatitis, and glossitis. Iron deficiency causes superficial glossitis.
- Ranula is a cyst of floor of mouth which is brilliantly transilluminant. Sometimes the cyst continues to enlarge and extends into neck below the angle of mandible. It is called plunging ranula.
- Median supramylohyoid sublingual dermoid is a midline swelling that occurs below the tongue. Lateral sublingual dermoid presents with a swelling in the lateral aspect of floor of mouth.
- Pleomorphic adenoma is the commonest salivary tumor typically found at the junction of hard and soft palate. The tumor is excised completely together with overlying mucosa.
- Squamous cell carcinoma of oral cavity is etiologically related to tobacco and alcohol habit and characterized by an irregular nonhealing ulcer. Other symptoms include odynophagia (painful swallowing), otalgia (pain in the ear), trismus, halitosis, toothache, and cervical lymphadenopathy.
- The surgery in squamous cell carcinoma of the oral cavity involves en bloc resection of tumor combined with radical neck dissection of lymph nodes. The radiotherapy techniques include external beam radiotherapy and Co-60; and brachytherapy using cesium-137 needles or iridium-192 wires. The chemotherapeutic drugs used are cisplatin, methotrexate, and bleomycin.
- White patches in the oral cavity are quite common and may have histological features of abnormal keratinization, hyperplasia or hypoplasia of epithelium, and disordered maturation (dysplasia). Dysplasia is a sign of possible malignant change.
- Lichen planus is a chronic inflammatory autoimmune disorder and the most common cause of persistent white patches in the oral cavity which commonly affects the cheek mucosa.
- Oral candidiasis or thrush is a type of infection of the oral cavity caused by *Candida albicans* and is characterized by a white pseudomembranous lesion closely adherent to oral mucosa. Candidiasis may be the first manifestation of HIV infection.
- Oral leukoplakia is a persistent white patch on the oral mucosa which does not disappear on rubbing. It is a premalignant condition and likely to turn into malignancy in 2–4% of patients. Hairy leukoplakia occurs on the lateral border of tongue and is a common finding in patients with HIV infection.
- Oral submucous fibrosis is a chronic progressive disease characterized by formation of fibrous bands beneath the oral mucosa. It is a common problem in India characterized by extra-articular ankylosis of temporomandibular joint.
- Dental ulcer of the tongue is caused by repeated trauma and is usually a painful, small elongated ulcer with sloping edge at the lateral border. It may become malignant if not treated in time. The treatment consists of removal of the cause, for example, rounding the sharp edge or point of the concerned tooth.
- Primary chancre is a painless ulcer usually on the tip of tongue. Snail-track ulcers are multiple superficial linear ulcers on the dorsum of tongue. Gummatous ulcer is a solitary oval or round ulcer in the midline of dorsum of tongue. It has punched-out edge and wash-leather slough in the floor.

(CONTD...)

KEY POINTS (...CONTD)

- Tuberculous ulcer is very painful and occurs near the tip of the tongue. It has watery granulation tissue in its floor.
- Carcinomatous ulcer of the tongue is a painless nonhealing ulcer commonly seen at the lateral border. It is irregular, hard, and granular with a heaped-up or everted edge that bleeds on touch. The lesions of posterior one-third are usually not visible but they can be palpated by a finger and can be seen with a pharyngeal mirror.
- Carcinoma tongue less than 1 cm in size is excised with 1 cm clearance all around. A tumor 1–2 cm in size is excised with 2 cm clearance all around (partial glossectomy). Radiotherapy can also be used.
- T2 tumor of the tongue is treated with hemiglossectomy. Large primary tumors (T3, T4) may be given preoperative radiotherapy to downstage the disease and then the resection is done. Advanced unresectable tumor of the tongue is treated by palliative radiotherapy and chemotherapy.
- Posterior growth in the tongue is better treated with radiotherapy, although it can also be removed by lip split and mandibulotomy. It carries a significant morbidity and mortality.
- If the mandible is involved in carcinoma tongue, a full procedure involving wide excision or hemiglossectomy, hemimandibulectomy, and radical neck dissection is done and this is called commando operation. The lost tongue may be reconstructed by deltopectoral flap, forehead flap, and pectoralis major flap.

SELF-ASSESSMENT

Long answer questions

1. Enumerate the cysts that can occur in the oral cavity. Describe the etiology, pathology, clinical features, diagnosis, and treatment of ranula.
2. Describe the etiology, pathology, clinical features, diagnosis, and treatment of carcinoma of oral cavity. What are the causes of white patches in the oral cavity?
3. Describe the etiology, pathology, clinical features, diagnosis, and treatment of oral leukoplakia.
4. Discuss the differential diagnosis and treatment of ulcers of tongue.
5. Describe the etiology, pathology, clinical features, diagnosis, and treatment of carcinoma of tongue.

Short answer questions

1. Aphthous ulcer
2. Ranula
3. Plunging ranula
4. Sublingual dermoid
5. TNM classification of carcinoma of cheek
6. Leukoplakia
7. Erythroplakia
8. Submucous fibrosis of cheek
9. Hemangioma of oral cavity
10. Ectopic salivary tumor
11. Perforation of palate

Multiple choice questions

1. Macrocheilia is
   - (a) Larger than normal opening of mouth
   - (b) Smaller than normal opening of mouth
   - (c) Enlargement of lip
   - (d) Enlargement of tongue
2. Which of the following is not true about aphthous ulcer?
   - (a) It is related etiologically to human papillomavirus 6
   - (b) It may be single or multiple
   - (c) It is a small superficial ulcer surrounded by a red halo
   - (d) It is a painless ulcer
3. All of the following facts are correct about ranula, except
   - (a) It is a swelling of floor of mouth
   - (b) It is bluish, soft, and cystic
   - (c) It is opaque to transillumination
   - (d) It is the result of submucosal extravasation of saliva from sublingual salivary gland

(CONTD...)

SELF-ASSESSMENT *(...CONTD)*

4. Ranula contains
   (a) Blood
   (b) Lymph
   (c) Salivary secretion
   (d) Sebaceous material
5. The site of occurrence of the ranula is
   (a) Floor of mouth
   (b) Upper lip
   (c) Cheek
   (d) Palate
6. Which of the following is the commonest site of occurrence of carcinoma oral cavity?
   (a) Cheek and gingivae
   (b) Palate
   (c) Tongue
   (d) Floor of mouth
7. Odynophagia is defined as
   (a) Difficulty in mastication
   (b) Painful swallowing
   (c) Difficulty in speech
   (d) Painful mastication
8. All of the following statements are true about carcinoma of oral cavity, except
   (a) It is usually an ulcerative lesion
   (b) The ulcer is irregular in shape and size
   (c) It is hard in consistency and bleeds on touch
   (d) It has an undermined edge
9. In TNM staging, T3 stands for
   (a) Tumor up to 2 cm in greatest dimension
   (b) Tumor 2–4 cm in greatest dimension
   (c) Tumor more than 4 cm in greatest dimension
   (d) Tumor invading the adjacent structures
10. In TNM staging, N2b stands for
   (a) Ipsilateral single node up to 3 cm
   (b) Ipsilateral single node 3–6 cm
   (c) Ipsilateral multiple nodes up to 6 cm
   (d) Bilateral or contralateral nodes up to 6 cm
11. Which of the following is the commonest cancer of the oral cavity?
   (a) Malignant melanoma
   (b) Transitional cell carcinoma
   (c) Squamous cell carcinoma
   (d) Adenocarcinoma
12. Which of the following diagnostic investigations is the most important in carcinoma of oral cavity?
   (a) CT scan
   (b) MRI
   (c) Biopsy
   (d) Orthopantomography
13. The most common site of metastasis of carcinoma of oral cavity is
   (a) Lungs
   (b) Liver
   (c) Bones
   (d) Upper cervical lymph nodes
14. What are the level II nodes of the neck?
   (a) Submandibular nodes
   (b) Upper jugular chain
   (c) Lower jugular chain
   (d) Nodes in posterior triangle
15. Which of the following is not true about the leukoplakia of oral cavity?
   (a) It is a persistent white patch on the oral mucosa
   (b) It is related to tobacco habit
   (c) Diagnosis is confirmed by biopsy
   (d) It is not a premalignant lesion
16. Which of the following is not true about submucous fibrosis of cheek?
   (a) It is characterized by the formation of fibrous tissue under the cheek mucosa
   (b) It is probably due to hypersensitivity to chilies, betel nut, and tobacco
   (c) It is always followed by cancer
   (d) It causes progressive limitation of opening of the mouth
17. Aglossia is defined as
   (a) Loss of sheen (moisture) of tongue
   (b) Congenital absence of tongue
   (c) Restriction of mobility of tongue
   (d) Atrophy of papillae of tongue
18. Which of the following lesions of the tongue is a manifestation of secondary syphilis?
   (a) Primary chancre
   (b) Syphilitic leukoplakia
   (c) Gumma
   (d) Snail-track ulcers

(CONTD...)

SELF-ASSESSMENT *(...CONTD)*

19. Which of the following lesions of tongue is a manifestation of tertiary syphilis?
    (a) Snail-track ulcers
    (b) Hutchinson's warts
    (c) Gummatous ulcer
    (d) Primary chancre
20. All of the following are the features of a tuberculous ulcer of tongue, except
    (a) It is situated on dorsum near circumvallate papillae
    (b) It is a painful shallow ulcer
    (c) It is soft and has unhealthy granulation tissue in the floor
    (d) It commonly occurs in patients of active laryngeal tuberculosis
21. Tuberculoma of tongue is
    (a) A type of malignant tumor
    (b) Tuberculous cold abscess
    (c) A mass of tuberculous granulation tissue
    (d) A type of tuberculous ulcer
22. The commonest site of ulcer on the tongue is
    (a) Near its lateral border
    (b) On the dorsum
    (c) On the undersurface
    (d) On posterior one-third
23. All of the following are true about a dental ulcer, except
    (a) It is caused by repeated trauma by a decayed tooth
    (b) It is situated on the lateral border of tongue
    (c) It never undergoes malignant transformation
    (d) It is a painful small ulcer with a sloping edge
24. A dental ulcer of tongue is usually treated by
    (a) Surgical excision of ulcer
    (b) Antibiotics
    (c) Antiseptic mouthwashes
    (d) Rounding of the sharpened or pointed tooth or extraction of related tooth
25. All of the following are true about a post-tussive ulcer, except
    (a) It is an ulcer of dorsum of tongue
    (b) The patient is usually a child having whooping cough
    (c) The ulcer is small and superficial
    (d) It occurs on the frenulum linguae of tongue
26. Which of the following is the commonest site of occurrence of carcinoma of tongue?
    (a) Dorsum of tongue
    (b) Lateral border
    (c) Undersurface
    (d) Posterior one-third
27. Which of the following is the usual carcinoma of tongue?
    (a) Mucoepidermoid carcinoma
    (b) Adenocarcinoma
    (c) Transitional cell carcinoma
    (d) Squamous cell carcinoma
28. The most common site of metastasis in carcinoma of tongue is
    (a) Lungs
    (b) Liver
    (c) Bones
    (d) Upper cervical lymph nodes
29. All of the following are precancerous conditions of carcinoma of tongue, except
    (a) Leukoplakia
    (b) Syphilitic glossitis
    (c) Sideropenic dysphagia
    (d) Geographic tongue
30. Ankyloglossia of carcinoma of tongue is due to
    (a) Atrophy of muscles of tongue
    (b) Infiltration of tongue musculature
    (c) Hypoglossal nerve palsy
    (d) Adhesions of tongue
31. Ankyloglossia is defined as
    (a) Restriction of movements of tongue, especially protrusion
    (b) Atrophy of one-half of the tongue
    (c) Restriction of movement of temporomandibular joint
    (d) Restriction of movements of soft palate
32. Tongue-tie is due to
    (a) Congenital shortening of frenulum linguae
    (b) Carcinoma of tongue
    (c) Hypoglossal nerve palsy
    (d) Plummer–Vinson syndrome
33. Macroglossia is
    (a) Opening of mouth larger than normal
    (b) Opening of mouth smaller than normal

(CONTD...)

SELF-ASSESSMENT (...CONTD)

(c) Chronic painless enlargement of tongue
(d) Small atrophic tongue

34. All of the following are true about hairy tongue, except
    (a) Tongue has a blackish thickened patch on its dorsum as if having bristly hair
    (b) It is probably due to pigment producing molds
    (c) It may occur in those who suck on antibiotic lozenges for a long period
    (d) It is a premalignant condition

35. What is the cause of hemiatrophy of tongue?
    (a) Plummer–Vinson syndrome
    (b) Ipsilateral hypoglossal nerve paralysis
    (c) Protein deficiency
    (d) Vitamin B deficiency

36. All of the following facts are true about an ectopic salivary tumor of the oral cavity, except
    (a) The oral cavity is one of the sites of occurrence of an ectopic salivary tumor
    (b) It arises from minor salivary glands
    (c) It occurs typically at the junction of soft and hard palate
    (d) It is a soft and tender swelling

37. The commonest site of occurrence of an ectopic salivary tumor in the oral cavity is
    (a) Lip
    (b) Cheek
    (c) Dorsum of tongue
    (d) Junction of hard and soft palate

38. Nasal regurgitation of food is a symptom of
    (a) Carcinoma of tongue
    (b) Perforation of palate
    (c) Hypoglossal nerve palsy
    (d) Ectopic salivary tumor of palate

Answers

1. (c) 2. (d) 3. (c) 4. (c) 5. (a) 6. (a) 7. (b) 8. (d) 9. (c) 10. (c) 11. (c) 12. (c) 13. (d) 14. (b) 15. (d) 16. (c) 17. (b) 18. (d) 19. (c) 20. (a) 21. (c) 22. (a) 23. (c) 24. (d) 25. (a) 26. (b) 27. (d) 28. (d) 29. (d) 30. (b) 31. (a) 32 (a) 33. (c) 34. (d) 35. (b) 36. (d) 37. (d) 38. (b)

Cleft Lip and Cleft Palate

18

Introduction

The cleft lip and cleft palate are the most common congenital abnormalities of orofacial region. They usually occur as isolated abnormalities, but may be associated with other congenital developmental defects such as Pierre Robin syndrome and Klippel–Feil syndrome.

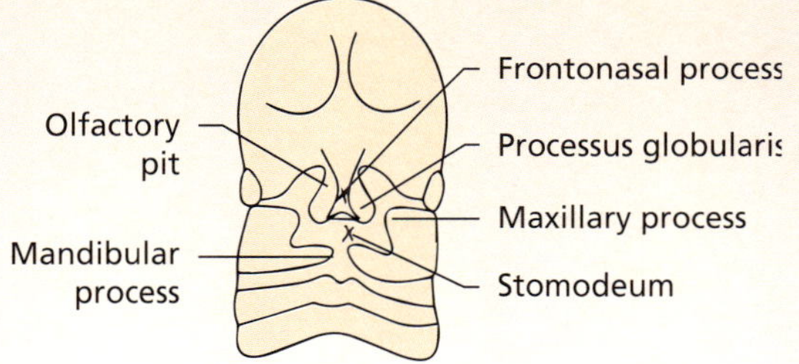

Figure 18.1 Development of face.

Development of face

About the sixth week of intrauterine life, a depression appears in the front of head called stomodeum or primitive mouth. Around it appear five processes—a frontonasal process at the cephalic end and a maxillary and a mandibular process on each side. The nose develops from the frontonasal process. All these processes coalesce to form the face including lips, alveolus, and palate and the coalescence process is completed in a brief period of 3 weeks (Fig. 18.1). Palate forms due to fusion of palatine shelves. Cleft lip is the result of disruption of muscles of upper lip and nasolabial region. Cleft palate is due to failure of fusion of two palatine shelves.

Incidence of clefts

- The incidence of cleft lip and palate is 1 in 600 live births, while that of cleft palate is 1 in 1000 live births. The relative incidence of these defects is as follows:
  - *Cleft lip*: 15%
  - *Cleft palate alone*: 40%
  - *Cleft lip and cleft palate*: 45%
- Overall these defects are more common in males but isolated cleft palate occurs more commonly in females than in males.
- In unilateral cleft lips, the left side is affected in 60% of patients.

Etiology

It is both genetic and environmental. The genetic factor is more significant in cleft lip and cleft palate combined than in isolated cleft palate where the environment factor plays a bigger role. The environmental factor includes maternal epilepsy and drugs, for example, steroids, diazepam, and phenytoin.

Surgical anatomy of cleft lip

Unilateral Cleft Lip

The nasolabial and bilabial muscle rings are disrupted on one side resulting in an asymmetrical deformity involving the external nasal cartilage with flaring of nose, nasal septum, and anterior maxilla (premaxilla). The defects affect the mucocutaneous tissues.

Bilateral Cleft Lip

The deformity is more pronounced but symmetrical. Both the superior muscular rings are disrupted on both sides producing flaring of nose, a protrusive premaxilla, and a small process of skin in front of premaxilla known as prolabium which is devoid of muscle.

Surgical anatomy of cleft palate

Hard palate is covered by special fibromucosa which is divided into three zones:

1. Palatal fibromucosa is in the center which is very thin and is directly below the nasal floor.
2. Maxillary fibromucosa is situated laterally. It is a thick layer and contains greater palatine neurovascular bundle.
3. Gingival fibromucosa lies more laterally adjacent to upper teeth.

The cleft palate occurs due to failure of fusion of two palatine shelves (Fig. 18.2):

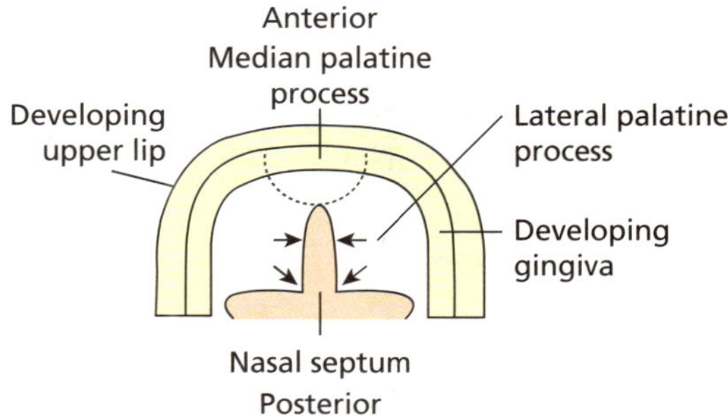

Figure 18.2 Development of secondary palate as seen from below.

- **Primary palate**: The primary palate consists of all structures in front of incisive foramen, that is, the alveolus and upper lip.
- **Secondary palate**: The secondary palate consists of the remainder of palate posterior to incisive foramen, that is, hard and soft palate.
- **Incomplete cleft palate**: When in the cleft of hard palate, the hard palate remains attached to the nasal septum and vomer, the cleft is incomplete.
- **Complete cleft palate**: When the nasal septum and vomer are completely separate from the palatine process, the cleft is complete.

Anatomy of Soft Palatal Cleft

The closure of velopharynx is achieved by five muscles working in a coordinated manner. It has a sort of sphincter mechanism. The components of velopharyngeal sphincter are soft palate, posterior pharyngeal wall, and lateral pharyngeal walls. The muscle fibers in the soft palate are transversely oriented with hardly any attachment to the hard palate. In a soft palatal cleft, the fibers are oriented anteroposteriorly inserting into posterior border of hard palate.

Classification

LAHSHAL System

The modern classification of cleft lip and palate is known as LAHSHAL system where the complete clefts of lip, alveolus, hard palate, and soft palate are labeled by capital letters, that is,

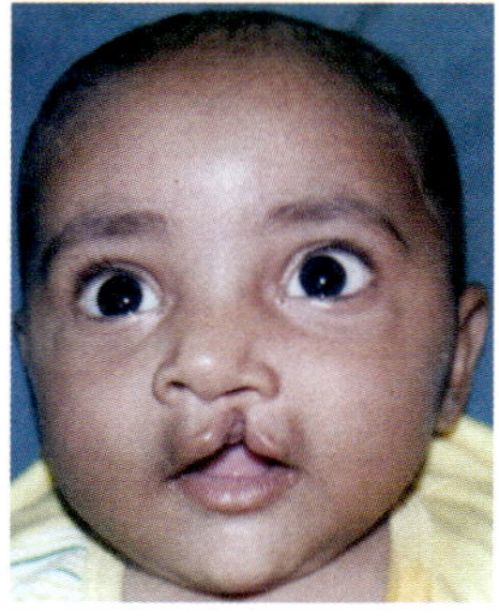

Figure 18.3 Unilateral incomplete cleft of upper lip (left). (Courtesy: Professor J.D. Rawat)

LAHSHAL is complete bilateral cleft lip and cleft palate, and lahSH means incomplete right unilateral cleft lip, alveolus, and hard palate with complete cleft of soft palate extending partly into left hard palate.

Anatomical Classification

- Cleft lip alone
  - Unilateral
  - Bilateral
  - Central (harelip)
  - Incomplete or complete (Figs 18.3 and 18.4)
    - Incomplete: The cleft does not extend into nasal floor.
    - Complete: The cleft extends into nasal floor.
  - Compound cleft lip: Cleft lip with cleft of alveolus

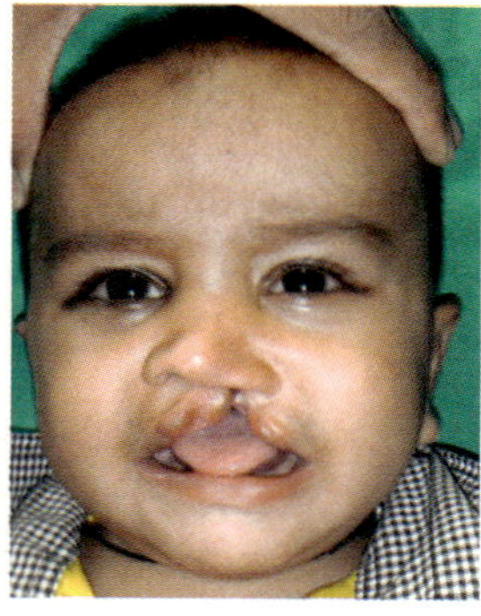

Figure 18.4 Unilateral complete cleft of upper lip (left). (Courtesy: Professor J.D. Rawat)

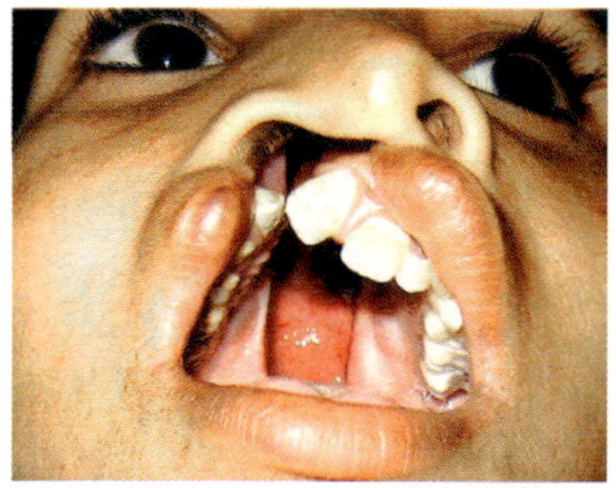

Figure 18.5 Complete cleft lip (right) with cleft palate. (Courtesy: Professor Surajit Bhattacharya)

- Cleft of primary palate (in front of incisive foramen) only
  - Complete (absence of premaxilla)
  - Incomplete (rudimentary premaxilla)
    - Unilateral
    - Bilateral
    - Median
- Cleft of secondary palate (behind incisive foramen) only
  - Complete (nasal septum and vomer are separated from palatine process)
  - Incomplete
  - Submucous
- Cleft of both primary and secondary palate
- Cleft lip and cleft palate together (Fig. 18.5)

Clinical features

The patient is brought with the problems mentioned in the subsequent text connected with these abnormalities.

Cosmetic Problem A cleft lip, apart from lip abnormality, produces deformity of alar cartilage and deviation of nasal skeleton. The nose becomes flat and wide (flaring of nose) on the side of the cleft. Bilateral clefts of lip may be associated with telecanthus in which the eyes are displaced laterally (Fig 18.6). A cleft of alveolus is associated with dental abnormalities and deformities. The cleft palate as such is not a cosmetic problem.

Feeding Difficulties A cleft palate interferes with swallowing of milk with escape of milk into the nose. A cleft baby finds it difficult to suckle the nipple due to interruption of oral sphincter in cleft

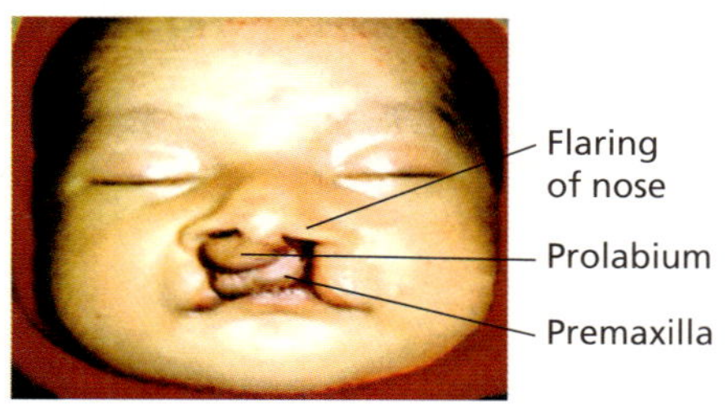

Figure 18.6 Bilateral cleft lip showing flaring more marked on the left side with prolabium and premaxilla. This patient has telecanthus also. (Courtesy: Professor Surajit Bhattacharya)

lip, and because of difficulty in creating negative pressure in the oral cavity due to cleft palate.

Speech Defect All clefts are associated with speech defect. Cleft lip patients have difficulty in speaking labials, for example, papa and mama. Cleft palate patients have difficulty with linguopalatals, for example, kho-kho, due to escape of air into the nose.

Hearing Abnormalities A cleft palate is usually associated with shorter eustachian tubes with straight eustachian canals allowing entry of milk into the middle ear producing middle ear infection and later impaired hearing.

Other Problems They include altered dentition or supernumerary teeth, recurrent respiratory tract infection, and hypoplasia of maxilla. Associated alveolar defect may be present in patients of complete cleft lip and cleft palate.

Management of cleft lip and cleft palate

Primary Treatment

The cleft lip can be detected by antenatal ultrasound 18 weeks after gestation except for isolated cleft palate. After its detection, parent counseling is required.

Feeding For feeding, enlarging the hole of the teat may be enough. Soft bottles (e.g., Mead Johnson) are good for these infants.

Airway Respiratory obstruction is usually seen in babies with Pierre Robin syndrome. It may be managed by nursing the baby prone, retained nasopharyngeal intubation, or labioglossopexy (surgical fixation of tongue to lower lip).

Surgical Treatment A well-planned and correctly done primary surgery gives good results with minimal need of secondary management.

Timing of Repair

The timing of repair of clefts is important for getting a good result which is described in Table 18.1.

Surgical Repair of Cleft Lip and Palate

The clefts of lip and palate are treated with surgical repair and the criteria to undertake surgery. Millard criteria—rule of "10"—are described in Box 18.1.

Table 18.1 Timing of repair of cleft lip and cleft palate

Type of cleft	Time of repair
Unilateral cleft lip	5–6 months
Bilateral cleft lip	4–5 months
Soft palatal cleft	6 months
Soft and hard palatal cleft	• Soft T at 6 months • Hard palate at 15–18 months
Unilateral cleft lip and palate	• Cleft lip and soft palate at 5–6 months • Hard palate and gum pad with or without lip revision at 15–18 months
Bilateral cleft lip and palate	• Cleft lip and soft palate at 4–5 months • Hard palate and gum pad with or without lip revision at 15–18 months

Box 18.1 Millard criteria—rule of "10"

- The baby should be 10 weeks old
- He/she should be 10 lb in weight
- He/she should have at least 10 g% hemoglobin
- Total leukocyte count (TLC) should be less than 10,000/mm^3

Surgical repair of cleft lip

After planning and proper marking, skin incisions are given to restore displaced tissues including skin, local muscles, and cartilage to their normal position. The muscular continuity is achieved by subperiosteal undermining of anterior maxilla. The horizontal fibers of orbicularis oris are sutured to achieve functional oral sphincter.

Surgical repair of cleft palate

It can be repaired by one- or two-stage palatoplasty. Two-stage closure encourages physiological narrowing of hard palatal cleft to minimize surgical dissection at the time of secondary procedure. Mucoperiosteal flaps are raised and stitched together in three layers—nasal mucosa, muscle layer, and palatal mucosa—with no tension and minimal scarring. The hook of pterygoid is broken to relax tensor palati to relieve tension on suture line.

Surgical Repair of Cleft Alveolus

It may require bone grafting to fill the bony defect.

Secondary Management

Following repair of the cleft, the patient is regularly examined by a multidisciplinary team to see for hearing, speech, dental development, and facial growth.

Hearing defects

- There is a high incidence of sensorineural and conductive hearing loss in these patients. Hence, they should all be assessed before 12 months of age by auditory brainstem responses (ABR) and tympanometry for sensorineural and conductive hearing loss, respectively.
- The sensorineural hearing loss is treated by a hearing aid. The conductive hearing loss is due to secretory otitis media and may require myringotomy.

Speech defects

- Regular speech assessment should be done to detect speech problems in the early stages. They include velopharyngeal incompetence and articulation problems.
- Velopharyngeal incompetence may be due to inadequate muscle repair and is characterized by nasal or hypernasal speech. The components of velopharyngeal sphincter are soft palate, posterior pharyngeal wall, and lateral pharyngeal walls. The articulation problems are due to compensatory mechanism to overcome velopharyngeal incompetence, or due to jaw, dental, or occlusal problems.
- The investigations to find the cause of speech defect include videofluoroscopy, nasal airflow studies (aerophonoscopy), and nasendoscopy.
- The speech problems are managed by speech and language therapy, secondary palatal surgery including intravelar veloplasty and pharyngoplasty, and speech training devices.

Dental problems

- Dental problems are very common in these patients. They are managed by dietary advice, fluoride supplements, and fissure sealants.
- Problems of eruption of teeth are common, for example, too many or too few teeth and cleft alveolus. They require appropriate treatment, that is, extraction or implantation.
- A well-maintained and disease-free dentition is an absolute prerequisite for orthodontic treatment which is done in two phases:
  - Mixed dentition (8–10 years) phase to expand the maxillary arches as a prelude to alveolar bone graft
  - Permanent dentition (14–18 years) phase to provide a normal-functioning dental occlusion (it may require surgical correction of a malpositioned or retrusive maxilla by maxillary osteotomy)

Secondary surgery

The results of cleft repair surgery depend on the quality of primary surgery. Hence, all those involved in the primary treatment must do their best. In spite of all the care, secondary surgery may be required from time to time as the need may be. The secondary surgical procedures are described in Box 18.2. The time schedule for the secondary surgeries is described in Box 18.3.

Box 18.2 Types of secondary surgeries in cleft lip and cleft palate patients

- Correction of defect of ala of nose
- Cleft lip revision
- Alveolar bone graft
  - Closure of oronasal fistula
  - Promote normal eruption of teeth
  - Placement of osseointegrated dental implant
- Secondary palatal procedures
  - Veloplasty
  - Pharyngoplasty
  - Closure of palatal fistula
- Orthognathic surgery
  - Maxillary advancement
  - Bimaxillary surgery
- Open septorhinoplasty
  - Improve nasal tip projection
  - Correct septal deformity
  - Relocation of alar cartilages

Box 18.3 Time schedule of secondary surgeries

- **Cleft lip revision**: 2 years after primary surgery
- **Pharyngoplasty**: 2 years of age (speaking time)
- **Orthodontic surgery**: Done in two phases:
  - *Mixed dentition*: 8–10 years
  - *Permanent dentition*: 14–18 years
- **Alveolar bone grafting**: Mixed dentition, that is, 8–10 years
- **Rhinoplasty**: After orthodontic surgery
- **Orthognathic surgery**: 16 years in a female, 19 years in a male

Complications of cleft surgery

Complications of cleft surgery include wound infection, bleeding, dehiscence, fistula formation, eversion or inversion of lip, hypertrophic scar, and absence of hair in a male at scar of lip repair.

Role of a dental surgeon

A dental surgeon plays a significant role in the management of patients of cleft lip and cleft palate:

- Initial examination of the patient and giving dietary advice and prescribing fluoride supplements and fissure sealants to have healthy teeth
- Orthodontic treatment in which the anatomical defects of upper alveolus are corrected: supernumerary teeth extracted, alveolar bone defect corrected by bone grafting, and arrangement made to replace missing teeth, and later on to provide a normal functioning dental occlusion
- Orthognathic surgery in which maxillary hypoplasia is corrected with maxillary osteotomies and bimaxillary surgery

Cephalometry

It is a two-dimensional radiographic study of various landmarks and imaginary lines on maxillofacial skeletal framework by taking a lateral and posteroanterior radiograph of facial skeleton.

Uses of Cephalometry

- Orthodontic diagnosis
- Classification of skeletal and dental abnormalities
- Planning and giving treatment to every individual patient of dentofacial abnormalities
- Evaluation of results of such treatment
- Predicting growth-related changes in maxillofacial structures

Technique

The radiography is done after putting the patient in a cephalometer with head adjusted in natural head position keeping the sagittal plane of head parallel with the film and radiograph is taken. Then another film is taken by putting the film in front of face parallel with coronal plane. A posteroanterior cephalogram is mainly used to assess the asymmetry of facial skeleton by drawing some lines on the radiograph (Fig. 18.7):

- A vertical line joining the midline of nose and chin and dental arch—midsagittal line
- A vertical line passing through the zygomatic arch on either side of midsagittal line
- A vertical line passing through the angle of mandible on either side
- Horizontal lines drawn along zygomatic plane, occlusal plane, extraorbital plane, and plane of lower border of mandible

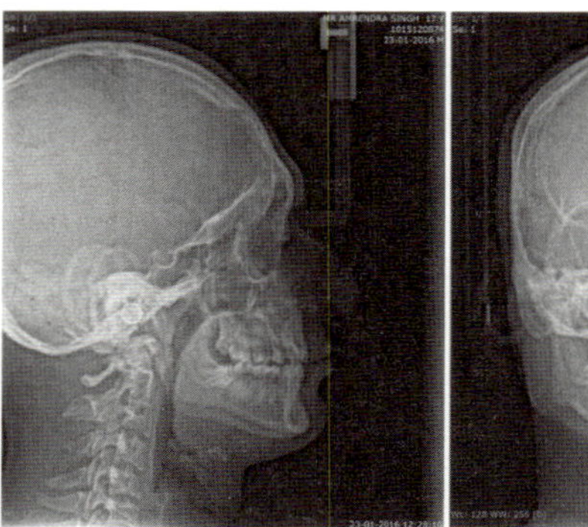
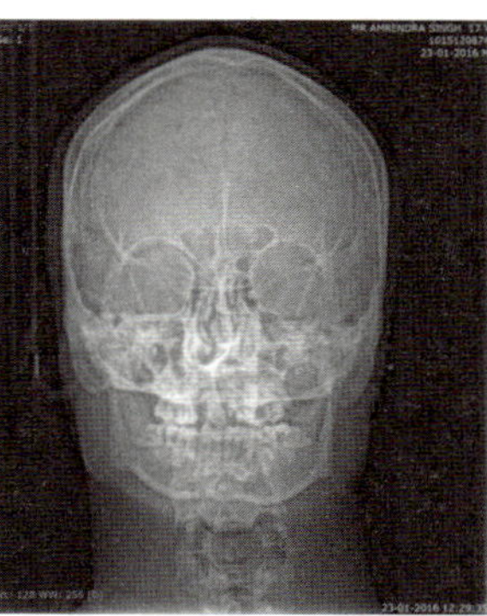

Figure 18.7 Cephalometrogram of a repaired cleft lip and cleft palate showing missing upper central incisors. (Courtesy: Dr. S.S. Sarkar, Sarkar Diagnostics)

KEY POINTS

- The cleft lip and cleft palate are the most common congenital abnormalities of orofacial region. They can occur alone or may be associated with other congenital developmental defects such as Pierre Robin syndrome and Klippel–Feil syndrome.
- In unilateral cleft lip, the nasolabial and bilabial muscle rings are disrupted on one side resulting in an asymmetrical deformity involving the external nasal cartilage, nasal septum, and anterior maxilla (premaxilla).
- In bilateral cleft lip, both the superior muscular rings are disrupted on both sides producing symmetrical deformity characterized by flaring of nose, protrusive premaxilla, and a small process of skin in front of premaxilla called prolabium which is devoid of muscle.
- In incomplete cleft lip, the cleft does not extend into nasal floor. In complete cleft lip, the cleft extends into nasal floor.
- The cleft palate occurs due to failure of fusion of two palatine shelves. If the hard palate remains attached to the nasal septum and vomer, the cleft is incomplete; if the nasal septum and vomer are completely separate from the palatine process, the cleft is complete.
- The modern classification of cleft lip and palate is known as LAHSHAL system where the complete clefts of lip, alveolus, hard palate, and soft palate are labeled by capital letters and incomplete clefts by small letters.
- Cleft lip causes cosmetic problems and difficulty in speaking labials. Cleft palate causes feeding difficulties, difficulty in pronouncing linguopalatals, and hearing abnormalities. Other problems in cleft patients include altered dentition or supernumerary teeth, recurrent respiratory tract infection, and hypoplasia of maxilla.
- Cleft lip can be detected by antenatal ultrasound 18 weeks after gestation except for isolated cleft palate.
- Unilateral cleft lip is treated in 4–5 months of age and bilateral cleft lip in 5–6 months of age. Soft

(CONTD...)

KEY POINTS (...CONTD)

palate clefts are treated at 6 months and hard palate clefts are treated between 15 and 18 months.

- Cleft lip is treated by surgery and must fulfill the Millard's rule of "10" criteria.
- Cleft palate can be repaired by one- or two-stage palatoplasty. Two-stage closure encourages physiological narrowing of hard palatal cleft to minimize surgical dissection at the time of secondary procedure.
- Cleft palate is usually associated with hearing problems, speech defects, and feeding difficulties. They need attention and proper treatment.
- Dental abnormalities are quite common in these patients. They are managed by dietary advice, fluoride supplements, fissure sealants, and orthodontic treatment.
- Secondary surgeries include correction of defect of ala of nose, cleft lip revision, alveolar bone grafting, secondary palatal procedures (veloplasty, pharyngoplasty, closure of palatal fistula), orthognathic surgery (correcting maxillary hypoplasia with maxillary osteotomies and bimaxillary surgery), and open septorhinoplasty.

SELF-ASSESSMENT

Long answer questions

1. Describe the etiology, surgical anatomy, clinical features, and treatment of cleft lip and cleft palate.
2. Describe the treatment of cleft palate. What is the role of a dental surgeon in its management?

Short answer questions

1. Development of face
2. Cleft lip
3. Cleft palate
4. Speech defect in cleft palate
5. Hearing problems in cleft lip and cleft palate
6. Dentoalveolar problems in cleft lip and cleft palate

Multiple choice questions

1. The incidence of cleft palate alone is
   (a) 4%
   (b) 14%
   (c) 20%
   (d) 40%
2. The incidence of cleft lip alone is
   (a) 1.5%
   (b) 15%
   (c) 20%
   (d) 25%
3. The incidence of cleft lip and cleft palate together is
   (a) 4.5%
   (b) 20%
   (c) 30%
   (d) 45%
4. Which one of the following facts is true about the cleft lip and cleft palate?
   (a) They have a right-sided preponderance
   (b) There is a female predilection for this anomaly
   (c) There is a female preponderance in isolated cleft palate
   (d) They occur equally in both the sexes
5. Cleft lip is caused by
   (a) Direct consequence of disruption of muscles of upper lip and nasolabial region
   (b) Failure of fusion of palatal shelves
   (c) Failure of median nasal process to make contact with frontal nasal process
   (d) All of the above
6. Prolabium has all of the following tissues, except
   (a) Skin
   (b) Muscle
   (c) Mucosa
   (d) Fibrocollagenous tissue

(CONTD...)

SELF-ASSESSMENT (...CONTD)

7. All of the following are the components of velopharyngeal sphincter, except
   (a) Palate
   (b) Adenoids
   (c) Posterior pharyngeal wall
   (d) Lateral pharyngeal walls
8. Associated alveolar defect is more likely to be present in
   (a) Incomplete isolated cleft lip
   (b) Bifid uvula
   (c) Incomplete cleft of soft palate
   (d) Complete cleft lip and cleft palate
9. An isolated cleft lip should be treated because of all of the following reasons, except
   (a) It causes cosmetic problem
   (b) It may cause feeding difficulties
   (c) It is dangerous to life
   (d) It causes difficulty in speaking labials, for example, papa and mama
10. An isolated cleft palate should be operated on because of the following reasons, except
   (a) It causes cosmetic problem
   (b) It is characterized by nasal regurgitation of feeds
   (c) Speech defect is always present
   (d) Middle ear infection is one of its complications
11. Cleft palate repair should be completed by
   (a) Six months of age
   (b) Twelve months of age
   (c) Eighteen months of age
   (d) Twenty-four months of age
12. Orthodontic treatment is essential for all of the following reasons, except
   (a) To do bone grafting at alveolar defect
   (b) To correct arch abnormalities and provide support to normal bone
   (c) To maintain the arch form and spaces during dental transition period
   (d) To maintain the arch form of the permanent dentition and replace the missing teeth
13. The best investigation for velopharyngeal insufficiency is
   (a) Nasendoscopy
   (b) Nasendoscopy and videofluoroscopy
   (c) Videofluoroscopy
   (d) CT scan
14. The displacement of medial canthi laterally is known as
   (a) Hypertelorism
   (b) Telecanthus
   (c) Hypotelorism
   (d) Epicanthus

Answers

1. (d) 2. (b) 3. (d) 4. (c) 5. (a) 6. (b) 7. (b) 8. (d) 9. (c) 10. (a) 11. (c) 12. (a) 13. (b) 14. (b)

Diseases of Temporomandibular Joint or Jaw Joint

19

Anatomy of temporomandibular joint

Temporomandibular joint (TMJ) is the articulation between the squamous part of temporal bone and the head of mandibular condyle (diarthrodial or freely movable joint). It is a complex joint because it involves two separate synovial joints having an intra-articular disc (meniscus) and both the joints function together in coordination (Figs 19.1 and 19.2).

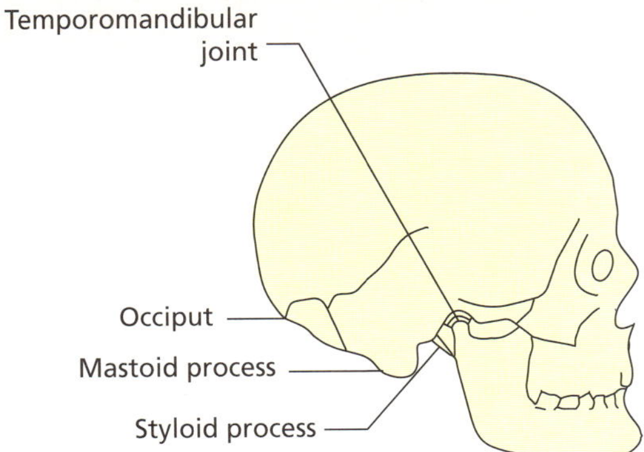

Figure 19.1 Anatomy of right temporomandibular joint.

Acute suppurative arthritis of temporomandibular joint

It is acute inflammation of TMJ with pus formation.

Etiopathogenesis It is caused by *Staphylococcus aureus*, *Streptococcus pyogenes*, and *Neisseria gonorrhoeae*. The bacteria enter the joint by the following routes:

- Local spread of infection from osteomyelitis of mandible (which has spread to condyle), middle ear infection, and rarely acute suppurative parotitis

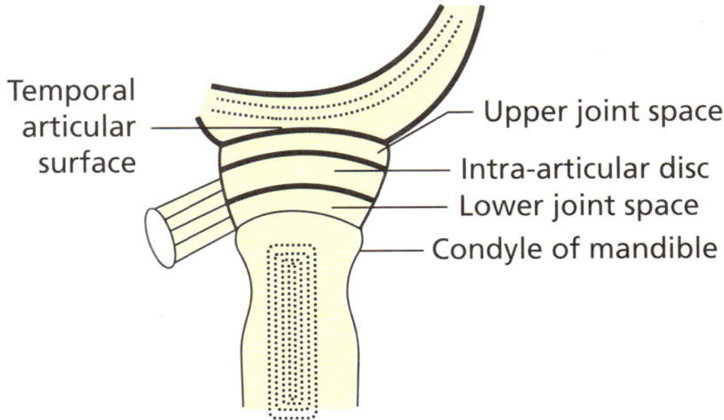

Figure 19.2 Appearance of temporomandibular joint in frontal section.

- Hematogenous spread of infection from a distant focus as occurs in pyemia

Clinical Features

- The patient presents with acute pain in the joint which increases with the movements of the jaw and is often referred upwards to the temple. The jaw is held stiff and slightly open.
- There may be swelling, redness, and tenderness in the preauricular and zygomatic regions.
- The pus may burrow deeply into the pterygoid fossa, upwards under the temporalis muscle, backwards into the external auditory meatus, or superficially to point on the skin surface.

Investigations The diagnosis can be confirmed by radiography, CT scan, and CT-guided needle aspiration. The aspirate is sent for culture and sensitivity. The blood shows polymorphonuclear leukocytosis and markedly raised erythrocyte sedimentation rate (ESR).

Treatment Broad-spectrum antibiotics, for example, co-amoxiclav, are started as early as possible and subsequently changed on receipt of culture and sensitivity report. If given early in adequate dose, the inflammation may resolve. If pus has formed, it is aspirated (Fig. 19.3a and b) or drained.

Complications This disease commonly ends in intra-articular ankylosis of jaw joint.

Ankylosis of temporomandibular joint

Ankylosis is chronic limitation or inability to open the mouth due to hypomobility or immobility of TMJ.

Types of Ankylosis

It is of two types: extra-articular and intra-articular.

Extra-Articular Ankylosis It results from lesions involving extra-articular structures. There is fibrosis and/or contracture of the soft tissues around the joint which follow gunshot injury; severe periarticular infections such as cancrum oris; destruction of mucosa of fauces or cheek by accidental, operative, or radiational injury; and osteomyelitis of mandible spreading into muscles of mastication. Submucous fibrosis of cheek also restricts the opening of mouth as the cheek loses its elasticity and stretchability.

Intra-Articular Ankylosis In this ankylosis, the pathology is inside the joint. The fusion of articular surfaces occurs by fibrous or osseous tissue (fibrous or bony ankylosis). It is usually a sequel of suppurative arthritis of jaw joint. Sometimes hemarthrosis may follow intra-articular fractures or fracture–dislocations of this joint.

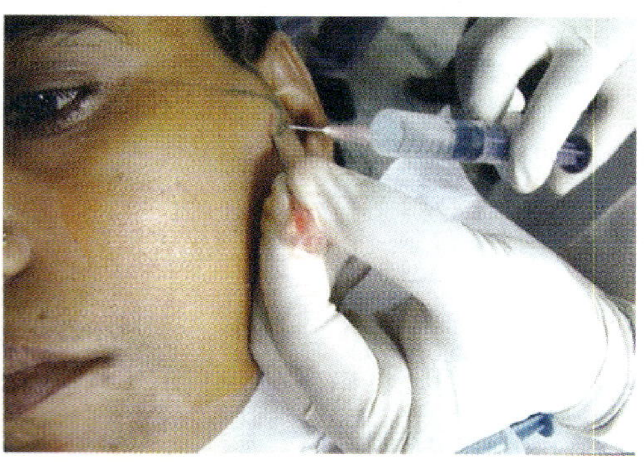

(a)

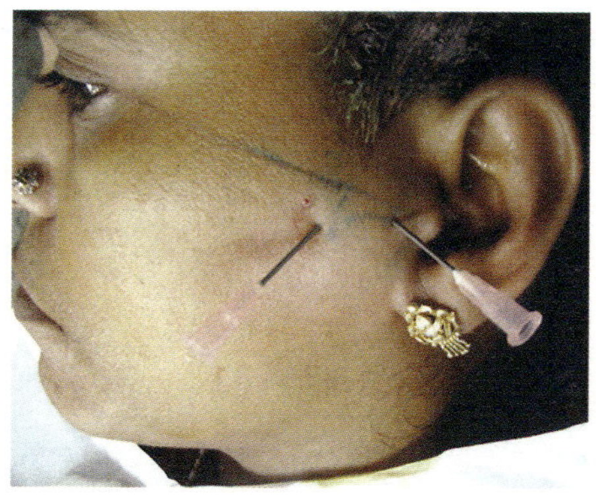

(b)

Figure 19.3 Aspiration and lavage of the left temporomandibular joint. (a) Needles in position for aspiration and lavage of left temporomandibular joint and (b) lavage of pus. (Courtesy: Professor Divya Mehrotra)

Etiology

Trauma The most common cause of ankylosis is trauma (26–75% of cases) leading to intra-articular fracture, dislocation, or bleeding. Prolonged immobilization of a condylar fracture, especially in children, results in ankylosis.

Infection It results in ankylosis in 44–68% of cases. The infection may be secondary to septicemia due to acute osteomyelitis and other systemic infections, or the infection may spread into this joint directly from adjacent areas, for example, otitis media, mastoiditis, and osteomyelitis of temporal bone.

Other Causes They include rheumatoid arthritis, osteoarthritis, and ankylosing spondylitis.

Clinical Features

It can occur at any age but most of the patients are children and young adults. The patient complains of difficulty in opening the mouth (Fig. 19.4). It is associated with oral sepsis and deformity of lower face. The nutrition is not impaired as the patient can swallow liquid food. As the mouth cannot be opened, cleaning the teeth is not possible. Hence, there is early onset of teeth decay. The extra-articular ankylosis permits slight degree of movement which is not present in the intra-articular type.

Unilateral ankylosis

The chin is receded with hypoplastic mandible on the affected side which has a concavity at the lower border. Cross-bite may be seen. In unilateral ankylosis, the chin deviates slightly on opening the mouth toward the side of ankylosis. Some degree of oral opening is possible. Interincisal opening varies depending on whether it is fibrous or bony ankylosis.

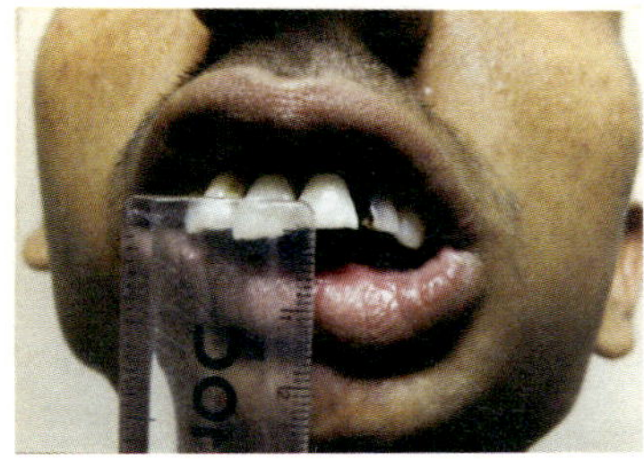

Figure 19.4 Ankylosis of temporomandibular joint (left). (Courtesy: Professor Divya Mehrotra)

Bilateral ankylosis

The patient presents with gradual reduction in opening of mouth. The chin is receded and atrophic, making the face bird-like (shrew-mouse appearance) (Fig. 19.5). The neck–chin angle may be reduced or almost completely absent. It happens when the ankylosis occurs during childhood. It is mostly due to failure of lower jaw to develop with age. Upper incisors are often protrusive with anterior open bite. Maxilla may be narrow. The oral opening may be reduced to zero. The gap between upper and lower teeth is measured when the patient tries to open the mouth fully.

Grading of Ankylosis

Normal interincisor distance is more than 3.5 cm (or three fingerbreadths).

- **Grade I ankylosis**: Between 3.0 and 3.5 cm
- **Grade II ankylosis**: Between 2.0 and 3.0 cm
- **Grade III ankylosis**: Less than 2 cm

Investigations

Radiography

- Orthopantomography will show both the joints which can be compared with each other.

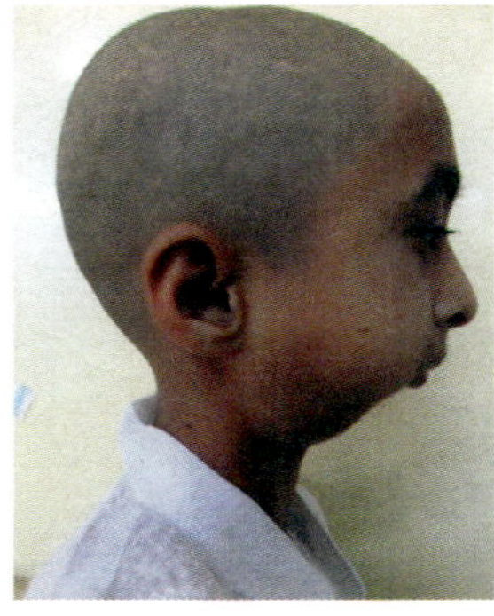

Figure 19.5 Shrew-mouse appearance of face in bilateral ankylosis of temporomandibular joint occurring in early life. (Courtesy: Professor Divya Mehrotra)

- Lateral oblique views will show the anteroposterior dimension of condylar mass. Elongation of coronoid process can be seen.

Posteroanterior radiography shows mediolateral extent of bony mass. It will also highlight the asymmetry in unilateral cases.

CT Scan

- It shows the full pathology of the lesion. It helps in planning surgical treatment (Figs 19.6 and 19.7).
- Fibrous ankylosis is characterized by reduced joint space with hazy appearance, but the normal anatomy of head and glenoid fossa can be appreciated.
- In bony ankylosis, the joint space is obliterated with abnormal bony tissue.

Complications of Ankylosis of Jaw

The complications of ankylosis of jaw include abnormal facial growth, speech impairment, malocclusion, poor oral hygiene, and carious and impacted teeth.

Treatment of Ankylosis

The main aim of treatment is to open the mouth so that oral hygiene can be maintained to prevent early teeth decay, and also a dental surgeon can do therapeutic work in the oral cavity if required.

Treatment of extra-articular ankylosis

- Regular, intermittent, and gradual stretching of contracted soft tissues with the help of wedge and screw dilators is the treatment of choice. It may fracture the front teeth.
- Excision of scar tissue around the joint and repair with pedicle or free grafting can also be performed to treat extra-articular ankylosis.
- Extra-articular arthroplasty of Esmarch: A wedge of mandible just in front of angle of mandible 2 cm broad at the lower margin and tapering to a point behind the last molar tooth is excised, and the jaw movements are started as early as possible.

Treatment of intra-articular ankylosis

A number of operative procedures are available to treat intra-articular ankylosis, as described in the subsequent text.

Condylectomy

- It is advocated to treat fibrous ankylosis where there is not much deformity of condylar head.
- Condylectomy is carried out via a preauricular incision, and horizontal osteotomy is done with a surgical burr at the level of condylar neck. Structures deep to the condylar neck are protected by using special condylar retractors. The condyle is removed after separating it from superior attachments. The stump of mandible should be smoothened.
- Unilateral condylectomy may cause deviation of mandible toward the same side on open-

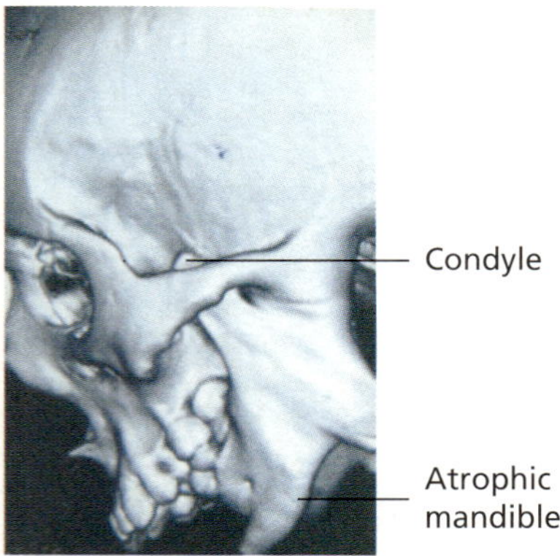

Figure 19.6 3D CT reconstruction of left temporomandibular joint region with ankylosis of joint with marked atrophy of mandible with over-riding maxilla. (Courtesy: Professor Divya Mehrotra)

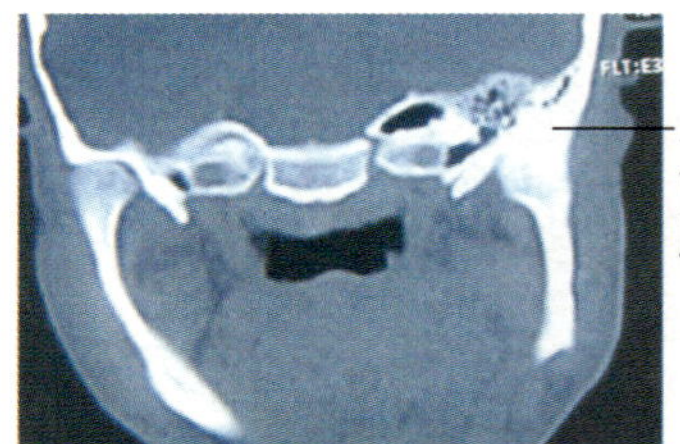

Figure 19.7 Coronal CT scan showing ankylosis of left temporomandibular joint.

ing the mouth while the bilateral procedure results in anterior open bite. To prevent this, an alloplastic material may be used to maintain joint space.

Gap Arthroplasty

- It is indicated in extensive bony ankylosis when a broad thick area of bone deposition obliterates the entire joint, sigmoid notch, and coronoid process.
- This procedure consists of two horizontal osteotomy cuts and removal of a bony wedge for creation of a gap between the roof of glenoid fossa and ramus. The gap must be at least 1 cm to prevent reankylosis.

Interpositional Arthroplasty

- It involves creation of a gap with insertion of autogenous or alloplastic barrier between the cut bony surfaces. A minimum gap of 0.5–1 cm should be kept between the graft and glenoid fossa. The interpositional materials used are described in Box 19.1.

Box 19.1 Interpositional materials used in gap arthroplasty

Autogenous materials	Alloplastic materials
• Cartilaginous grafts	• Tantalum foil
• Temporal muscle grafts	• Stainless steel
• Temporal fascia	• Titanium
• Fascia lata	• Silastic
• Dermis	• Teflon
	• Acrylic

Complications of Ankylosis Surgery

The complications of TMJ ankylosis surgery are of three types and are described in Table 19.1.

After treatment, this problem can recur. The causes of recurrence are described in Box 19.2.

Box 19.2 Causes of recurrence of ankylosis

- Inadequate gap between the articular surfaces
- Inadequate excision of ankylotic mass
- Fracture of costochondral graft
- Loosening of graft due to inadequate fixation
- Inadequate coverage of glenoid fossa surface by interpositional graft
- Inadequate postoperative physiotherapy

Trismus

Trismus is defined as difficulty in opening the mouth due to spasm of muscles of mastication (lock jaw).

Causes of Trismus

The causes of trismus are listed in Box 19.3.

The cause of trismus is identified by clinical features of the patient and investigations and treated accordingly.

Table 19.1 Complications of ankylosis surgery

Anesthetic complications	Intraoperative complications	Postoperative complications
• Difficult intubation • Aspiration of blood, throat secretions during extubation • Airway obstruction after extubation	• Hemorrhage • Injury to external auditory meatus • Injury to zygomatic and temporal branches of facial nerve • Injury to glenoid fossa with entry into middle cranial fossa • Injury to auriculotemporal nerve (Frey's syndrome) • Injury to parotid gland • Injury to teeth during opening of jaw with a jaw stretcher	• Wound infection • Open bite deformity • Recurrence of ankylosis (Box 19.2)

Box 19.3 Causes of trismus

- Tetanus: A characteristic early symptom of this disease
- Acute suppurative arthritis of temporomandibular joint
- Infection spreading into the muscles of mastication from acute osteomyelitis of mandible, parotitis
- Reflex spasm due to infected or impacted molar, irritative ulcer on the gum, tongue, or floor of mouth, and dental and peritonsillar abscess and cancer of fauces with secondary infection
- Functional (hysterical spasm)
- Trismus nascentium in infants at birth

Dislocation of temporomandibular joint

It is the displacement of articular surfaces of TMJ. It is of many types: acute anterior dislocation, other types of acute dislocations, and habitual or recurrent dislocation.

Acute Anterior Dislocation of Temporomandibular Joint

The mandible may get dislocated at TMJ when the condyle of mandible slips forward on or over the articular eminence (anterior dislocation) of articular surfaces.

Etiology

Predisposing factors include laxity of ligaments, capsule, and abnormal skeletal anatomy.

The causes of anterior dislocation are given in the subsequent text.

Extrinsic or Iatrogenic Causes

- Blow on the chin when the mouth is open
- Use of mouth gag during general anesthesia
- Dental extractions and operations, especially those performed under general anesthesia when the local muscles are relaxed

Intrinsic or Self-Induced Causes

- Excessive yawning, vomiting, sighing or laughing loudly, or opening mouth too widely for eating
- Hysterical fits

Clinical features

The dislocation of mandible is most frequent in middle-aged women. It may be unilateral or bilateral, the bilateral being twice more common than unilateral.

Unilateral Dislocation It is characterized by difficulty in speaking, mastication, and swallowing, and profuse drooling of saliva. The jaw is displaced toward the opposite side and mouth remains partly open. A hollow is visible and palpable immediately in front of tragus and the condyle is seen and palpable in a somewhat anterior position.

Bilateral Dislocation The mouth is fixed in partly open position, hollows are palpable in front of both tragi, and both the condyles are anteriorly positioned.

Diagnosis

The diagnosis is clinical; hence, usually no investigations are required. However, radiography may be done to confirm the diagnosis.

Treatment

Manipulative Reduction The dislocation is reduced by manipulation without anesthesia, under local anesthesia, or under general anesthesia as required. The thumbs of operator should be covered with gauze to prevent injury during manipulation as sudden reduction may injure them. The dislocation is reduced by pressing the thumbs on lower molar teeth and rotating the body of mandible upwards with fingers of both hands at the same time. For first-time dislocation, no retentive apparatus is required.

Retentive Apparatus If there is a delay of 1 or 2 days or it is a second or third dislocation, gold bands applied to an upper and a lower premolar may be tied together with silk just so tight as to prevent the mouth being opened more than 1 cm. They are kept for 2–3 weeks.

Treatment of irreducible dislocation

It is a rare problem which is of two types:

1. Locking of coronoid process against maxilla: It is reduced by opening the mouth more widely, may be under general anesthesia which permits its reduction.
2. Meniscus becoming detached anteriorly from the capsule and folding backwards to fill the glenoid cavity. It is treated by excision of meniscus and open reduction.

Other types of acute dislocations

Rarely the head of mandible is dislocated in other directions and depending on the direction of dislocation of head, the dislocation can be of the types given in the subsequent text.

Posterior Dislocation It occurs from a blow on the chin of an elderly edentulous person who has lost the angle between the body and the ramus of the mandible. The tympanic plate of auditory meatus is fractured and the condyle goes backwards. The chin attains a receded position. In unilateral dislocation, the chin deviates to the affected side. The condyle blocks the external auditory meatus.

Medial or Lateral Dislocation It can occur when the neck of condyle is fractured.

Upward Dislocation It is very rare. It occurs from a blow on the point of chin in edentulous persons or at least in those who have lost their molars. The glenoid fossa is fractured and the condyle enters the middle cranial fossa.

These dislocations, truly speaking, are fracture–dislocations. They are usually treated by open reduction.

Habitual or Recurrent Dislocation or Subluxation

It is characterized by repeated episodes of dislocation where there is abnormal anterior excursion of the condyles beyond the articular eminence which the patient is able to manipulate back to normal position. It is also known as hypermobility or chronic subluxation.

Etiology

- **Etiological triad**: The triad of ligamentous and capsular flaccidity, shallowness of articular eminence, and trauma is well recognized in the genesis of recurrent dislocation.
- **Predisposing factors**: In such predisposed persons, the acts of yawning, laughing, and vomiting may precipitate dislocation. It may also occur in epilepsy, dystrophia myotonica, and Ehlers–Danlos syndrome.

Clinical features

The patient is usually a young adult who presents with recurrent locking of the jaw at a certain degree of opening of mouth. It has all the signs and symptoms of acute dislocation except that the mouth is less open, there is lesser pain with each succeeding episode, and reducing is easy and often self-effected.

Treatment

The treatment methods are:

- Limiting the oral opening by prefabricated splint to the maxillary and mandibular arches may be helpful.
- Intra-articular injections of sclerosing agent may be used but the result is short lived.
- Capsulorrhaphy or capsule tightening procedure is effective over a short period.
- Creation of a mechanical obstacle in the region of articular eminence, for example, putting a graft taken from zygoma over the eminence to increase its size and height. It is an effective operation but may limit the movement as the height of eminence is increased.
- Excision of meniscus: It is simpler, equally effective, and more physiological than previous operations. It allows the condyle to slip deeply into glenoid with no limitation of movement.
- High condylectomy above the attachment of lateral pterygoid may be performed.

KEY POINTS

- Temporomandibular joint (TMJ) is the articulation between the squamous part of temporal bone and the head of mandibular condyle (diarthrodial or freely movable joint).
- Acute suppurative arthritis of TMJ is characterized with acute pain in the joint, swelling, redness, and tenderness in the preauricular and zygomatic regions. It is treated by antibiotics and pus aspiration with lavage of the joint.
- Ankylosis of TMJ is chronic limitation or inability to open the mouth. It of two types: extra-articular ankylosis results from fibrosis and/or contracture of the soft tissues around the joint. Intra-articular ankylosis results from fusion of articular surfaces by fibrous tissue (fibrous ankylosis) or osseous tissue (bony ankylosis) due to suppurative arthritis of jaw or intra-articular fractures of the joint.
- The main effects of ankylosis of TMJ are early teeth decay and failure of lower jaw to develop if ankylosis occurs during early life, resulting in a shrew-mouse appearance.
- The treatment of extra-articular TMJ ankylosis includes stretching of contracted soft tissues, excision of scar tissue around the joint, and repair with pedicle or free grafting and extra-articular arthroplasty of Esmarch.
- Intra-articular ankylosis is treated by condylectomy, gap arthroplasty, or interpositional arthroplasty.
- Recurrence of TMJ ankylosis is an important complication which is due to inadequate excision of ankylotic mass, fracture or loosening of the graft, inadequate coverage of glenoid fossa by interpositional graft, and inadequate postoperative physiotherapy.
- Trismus is defined as difficulty in opening the mouth due to spasm of muscles of mastication (lock jaw). Causes include infections (tetanus), trauma, reflex muscular spasm, etc. Trismus is treated by removal of cause.
- Anterior dislocation of TMJ is the most common type of dislocation which occurs when the condyle of mandible slips forward on or over the articular eminence.
- Acute dislocation of TMJ is characterized by difficulty in speaking, mastication, and swallowing, and profuse drooling of saliva. It is treated by manipulative reduction. If it recurs, reduction is followed by application of a retentive apparatus.
- In bilateral dislocation of TMJ, the mouth is fixed in a partly open position with hollows palpable in front of both tragi. Condyle is displaced anteriorly and can be palpated anterior to the hollow.
- Habitual or recurrent dislocation or subluxation of TMJ is characterized by repeated episodes of dislocation which the patient is able to manipulate back to normal position. It is also known as hypermobility or chronic subluxation.
- Treatment methods of recurrent dislocation of TMJ are limiting the oral opening by prefabricated splint, intra-articular injections of sclerosing agent, capsule tightening procedure, creation of a mechanical obstacle in the region of articular eminence, excision of meniscus, and high condylectomy above the attachment of lateral pterygoid.

SELF-ASSESSMENT

Long answer questions

1. What are the causes of ankylosis of temporomandibular joint? Describe the treatment of a patient with unilateral bony ankylosis of this joint.
2. What are the causes of dislocation of temporomandibular joint? What are the types of dislocation? Discuss the causes, symptoms and signs, and treatment of recurrent dislocation.

Short answer questions

1. Acute suppurative arthritis of temporomandibular joint
2. Ankylosis
3. Trismus
4. Recurrent dislocation of temporomandibular joint

(CONTD...)

SELF-ASSESSMENT *(...CONTD)*

Multiple choice questions

1. All of the following are the features of acute suppurative arthritis of temporomandibular joint, except
   (a) It is caused by *Staphylococcus aureus, Streptococcus pyogenes*, and *Neisseria gonorrhoeae*
   (b) The bacteria enter the joint by local spread or bloodstream
   (c) It is characterized by local pain, swelling, and difficulty in the movements of the jaw
   (d) It never leads to ankylosis of TMJ
2. The most important diagnostic investigation in acute suppurative arthritis of TMJ is
   (a) Plain radiography
   (b) CT scan
   (c) Blood culture
   (d) CT-guided needle aspiration and culture of aspirate
3. The most common complication of suppurative arthritis of TMJ is
   (a) Cavernous sinus thrombosis
   (b) Septicemia
   (c) Extradural abscess
   (d) Ankylosis of TMJ
4. Which of the following facts is not true about TMJ ankylosis?
   (a) It is chronic limitation or inability to open the mouth
   (b) It is of two types: extra-articular and intra-articular
   (c) The patient becomes weak and emaciated due to lack of nutrition
   (d) It leads to early teeth decay
5. All of the following are the features of extra-articular ankylosis, except
   (a) The cause of ankylosis is not in the joint but around it
   (b) It permits some degree of movement
   (c) X-ray shows deposit of osteoid tissue in the joint
   (d) It is treated by removal of cause or Esmarch's operation
6. The intra-articular ankylosis is characterized by all of the following features, except
   (a) The cause of ankylosis is inside the joint
   (b) It does not permit any movement of the jaw
   (c) The joint is normal on radiography
   (d) It is treated by arthroplasty
7. Bird-like face or shrew-mouse appearance is seen
   (a) If bilateral intra-articular ankylosis occurs during childhood
   (b) When bilateral extra-articular occurs in adulthood
   (c) When unilateral intra-articular ankylosis occurs during adulthood
   (d) When bilateral intra-articular ankylosis occurs during adulthood
8. Which is the commonest dislocation of TMJ?
   (a) Posterior dislocation
   (b) Anterior dislocation
   (c) Superior dislocation
   (d) Medial dislocation
9. Which one of the following is a true dislocation and not a fracture–dislocation?
   (a) Anterior dislocation
   (b) Posterior dislocation
   (c) Superior dislocation
   (d) Medial dislocation
10. Anterior dislocation of TMJ occurring for the first time is treated by
    (a) Manipulative reduction
    (b) Manipulative reduction and use of retentive apparatus
    (c) Open reduction
    (d) Open reduction with excision of meniscus
11. In which dislocation of TMJ is excision of meniscus required?
    (a) Anterior dislocation occurring for the first time
    (b) Anterior dislocation occurring for the second time
    (c) Irreducible dislocation due to locking of coronoid process against maxilla
    (d) Irreducible dislocation due to detached meniscus filling the glenoid

(CONTD...)

SELF-ASSESSMENT (...CONTD)

12. The treatment of choice for recurrent dislocation is
    (a) Manipulative reduction
    (b) Manipulative reduction and use of retentive apparatus
    (c) Capsule tightening procedure or capsulorrhaphy
    (d) Creation of a mechanical obstacle in the region of articular eminence by bone grafting

Answers

1. (d) 2. (d) 3. (d) 4. (c) 5. (c) 6. (c) 7. (a) 8. (b) 9. (a) 10. (a) 11. (d) 12. (d)

Diseases of Salivary Glands

20

Anatomy of salivary glands

There is a pair of each of three salivary glands on either side of oral cavity, that is, parotid, submandibular, and sublingual. They are ectodermal in origin.

Parotid Gland

The parotid salivary gland is a bilobed structure situated in front of the ear (Fig. 20.1). The facial nerve and its branches (pes anserinas) and superficial temporal artery run between the deep and the superficial lobes. It is drained by Stensen's duct which runs anteriorly on the surface of buccinator below the buccal branch of facial nerve into the mouth with its opening situated at the level of crown of upper second molar inside the cheek. The lower part of the gland tapers to a blunt apex and extends into the neck and is called tail of the gland.

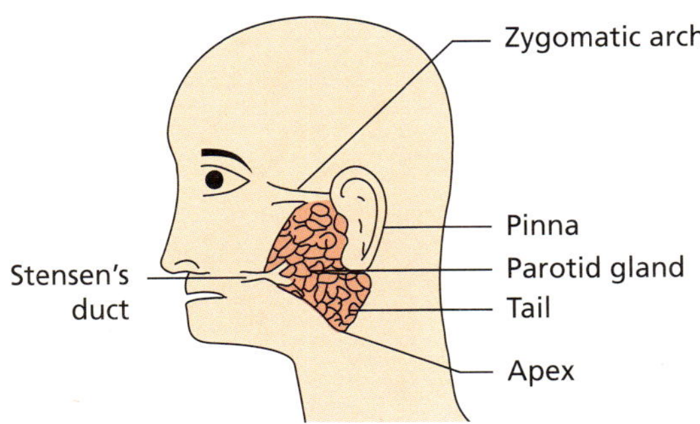

Figure 20.1 Anatomy of parotid.

It receives its blood supply from external carotid artery and drains into external jugular vein. The lymphatic drainage occurs into parotid lymph glands which are partly extraglandular and partly intraglandular and finally into deep cervical lymph nodes.

Submandibular and Sublingual Glands

The submandibular salivary gland is an ovoid structure lying partly hidden by the angle of mandible. It is drained by Wharton's duct in the floor of mouth by the side of frenulum linguae.

The lingual nerve and submandibular ganglion are related to its upper pole and the hypoglossal nerve is deep to it. The facial artery emerges from under the surface of stylohyoid, and enters the gland from its posterior and deep surface, reaching its lateral surface crossing the lower border of mandible to enter the face.

The venous drainage occurs by anterior facial vein and lymphatic drainage into submandibular lymph nodes.

The sublingual salivary gland lies in the floor of mouth anteriorly under the mucosa and drains directly into the oral cavity (Fig. 20.2).

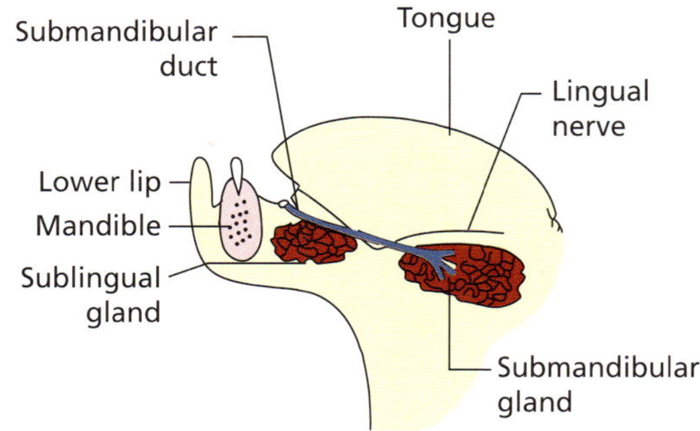

Figure 20.2 Anatomy of sublingual and submandibular salivary glands.

Minor or Ectopic Salivary Glands

Besides the above-mentioned glands, there are hundreds of minor salivary glands widely distributed in the mucosa of lips, cheeks, palate and uvula, floor of the mouth, tongue, and peritonsillar region. A few are found in the nasopharynx, paranasal sinuses, larynx, trachea, bronchi, and lacrimal glands. They maintain resting levels of saliva necessary for moisturizing, lubrication, cleansing, digestion, and immunological protection of oral environment.

1. INFECTIVE AND INFLAMMATORY DISORDERS

Acute bacterial sialadenitis (parotid abscess)

It is acute bacterial inflammation of salivary glands which usually affects the parotid gland and may sometimes affect the submandibular gland also, resulting in suppuration.

Etiology

- The most common bacterium responsible for infection is *Staphylococcus aureus*. Other organisms include streptococci, *Escherichia coli*, and anaerobes. From the oral cavity, they usually enter the parotid through the Stensen's duct.
- The predisposing factors include dry mouth, dehydration, salivary ductal obstruction (stone, stricture), salivary stasis or decreased secretion, and poor oral hygiene.

Clinical Features

- It may occur in a sick person with dehydration and poor oral hygiene or in postoperative phase as a complication of poor nursing care. It may also occur in an elderly who is taking diuretics or is dehydrated.
- The patient presents with pain, swelling, redness, and tenderness in the parotid region. There may be fever, malaise, and trismus.
- The parotid is covered by a thick and tough parotidomasseteric fascia; hence, the parotid abscess does not show any fluctuation until very late (Fig. 20.3). The orifice of the duct may be inflamed and may exude pus.

Investigations

The blood shows polymorphonuclear leukocytosis. The abscess can be imaged by ultrasonography and aspirated to confirm the presence of pus which is sent for culture and sensitivity.

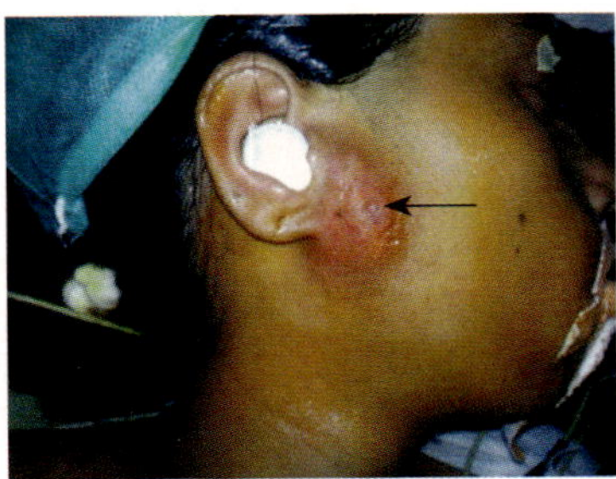

Figure 20.3 Parotid abscess which has involved the overlying skin. (Courtesy: Professor Sandeep Tewari)

Complications

The complications of acute bacterial sialadenitis include septicemia, trismus, and rupture into the external auditory canal.

Treatment

Antibiotics The patient is given nafcillin 1 g intravenously every 4–6 hours to start with followed by oral dicloxacillin, amoxicillin–clavulanate, or ampicillin–sulbactam. Suitable changes are made when culture report comes. The antibiotics are given for 10 days.

Incision and Drainage If the swelling does not subside, the abscess is drained by a vertical incision made in front of tragus (Blair's incision) followed by a transverse incision in the parotid fascia to protect the facial nerve. One should not wait for fluctuation to avoid complete loss of parotid parenchyma and function. Image-guided catheter drainage may be done.

Supportive Measures The salivary flow is increased by proper hydration, warm compression, and sialogogues (lemon drops). If there is a cause, it should be removed and oral hygiene should be maintained by chlorhexidine mouth washes.

Viral sialadenitis

Mumps is the most common type of viral sialadenitis. Cytomegalovirus (CMV) is the second most common cause of acute viral sialadenitis and may mimic infectious mononucleosis clinically.

Mumps

Etiology Mumps is caused by paramyxovirus that spreads by respiratory droplets. It has an incubation period of 14–21 days and occurs mostly in children.

Glands Involved Parotid is the most commonly affected salivary gland. Other salivary glands may be involved in 10% of cases.

Clinical Features The patient presents with parotid pain, tenderness, edema, and swelling. Usually one parotid is affected first followed by the involvement of other. Unilateral disease occurs in 25% of cases. Stensen's duct orifice may be red and swollen. The parotid glands return to normal within a week.

Diagnosis The diagnosis can be confirmed by isolating the virus from the swab of the parotid duct.

Complications Testicular swelling and tenderness occur in 75% of cases 7–10 days after the onset of parotitis. It may be followed by testicular atrophy.

Treatment It is symptomatic including isolation of patient until the swelling subsides. It is a preventable disease and can be prevented by live virus vaccination.

Chronic sialadenitis

It is a chronic or recurrent inflammation of parotid and submandibular salivary glands. It is more common in submandibular than in parotid gland.

Etiology It may develop as a result of acute bacterial or viral sialadenitis. There may be a history of ductal obstruction.

Pathology Recurrent inflammation leads to destruction and fibrosis of acini with ductal ectasia. It reduces the salivary flow which creates a cycle of ascending sialadenitis, ductal ectasia, acinar atrophy, fibrosis, and obstruction.

Clinical Features It is characterized by recurrent local pain and swelling during eating which reduces gradually after eating is over.

Diagnosis Sialography, which is a radiographic visualization of salivary ductal system after injecting a radio-opaque dye in the salivary ducts, shows multiple sites of obstruction and dilatation.

Treatment It consists of sialogogues (e.g., lemon balls and chewing gum), adequate oral hydration, and a course of amoxicillin–clavulanate or cephalexin. Other drugs are clindamycin, cefoxitin, nafcillin, or vancomycin plus metronidazole. The persistent disease is treated by excision of the affected salivary gland.

2. SALIVARY GLAND TUMORS

Classification

The classification of salivary gland tumors is described in Box 20.1.

Box 20.1 Classification of salivary gland tumors

Benign tumors

- Pleomorphic adenoma or mixed tumor
- Adenolymphoma (Warthin's tumor)
- Oncocytoma
- Basal cell adenoma (rare)

Malignant tumors

- Mucoepidermoid carcinoma
- Adenoid cystic carcinoma
- Acinic cell carcinoma
- Adenocarcinoma
- Malignant mixed tumor
- Squamous cell carcinoma
- Undifferentiated carcinoma

Incidence

- The tumors of salivary glands constitute 5% of head and neck tumors and affect major salivary glands five times more commonly than minor ones.
- Eighty percent of salivary tumors occur in the parotids of which 80% are benign and 80% of these are pleomorphic adenomas.

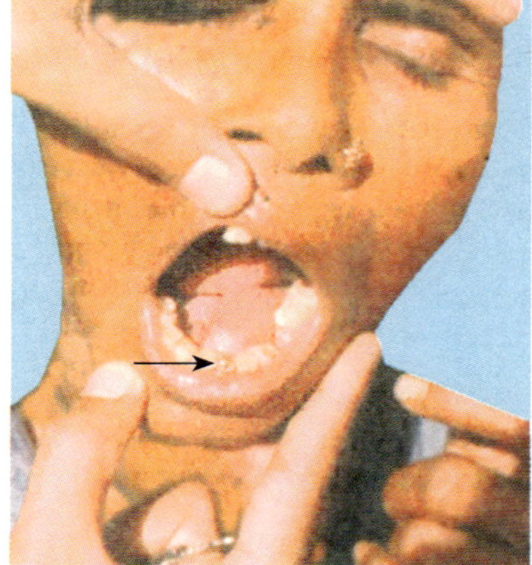

Figure 20.4 Sublingual salivary tumor.

- Fifteen percent of salivary tumors affect the submandibular gland of which 50% are benign and 95% of these are pleomorphic adenomas.
- Five to ten percent of tumors occur in minor salivary glands. Of these, only 10% are benign. Sublingual salivary tumors are very rare (Fig. 20.4).

Pleomorphic adenoma

Pleomorphic adenoma is the most common salivary tumor which accounts for 80% of parotid tumors and 50% of all salivary gland tumors.

Pathology

Pleomorphic adenoma has both stromal and epithelial components. Grossly it contains

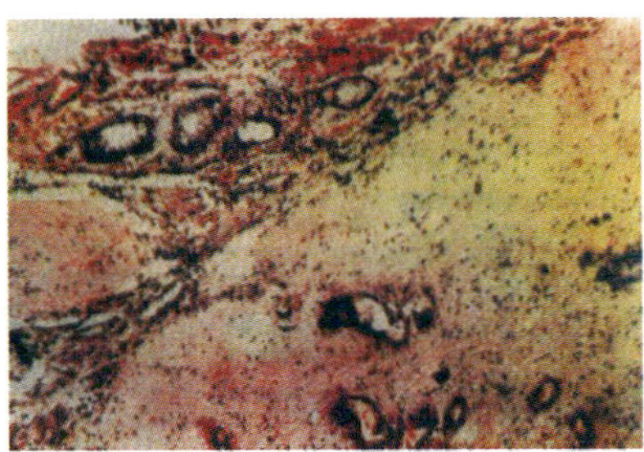

Figure 20.5 Microscopic picture of pleomorphic adenoma of parotid showing a variegated appearance consisting of acini and myxomatous and chondroid tissue. (Courtesy: Professor P.K. Agarwal)

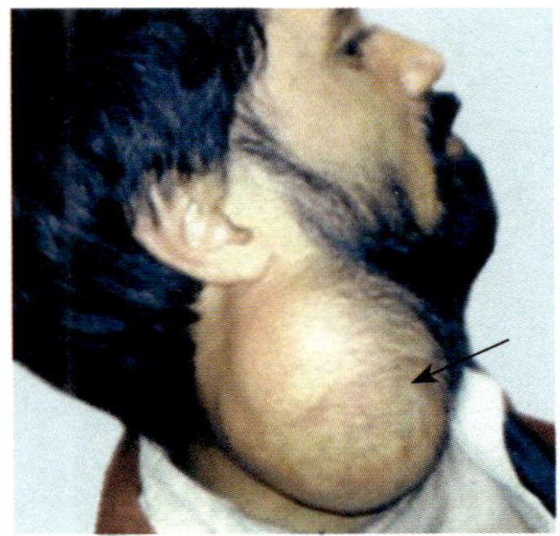

Figure 20.7 Pleomorphic adenoma of right submandibular salivary gland. The ear lobule is normal.

cartilage, cystic spaces, and solid tissues. It is an encapsulated tumor but may have pseudopods that may extend beyond the main limit of tumor. Commonly it involves the superficial lobe. It may occur in the deep lobe when it is in relation to styloid process, mandible, styloglossus, and stylopharyngeus muscles. Microscopically it reveals epithelial cells, myoepithelial cells, mucoid material with myxomatous changes, and cartilage/pseudocartilage (Fig. 20.5).

Clinical Features

- It is more common in women than in men (3:1) with a peak incidence in the fourth and fifth decades.
- The patient presents with a painless, smooth or lobulated, firm, mobile, and nontender swelling in the parotid region (Fig. 20.6) which cannot be moved above the zygomatic bone (it is called curtain sign as the deep fascia covering the parotid is attached above to zygomatic arch preventing the movement of parotid swelling up). The ear lobule may be lifted. The facial nerve is normal.
- It may affect the submandibular salivary gland (Fig. 20.7). Here the ear lobule is not lifted.
- Deep lobe tumor: The patient may present with dysphagia. Usually there is no external swelling but it is present in lateral wall of pharynx displacing the posterior pillar and the soft palate. It is examined by bidigital palpation.

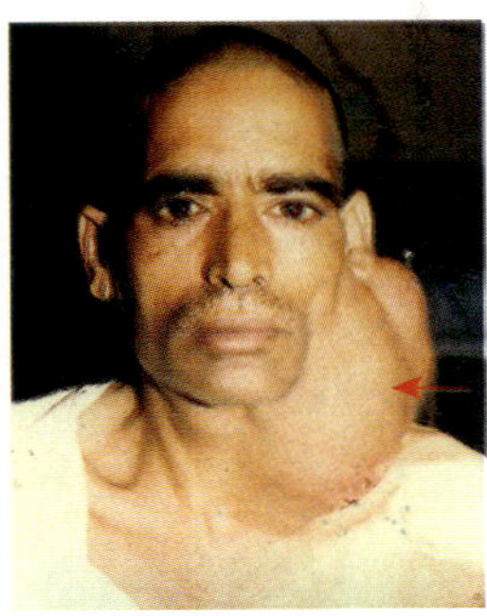

Figure 20.6 Pleomorphic adenoma of left parotid.

Malignant Transformation

A long-standing pleomorphic adenoma may turn into a carcinoma. Its features are enumerated in Box 20.2.

Box 20.2 Features of malignant transformation of a pleomorphic adenoma

- Recent increase in size
- Appearance of pain and nodularity
- Fixity to skin, ulceration
- Fixity to masseter
- Involvement of facial nerve
- Enlargement of neck lymph nodes
- Restriction of movements of mandible

Investigations

- Biopsy should never be done as there are increased chances of seedling and recurrence.
- FNAC can be done but its track must be excised at the time of excision of the tumor.

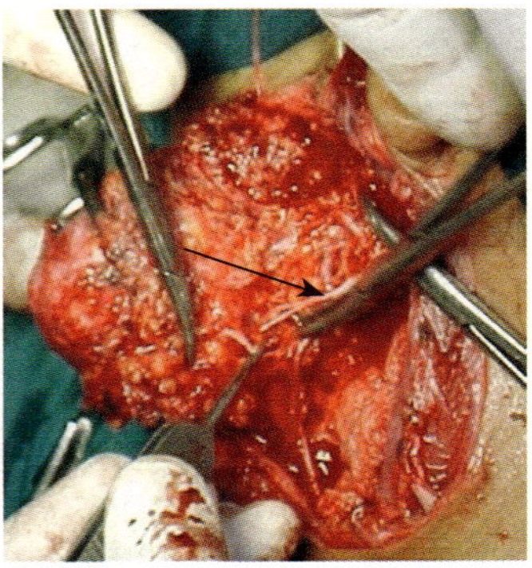

Figure 20.8 Superficial parotidectomy—branches of facial nerve are seen in the operative field. (Courtesy: Professor Sandeep Kumar)

- CT scan/MRI can be done to see the status of deep lobe, local extension, and lymphatic spread. MRI reveals neurovascular invasion, if any.

Treatment

Parotid Tumor

- A tumor of superficial lobe is excised by superficial parotidectomy in which the parotid superficial to facial nerve is completely removed (Fig. 20.8). The facial nerve is protected from injury during dissection.
- A tumor of deep lobe is removed by total conservative parotidectomy retaining the facial nerve. The types of parotidectomy are given in Box 20.3.

Box 20.3 Types of parotidectomy

- **Superficial parotidectomy**: Removal of superficial lobe of parotid, superficial to facial nerve
- **Total conservative parotidectomy**: Removal of both superficial and deep lobes of parotid with preservation of facial nerve
- **Radical parotidectomy**: Removal of both lobes of parotid with facial nerve, fat, fascia, muscles (masseter, pterygoids, and buccinator), and lymph nodes, done in carcinoma of parotid
- **Suprafacial parotidectomy**: Local resection of lower pole of parotid where all branches of facial nerve need not be dissected

- Enucleation of the tumor should never be done as it may leave behind the tumor as pseudopods.
- Recurrence occurs in 5% of cases and it is due to spillage, improper technique, inadequate margin of excision, retained pseudocapsule, and multicentricity.

Submandibular Tumor It is excised by a submandibular incision below the angle of mandible given in one of the skin creases protecting the cervical branch of facial nerve and facial artery. The whole gland containing the tumor is excised.

Adenolymphoma (Warthin's tumor, papillary cystadenolymphomatosum)

Site It is not a lymphoma, but a benign tumor that occurs only in parotid, usually in the lower pole.

Pathology It consists of a double layer of columnar epithelium with papillary projections into cystic spaces with lymphoid tissue in the stroma.

Predisposing Factors It is etiologically related to smoking and radiation exposure.

Clinical Features The patient is usually an elderly male who presents with a slow-growing, smooth, soft, cystic, and fluctuant swelling in the lower pole. It is often bilateral.

Diagnosis The diagnosis can be confirmed by ^{99m}Tc pertechnetate scan which shows a "hot spot" and FNAC.

Treatment It is treated by superficial parotidectomy. This tumor does not turn into malignancy. One should never try to enucleate it as it is very much likely to rupture with spillover of tumor cells.

Adenolymphoma must be differentiated from a pleomorphic adenoma and their differences are described in Table 20.1.

Table 20.1 Differences between adenolymphoma and pleomorphic adenomas

Features	Adenolymphoma (Warthin's tumor)	Pleomorphic adenoma
Age	Elderly male	Middle-aged people
Side	Often bilateral	Usually unilateral
Site	Parotid salivary gland only	Can affect any salivary gland
Swelling	Smooth, soft, cystic swelling usually in lower pole	Smooth or lobulated, firm and solid swelling
^{99m}Tc pertechnetate scan	Hot spot at the site of tumor	Negative
Malignant transformation	Does not occur	Can occur
Treatment	Superficial parotidectomy	Superficial parotidectomy
Recurrence	Rare	More likely
Histopathology	Double layer of columnar epithelium with papillary projections into cystic spaces with lymphoid stroma	Epithelial cells, myoepithelial cells, mucoid material with myxomatous changes, and cartilage/pseudocartilage

Oncocytoma (oxyphil adenoma)

It is a rare tumor which is common in parotid, but can rarely arise from submandibular salivary gland. Oncocytoma is a small tan-colored encapsulated tumor. Microscopically it shows large oncocytes with swollen granular cytoplasm. It is treated by excision.

Basal cell adenoma

It is a rare benign tumor that contains isomorphic basaloid cells with basal layer and basement membrane. Basal cell adenoma is common in minor salivary glands and looks like a lymph node. It is treated by excision.

Mucoepidermoid carcinoma

- It is the commonest malignant tumor of parotid and the second commonest malignant tumor of submandibular and sublingual salivary glands. It can occur in minor salivary glands, especially of palate.
- Mucoepidermoid carcinoma contains malignant epidermoid and mucus-secreting cells. It is of three grades: low grade (mucous cells only), intermediate grade (clear cells), and high grade (epidermoid cells). The high-grade type has a high propensity for distant spread.
- It is excised widely with related lymph nodes in continuity. It may recur after treatment, especially a high-grade tumor.

Adenoid cystic carcinoma (cylindromatous carcinoma)

- It is the second most common malignant tumor of salivary glands and the most common tumor of submandibular and sublingual salivary glands. Fifty percent of tumors occur in minor salivary glands, especially of palate.
- Microscopically it is of three types: cribriform, tubular, and solid. It is a slow-growing but highly malignant tumor with a remarkable propensity for recurrence.
- It has a high propensity for perineural spread along mandibular and maxillary divisions of trigeminal nerve and facial nerve and may reach Gasserian ganglion, pterygopalatine ganglion, and cavernous sinus. Hematogenous spread can occur into the lungs, bones, and liver.

- Treatment consists of excision of tumor with radiation therapy for microscopic disease that is assumed to exist at the periphery of tumor.

Acinic cell carcinoma

It is a rare tumor that is derived from serous acinar cells and is found almost exclusively in parotid. The patient is commonly an elderly female.

Adenocarcinoma

It is an uncommon tumor that is common in children and occurs equally in both the sexes.

Malignant mixed tumor

It is of two types: carcinoma ex pleomorphic adenoma and primary malignant mixed tumor. It constitutes 10% of salivary malignant tumors and consists of epithelial and mesenchymal elements.

Squamous cell carcinoma

It is a rare tumor and accounts for 1% of all salivary cancers. It is common in men and occurs in the sixth and seventh decades of life. Parotid is the commonest site and it never occurs in minor salivary glands. It arises from the ductal system.

Clinical Features

The patient presents with a swelling of insidious onset which grows rapidly and may attain a large size. It is hard and nodular, and often involves the facial nerve, skin, and cervical lymph nodes. Involvement of facial nerve indicates malignancy. The carcinoma may invade the adjacent jaw and masticatory muscles.

TNM Staging

TNM staging of squamous cell carcinoma of salivary glands is given in Box 20.4.

Box 20.4 TNM staging of squamous cell carcinoma of salivary glands

- **T—tumor size**
  - *T1*: Tumor <2 cm without extraparenchymal spread
  - *T2*: Tumor 2–4 cm without extraparenchymal spread
  - *T3*: Tumor >4 cm, or with extraparenchymal spread but no facial nerve involvement
  - *T4*
    - T4a: Spread to facial nerve, skin, mandible, ear canal
    - T4b: Spread to base of skull, pterygoid plates, and encasement of external carotid artery
- **N—nodal involvement**
  - *N1*: Single ipsilateral node <3 cm
  - *N2a*: Single ipsilateral node 3–6 cm
  - *N2b*: Multiple ipsilateral nodes <6 cm
  - *N2c*: Bilateral or contralateral nodes <6 cm
  - *N3*: Single node >6 cm
- **M—metastasis**
  - *M0*: No distant metastasis
  - *M1*: Distant metastasis present

Investigations

- **Laboratory studies**: Blood is examined for hemoglobin, counts, ESR, sugar, urea, creatinine, and others as required.
- **Biopsy**: Open biopsy must not be done. FNAC may be done but the needle track must be excised at the time of operation.
- **CT scan**: It is done to see the extent of disease, that is, deep lobe involvement, involvement of bone, and extension into the base of skull and parapharyngeal space. Bony changes in the foramina and fissures of skull are signs of perineural spread.
- **MRI**: It can also be used to study the extent of tumor and perineural extension, the signs of which include replacement of perineural fat with tumor, contrast (gadolinium) enhancement, and increased size of the nerve.
- **FNAC**: It provides cytological diagnosis. Open biopsy should not be done. The enlarged cervical lymph nodes can also be studied by FNAC.

Treatment of Carcinoma of Salivary Glands

Surgery

- Low-grade T1, T2, and T3 tumors of parotid are treated by total conservative parotidectomy. The complications of parotidectomy are described in Box 20.5.

Box 20.5 Complications of parotidectomy

- Bleeding
- Wound infection
- Flap necrosis
- Frey's syndrome
- Facial nerve palsy
- Numbness of ear lobule
- Sialocele

- T4, high-grade tumors and squamous cell carcinoma are treated by radical parotidectomy which includes facial nerve sacrifice, and may be resection of skin, mandibular ramus, temporal bone masseter muscle, and infratemporal fossa dissection. The facial nerve can be reconstructed using a nerve graft taken from great auricular nerve or sural nerve. All branches except buccal branch are repaired using cable graft. Nerve grafting is not a contraindication for radiotherapy in future.
- If neck nodes are involved, modified radical neck dissection (MRND) is done.
- A submandibular salivary carcinoma is treated with total submandibular gland removal with modified radial neck dissection.

Management of Facial Nerve in the Surgery of Parotid Tumors Details of the facial nerve management in surgery of parotid tumors are given in Box 20.6.

Box 20.6 Management of facial nerve in surgery of parotid tumor

- Saved in all benign tumors by careful dissection
- Saved in malignant tumors if possible by peeling the tumor off the nerve with use of post-operative radiotherapy for microscopic residual disease
- Gross nerve involvement (the nerve is sacrificed proximally to get a cancer free margin which may need temporal bone resection and simultaneous nerve grafting)
- Facial nerve rehabilitation
  - Protection of cornea from exposure keratitis including lateral tarsorrhaphy
  - Maintenance of oral competence
  - Operative rehabilitation by static facial slings, dynamic muscular slings, and delayed innervation procedures

Radiotherapy Usually postoperative external radiotherapy is given in all carcinomas. But it is more useful in adenoid cystic and squamous cell carcinomas. It is delayed for 6 weeks if nerve grafting is done. It improves the results and reduces the chances of recurrence. In large tumors, preoperative radiotherapy is given to reduce the size of tumor (to downgrade) to make it better operable.

Chemotherapy In malignant tumors, chemotherapy may also be combined with other treatments, but it is less effective. The drugs include 5-FU, cisplatin, doxorubicin, epirubicin, and cetuximab.

Minor salivary gland tumors

Incidence These tumors constitute 10% of salivary tumors. The palate is the commonest site where 40% tumors occur. Ten percent of these tumors are benign and are pleomorphic adenomas, and 90% are malignant and are mostly adenoid cystic carcinomas.

Clinical Features They present as a firm or hard swelling with or without ulceration over the summit. A malignant tumor may extend into palate, maxilla, and pterygoids and may involve the lymph nodes of neck.

Diagnosis The diagnosis is confirmed by biopsy. CT scan may be required.

Treatment A tumor less than 1 cm in size is excised with 1 cm clearance margin. If the tumor is more than 1 cm wide, excision is done. The palatal wound is left open to granulate and epithelize. If the bony palate is involved, it is also excised and the defect is closed by a flap or dental palate.

3. OTHER DISEASES OF THE SALIVARY GLANDS

Sialolithiasis

Sialolithiasis is stone formation in the salivary glands/ducts.

Etiology

Salivary calculi are both a cause and a consequence of chronic sialadenitis. They develop due to deposition of salts dissolved in saliva on an organic nidus of mucus or cellular debris. The calculi are more common (80%) in the submandibular salivary gland because its secretion is viscous and contains more calcium, and drains against gravity causing stasis.

Pathology

The stones are usually small and composed of organic calcium and sodium phosphate deposited on an organic nucleus. Their composition is same as that of dental tartar. They are usually present in the ductal system causing obstruction which may result in acute or chronic sialadenitis.

Clinical Features

Submandibular Calculi

- Eighty percent of salivary calculi occur in the submandibular gland (duct). They can occur at any age.
- The patient presents with painful swelling of the gland especially during meals and may report extrusion of gravel from the duct.
- The submandibular gland may be swollen, smooth, and tender. The stone is usually palpable or visible in the floor of mouth on one side (Fig. 20.9). There is decreased salivary flow from the duct.

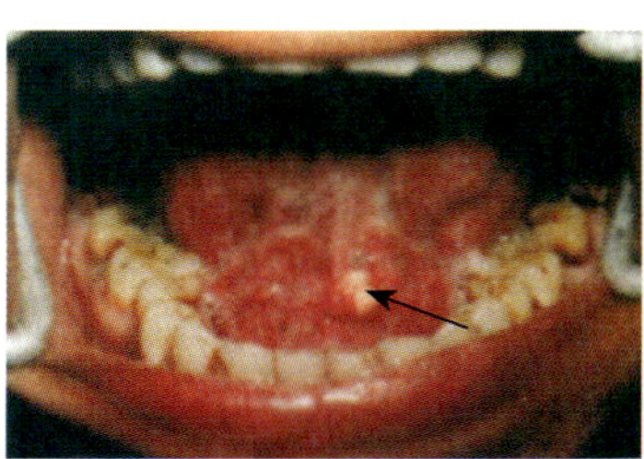

Figure 20.9 Two small pale yellow salivary calculi seen at the orifice of left submandibular salivary duct in the floor of mouth. (Courtesy: Professor R.M. Mathur)

Investigations

Intraoral radiography (dental) occlusion films may show radio-opaque stones in 80% of cases (Fig. 20.10). Ultrasonography may be used. Radiolucent stones may be seen by sialography.

Parotid Calculi

- The patient is usually more than 30 years of age and presents with a painful parotid swelling of one whole gland of sudden onset as soon as he/she starts taking meals. It is associated with a sensation of dryness in the cheek on the same side.
- After some time, there is a gush of salty or foul-smelling liquid into the mouth with relief

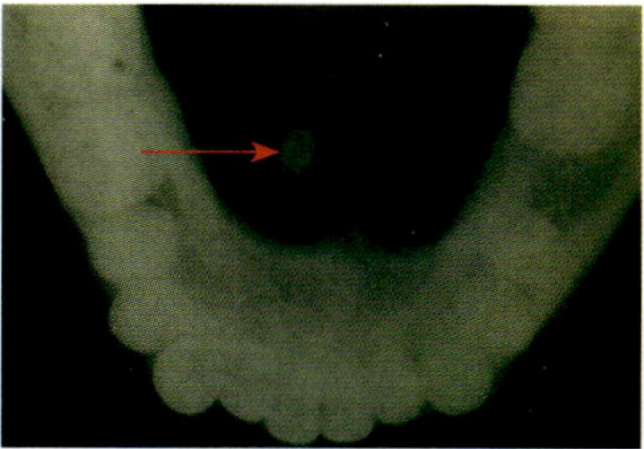

Figure 20.10 Radiograph of floor of mouth showing a small oval radio-opaque shadow on the right side of midline due to a stone in the submandibular salivary duct.

from pain and swelling. The duct orifice may have redness and may be pouting. The tip of the stone may sometimes be visible.

Investigations of Parotid Calculi The parotid calculi are difficult to image by radiography as they are small and overlapped by facial skeleton. They may be seen by ultrasound, CT scan, or sialography.

Treatment

Submandibular Stone A stone close to the duct orifice is removed by ductal dilatation and manipulation (Fig. 20.11). A palpable submandibular duct stone is removed by making a longitudinal incision on the duct. The incised duct need not be sutured. A stone in the hilum of gland is treated by submandibular gland excision.

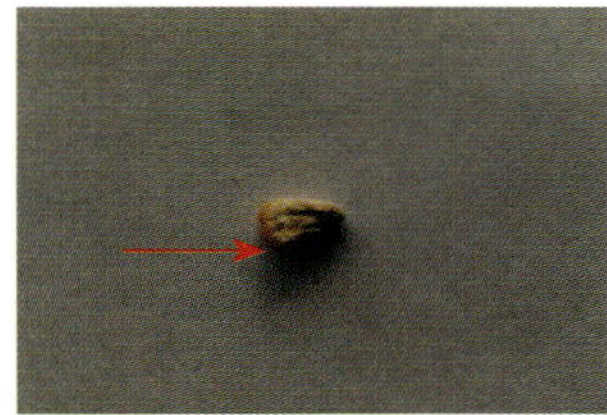

Figure 20.11 Stone removed from the submandibular salivary duct.

Parotid Stone A stone near the duct orifice can be removed by meatal dilatation and manipulation. A stone in the gland is treated by parotidectomy.

Frey's syndrome (auriculotemporal syndrome)

Etiopathogenesis It is a complication of operations on the parotid and occurs in 10% of cases. It follows injury to the auriculotemporal nerve wherein the postganglionic parasympathetic fibers from the otic ganglion unite with sympathetic fibers from superior cervical ganglion supplying the overlying skin.

Clinical Features The patient presents with flushing, sweating, erythema, pain, and hyperesthesia of the skin of parotid region supplied by auriculotemporal nerve during eating when salivation is stimulated.

Diagnosis

- **Starch–iodine test**: The involved skin is painted with iodine and dried. Dry starch powder sprinkled over this area will become blue when sweating occurs during eating.

Treatment It is symptomatic and reassurance. Most of the patients recover within 6 months.

- Antiperspirant such as aluminum chloride may be used.
- Only a few patients require surgical division of the tympanic branch of glossopharyngeal nerve below the round window of middle ear (Jacobson nerve).

Injection of botulinum toxin into the affected skin may give relief.

Prevention Frey's syndrome can be prevented by placing muscle, fascial flap, or an artificial membrane under the skin during closure of the wound after parotidectomy.

Parotid salivary fistula

Parotid salivary fistula is an abnormal opening in the parotid region which discharges watery fluid that increases at the time of meals (sialorrhea).

Causes The causes of a parotid salivary fistula are:

- Postoperative fistula may follow drainage of a parotid abscess and superficial parotidectomy.
- Traumatic fistula may follow penetrating injuries of the parotid region.

Types Anatomically the fistula is of two types: gland fistula and duct fistula.

Clinical Features

- **Gland fistula**: It produces some moisture of the overlying skin.
- **Duct fistula**: It presents with free flow of saliva on the skin during meals or when the patient smells or thinks of food. The skin around the opening may be excoriated.

Diagnosis The communication of the fistula with the main duct or a ductule can be seen by sialography. It will also reveal if the ductal system has obstruction.

Treatment

- A small fistula may heal by itself with time. Pro-Banthine 50 mg four times daily may be helpful.
- A large fistula is repaired on a fine nylon splint (Newman and Seabrook's operation). If it fails, avulsion of auriculotemporal nerve may be done as it reduces the salivary secretion markedly.

Xerostomia

Xerostomia is a symptom characterized by dryness of mouth due to lack of salivary secretion. It results in difficulty in mastication and swallowing and early teeth decay.

Etiology The etiology of xerostomia is described in Table 20.2.

The investigations and treatment depend on the cause of this symptom.

Sjogren's syndrome (sicca syndrome)

Sjogren's syndrome is an autoimmune disorder causing progressive destruction of lacrimal and salivary glands characterized by a varying degree of dryness of eyes (xerophthalmia) and dryness of mouth (xerostomia).

Types It can occur in isolation ("primary" Sjogren's syndrome), or in association with another similar disease, for example, rheumatoid arthritis, systemic lupus erythematosus (SLE), and primary biliary cirrhosis.

Pathology There is progressive lymphocyte and plasma cell infiltration of the lacrimal and salivary glands.

Clinical Features

- Most of the patients (90%) are women with an average age of 50 years.
- Dryness of the eyes (keratoconjunctivitis sicca) and dryness of the mouth are the most common features.
- Burning, itching, and a sensation of foreign body (e.g., grain of sand) in the eyes are common symptoms. Dryness of mouth results in severe dental caries.

Investigations

- Blood examination shows polyclonal hypergammaglobulinemia, rheumatoid factor positivity (70%), and antinuclear antibodies (95%).
- Antibodies against the cytoplasmic antigens SS-A and SS-B are often present.
- Other investigations include Schirmer's test (measurement of volume of tears) and lip

Table 20.2 Etiology of xerostomia

Causes	Examples
Salivary gland diseases	• Congenital aplasia • Sjogren's syndrome • Diffuse sialadenitis • Radiation injury to salivary tissue
Systemic diseases reducing salivary secretion	• Aging • Dehydration • Diabetes mellitus • Uremia • Rheumatoid arthritis
Drugs	• Atropine • MAO inhibitors • Tricyclic antidepressants
Local lesions of oral cavity	• Mouth breathing • Radiation injury to oral mucosa
Psychogenic xerostomia	—

biopsy which shows lymphoid foci in minor salivary glands.

Complications The complications of this syndrome include accelerated dental caries, oral candidiasis, destructive periodontal disease, and lymphoma.

Treatment

- The treatment is symptomatic and supportive as the cause is not known.
- Frequent use of artificial tears relieves ocular symptoms. Topical ocular 0.05% cyclosporin also gives relief. The mouth should be kept wet by sipping water frequently or using sugar-free chewing gums and hard candies. Pilocarpine 5 mg four times daily and acetylcholine derivative cevimeline 30 mg orally three times daily may give relief.

Salivary gland trauma

The injuries to salivary glands are uncommon.

Etiology They may be injured by blunt or penetrating trauma. Injury to the parotid may be associated with injury to facial nerve, Stensen's duct, local soft tissues, mandible, or zygoma.

Clinical Features Lacerations of Stensen's duct may occur with facial lacerations posterior to the anterior edge of masseter muscle and result in simultaneous injury to the buccal branch of facial nerve.

Treatment

- The severed Stensen's duct is repaired over a small polythene catheter using fine interrupted sutures.
- All lacerations in the parotid region must be examined for facial nerve injury. If nerve injury is suspected, each of the five major branches is assessed by observing voluntary movements and response to nerve excitability testing.
- Facial nerve injuries anterior to a vertical line drawn from the lateral canthus of the eye generally do not require exploration as the nerve regenerates spontaneously. But some surgeons advocate microscopic repair to prevent synkinesis.
- The nerve is explored by a parotidectomy incision and repaired with the help of an operating microscope by anastomosing the cut ends with 10-0 monofilament suture. Lost nerve segments are made up by grafts obtained from great auricular or sural nerve.
- A contaminated wound, for example, a gunshot wound, is explored and debrided, and the proximal and distal cut ends are tagged with metal clips and then delayed repair is done when the wound becomes clean within 30 days.

Swellings of parotid region

The swellings in the parotid region are quite common. The causes of swellings of parotid region are described in Box 20.7.

Box 20.7 Swellings of parotid region

- **Nonspecific swellings**
  - Enlarged lymph nodes
  - Sebaceous cyst
  - Tumors, for example, papilloma, lipoma, hemangioma, neurofibroma
- **Specific swellings**
  - Swellings of parotid salivary gland
    - Swellings of the whole gland
      - Acute bacterial parotitis (parotid abscess)
      - Mumps
      - Distended gland due to calculus obstruction of Stensen's duct
    - Localized swellings
      - Pleomorphic adenoma
      - Carcinoma
      - Adenolymphoma
      - Cyst
  - Swellings of ascending ramus of mandible
    - Ameloblastoma
    - Osteosarcoma

The differential diagnosis of swellings of the parotid region is described in the subsequent text.

Enlarged Lymph Nodes There are two groups of lymph nodes in this region: preauricular and parotid. The preauricular lymph nodes are superficial to parotidomasseteric fascia and the parotid lymph nodes are deep to it. They are enlarged in acute lymphadenitis, tuberculosis, and metastatic disease. Acute lymphadenitis is characterized by painful, soft, and tender enlarged lymph nodes of short duration with a focus of acute infection in the drainage area, for example, scalp infection and acute external otitis.

Tuberculous lymphadenitis is seen in the young. The nodes are moderate in size, firm, nontender, and matted. Metastatic nodes are usually seen in an elderly person. They are hard and mobile or fixed with a primary cancer situated in the drainage area.

Sebaceous Cyst It is a hemispherical slow-growing swelling, soft, and nontender, and has a punctum on the top.

Tumors

- Papilloma is a small, pale, soft, and branched swelling like a small plant. Lipoma is soft, lobulated or smooth, and nontender, and has an edge which slips under the finger.
- Hemangioma is a bluish, soft, nontender, and compressible swelling.
- Neurofibroma is a firm or hard ovoid swelling which if pressed may cause tingling in the supply area of the affected nerve.

Specific Swellings

Acute Bacterial Parotitis (Parotid Abscess)

- The patient is usually a debilitated person who is suffering with a major illness or has undergone a major operation and presents with pain and swelling in the parotid region of a short duration associated with fever.
- The pain is a continuous throb which radiates to the ear and the side of the head. The whole of the parotid gland is swollen, smooth, hot, very tender, and brawny. The orifice of the Stensen's duct may have a bead of pus or signs of acute inflammation.

Mumps (Viral Parotitis)

- The patient is usually a young person who has pain, fever, and bilateral parotid swelling of acute onset.
- The parotids swell one after the other. The swellings are mild to moderate in size, smooth, firm, and tender. There may be edema of the parotid region which may extend down into the neck giving the patient a double chin appearance.

Distended Gland due to Calculus Obstruction of Stensen's Duct

- The patient is usually a middle-aged person who presents with recurrent attacks of painful swelling of whole parotid of acute onset at the time of meals. It is associated with dryness of mouth on that side
- The swelling is smooth, tender, and soft or tense. The orifice of the Stensen's duct may be edematous and sometimes may have the projecting tip of the stone.
- The attack is followed by remission of swelling after sometime, often sudden with a gush of salty or foul-smelling liquid into the mouth.

Pleomorphic Adenoma (Mixed Parotid Tumor)

- The patient is usually a middle-aged person who presents with a painless, slow-growing swelling of insidious onset. It is situated a little in front of and above the angle of mandible.
- It is smooth or lobulated, firm, mobile, and nontender. The ear lobule is displaced upwards and outwards. The facial nerve and lymph nodes are normal.

Carcinoma of Parotid

- The patient is usually a middle-aged or elderly person who presents with a rapidly growing swelling in the parotid region.
- It is irregular, hard, and ill-defined, and may be fixed. The facial nerve is paralyzed partially or completely. The regional lymph nodes may be enlarged.

Adenolymphoma (Warthin's Tumor)

- The patient is usually an elderly person, more commonly a male, who presents with a slow-growing, smooth, soft, cystic, opaque, and nontender swelling arising from the lower pole. It is often bilateral.

Cyst

- Rarely a cyst is encountered in the parotid region. It is smooth, soft or tense, nontender, and a translucent swelling.

Ameloblastoma of Ascending Ramus of Mandible

- The patient is usually in the fourth to fifth decade of life and presents with a painless, slow-growing swelling near the angle of mandible which attains a large size extending into the vertical ramus.
- It is smooth, hard, and nontender with intact inner table. It may have egg-shell crackling. The ear lobule, facial nerve, and lymph nodes are normal.

Osteosarcoma of Ascending Ramus of Mandible

- The patient is usually young and presents with a painful, rapidly growing swelling of recent onset.
- The swelling is smooth, hard, or variable in consistency. The inner table of mandible is also expanded. The ear lobule, the facial nerve, and lymph nodes are normal.

Investigations

They include blood counts, examination of swab of Stensen's duct (mumps), ultrasonography, CT scan, biopsy (not in a pleomorphic adenoma), and ^{99m}Tc pertechnetate scan.

Treatment

- Acute bacterial parotitis is treated with intravenous broad-spectrum antibiotics, hydration, maintenance of oral hygiene, and measures to increase salivary flow. If there is no relief within 24 hours, surgical decompression is required.
- Mumps is given symptomatic and supportive treatment.
- Stone in the Stensen's duct is removed.
- Pleomorphic adenoma is excised by superficial parotidectomy. A carcinoma of parotid is treated by total or radical parotidectomy depending on the extent of disease. Facial nerve may require grafting. Postoperative radiotherapy is required in larger and high-grade cancers. Adenolymphoma is excised.
- Ameloblastoma is treated by resection of tumor and reconstruction of the jaw. Osteosarcoma is first treated by chemotherapy followed by resection.

KEY POINTS

- Acute bacterial sialadenitis (parotid abscess) is caused by *Staphylococcus aureus* and occurs in a sick person with poor oral hygiene. It presents with pain, swelling, redness, and tenderness in the parotid region and the orifice of the Stensen's duct may be inflamed and may exude pus. Fluctuation is a late sign. It is treated by early removal of pus.
- Mumps is the most common type of viral sialadenitis. Cytomegalovirus (CMV) is the second most common cause of acute viral sialadenitis. It may be followed by testicular atrophy.
- Chronic sialadenitis is a chronic or recurrent inflammation, more common in submandibular salivary gland. It is treated by sialogogues, antibiotics, and persistent disease by excision of the salivary gland.
- The tumors of salivary glands constitute 5% of head and neck tumors and affect major salivary glands five times more commonly than minor ones. Eighty percent of salivary tumors occur in the parotids of which 80% are benign and 80% of these are pleomorphic adenomas.
- Pleomorphic adenoma presents as a painless, smooth or lobulated, and firm swelling of parotid region with normal facial nerve. It should not be biopsied and treated by superficial parotidectomy saving the facial nerve.
- Warthin's tumor is a benign neoplasm of the parotid. The diagnosis can be confirmed by ^{99m}technetium pertechnetate scan which shows a "hot spot." It is treated by superficial parotidectomy.
- Mucoepidermoid carcinoma is the commonest malignant tumor of parotid and the second commonest malignant tumor of submandibular and sublingual salivary glands. It can occur in minor salivary glands, especially of palate.
- Adenoid cystic carcinoma is the second most common malignant tumor of salivary glands and the most common tumor of submandibular and

(CONTD...)

KEY POINTS (...CONTD)

sublingual salivary glands. Fifty percent of tumors occur in minor salivary glands, especially of palate. It has a high propensity for perineural spread.

- Squamous cell carcinoma is most common in parotid gland. Low-grade T1, T2, and T3 tumors of parotid are treated by total conservative parotidectomy. T4 and high grade tumors are treated by radical parotidectomy. The facial nerve can be reconstructed using a nerve graft taken from great auricular nerve or sural nerve.
- The salivary calculi are more common in the submandibular salivary gland. The stone is usually palpable or visible in the floor of mouth on one side. A stone close to the duct orifice is removed by ductal dilatation and manipulation and a stone in the hilum is treated by excision of the gland.
- A parotid calculus presents as a painful parotid swelling of one whole gland of sudden onset with dryness of ipsilateral cheek as soon as the patient starts taking meal.
- Frey's syndrome is a complication of operations on the parotid characterized by flushing, sweating, erythema, pain, and hyperesthesia of the skin supplied by auriculotemporal nerve during eating when salivation is stimulated.
- Xerostomia is a symptom characterized by dryness of mouth due to lack of salivary secretion. It results in difficulty in mastication and swallowing and early teeth decay.
- Sjogren's syndrome is an autoimmune disorder causing progressive destruction of lacrimal and salivary glands characterized by a varying degree of dryness of eyes (xerophthalmia) and dryness of mouth (xerostomia).
- Facial nerve injury is repaired by anastomosing the cut ends with 10-0 monofilament suture. Lost nerve segments are made up by grafts obtained from great auricular or sural nerve.

SELF-ASSESSMENT

Long answer questions

1. Describe the pathology, clinical features, investigations, and treatment of pleomorphic adenoma of parotid gland. Classify the tumors of parotid gland.
2. Describe the types, clinical features, and treatment of carcinoma of parotid.
3. Describe the differential diagnosis of parotid gland swellings. Briefly mention their treatment.

Short answer questions

1. Ectopic salivary glands
2. Warthin's tumor
3. Adenoid cystic carcinoma
4. Mucoepidermoid carcinoma
5. Salivary calculus
6. Calculus in Wharton's duct
7. Frey's syndrome
8. Sjogren's syndrome

Multiple choice questions

1. Salivary glands are derived from
   (a) Endoderm
   (b) Ectoderm
   (c) Mesoderm
   (d) Mixed origin
2. What is the number of main salivary glands?
   (a) 4
   (b) 8
   (c) 2
   (d) 6
3. Submandibular salivary gland is drained by
   (a) Wharton's duct
   (b) Stensen's duct
   (c) Duct of Wirsung
   (d) Duct of Santorini
4. Parotid gland is drained by
   (a) Stensen's duct
   (b) Wharton's duct
   (c) Duct of Santorini
   (d) Duct of Wirsung

(CONTD...)

SELF-ASSESSMENT *(...CONTD)*

5. What is the relationship of buccal branch of facial nerve with the Stensen's duct?
   (a) Above the duct
   (b) Below the duct
   (c) Superficial to duct
   (d) Deep to duct
6. All of the following features are correct about the Stensen's duct, except
   (a) It runs anteriorly on the surface of masseter
   (b) It lies superior to buccinator
   (c) It passes through buccinator
   (d) It opens inside the cheek opposite the crown of upper second molar
7. Which of the following statements is false about parotid abscess?
   (a) It is due to dry mouth and poor oral hygiene
   (b) The most common causative organism is *Staphylococcus aureus*
   (c) Infection enters the gland usually by bloodstream
   (d) Fluctuation is a late sign
8. Which of the following facts is not true about the viral parotitis?
   (a) It is usually caused by mumps virus
   (b) It commonly occurs in children
   (c) Painless unilateral parotid swelling is its main symptom
   (d) It may lead to testicular atrophy
9. Sialography is defined as
   (a) Plain radiographic visualization of salivary glands
   (b) Visualization of salivary glands by CT scan
   (c) Radiographic visualization of ductal system of a salivary gland by injecting radiographic contrast into its duct
   (d) Imaging of salivary glands by MRI
10. Sialogogue is a drug that
    (a) Stimulates salivary secretion
    (b) Reduces salivary secretion
    (c) Relieves pain of salivary gland inflammation
    (d) Sterilizes infected saliva
11. The commonest tumor of salivary gland is
    (a) Mucoepidermoid carcinoma
    (b) Warthin's tumor
    (c) Pleomorphic adenoma
    (d) Oncocytoma
12. The commonest site of tumor in the parotid is
    (a) Accessory parotid
    (b) Deep lobe
    (c) Neck of gland
    (d) Tail of gland
13. Which of the following facts is not true about pleomorphic adenoma?
    (a) It is the most common salivary tumor
    (b) It accounts for 80% of parotid tumors
    (c) It is always associated with facial nerve palsy
    (d) It recurs if treated by enucleation
14. A pleomorphic adenoma of parotid is treated by
    (a) Enucleation of the tumor
    (b) Superficial parotidectomy
    (c) Total parotidectomy
    (d) Total parotidectomy with block dissection of cervical lymph nodes
15. Which of the following features is not true about Warthin's tumor?
    (a) It is the second common tumor of parotid gland
    (b) It is five times more common in men than in women
    (c) It is a malignant tumor
    (d) It has papillary cystic patterns with a marked lymphatic component
16. Warthin's tumor usually occurs in
    (a) Submandibular salivary gland
    (b) Parotid gland
    (c) Sublingual gland
    (d) Ectopic salivary glands
17. Which one of the following is the commonest malignant tumor of parotid?
    (a) Acinic cell carcinoma
    (b) Adenoid cystic carcinoma
    (c) Mucoepidermoid carcinoma
    (d) Primary squamous cell carcinoma
18. A T2 carcinoma of parotid means
    (a) Tumor up to 2 cm in size
    (b) Tumor 2–4 cm in size
    (c) Tumor 4–6 cm in size
    (d) Tumor more than 6 cm in size

(CONTD...)

SELF-ASSESSMENT *(...CONTD)*

19. The commonest site of a salivary stone is
    (a) Parotid gland
    (b) Wharton's duct
    (c) Sublingual gland
    (d) Stensen's duct
20. The dominant chemical constituent of a salivary stone is
    (a) Organic calcium and sodium phosphate
    (b) Calcium oxalate
    (c) Cholesterol
    (d) Urate
21. Frey's syndrome usually follows
    (a) Drainage of a parotid abscess
    (b) Excision of submandibular salivary gland
    (c) Excision of an ectopic salivary tumor
    (d) Removal of a stone from Wharton's duct
22. Sjogren's syndrome is characterized by all of the following, except
    (a) It is an autoimmune disorder
    (b) The salivary glands are progressively destroyed
    (c) Xerostomia is a classical symptom
    (d) The moisture of conjunctival sac is normal

Answers

1. (b) 2. (d) 3. (a) 4. (a) 5. (b) 6. (b) 7. (c) 8. (c)
9. (c) 10. (a) 11. (c) 12. (d) 13. (c) 14. (b) 15. (c)
16. (b) 17. (c) 18. (b) 19. (b) 20. (b) 21. (a) 22. (d)

Diseases of Pharynx

21

Surgical anatomy

Pharynx is a conical fibromuscular tube forming the upper part of aerodigestive tract having three constrictors—superior, middle, and inferior—in its wall. It is 12–13 cm long and extends from the base of skull to the lower border of cricoid cartilage where it is continuous with esophagus. The pharyngoesophageal junction is 1.5 cm wide and is the narrowest part of digestive tract. Anatomically the pharynx is divided into three parts: nasopharynx, oropharynx, and hypopharynx (laryngopharynx) (Fig. 21.1).

Nasopharynx (Pars Nasalis) It is the uppermost part that extends from the base of skull to the palate. It acts as a conduit of air from nose to oropharynx (and then to larynx). It has Eustachian tubes opening in its lateral wall (Fig. 21.1).

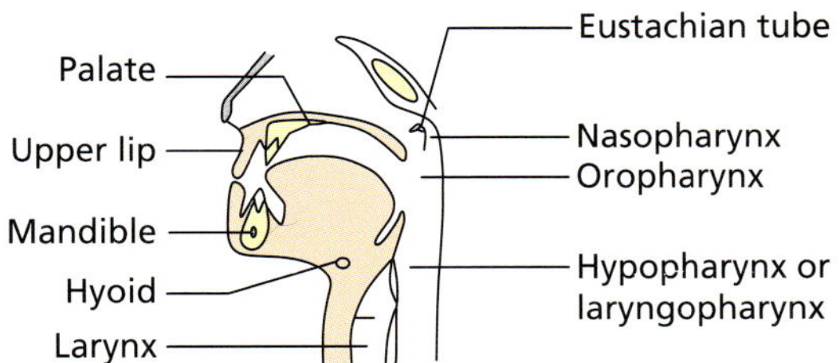

Figure 21.1 Anatomy of pharynx.

Oropharynx It extends from the level of palate above to the lingual surface of closed epiglottis below. Oropharynx acts as a conduit for the passage of air (from back to front) and food (from front to back) and helps in the pharyngeal phase of deglutition. It has Waldeyer's ring in its wall which helps in local defense (Fig. 21.2).

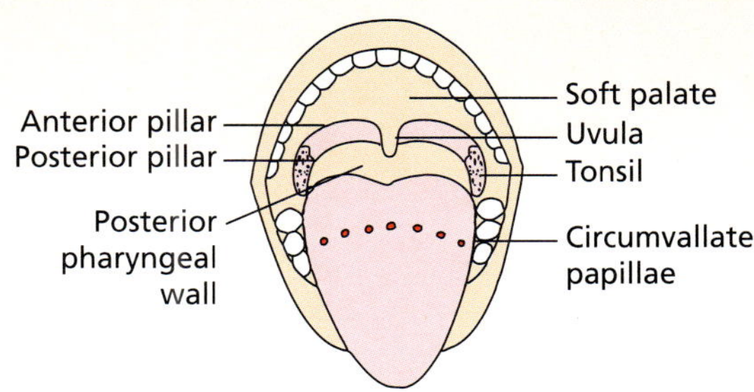

Figure 21.2 Anatomy of oropharynx.

Laryngopharynx (Pars Laryngea) It is the part of pharynx located behind the larynx which opens into its anterior wall. It is alimentary and respiratory in function except below the opening of larynx where it is only alimentary.

1. INFLAMMATIONS AND INFECTIONS

Acute pharyngitis

It is acute inflammation of pharyngeal mucosa caused by a variety of viruses, bacteria, fungi, and *Chlamydia trachomatis*.

Etiology

- Viral pharyngitis is more common. It is caused by a large number of viruses, especially adenoviruses and rhinoviruses.
- Bacterial pharyngitis is caused by group A β-hemolytic *Streptococcus* (GABHS), *Haemophilus influenzae*, *Moraxella catarrhalis*, *Neisseria gonorrhoeae*, and coagulase-positive staphylococci. Acute GABHS infection is important as it may lead to subsequent complications such as rheumatic fever and glomerulonephritis.

Clinical Features

- It is characterized by varying degrees of fever, malaise, pain in the throat (sore throat) and dysphagia (odynophagia), redness, and edema, and may be an occult membrane present in the throat.
- The viral pharyngitis is generally mild and accompanied by rhinorrhea and hoarseness while the bacterial pharyngitis is more severe, except gonococcal which is mild.
- The cervical lymph nodes may be enlarged and tender.
- The symptoms and signs most suggestive of GABHS pharyngitis are described in Box 21.1.

Box 21.1 Clinical features of GABHS pharyngitis

Centor criteria

- Fever over 38°C
- Tender upper cervical lymphadenopathy
- Lack of cough
- Pharyngotonsillar exudate

Investigations

- Blood shows polymorphonuclear leukocytosis in bacterial pharyngitis.
- A single swab throat culture is 90–99% sensitive for GABHS infection. Failure to get bacterial growth is suggestive of viral pathology.

Complications

The infection may spread and may cause retropharyngeal and parapharyngeal abscesses.

Treatment

- Symptomatic treatment includes warm saline gargles, and analgesic and anti-inflammatory agents such as aspirin or acetaminophen. In severe cases, anesthetic gargles and lozenges (e.g., benzocaine) may provide additional relief.
- The antibiotics of choice include penicillin V potassium 250 mg orally three times daily or 500 mg twice daily for 10 days, or cefuroxime axetil 250 mg orally twice daily for 5–10 days. Other effective antibiotics include erythromycin, cefpodoxime, and azithromycin.

Gonococcal Pharyngitis

It occurs following ororeceptive intercourse with an infected person. It is treated with a single dose of intramuscular ceftriaxone or oral cefixime.

Diphtheritic Pharyngitis

- **Etiology**: It is caused by *Corynebacterium diphtheriae*.
- **Clinical features**: The patient presents with low-grade fever, odynophagia, and a gray tonsillar pseudomembrane associated with fetid odor. It bleeds if one tries to remove the membrane. It may spread to larynx producing acute laryngeal obstruction.

- **Diagnosis**: The diagnosis is confirmed by culture of throat swab.
- **Treatment**: It is treated by diphtheria antitoxin (20,000–1,00,000 units) and penicillin 250 mg orally four times daily or erythromycin 500 mg four times daily for 14 days. Removal of membrane by direct laryngoscopy or bronchoscopy may be required to prevent airway obstruction.

Infectious Mononucleosis

- **Etiology**: It occurs in children and young adults and is caused by Epstein–Barr virus.
- **Clinical features**: It is characterized by shaggy, white-purple tonsillar exudate often extending into nasopharynx, a pharyngeal pseudomembrane, laryngeal edema, marked lymphadenopathy, and hepatosplenomegaly.
- **Diagnosis**: A positive heterophile agglutination test or elevated anti-EBV titer is corroborative.
- **Treatment**: The treatment is symptomatic with acetaminophen or other nonsteroidal anti-inflammatory drugs (NSAIDs) and warm saline throat gargles three or four times daily. Acyclovir decreases viral shedding but shows no clinical benefit.

Chronic pharyngitis

It is a comprehensive term which includes many chronic irritative and inflammatory conditions of pharynx characterized by discomfort in the throat.

Etiology

- Persistent infection of tonsils, nose, and sinuses with constant trickling of exudate into pharynx
- Mouth breathing resulting in persistent dryness of pharynx
- Chronic smoking and alcoholism
- Exposure to environmental pollutants such as smoke and dust

Types of Chronic Pharyngitis

Chronic pharyngitis is of three types which are described in Table 21.1.

Diagnosis

The diagnosis is mostly clinical but blood counts and examination of throat swab may be done. Sometimes pharyngoscopy and, may be, biopsy are indicated.

Complications

The complications include persistent speech defect and the spread of infection to the retropharyngeal and parapharyngeal spaces. It may act as a focus of infection for the spread of infection anywhere in the body. It does not predispose for carcinogenesis.

Treatment

- Removal of etiological factors, steam inhalation, and warm saline gargles are effective.

Table 21.1 Types and clinical features of chronic pharyngitis

Type	Symptoms	Appearance of pharyngeal mucosa
Simple chronic pharyngitis	Feeling of dryness, discomfort, and presence of phlegm in the throat	Pharyngeal mucosa is chronically inflamed
Chronic hyperplastic pharyngitis	• The patient feels a compulsion to repeatedly clean the throat and gagging • There is early tiredness of voice	Posterior pharyngeal mucosa is thickened and granular. It may be red or grayish red with venous telangiectasis
Chronic atrophic pharyngitis	• The patient has a continuous desire to clear the throat • May be associated with atrophic rhinitis	Posterior pharyngeal wall is dry and glazed with tough crusts or tenacious secretion

- Mandl's throat paint may be applied locally to provide a protective film for the dry mucosa.
- The lymphoid granules of posterior pharyngeal wall are treated with a chemical or electrocautery.

Acute tonsillitis

It is acute inflammation of tonsils caused by a variety of viruses and bacteria and characterized by pain in the throat, fever, and malaise.

Types of Acute Tonsillitis

Acute tonsillitis is of four types which are described in Table 21.2.

Etiology

The causative organisms include a variety of viruses, for example, influenza A, B, and C, parainfluenza, and adenovirus; and bacteria, for example, GABHS, staphylococci, *H. influenzae*, and pneumococcus.

Clinical Features

- It commonly occurs in children younger than 10 years of age and is characterized by pyrexia, sore throat, odynophagia, referred otalgia, and malaise.
- The tonsils are red, enlarged, and edematous. The tonsillar crypts may be filled with yellowish purulent exudate (follicular tonsillitis), or the tonsils may be covered with a yellowish white membrane (membranous tonsillitis).
- The tongue is coated, and the jugulodigastric lymph nodes may be enlarged and tender.

Investigations

- Blood may have polymorphonuclear leukocytosis.
- Culture of the throat swab is indicated to identify the causative organism and to find its sensitivity to antibiotics.

Complications

The complications of acute tonsillitis include peritonsillar abscess, septicemia, rheumatic fever, and acute glomerulonephritis.

Treatment

- **Symptomatic measures**: These include bed rest, warm saline gargles, analgesics and antipyretics, and antibiotics.
- **Antibiotics**: Penicillin V potassium 250 mg orally three times daily or 500 mg twice daily for 10 days or cefuroxime axetil 250 mg orally twice daily for 5–10 days. Other antibiotics include erythromycin, cefpodoxime, cefuroxime, and azithromycin.

Chronic tonsillitis

It is chronic inflammation of tonsils which may follow recurrent attacks of acute tonsillitis when the tonsils do not return to their normal healthy status.

Etiology A mixed flora of aerobic and anaerobic bacteria usually causes it. *H. influenzae* and GABHS play a major role.

Clinical Features The patient presents with recurrent sore throat and cough may be associated with bad breath (halitosis) and bad taste in

Table 21.2 Types of acute tonsillitis

Type	Clinical features
Acute catarrhal tonsillitis	Superficial inflammation of tonsils usually caused by viral infection
Acute follicular tonsillitis	White or yellow exudate at the mouth of crypts
Acute parenchymatous tonsillitis	Acute inflammation involving the whole tonsils
Acute membranous tonsillitis	Formation of a dirty white membrane of exudates on the medial surface of tonsils

Table 21.3 Types of chronic tonsillitis

Type of chronic tonsillitis	Characteristics
Chronic follicular tonsillitis	Debris or cheesy material present at the opening of crypts
Chronic hypertrophic (parenchymatous) tonsillitis	Gross enlargement of tonsils due to lymphoid hyperplasia
Chronic fibrotic tonsillitis	Small and fibrotic tonsils

mouth. It may be associated with upper cervical lymphadenopathy. It is of three clinicopathological types as described in Table 21.3.

Diagnosis The diagnosis is mostly clinical but blood counts and examination of throat swab taken from tonsils may be done. Fine needle aspirate of tonsils may be cultured.

Complications Include persistent throat discomfort especially during speaking, local spread of infection, and chronic halitosis (a social problems). It has nothing to do with carcinogenesis.

Treatment

- It includes warm saline gargles and intermittent courses of antibiotics depending on the culture and sensitivity report. Tonsillectomy is done if there are four to six documented episodes of acute tonsillitis per year, three to four attacks in each of the preceding 2 years, or three attacks in each of the preceding 3 years.

Peritonsillar abscess (quinsy)

It is the collection of pus around the tonsil.

Etiology When the infection from tonsillitis penetrates the tonsillar capsule and involves the surrounding tissue, it results in peritonsillar cellulitis and abscess. The pus collects beyond the tonsillar tissue into the space between the anterior and posterior tonsillar pillars and the soft palate. The pus formation in this space is frequently associated with *Streptococcus pyogenes* infection.

Clinical Features

- The patient presents with fever, severe sore throat, odynophagia, and malaise. The mouth remains open with saliva dribbling all the time.
- The patient talks as if there is a hot potato in the mouth ("hot potato voice"). The anterior tonsillar pillar is edematous and bulging.

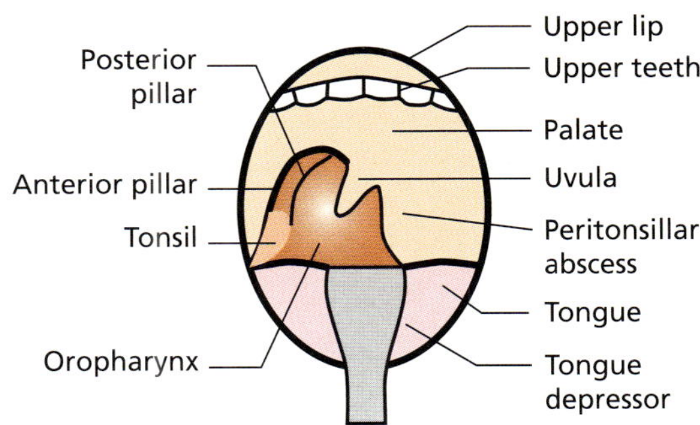

Figure 21.3 Left peritonsillar abscess.

- The soft palate and uvula are displaced medially or to the opposite side (Fig. 21.3).

Diagnosis The diagnosis can be confirmed by aspirating pus from the peritonsillar swelling just superior and medial to the upper pole of the tonsil.

Complications The complications of peritonsillar abscess include local spread of infection with submandibular cellulitis, edema of larynx, bacteremia, toxemia, and pyemia.

Treatment

- The patient is given a dose of parenteral amoxicillin (1 g), amoxicillin–sulbactam (3 g), or clindamycin (600–900 mg).
- The pus is aspirated with a 19-gauge or 21-gauge needle passed medial to upper last molar not deeper than 1 cm as the internal carotid artery may be situated more medially than its normal site and pass posterior and deep to the tonsillar fossa.
- Less severe disease is treated for 7–10 days with oral antibiotics including amoxicillin 500 mg three times a day, amoxicillin–clavulanate 875 mg twice daily, or clindamycin 300 mg four times daily.
- Drainage: The pus may be removed by an incision through the anterior tonsillar pillar.

- Tonsillectomy: To drain the pus and to prevent recurrence, it may be appropriate to do immediate tonsillectomy (quinsy tonsillectomy). Other advantages of this approach are quick relief, greater technical simplicity, lesser bleeding, and shorter hospital stay.

Adenoid hyperplasia (hypertrophy)

Anatomy of Adenoids The nasopharyngeal tonsils (adenoids) are situated at the posterior wall and roof of nasopharynx. They consist of lymphoid tissue which is covered by ciliated columnar epithelium. They are normally present at birth and enlarge up to the age of 6 years. Then they start regressing and disappear by about 12 years of age. Sometimes residual adenoids may be seen even in adults.

Etiology Adenoid hyperplasia usually follows recurrent attacks of rhinitis and tonsillitis.

Clinical Features

- Adenoid hyperplasia usually occurs in children and presents with upper airway (nasopharyngeal) obstruction, nasal discharge, recurrent pain in the ear with diminished hearing, ear discharge, and toneless speech that loses the nasal tinge.
- In chronic cases, due to mouth breathing the face has a dull expression with open mouth and depressed cheeks (adenoid facies). The nasal alae become pinched and indrawn. The palate is usually high arched. During sleep, these patients may experience episodes of hypopnea and periods of cessation of naso-oral airflow for longer than 10 seconds, persistent chest wall movement, and subsequent hypoxia and hypercapnia.
- The obstructive sleep apnea syndrome is characterized by frequent arousals during sleep and also some signs such as weight loss, behavioral changes, learning disabilities, daytime somnolence, and enuresis.

Investigations

- X-ray of the face, lateral view, shows the soft-tissue shadow of enlarged adenoids (Fig. 21.4).

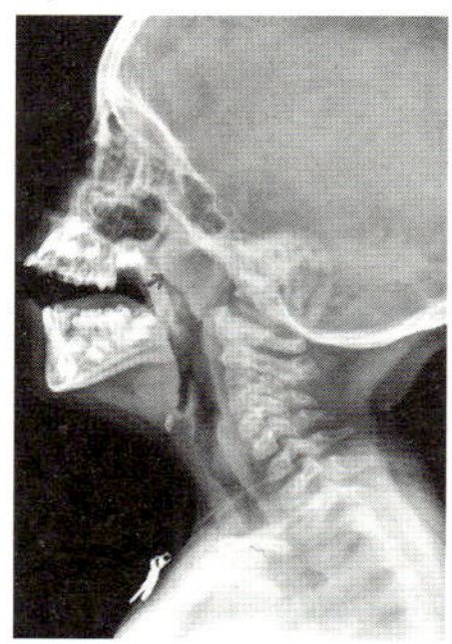

Figure 21.4 Lateral view of head and face showing soft-tissue shadow of enlarged adenoids. (Courtesy: Dr. S.S. Sarkar, Sarkar Diagnostics)

- The nasopharyngoscopy shows the lesion.

Complications These include nasopharyngeal obstruction, Eustachian tube obstruction, and hearing problems.

Treatment

- It is treated with hot saline gargles, oral antihistaminics and decongestants, and intermittent courses of antibiotics.
- When the nasopharyngeal obstruction is marked and is not relieved by the above-mentioned measures, adenoidectomy (with tonsillectomy) is indicated.

Isolated Adenoid Hypertrophy

Rarely isolated adenoid hypertrophy occurs. It is secondary to physiological enlargement of adenoids or chronic viral nasopharyngitis. It is treated by adenoidectomy.

Tonsillectomy

The excision of tonsils is one of the commonest operations done by an ENT surgeon.

Indications

Complete removal of tonsils is preferred to wedge biopsy when the squamous cell carcinoma is a possibility. In lymphoma, tonsils are removed for staging of disease. The tonsils are removed under general anesthesia by dissection method. The indications of tonsillectomy are described in Box 21.2.

Box 21.2 Indications of tonsillectomy

- **Absolute indications**
  - Sleep apnea, chronic upper respiratory obstruction, cor pulmonale due to tonsillar disease
  - Tonsillar tumors
- **Relative indications**
  - Recurrent acute tonsillitis
  - Chronic tonsillitis
  - Peritonsillar abscess
  - Tonsillitis causing febrile convulsions
  - Diphtheria carriers
  - Systemic disease caused by group A β-hemolytic *Streptococcus*

Surgical technique

The patient lies supine with neck extended. The mouth is opened fully and kept open with a Boyle–Davis mouth gag. The tonsil is grasped at the upper pole with tonsil-holding forceps and removed by dissection. All the bleeding points are controlled by pressure, coagulation, and ligation.

Complications of tonsillectomy

Complications of tonsillectomy are due to anesthesia and operation and they are described in Box 21.3. Hemorrhage is the most common immediate postoperative complication but it is rare.

Box 21.3 Complications of tonsillectomy

- **Complications due to anesthesia**
  - Traumatic intubation
  - Cardiopulmonary arrest
  - Malignant hyperthermia
- **Complications due to surgery**
  - Hemorrhage
  - Infection
  - Pain, otalgia
  - Airway obstruction
  - Velopharyngeal incompetence

Parapharyngeal abscess

It is the collection of pus in the parapharyngeal space due to extension of infection from the tonsils.

Surgical Anatomy of Parapharyngeal Space

It is a cone-shaped space situated below the base of skull and lateral to the pharynx. It is bounded above by petrous portion of temporal bone, medially by superior constrictor covered by buccopharyngeal fascia, laterally by pterygoid muscles and mandible, anteriorly by pterygomandibular raphe, posteriorly by apposition of buccopharyngeal and prevertebral fasciae, and inferiorly it extends up to hyoid bone. The styloid process divides the parapharyngeal space into anterior and posterior compartments.

Etiology

Infection in this space comes from peritonsillar abscess, deep parotid abscess, infected third molar root, penetrating injuries, and petrositis.

Clinical Features

The patient is usually a child who presents with local pain, fever, chills, odynophagia, and significant general malaise of acute onset. The signs of involvement of posterior compartment are bulge of lateral pharyngeal wall behind the posterior pillar, paralysis of last four cranial nerves and sympathetic chain, and swelling in the parotid region.

Parapharyngeal abscess has to be differentiated from a peritonsillar abscess as described in Table 21.4.

Diagnosis

The abscess can be imaged by ultrasonography, CT scan, or MRI.

Table 21.4 Differences between parapharyngeal abscess and peritonsillar abscess

Features	Parapharyngeal abscess	Peritonsillar abscess
External swelling	Swelling behind the angle of mandible or swelling in parotid region	No external swelling
Internal swelling	Tonsil pushed medially in anterior compartment abscess, and the lateral pharyngeal wall behind posterior pillar is pushed medially in posterior compartment abscess	Swelling of tonsil anterior to posterior tonsillar pillar
Edema of soft palate	Minimal	Marked
Uvula	In midline	Deviated to opposite side

Complications

Complications include edema of larynx and acute laryngeal obstruction, jugular vein thrombophlebitis, spread of infection into other neck spaces, and carotid artery erosion.

Treatment

An early abscess may subside with intravenous antibiotics including metronidazole. A late abscess which is pointing into oropharynx is drained into pharynx with a blunt instrument or with a gloved finger. It is done under general anesthesia given by an expert anesthetist with good illumination and arrangement for prompt suction of pus from the pharynx.

Retropharyngeal abscess

It is collection of pus in the retropharyngeal space between the posterior wall of pharynx and the vertebral column (Fig. 21.5).

Surgical Anatomy

There are two fascial spaces behind the pharynx, one anterior space between the buccopharyngeal fascia covering the posterior wall of pharynx and the prevertebral fascia covering the cervical vertebral column. It extends from base of skull up to bifurcation of trachea. A fibrous raphe in the midline divides it into two lateral compartments containing retropharyngeal lymph nodes. The other is prevertebral space that is bounded anteriorly by prevertebral fascia and posteriorly by vertebral bodies. It extends from the base of skull to the coccyx.

Acute Retropharyngeal Abscess

Etiology It occurs following pyogenic infection of retropharyngeal lymph nodes. These nodes are present in the infants younger than 3 years of age. Then they atrophy with age. Infection into these nodes spreads from tonsils, nasopharynx, oropharynx, and paranasal sinuses.

Clinical Features

- It is most commonly seen in children younger than 1 year of age and characterized by severe malaise, neck rigidity, dysphagia, drooling, croupy cough, altered cry, and marked dyspnea which may be the most prominent symptom. It may be associated with febrile convulsions and vomiting. On examination, the

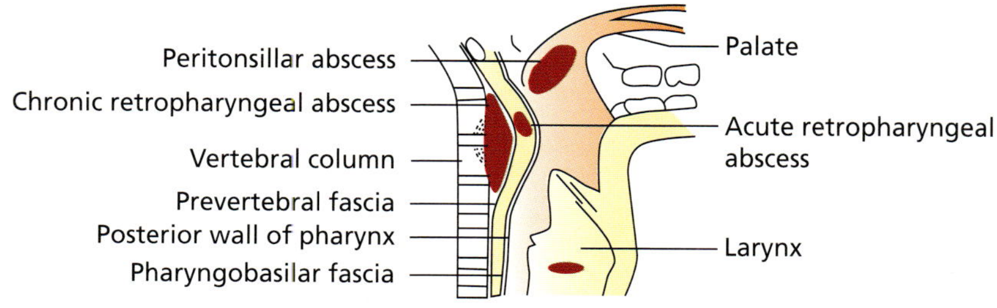

Figure 21.5 Anatomy of retropharyngeal abscesses.

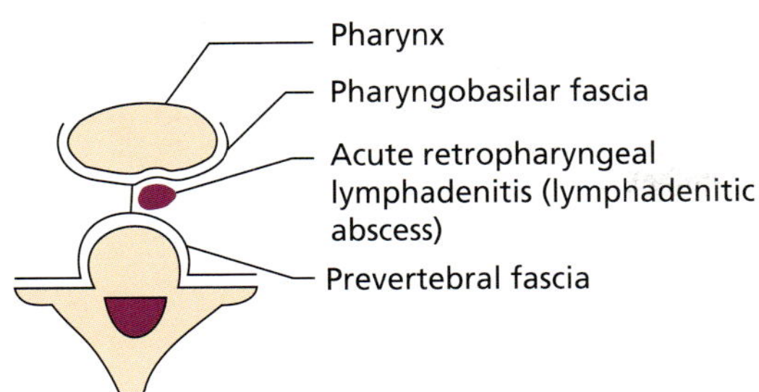

Figure 21.6 Anatomy of acute retropharyngeal abscess.

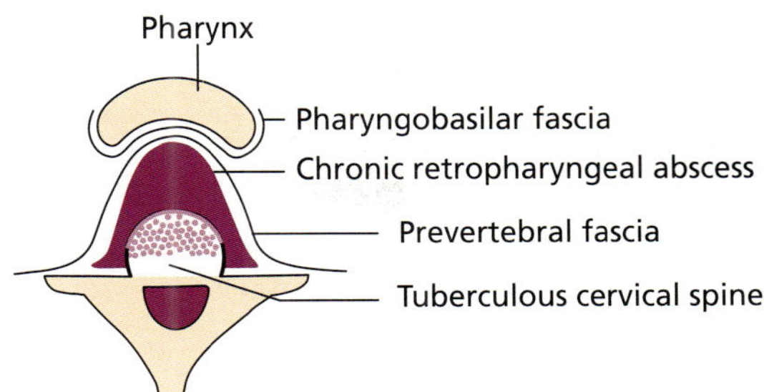

Figure 21.7 Anatomy of chronic retropharyngeal abscess.

posterior wall of pharynx is red and swollen usually on one side of midline (Fig. 21.6). The abscess may be pointing out on the thinned mucosa.

- Sometimes a foreign body such as a fish bone may perforate the posterior wall of pharynx and produce an abscess. This type of abscess occurs in older children and young adults.

Investigations Radiograph of the neck, lateral view, reveals widening of retropharyngeal soft-tissue shadow. At the level of C2, the widening is greater than 7 mm. CT scan delineates the lesion exactly.

Complications The complications of acute retropharyngeal abscess include pharyngeal obstruction, odynophagia, spread of infection, and rupture with aspiration of pus into larynx.

Treatment The treatment is started with intravenous antibiotics. An early lesion may resolve with this treatment. If it does not, it is drained in head-down position by thrusting a pair of dressing forceps guided by a finger into the abscess and the pus is sucked out quickly at the same time. Airway obstruction may require management.

Chronic Retropharyngeal Abscess (Prevertebral Abscess)

Etiology It is a collection of pus behind prevertebral fascia and in front of vertebral column (Fig. 21.7) that is usually due to tuberculosis of upper cervical spine (caries spine).

Clinical Features The patient is usually a young adult who has a swelling in the posterior wall of pharynx of insidious onset. It is soft, cystic, and nontender in the center. There may be pain in the neck with restricted mobility of cervical spine. In addition, there may be fullness behind the sternomastoid muscle on one side.

Investigations X-ray of cervical spine shows bone destruction and loss of normal curvature of spine. The spine may be unstable. Hence, excess manipulation may lead to serious neurological complications. MRI shows better details of the disease (Fig. 21.8). Pus may be aspirated and examined bacteriologically.

Treatment It is treated with antituberculous drugs. The abscess may require evacuation which is done by a neck incision. It is not evacuated through the mouth for fear of secondary infection.

The differences between acute and chronic retropharyngeal abscesses are described in Table 21.5.

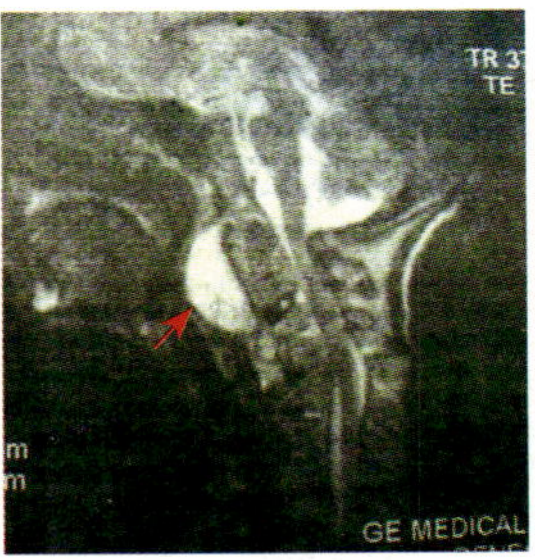

Figure 21.8 Sagittal MRI of upper neck and lower face showing a retropharyngeal abscess due to tuberculosis of upper cervical spine.

Table 21.5 Differences between acute and chronic retropharyngeal abscesses

Features	Acute retropharyngeal abscess	Chronic retropharyngeal abscess
Definition	Accumulation of pus behind the pharynx in front of prevertebral fascia	Accumulation of pus behind the pharynx behind prevertebral fascia
Etiology	Acute pyogenic infection of retropharyngeal lymph nodes	Tuberculosis of upper cervical vertebral column
Site of swelling	Posterior pharyngeal wall by the side of midline	Posterior pharyngeal wall in midline
Clinical features	• Child younger than 1 year of age with malaise, neck rigidity, dysphagia, drooling, croupy cough, altered cry, and marked dyspnea • Swelling in posterior wall of oropharynx by the side of midline. Pus may point out on thinned mucosa	• Young adult with low-grade fever, neck pain, and restricted mobility • Swelling in center of posterior wall of pharynx which is soft, cystic, and nontender • Signs of tuberculosis of upper cervical vertebral column present
Investigations	Blood shows polymorphonuclear leukocytosis	• Blood shows lymphocytosis and raised ESR • X-ray or MRI of cervical spine shows tuberculosis of upper cervical vertebrae
Treatment	• Intravenous antibiotics—an early lesion may resolve • Drainage per orally in head-down position with a dressing forceps guided by a finger	• Antituberculous drugs • Evacuation of pus by a neck incision

ESR, erythrocyte sedimentation rate.

2. TUMORS

Juvenile angiofibroma (nasopharyngeal angiofibroma)

It is the most common benign tumor of nasopharynx seen in adolescents having immature fibroblasts and thin-walled blood vessels and characterized by profuse epistaxis and nasal obstruction.

Etiology

It is not known. It is a hormone-dependent tumor which is stimulated by testosterone, and its in vitro growth is inhibited by antiandrogens such as cyproterone and flutamide.

Pathology

- It is a rounded globular tumor arising from a peduncle or a broad base which is attached to the lateral wall of nasopharynx. It is deep red or varied pinkish gray in color. The consistency is usually spongy or rubbery.
- Microscopically it consists of connective tissue stroma containing immature fibroblasts and thin-walled blood vessels having a single layer of endothelium.
- It is a locally invasive tumor that does not have a capsule and does not produce metastases. It spreads locally with finger-like projections into nasal cavity, paranasal sinuses, infratemporal and pterygopalatine fossae, orbit, and skull.

Clinical Features

The patient is usually an adolescent male (10–20 years) who presents with profuse epistaxis and nasal obstruction. Other symptoms include rhinorrhea, hyponasality of speech, otalgia, and facial swelling (Fig. 21.9).

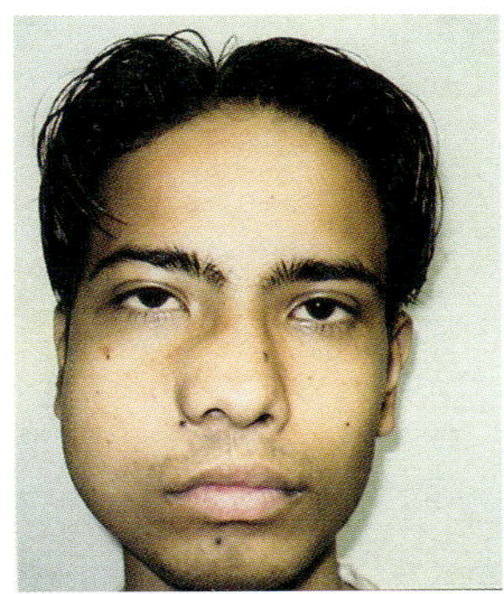

Figure 21.9 Angiofibroma of right nasopharynx extending into ethmoid and sphenoid causing swelling of right cheek. (Courtesy: Professor Surajit Bhattacharya)

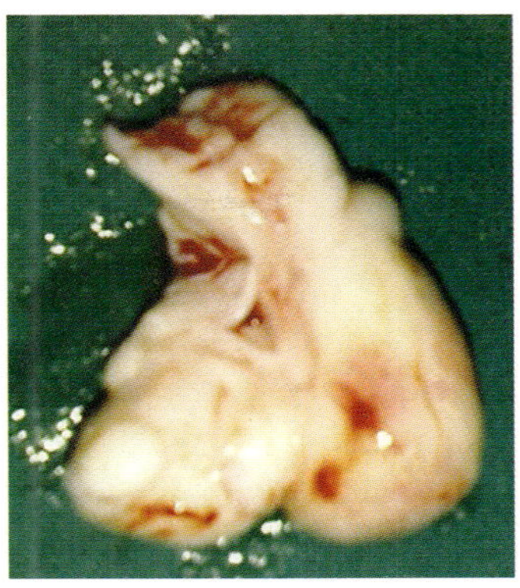

Figure 21.11 Excised nasopharyngeal angiofibroma. (Courtesy: Professor S.P. Agarwal)

Investigations

- Radiography of paranasal sinuses, lateral view and Water's view, may show the soft-tissue shadow and bony erosion.
- X-ray of base of skull should also be done to see local extension.
- CT scan shows the extent of tumor (Fig. 21.10).
- Carotid angiography reveals the vascularity of the tumor.
- Biopsy as a rule should not be done as it may cause profuse uncontrollable bleeding.

Treatment

- Preoperative arterial embolization of the tumor and estrogen therapy reduces the blood supply of the tumor and then it can be surgically removed (Fig. 21.11).
- A tumor confined to nasopharynx can be removed by transpalatal approach.
- Large tumors extending into nasal cavity, maxillary sinus, ethmoid, or sphenoidal sinus are excised by lateral rhinotomy and transpalatal or Caldwell-Luc approach or both.
- Radiotherapy can be given as it is a moderately radio-responsive tumor. A dose of 3000–5000 rad if given preoperatively reduces its vascularity.

Carcinoma of nasopharynx

It is not a common cancer, but it is more prevalent in China and Southeast Asia with an incidence of

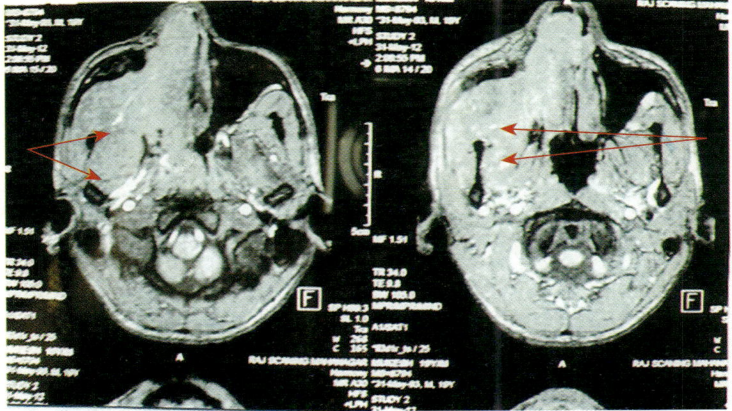

Figure 21.10 Axial CT scan showing nasopharyngeal angiofibroma extending into maxilla, ethmoid, and sphenoid. (Courtesy: Professor Surajit Bhattacharya)

about 18% of all tumors. In India, it constitutes about 0.5% of all cancers and has a high incidence in northeastern states probably due to their Mongoloid origin.

Etiology

- It is not exactly known. The people of Mongoloid origin are more susceptible to this cancer.
- A genetically determined susceptibility allows the Epstein–Barr virus infection in early life. This tumor is associated with elevated IgA antibody to the viral capsid antigen to this virus.
- Environmental factors such as ingestion of salted fish, smoke from burning incense, and raw tobacco may contribute to its etiology.

Pathology

About 85% of tumors are squamous cell carcinomas. Less common cancers include lymphoepithelioma, adenocarcinoma, mucosal melanoma, sarcoma, and non-Hodgkin lymphoma. The tumor is usually poorly differentiated and may have significant lymphoid infiltration when it is known as lymphoepithelioma.

Modes of Spread

- Local spread occurs into the nasal cavity, Eustachian tube, orbit, parapharyngeal space, and cranium.
- The lymphatic spread occurs into upper jugular and posterior triangle lymph nodes.
- Hematogenous spread is rare and involves lungs, liver, and bones.

Clinical Features

Most of the tumors arise from the fossa of Rosenmuller, other sites of occurrence being roof and posterior wall. It is most commonly seen in the fifth to seventh decades of life with a male/female ratio 3:1, initially with nonspecific symptoms mimicking those of rhinitis or sinusitis. The symptoms and signs are classified into four groups and described in Table 21.6.

Any adult with persistent unilateral nasal symptoms or otitis media of recent onset should be thoroughly evaluated for this tumor with nasal endoscopy and nasopharyngoscopy.

Investigations

Rhinoscopy Anterior rhinoscopy shows a red and friable mass in nasopharynx which bleeds on touch. Posterior rhinoscopy also shows the lesion. The palate may be pushed downwards and forwards.

Radiography Radiography of face and lateral view of skull may show the soft-tissue shadow of the tumor and local bony erosion.

Biopsy It is done with a needle forceps introduced through the nose while the nasopharynx is seen by a mirror inserted through the mouth, aided by a Jacques catheter for putting traction on palate.

Table 21.6 Signs and symptoms of carcinoma of nasopharynx

Symptomatic group	Description of symptoms
Nasal symptoms	• Slight intermittent epistaxis with small clots • Nasal speech • Nasal obstruction • Profuse mucoid or mucopurulent discharge
Aural symptoms	• Unilateral deafness with pain in the ear • Otitis media due to Eustachian tube obstruction
Cervical lymphadenopathy	• May be the first clinical manifestation of this disease • Present in 60–70% of patients
Cranial nerve involvement	• Pain in trigeminal nerve distribution • Present in 38% of patients due to intracranial spread of this tumor

CT Scan/MRI They are done to see the extent of tumor. MRI is the best imaging method to delineate the extent of the disease and plan appropriate surgery and radiation.

T Staging

The T staging of carcinoma of nasopharynx is given as follows:

- **Tis**: Carcinoma is present in situ.
- **T1**: Tumor confined to one site or no tumor is visible but random biopsy is positive.
- **T2**: Tumor involves two sites (posterosuperior and lateral walls).
- **T3**: Tumor has extended to oropharynx or nasal cavity.
- **T4**: There is involvement of skull or cranial nerve/nerves.

Treatment

- Early disease is treated with megavoltage radiotherapy, 200 rad/day for 5 days a week with a total dose of 6000–7000 rad.
- Advanced disease is treated with concurrent radiation and cisplatin followed by adjuvant chemotherapy with cisplatin and 5-fluorouracil.
- Locally recurrent disease is treated with repeat irradiation or surgery.

Prognosis

In early disease, the 3-year survival rates are more than 75%, and in advanced disease they are 30–50%.

Tumors of tonsil

Many types of tumors are known to affect tonsils, but the common tumors are carcinoma and lymphoma (NHL type).

- **Clinical features**: The patient presents with a unilateral tonsillar lesion. The carcinoma presents as an ulcerated hard lesion, while the lymphoma presents with a firm painless mass.
- **Diagnosis**: The diagnosis is confirmed by biopsy. The extent of the lesion is determined by CT scan or MRI.
- **Treatment**: Early carcinoma is treated with radiotherapy, and late carcinoma with chemoradiation. The neck nodes are treated with radiotherapy or removed by block dissection. The lymphoma is first staged and then treated with radiotherapy and chemotherapy.
- **Prognosis**: Prognosis of malignant tumors of the tonsil is bad with poor 5-year survivals.

Carcinoma of oropharynx

Anatomy of Oropharynx The oropharynx extends from the palate above to the apex of epiglottis below. It includes soft palate, tonsils, tonsillar pillars, posterior pharyngeal wall, posterior one-third of tongue, and lingual surface of epiglottis. It is lined by stratified squamous epithelium.

Etiology Excessive and long-term use of tobacco and alcohol is related etiologically to this cancer.

Pathology The squamous cell carcinoma is the most common type which is not as well differentiated as oral carcinoma. Deep infiltration is common. Other cancers include adenoid cystic carcinoma, adenocarcinoma, lymphoepithelioma, and lymphoma (NHL type).

Mode of Spread This cancer spreads by lymphatic route and local infiltration.

- The posterior wall cancers drain bilaterally to jugular chain nodes (levels II, III, and IV) and retropharyngeal nodes of Ranvier.
- The cancers of tonsillar region drain primarily to upper and midjugular chain of lymph nodes and to submandibular nodes (levels I, II, and III).
- The nodes in the posterior triangle become involved following involvement of jugular chain nodes.

- The overall incidence of lymph node involvement is about 70%. Bilateral lymph node metastases occur in 50% of cases.
- Local spread: Carcinoma of pharyngeal tongue may spread laterally to involve the mandible, anteriorly to involve the oral tongue, and inferiorly to involve the vallecula and supraglottic larynx. Carcinoma of the tonsillar region readily extends into the mandible. It may infiltrate the pterygoid muscles producing trismus.

Clinical Features

- This cancer occurs commonly in middle-aged and elderly people, more commonly males.
- It is usually symptomless in the beginning, and the symptoms occur as the disease advances.
- It is characterized by persistent sore throat which may be accompanied by persistent otalgia. The patient may present with enlarged neck nodes. Other symptoms include a vague sensation of throat irritation, restriction of tongue motion ("hot potato voice"), odynophagia, and bleeding. The tumor may be visible and/or palpable on oropharyngeal examination.

Investigations The diagnosis is confirmed by endoscopy and biopsy. CT scan or MRI may be done to determine the extent of the disease.

Staging of Disease

- **T1**: Tumor up to 2 cm in the greatest dimension
- **T2**: Tumor 2–4 cm in the greatest dimension
- **T3**: Tumor more than 4 cm in the greatest dimension
- **T4**: Invasion of the tumor in adjacent structures, for example, cortical bone, deep muscles of tongue, larynx, maxillary sinus, and skin

Treatment

- T1 and T2 tumors can be treated with surgery or radiotherapy with similar results. In this stage, the tumor is diagnosed less commonly.
- T3 and T4 tumors are treated by a combination of radiotherapy and surgery. It may be combined with chemotherapy (5-FU and cisplatin). The operative defects are repaired with skin grafts, pedicled myocutaneous flaps, or free flaps.

Prognosis Five-year survival rates of this tumor are: stage I, 80–90%; stage II, 65–75%; stage III, 40–50%; and stage IV, 30%.

Carcinoma of hypopharynx

Surgical Anatomy of Hypopharynx

The hypopharynx extends from apex of epiglottis above to lower border of cricoid below. It includes pyriform sinuses situated lateral to larynx, postcricoid region lying immediately behind larynx, posterior pharyngeal wall, and the marginal area where the medial wall of pyriform sinus and the false vocal cords meet superiorly at aryepiglottic fold. It is lined by stratified squamous epithelium.

Etiology

The exact cause of this cancer is not known but it is etiologically related to excessive consumption of tobacco and alcohol. Postcricoid carcinoma commonly occurs in women suffering with Plummer–Vinson syndrome.

Pathology

More than 95% of hypopharyngeal cancers are squamous cell carcinoma which is an infiltrating ulcerative lesion. The incidence of poorly differentiated cancers is higher here than in other regions. The common sites of occurrence of this cancer are pyriform sinus and postcricoid region.

Clinical Features

In early disease, there are no symptoms and signs. Hence, the patient presents late with nonspecific symptoms with discomfort, difficulty in swallowing, huskiness of voice, halitosis, and blood-tinged sputum. The patient may present with cervical lymph node metastasis which may be the first symptom.

T Staging

- **T1**: Tumor is limited to one subsite of hypopharynx.
- **T2**: Tumor involves more than one subsite or an adjacent site without fixation of hemilarynx.
- **T3**: Tumor involves more than one subsite or an adjacent site with fixation of hemilarynx.
- **T4**: Tumor invades adjacent structures, for example, cartilages of larynx or soft tissues of neck.

Carcinoma of Pyriform Sinus of Hypopharynx

The carcinoma of pyriform sinus constitutes about 60% of all hypopharyngeal tumors. It is commonly seen in patients 40–60 years of age with a male:female ratio of 8:1.

- **Mode of spread**: This area has a rich lymphatic supply; hence, these tumors have a 75% incidence of regional lymphatic metastases to deep jugular cervical lymph nodes (levels II, III, and IV). Local spread may occur into the ala of thyroid cartilage. Distant spread occurs to liver, lung, and bones in 25% of cases usually after 12–24 months.
- **Clinical features**: Because of poor sensory supply, pain is not an important symptom. Hence, the patient presents late. More than 40% of patients present with lymph node metastases. Subsequently the patient may present with pricking sensation on swallowing liquids, dysphagia, referred otalgia, hoarseness of voice, difficulty in breathing, fetid smell from mouth, and blood-tinged sputum. The cervical lymph nodes may be palpable between mastoid and angle of mandible.
- **Investigations**: Endoscopy may show an ulcerative or proliferative lesion which must be biopsied at the same time. The earliest sign is pooling of saliva in pyriform fossa.

Carcinoma of Postcricoid Area of Hypopharynx

This cancer occurs at pharyngoesophageal junction and constitutes about 30% of all laryngopharyngeal malignancies.

- **Etiology**: It is etiologically related to Plummer–Vinson syndrome. Hence, it is preventable by timely treatment of this syndrome.
- **Mode of spread**: It is usually an ulcerative lesion and infiltrates the local tissues causing obstruction of esophageal inlet, and may involve paratracheal lymph nodes. Later on, neck nodes of both sides are involved.
- **Clinical features of carcinoma of hypopharynx**: The patient presents with progressive dysphagia leading to malnutrition and weight loss. Other symptoms include referred otalgia, hoarseness of voice, and absence of laryngeal crepitus.
- **Investigations**: Laryngoscopy reveals pooling of saliva in pyriform sinus and sometimes a tumor or widening of postcricoid space. Blood shows iron deficiency anemia. Barium swallow shows holdup of barium at esophageal inlet. Endoscopic biopsy confirms the diagnosis.

Treatment of Carcinoma of Hypopharynx

It is treated by total laryngopharyngectomy with gastric pull-up for reconstruction of food passage. An early lesion can be treated by radiotherapy.

Prognosis

Overall prognosis of carcinoma of hypopharynx is poor because of its site and late diagnosis.

3. OTHER DISEASES OF THE PHARYNX

Foreign bodies in pharynx

Types of Foreign Bodies A variety of foreign bodies may be lodged in pharynx. They may be irregular or regular in shape.

- Irregular foreign bodies are likely to be lodged in vallecula or pyriform sinuses.
- Regular or smooth foreign bodies are commonly lodged at pharyngoesophageal junction, especially in children.

Clinical Features The patient presents with dysphagia, odynophagia, or aphagia. In a young child or infant, drooling is a characteristic sign. Dyspnea, wheezing, or persistent cough may occur due to obstruction of larynx. If the food passage is penetrated by a sharp foreign body such as a pin or fish bone, subcutaneous emphysema and later cellulitis of neck occurs.

Investigations

- Radiography of neck reveals radio-opaque foreign bodies.
- Barium swallow may be required to image radiolucent foreign bodies.

Treatment

- Oropharyngeal foreign bodies can be removed with a curved hemostat.
- Hypopharyngeal foreign bodies can be removed endoscopically under general anesthesia.

Pharyngeal pouch or Zenker's diverticulum

It is the protrusion of pharyngeal mucosa through the Killian's dehiscence which is a weak area in the posterior wall of pharynx between the oblique fibers of thyropharyngeus and the transverse fibers of cricopharyngeus at the lower end of inferior constrictor of pharynx (Fig. 21.12). It is a pulsion diverticulum that results from transient incomplete opening of pharyngoesophageal junction or upper esophageal sphincter.

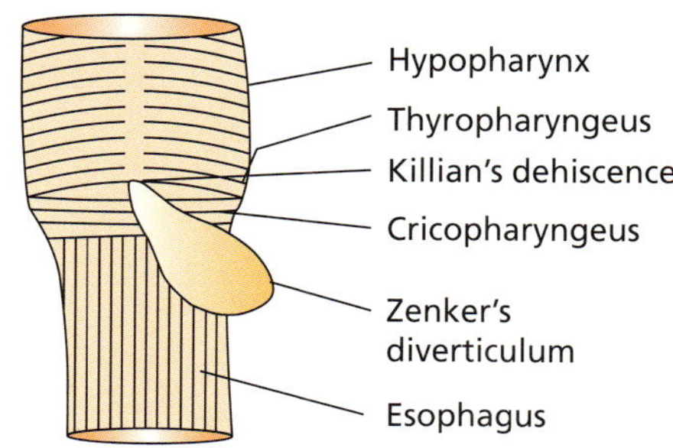

Figure 21.12 Anatomy of pharyngeal pouch (Zenker's diverticulum).

Stages of Pharyngeal Diverticulum

- **Stage 1**: Small diverticulum pointing toward the vertebral column. It is asymptomatic and incidentally diagnosed by barium meal.
- **Stage 2**: Large globular diverticulum with vertical mouth. It causes regurgitation, violent cough, dysphagia, and repeated respiratory infection.
- **Stage 3**: Large globular diverticulum which has gone down because of weight of contents. Its mouth is horizontal. It presents with dysphagia.

The stages of pharyngeal diverticulum are described in Figure 21.13.

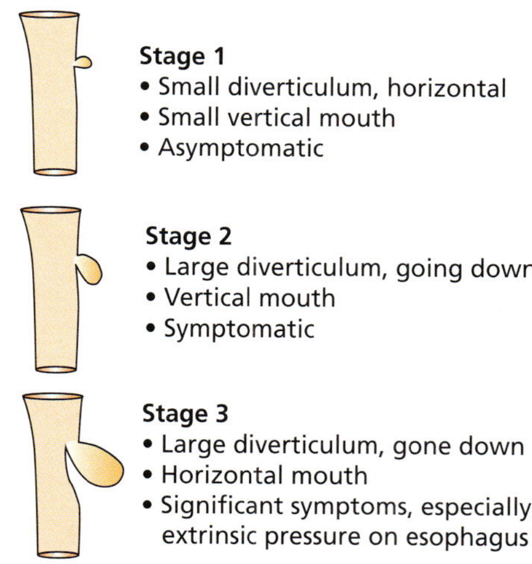

Figure 21.13 Stages of a pharyngeal diverticulum.

Clinical Features

- It usually occurs after 60 years of age and is twice more common in men than in women.
- Initially it is asymptomatic when it may be discovered during radiographic examination of pharynx.
- In the early phase of disease, the patient complains of something in throat (globus) or slight regurgitation on swallowing.
- As the disease advances, there is regurgitation of undigested food sometimes hours after a meal, especially when the patient bends down or turns over in bed at night. The patient may wake up at night with a feeling of tightness in the throat and a bout of coughing.
- As the diverticulum enlarges, there may be gurgling noise in the neck during meals and it may be visible as a swelling. The swelling may increase when the patient drinks or takes some food. It may cause dysphagia.
- There is a soft swelling in the neck usually on its left side. If it is pressed, there is gurgling noise and regurgitation of food or frothy saliva in the mouth.

Investigations

Radiography

- Plain X-ray of neck may show a gas shadow and fluid level in the neck.
- Barium swallow shows the pouch.
- The videofluoroscopic study reveals pharyngeal contraction waves and the integrity of upper esophageal sphincter.

Endoscopy It must not be done as it may perforate the diverticulum.

Complications

They include diverticulitis, peridiverticulitis, peridiverticular abscess (Fig. 21.14), cellulitis of neck, mediastinal spread of infection, and fistula.

Treatment

- An asymptomatic diverticulum does not need any treatment.
- A symptomatic diverticulum is excised (diverticulectomy) by an oblique left cervical incision parallel to anterior border of sternomastoid or transverse incision centered over cricoid. Before closing the wound, cervical esophagomyotomy is done. The complications of operation include wound infection, mediastinitis, pharyngeal fistula, and stenosis of upper esophagus.
- Dohlman's or Steiffert's procedure: Endoscopic division of septum by diathermy and stapling of the partition wall between esophagus and pouch is the recent method of treatment of a pharyngeal diverticulum.

Dysphagia

Dysphagia is a symptom characterized by difficulty in swallowing. It is mostly caused by some type of obstruction of upper food passage. It

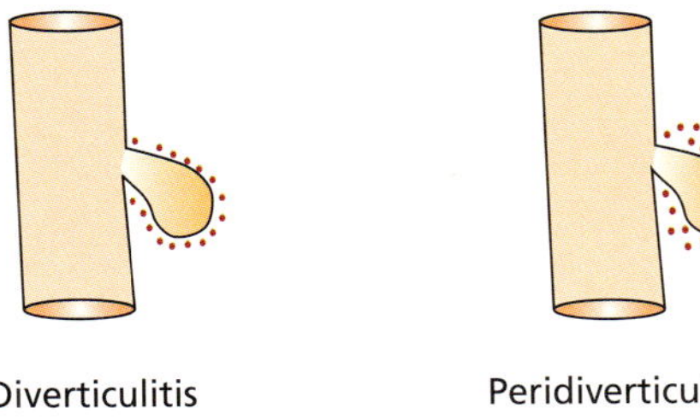

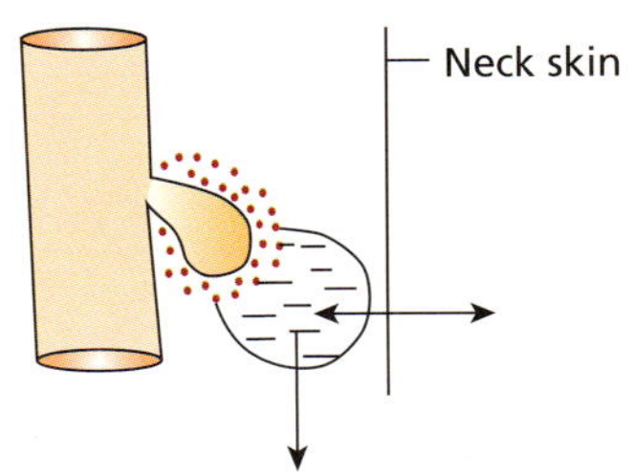

Figure 21.14 Complications of a pharyngeal diverticulum.

has to be differentiated from odynophagia which is pain during deglutition which may also make swallowing difficult.

Etiology

To complete the act of swallowing, two things are required:

- The food passage must be patent.
- The neuromuscular forces of deglutition must be normal.

The dysphagia due to defects in the above-mentioned requirements are described in Box 21.4.

Box 21.4 Causes of dysphagia

- **Defects of food passage**
  - In the lumen: Impacted foreign body, for example, artificial denture, a large bolus of food, coins, mango seed, and others
  - In the wall
    - Inflammations: Peritonsillar abscess, acute esophagitis (they cause odynophagia)
    - Carcinoma of posterior one-third of tongue, pharynx, and esophagus
    - Esophageal stricture
  - Outside the wall
    - Large tumors of cervical lymph nodes, thyroid, and mediastinum
    - Pharyngeal pouch (Zenker's diverticulum)
    - Aneurysm of thoracic aorta
    - Paraesophageal hiatus hernia
- **Deficiency of neuromuscular forces of deglutition**
  - Spasm of food passage: Plummer–Vinson syndrome, achalasia cardia
  - Neurological disorders, for example, bulbar palsy
  - Infections, for example, tetanus, rabies

Clinical Diagnosis

- **Age**: Dysphagia due to carcinoma of food passage occurs mostly in middle-aged and elderly people.
- **Sex**: Plummer–Vinson syndrome is a disease of middle-aged women.
- **Onset**: Sudden onset of dysphagia is seen in impacted foreign body in food passage while dysphagia of gradual onset is seen in esophageal carcinoma and stricture.
- **Site of obstruction** may be told by the patient.
- Presence of a **visible and/or a palpable lump** in the neck in the vicinity of food passage, for example, a large goiter, lymph node mass, and pharyngeal pouch, helps in the diagnosis.

Investigations

- Esophagoscopy and biopsy, when indicated, confirm the diagnosis in most of the cases. They should not be done in pharyngeal pouch.
- Barium swallow is sometimes required, especially where the facilities for endoscopy are not available or when endoscopy is contraindicated, for example, pharyngeal pouch. It shows the site and nature of obstruction in most of the cases.
- Esophageal manometry is required in motility disorders.

Complications

Dysphagia may be associated with some pulmonary complication because of reflux of esophageal contents into the lungs.

Clinical Features and Treatment of Common Causes of Dysphagia

Foreign Body in Food Passage

- The patient has dysphagia of acute onset and a history of swallowing a foreign body.
- The diagnosis is confirmed by radiography and/or endoscopy.
- The foreign bodies are removed with the help of an endoscope. Rarely an open operation is required.

Stricture of Esophagus

- The patient presents with chronic dysphagia of a long duration. A history of swallowing a corrosive or gastroesophageal reflux is present.

- The diagnosis is confirmed by esophagoscopy and/or barium swallow which reveal the smooth narrowing of esophagus with proximal dilatation.
- The strictures are dilated endoscopically or reconstructed.

Carcinoma of Esophagus

- The patient is usually a middle-aged or elderly person who complains of oppression and heaviness behind the sternum during meals and dysphagia which is steadily progressive. Initially it is for solid foods and finally for liquids also (total dysphagia).
- Barium swallow shows irregular narrowing with shouldering and without much proximal dilatation (rat-tail deformity). Esophagoscopy and biopsy confirm the diagnosis.
- It is treated by resection of affected esophagus. In an unresectable cancer, the patency of esophagus is provided by endoscopic stenting.

Achalasia Cardia

- The patient is usually a woman of about 40 years of age who complains of regurgitation of food several hours after meal. There is dysphagia which is more for liquids than for solids.
- Barium swallow shows enormous dilatation, maybe with tortuosity (sigmoid esophagus) with smooth narrowing and termination at lower end and lack of fundal gas in the stomach.
- It is treated by endoscopic dilatation or cardiomyotomy (Heller's operation).

Plummer–Vinson Syndrome

- The patient is usually a middle-aged woman who has dysphagia associated with glossitis and anemia. The tongue is smooth, pale, and devoid of papillae. The lips and corners of mouth are often cracked. The fingernails are concave like a spoon (koilonychia).
- The blood shows microcytic hypochromic anemia and low serum iron (normal being 9–27 mmol/L). The endoscopy shows narrowing at pharyngoesophageal junction with webs.
- It is treated by correction of iron deficiency anemia and endoscopic dilatation.

If not treated, it may result in a postcricoid carcinoma.

Pharyngeal Pouch (Zenker's Diverticulum)

- The patient is usually a male older than 50 years of age who initially complains of regurgitation of undigested food at an unpredictable time or after changing sides in bed at night. Sometimes the patient may wake up from sleep with a feeling of choking followed by severe cough. When the pouch enlarges in size, it produces dysphagia by extrinsic pressure. When the patient swallows some liquid, the pouch enlarges with gurgling noise in the neck.
- Barium study with thin barium reveals the pouch in the neck.
- This lesion (Zenker's diverticulum) is excised or treated endoscopically.

KEY POINTS

- Pharyngitis is mostly a viral infection. Bacterial pharyngitis caused by group A β-hemolytic *Streptococcus* (GABHS) is important as it may be complicated by rheumatic fever and glomerulonephritis.
- Tonsillitis is the commonest types of throat infection caused by a variety of viruses and bacteria characterized by throat pain and swollen red tonsils.
- Peritonsillar abscess (quinsy) is a collection of pus around the tonsil and characterized by throat pain, swelling of tonsil, and displacement of uvula to the opposite side. The administration of antibiotics, pus drainage, and tonsillectomy are the treatment methods.
- Parapharyngeal abscess occurs due to spread of infection from peritonsillar abscess, deep parotid abscess, infected third molar root, penetrating injuries, and petrositis.
- Retropharyngeal abscess is collection of pus in the retropharyngeal space between the posterior wall of pharynx and the vertebral column. It is of two types: acute and chronic.

(CONTD...)

KEY POINTS *(...CONTD)*

- Acute retropharyngeal abscess occurs following pyogenic infection of retropharyngeal lymph nodes and is characterized by red swollen posterior pharyngeal wall of one side of midline.
- Chronic retropharyngeal abscess (prevertebral abscess) is characterized by pain in the neck with restricted mobility of cervical spine, fullness behind the sternomastoid muscle on one side, and swelling in posterior pharyngeal wall in midline.
- Juvenile angiofibroma is the most common locally invasive benign tumor of nasopharynx. It manifests with profuse epistaxis and nasal obstruction. Biopsy is not done in this tumor for fear of severe bleeding. It is excised.
- Carcinoma of nasopharynx is mostly a squamous cell carcinoma. Most of the tumors arise from the fossa of Rosenmuller with early presentation of slight intermittent epistaxis with small clots. Any adult with persistent unilateral nasal symptoms or otitis media of recent onset should be thoroughly evaluated for this tumor. Radiotherapy is the mainstay of treatment.
- Squamous cell carcinoma is the most common type of oropharyngeal carcinoma characterized by persistent sore throat which may be accompanied by persistent otalgia. T1 and T2 tumors can be treated with surgery or radiotherapy. T3 and T4 tumors are treated by a combination of radiotherapy and surgery.
- More than 95% of hypopharyngeal cancers are squamous cell carcinoma which is an infiltrating ulcerative lesion. The common sites of occurrence of this cancer are pyriform sinus (60%) and postcricoid region; the former has non-specific symptoms and the latter dysphagia. It is treated by radiotherapy or laryngopharyngectomy.
- Foreign bodies may be lodged in pharynx leading to dysphagia, odynophagia, or aphagia. In a young child or infant, drooling is a characteristic sign.
- Zenker's diverticulum is the protrusion of pharyngeal mucosa through the Killian's dehiscence characterized by regurgitation of undigested food and gurgling noise in the neck during meals which may be visible as a swelling. It is treated by excision or endoscopic division of septum.
- Dysphagia is difficulty in swallowing and odynophagia is pain during deglutition which may also make swallowing difficult.
- Sudden onset of dysphagia is seen in impacted foreign body in food passage while dysphagia of gradual onset is seen in esophageal carcinoma and stricture. Esophagoscopy and biopsy, when indicated, confirm the diagnosis in most of the cases. Treatment is removal of the cause.
- Plummer–Vinson syndrome occurs usually in a middle-aged female characterized by dysphagia, iron deficiency anemia, koilonychia, cheilosis, and atrophy of papillae of tongue. These patients may subsequently develop a postcricoid carcinoma. It is treated by correction of iron deficiency anemia and dilatation.

SELF-ASSESSMENT

Long answer questions

1. Describe the etiology, pathology, clinical features, complications, and treatment of acute tonsillitis.
2. What is dysphagia? Describe its causes, diagnosis, and treatment.

Short answer questions

1. Quinsy
2. Adenoids
3. Tonsillectomy
4. Retropharyngeal abscess
5. Pharyngeal diverticulum
6. Plummer–Vinson syndrome

Multiple choice questions

1. Eustachian tube opens into
   (a) Lateral wall of nasopharynx
   (b) Posterior wall of nasopharynx
   (c) Posterior wall of oropharynx
   (d) Lateral wall of oropharynx

(CONTD...)

SELF-ASSESSMENT *(...CONTD)*

2. The laryngeal opening is situated in
   (a) Anterior wall of oropharynx
   (b) Lateral wall of oropharynx
   (c) Anterior wall of hypopharynx
   (d) Posterior wall of hypopharynx
3. Pharynx has
   (a) Two constrictors
   (b) Three constrictors
   (c) Four constrictors
   (d) Five constrictors
4. What is the lower limit of oropharynx?
   (a) Base of tongue
   (b) Tonsils
   (c) Lingual surface of closed epiglottis
   (d) Base of epiglottis
5. Which of the following facts is not true about juvenile angiofibroma of nasopharynx?
   (a) It is a benign tumor of nasopharynx
   (b) It is a hormone-dependent tumor stimulated by testosterone
   (c) It does not have a capsule
   (d) Biopsy should be done to confirm the diagnosis
6. Quinsy is a collection of pus in
   (a) Between the anterior and posterior tonsillar pillars into the soft palate
   (b) Parapharyngeal space
   (c) Retropharyngeal space anterior to prevertebral fascia
   (d) Retropharyngeal space behind prevertebral fascia
7. All of the following are the features of a juvenile angiofibroma, except
   (a) It is a very vascular tumor
   (b) It commonly occurs in adolescent males
   (c) Epistaxis is a rare symptom of this tumor
   (d) Carotid angiography may be done to evaluate its blood supply
8. All of the following features are true about carcinoma of nasopharynx, except
   (a) The tumor originates mostly in fossa of Rosenmuller
   (b) Elevated Epstein–Barr virus titer is found in a large number of cases
   (c) Slight intermittent epistaxis is one of the early symptoms
   (d) It usually spreads to lungs by hematogenous route
9. The carcinoma of oropharynx is usually
   (a) An adenocarcinoma
   (b) A transitional cell carcinoma
   (c) A basal cell carcinoma
   (d) A squamous cell carcinoma
10. All of the following are true about oropharyngeal carcinoma, except
    (a) It is etiologically related to long-term use of tobacco and alcohol
    (b) Metastases usually occur in the brain by hematogenous spread
    (c) It is more common in males than in females
    (d) It is characterized by persistent sore throat
11. A T3 cancer of oropharynx means
    (a) Tumor up to 2 cm in size
    (b) Tumor 2–4 cm in size
    (c) Tumor invading adjacent structures
    (d) Tumor more than 4 cm in size
12. The 5-year survival rate in T1 oropharyngeal carcinoma is
    (a) 85%
    (b) 75%
    (c) 65%
    (d) 55%
13. The most common site of metastases of oropharyngeal carcinoma is
    (a) Cervical lymph nodes
    (b) Lungs
    (c) Bones
    (d) Liver
14. The pyriform fossae are included in
    (a) Nasopharynx
    (b) Oropharynx
    (c) Hypopharynx
    (d) Larynx
15. Hypopharynx is lined by
    (a) Columnar epithelium
    (b) Squamous epithelium
    (c) Transitional epithelium
    (d) Cuboidal epithelium

(CONTD...)

SELF-ASSESSMENT *(...CONTD)*

16. Which of the following statements is false about carcinoma of hypopharynx?
    (a) It is etiologically related to excessive use of tobacco and alcohol
    (b) Most of the patients are young adults
    (c) It is usually a squamous cell carcinoma
    (d) The usual mode of spread is by lymphatics to cervical lymph nodes
17. Histologically a hypopharyngeal carcinoma is usually a
    (a) Squamous cell carcinoma
    (b) Transitional cell carcinoma
    (c) Basal cell carcinoma
    (d) Adenocarcinoma
18. The diagnosis of carcinoma of hypopharynx is confirmed by
    (a) Endoscopic biopsy
    (b) Barium swallow
    (c) CT scan
    (d) MRI
19. The 5-year survival rate of carcinoma of hypopharynx is
    (a) 30%
    (b) 40%
    (c) 50%
    (d) 60%
20. A pharyngeal diverticulum is defined as
    (a) Mucosal herniation of nasopharynx
    (b) Herniation of lining of oropharynx
    (c) Anterior herniation of mucosa of hypopharynx
    (d) Protrusion of mucosa through Killian's dehiscence
21. Killian's dehiscence is defined as
    (a) A weak area in the posterior wall of lower end of pharynx between two sets of fibers of inferior constrictor of pharynx
    (b) A weak area in the posterior wall of oropharynx
    (c) A weak area in the lateral wall of oropharynx
    (d) A weak area in the roof of nasopharynx
22. Which of the following statements is false about pharyngeal pouch?
    (a) It is pulsion diverticulum
    (b) It is usually seen in elderly persons
    (c) It may cause gurgling during meals in the neck with the appearance of a swelling
    (d) The diagnosis is usually confirmed by endoscopy
23. Dysphagia is defined as
    (a) Painful swallowing
    (b) Difficulty in swallowing
    (c) Difficulty in mastication of food
    (d) Lack of salivary secretion
24. Odynophagia is a symptom characterized by
    (a) Painful swallowing
    (b) Difficulty in swallowing
    (c) Difficulty in mastication
    (d) Lack of salivary secretion
25. All of the following statements are true about dysphagia, except
    (a) It is defined as difficulty in swallowing
    (b) It can be caused by accidental swallowing of an artificial denture
    (c) Tetanus can never cause dysphagia
    (d) The diagnosis is confirmed by esophagoscopy
26. All of the following are true about dysphagia, except
    (a) From partial it may become total dysphagia
    (b) It may be caused by carcinoma of esophagus
    (c) Stricture of esophagus produces dysphagia of chronic onset
    (d) It is never associated with some pulmonary complication
27. All of the following facts are true about esophageal stricture, except
    (a) It is fibrous narrowing of esophagus
    (b) It causes dysphagia of acute onset
    (c) Swallowing of a corrosive is one of its important causes
    (d) It is treated by endoscopic dilatation or reconstruction
28. All of the following statements are true about carcinoma of esophagus, except
    (a) It is a disease of young males in the second decade of life

(CONTD...)

SELF-ASSESSMENT *(...CONTD)*

(b) It causes progressive dysphagia
(c) The diagnosis is confirmed by esophagoscopy and biopsy
(d) It is treated by resection and anastomosis

29. All of the following statements are true about achalasia cardia, except
(a) The patient is usually a woman about 40 years of age
(b) There is dysphagia more for solids than for liquids
(c) The diagnosis is confirmed by barium swallow and endoscopy
(d) It is treated by cardiomyotomy

30. Plummer–Vinson syndrome has all of the following features, except
(a) Atrophy of papillae of tongue
(b) High serum iron
(c) Dysphagia
(d) Koilonychia

31. Koilonychia is defined as
(a) Spoon-shaped nails
(b) Convex nails
(c) Nails with white ridges
(d) Brittle nails

32. The normal serum iron level is
(a) 7–8 mmol/L
(b) 9–27 mmol/L
(c) 28–31 mmol/L
(d) 32–35 mmol/L

33. All of the following facts are true about Plummer–Vinson syndrome, except
(a) The patient is usually a middle-aged female who presents with dysphagia
(b) The patient has microcytic hypochromic anemia
(c) The nails are normal
(d) It may lead to postcricoid carcinoma of pharynx

Answers

1. (a) 2. (c) 3. (b) 4. (c) 5. (d) 6. (a) 7. (c) 8. (d) 9. (d) 10. (b) 11. (d) 12. (b) 13. (a) 14. (c) 15. (b) 16. (b) 17. (a) 18. (a) 19. (a) 20. (d) 21. (a) 22. (d) 23. (b) 24. (a) 25. (c) 26. (d) 27. (b) 28. (a) 29. (b) 30. (b) 31. (a) 32. (b) 33. (c)

Diseases of Larynx

22

Surgical anatomy

Larynx is situated in the front of hypopharynx opposite the third to sixth cervical vertebrae. It is a hollow tube made up of cartilages, for example, thyroid and cricoid cartilages and rings of trachea in which the cricoid is the only complete cartilaginous ring, muscles, membranes, and connective tissue (Fig. 22.1) with an inner lining of squamous epithelium. The cavity of larynx has a vestibule, a ventricle (sinus of larynx), and subglottic space. The most important structure inside the larynx is vocal cords which are two pearly white sharp bands extending from the middle of thyroid cartilage anteriorly to the vocal processes of arytenoids posteriorly (Fig. 22.2). Larynx moves up during deglutition to protect the airway from the accidental entry of food and drinks. It can be moved from side to side passively producing a grating sensation called laryngeal crepitus. The functions of larynx are described in Box 22.1.

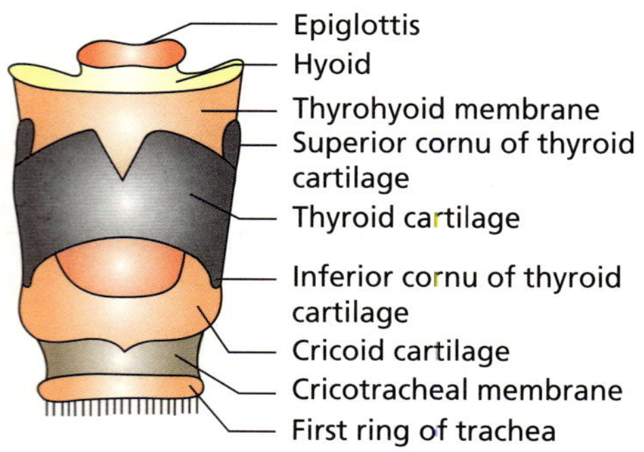

Epiglottis
Hyoid
Thyrohyoid membrane
Superior cornu of thyroid cartilage
Thyroid cartilage
Inferior cornu of thyroid cartilage
Cricoid cartilage
Cricotracheal membrane
First ring of trachea

Figure 22.1 Larynx from the front.

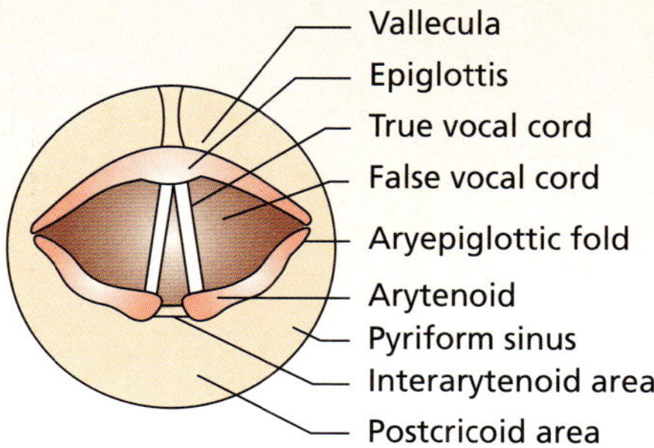

Figure 22.2 Laryngoscopic appearance of larynx.

Box 22.1 Functions of larynx

- To provide a conduit for breathing
- To protect lower airway by closure of laryngeal inlet and cough reflex
- Phonation, mainly by vibration of vocal cords
- To help in respiratory function by regulation of flow of air to and from the lungs

1. TRAUMA OF LARYNX

Laryngeal trauma

The laryngeal injuries are not uncommon and some of them may be dangerous to life.

Etiology

The most common cause of laryngeal trauma is an automobile accident. Other causes are listed as follows:

- **Iatrogenic injury**
  - Prolonged intubation
  - Inappropriate tracheostomy
  - Laryngotomy and cricothyroidotomy
- **Accidental injury**
  - Automobile accidents (in passengers in the front seat, there occurs hyperextension of neck and then compression or crushing of larynx between dashboard and cervical vertebral column)
  - Blows on the front of neck, for example, fan belt of a thrasher
  - Strangulation of neck
  - Cut throat by a sword or wire
- **Laryngeal burns**
  - Inhalation of corrosive gases, very hot air, steam
  - Swallowing of corrosives

Pathology

The most common injury is vertical fracture of thyroid cartilage with or without fracture of cricoid cartilage especially in people over the age 40 years which occurs due to loss of elasticity and calcification. An unreduced fracture of cricoid may result in subglottic stenosis. Escape of air into tissues around larynx may cause subcutaneous emphysema, pneumomediastinum, and pneumothorax. The laryngeal trauma may pose a threat to life by disturbing respiration. The pathological types of laryngeal trauma are described in Box 22.2.

Box 22.2 Types of laryngeal trauma

- Laceration of larynx
- Hemorrhage in and around larynx
- Fracture of hyoid bone, cartilaginous framework of larynx
- Dislocation of cricoarytenoid joint and cricothyroid joint
- Traumatic edema of laryngeal mucosa
- Detachment of larynx from the trachea

Clinical Features

Following trauma, the patient presents with pain in front of neck, difficulty in breathing, cough, and hemoptysis. On examination, there may be swelling, abrasions, bruising, and lacerations in the neck. On palpation, there may be tenderness, crepitus of emphysema, and fracture and may be a gap between fractured fragments or two cartilages. The clinical features of laryngeal trauma are described in Box 22.3.

Box 22.3 Clinical features of laryngeal trauma

- Respiratory distress
- Swelling of neck and crepitus due to subcutaneous emphysema
- Dysphonia or aphonia
- Stridor
- Cough, hemoptysis, odynophagia
- Loss of laryngeal prominence (Adam's apple)

Investigations

- **Radiography**: Radiography of neck, especially lateral view, shows subcutaneous emphysema and fracture and displacement of cartilages.
- **Laryngoscopy**: If the condition of the patient permits, laryngoscopy is done. Direct and indirect laryngoscopies can be done but the

indirect one is simpler, safer, and easier. The findings include edema of laryngeal mucosa, hemorrhages, and inward pushing of laryngeal framework. The direct laryngoscopy shows the inside of larynx better.

Complications

The complications of laryngeal trauma and its treatment include laryngeal stenosis, recurrent laryngeal nerve paralysis, perichondritis, laryngeal web formation, and vocal cord fixation.

Treatment

- **Airway patency**: The airway must be kept patent and clear. It may require direct laryngoscopy, intubation, or tracheostomy. If a high tracheostomy or cricothyroidotomy has been performed in emergency, it should be revised as soon as possible to the third or fourth tracheal ring to prevent vocal cord paralysis and subglottic stenosis.
- **General measures**: The general measures include cool mist insufflation, intravenous fluids, broad-spectrum antibiotics (e.g., cefazolin), and parenteral corticosteroids to reduce edema.
- **Surgical treatment**: The penetrating injuries are explored urgently. The severe injuries require open reduction with stabilization of all cartilaginous, mucosal, and soft-tissue defects with internal fixation with a soft stent.

Vocal nodules (singer's nodes)

Etiopathogenesis These are small rounded elevations situated at the junction of anterior one-third and posterior two-thirds of true vocal cords in singers who use high-intensity sounds for a long period. The pathogenesis is described in Box 22.4.

Box 22.4 Etiopathogenesis of vocal nodules

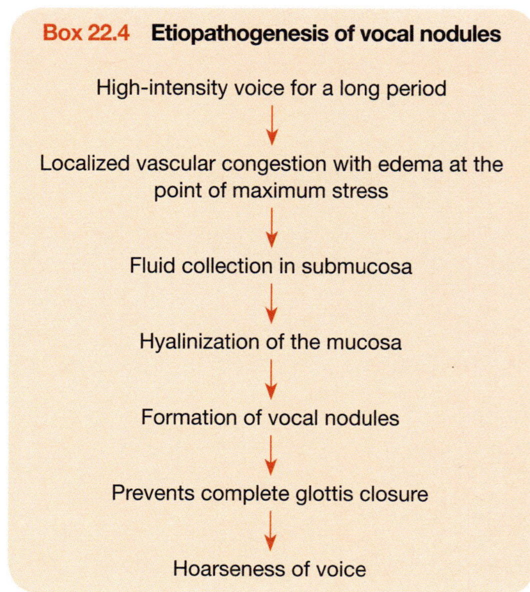

Clinical Features

- This condition is seen in male children, young adult women, teachers, singers, and screamers who present with recurrent attacks of dysphonia and chronic hoarseness.
- A singer has decreased range of high notes and loss of flexibility of voice and vocal fatigue.

Investigations

- Laryngoscopy shows the nodules (Fig. 22.3).
- Stroboscopy reveals the situation of vocal nodules at the point of maximum vibrations.

Treatment It includes voice therapy, endoscopic microlaryngeal surgical excision, or laser excision.

Vocal cord paralysis

Vocal cord paralysis is not an uncommon problem. It affects breathing and speech. Hence, it requires mention.

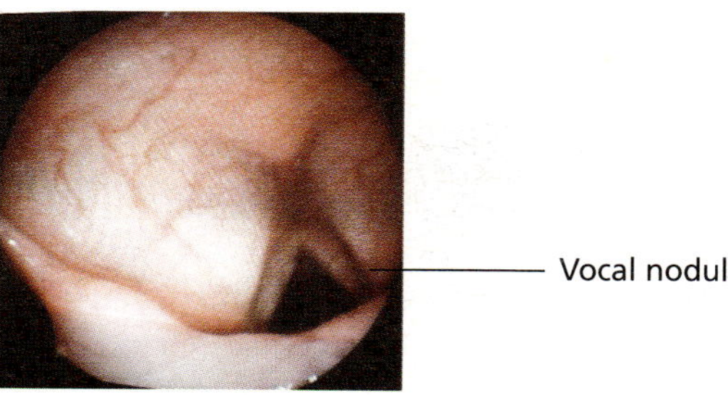

Figure 22.3 Laryngoscopy showing nodules of vocal cord. (Courtesy: Professor S.P. Agarwal)

Etiology

Vocal cord paralysis may occur from a lesion or damage to the vagus nerve or recurrent laryngeal nerve but in most cases it results from injury to the laryngeal nerves during thyroid surgery. In many cases, the cause of paralysis is not known (idiopathic when it may be viral mononeuropathy). The paralysis of vocal cords manifests as vocal cord immobility. The vocal cords may also become immobile due to causes other than palsy. The causes of vocal cord paralysis/immobility are described in Table 22.1.

Pathophysiology

The recurrent laryngeal nerves are the primary innervators of the abductors and the adductors of the vocal cords, while the superior laryngeal nerves supply the cricothyroid muscles of larynx.

- Recurrent laryngeal nerve injury results in paralysis of vocal cords in paramedian position 2–3 mm lateral to midline.
- Combined injury to recurrent and superior laryngeal nerves paralyzes the vocal cords in intermediate position several millimeters lateral to paramedian position.

Clinical Features

- Unilateral left vocal cord paralysis is most common. It produces breathy hoarseness with varying amounts of aspiration of liquids, vocal fatigue, and dysphagia.
- Bilateral vocal cord paralysis usually causes inspiratory and expiratory stridor, if acute. If it is of insidious onset, it may be asymptomatic at rest and causes dyspnea on exertion.

Investigations

Radiology

- Chest X-ray may be of help in finding the cause of vocal cord palsy.
- CT scan with contrast from skull base to aortopulmonary window (the span of recurrent laryngeal nerve) is done if no other cranial nerve is involved. MRI is done if other cranial nerve deficits or high vagal weakness with paralysis of palate is noted to see the brain and brainstem.

Stroboscopy Stroboscopic examination of the vocal cords is done to find their vibratory pattern.

Treatment

Spontaneous Recovery When no cause is found or paresis follows an operation in which the nerve was not divided, spontaneous recovery occurs with time, usually within a year.

Treatment of Unilateral Paralysis

- Persistent paralysis is treated by medialization of paralyzed cord in order to create a stable platform for vocal cord vibration. It is done by injection laryngoplasty using Teflon, Gelfoam, fat, or collagen. Teflon is the only permanent injectable material, but it may result in granuloma formation in vocal cords in some patients. Temporary injectable materials, for example, collagen or fat, provide excellent

Table 22.1 Etiology of vocal cord paralysis

Unilateral paralysis	Bilateral paralysis	Vocal cord immobility (not related to paralysis)
• **Recurrent laryngeal nerve paralysis** – Operations on thyroid – Carcinoma of thyroid – Other neck operations, for example, anterior discectomy and carotid endarterectomy – Apical lung cancer • **Vagus nerve paralysis** – Tumors of skull base involving 9th, 10th, and 11th cranial nerves, and during surgical treatment of these tumors	• Thyroid surgery • Esophageal carcinoma • Ventricular shunt malfunction	• Cricothyroid arthritis secondary to advanced rheumatoid arthritis • Intubation injuries • Glottic and subglottic stenosis • Carcinoma of larynx

temporary restoration of voice and can be injected under local or general anesthesia.

- In permanent paralysis, formal medialization thyroplasty can be done by creating a small window in the thyroid cartilage and placing a silastic implant between the thyroarytenoid muscle and the inner table of thyroid cartilage that displaces the soft tissues and arytenoids medially.

Treatment of Bilateral Paralysis It may be acute-onset palsy or insidious-onset palsy.

- The acute-onset palsy causes airway obstruction that requires emergency intervention to create an airway (tracheostomy). The goal of intervention is creation of a safe airway with minimal reduction in voice quality and airway protection from aspiration.
- For managing insidious-onset palsy, a number of vocal cord lateralization procedures are available to manage this problem and remove the tracheostomy tube.

Foreign bodies in airway

A foreign body when placed in the mouth may be suddenly aspirated into the airway during cough or sudden movements. It results in violent cough but it may not be thrown out due to spasmodic closure of larynx.

Etiology

- In children, a variety of foreign bodies including seeds, beans, pins, and tiny toys may be aspirated into the airway.
- In adults, large poorly chewed pieces of food are the most common foreign bodies. They can impact into trachea, bronchi, and larynx, in that order.

Clinical features

- A large foreign body may lodge in the supraglottic area or glottis and produce urgent respiratory distress.
- Small foreign bodies commonly lodge in right main bronchus producing unilateral wheezing or chronic cough in children not responding to treatment.
- If a foreign body is lodged in larynx, there is immediate pain in the neck, laryngospasm, dyspnea, and inspiratory stridor proportionate to the degree of laryngeal obstruction. In partial obstruction, the patient can exchange air and can cough. In complete obstruction, the patient is aphonic, is unable to cough or exchange air, and is clutching his/her neck.

Diagnosis

A radio-opaque foreign body can be imaged by radiography but radiography is done if the patient is fit for it.

Treatment

- **Heimlich maneuver**: The patient is held from behind with both arms around lower thorax and a series of sudden manual thrusts of compression are applied at thoracoabdominal junction. It may lead to sudden violent expiration which may throw the foreign body out.
- **Endoscopic removal**: In the cases with partial obstruction, the foreign body is removed with the help of a direct laryngoscope and alligator forceps.

2. INFLAMMATIONS AND INFECTIONS

Laryngitis

It is the inflammation of larynx due to infection and other causes. It is of many types as described below.

Acute Laryngitis

Etiology It usually occurs in association with a general viral upper respiratory tract infection caused mainly by rhinoviruses, respiratory syncytial virus, and adenoviruses. It is usually a self-limiting problem. If the hoarseness of voice persists for more than a few days, the possibility of secondary bacterial invasion by *Moraxella catarrhalis*, *Haemophilus influenzae*, and *Streptococcus pneumoniae* must be considered.

Clinical Features Hoarseness, cough, and odynophagia are often marked with minimal edema or marked edema of the true vocal cords.

Treatment It consists of vocal rest, hydration, humidification, and erythromycin, cefuroxime, or amoxicillin–clavulanate. Oral or intramuscular corticosteroids may be given in some cases of professional vocalists to speed recovery but it may result in bleeding from inflamed vocal folds.

Chronic Nonspecific Laryngitis

Etiology It is chronic inflammation of larynx which is related to many causative factors, that is, voice misuse, chronic smoking, inhalation of vocal irritants, gastroesophageal reflux (GOR), and alcoholism.

Types It is of two types:

1. **Chronic nonhyperplastic laryngitis**: It is characterized by chronic diffuse inflammation of true vocal cords, ventricular bands, interarytenoid area, and root of epiglottis.
2. **Chronic hyperplastic laryngitis**: It is characterized by diffuse symmetrical or localized epithelial hyperplasia, metaplasia, keratinization, edema, and round cell infiltration of the mucosa. The pseudostratified ciliated squamous epithelium changes to squamous epithelium and the squamous epithelium of vocal cords becomes keratinized.

Clinical Features

- The patient is around 50 years of age, more commonly a male, and presents with hoarseness of voice of long duration.
- Other symptoms include tiredness or weakness of voice, dryness, and tickling sensation in the throat.
- The patient tries to repeatedly clear his/her throat; cough may be present and a little gelatinous mucus may be expectorated.

Laryngoscopy It shows the following findings:

- **Chronic nonhyperplastic laryngitis**: It is characterized by diffuse symmetrical chronic inflammation of true vocal cords, ventricular bands, interarytenoid area, and root of epiglottis. There is diffuse generalized edema and hyperemia.
- **Chronic hyperplastic laryngitis**: In early disease, only true vocal cords are involved. Later on, whole of the larynx is involved. Initially there is capillary injection and edema of vocal cords. Later on, keratinization occurs and then the vocal cords may become gray, irregular, bulky, and nodular.

Complications The complications of laryngitis include edema of larynx, local spread of infection, and persistent damage to voice.

Treatment

- Remove the cause, for example, avoid smoking and alcohol, and voice abuse.
- Other measures include mucolytic and mucokinetic expectorants, speech therapy, and medicated steam inhalations.
- The hyperplastic laryngitis may require removal of all or most of the diseased epithelium by stripping.

Chronic Specific Laryngitis—Laryngeal Tuberculosis

It is an uncommon type of laryngitis but still occurs in our country.

Etiology It is usually secondary to active pulmonary tuberculosis in which the laryngeal mucosa gets infected by mycobacteria-rich sputum.

Clinical Features Most of the patients are young and present with hoarseness and weakness of voice, laryngeal pain, dysphagia, and referred otalgia. This disease has three stages which are described in Table 22.2.

Investigations

- X-ray of the chest is invariably positive for active pulmonary tuberculosis.
- The sputum is sent for smear and culture for *Mycobacterium tuberculosis*. It is likely to be positive.

Table 22.2 Clinical features and laryngoscopic findings in laryngeal tuberculosis

Stage	Clinical features	Laryngoscopic findings
Stage I	Frequent attacks of hoarseness of voice when it is associated with dysphagia especially for fluids for which there is no pharyngeal cause	Pallid laryngeal mucosa from edema and interarytenoid swelling due to inflammation
Stage II	• Increasing pain on swallowing fluids (odynophagia) which may be referred to the ears • Troublesome cough which may be sometimes painful	• Ulceration of one or both vocal cords giving "mouse-nibbled appearance" • Pale superficial ulceration of posterior surface of epiglottis
Stage III	Weak voice with almost incessant coughing with distressing pain	Perichondritis and necrosis of laryngeal cartilages, that is, arytenoids, epiglottis, and rarely other cartilages

- Laryngoscopy shows changes in the larynx with findings depending on the stage of the disease (Table 22.2).

Treatment It includes antituberculous drugs, vocal rest, and symptomatic treatment of cough and pain.

Laryngopharyngeal reflux

Etiology GOR can occur in the larynx (laryngopharyngeal reflux) and can cause chronic hoarseness.

Clinical Features Symptoms include chronic hoarseness of voice, throat discomfort, chronic cough, a sensation of postnasal drip, esophageal spasm, and asthma in some patients.

Diagnosis Before diagnosing this condition, other causes of hoarseness must be excluded by laryngoscopy. The diagnosis is mostly clinical as only around 50% of patients with laryngeal acid exposure have typical symptoms of heartburn and regurgitation. Furthermore, most of the patients do not meet the criteria for GOR by pH probe testing.

Treatment It is treated with modifications of diet, going to bed at night at least 3 hours after dinner, elevation of head end of bed by 6 inches, and full-strength proton pump inhibitor, for example, omeprazole 40 mg twice daily for a minimum of 3 months. Nonresponders should be evaluated with a double pH probe (proximal and distal esophageal probes).

Vocal cord polyp

Etiology These lesions occur on the true vocal cords in patients who use their voice too loudly for longer periods. It results in rupture of submucosal capillaries with extravasation of blood and accumulation of fluid. Polyp results from organization and hyalinization of this accumulation.

Clinical Features There is rapid onset of hoarseness during extreme vocal abuse.

Laryngoscopy It reveals a single nodule larger than vocal nodules but at the same position. It is soft, smooth, dark, hemorrhagic, and often pedunculated.

- On phonation, the polyp may come on cord's upper surface to which it is attached and cause negligible interference with phonation.
- If it is pedunculated, it moves up and down with respiration.

The differences between a vocal cord polyp and vocal cord nodules (singer's nodes) are described in Table 22.3.

Table 22.3 Differences between a vocal cord polyp and vocal nodules

Features	Vocal cord polyp	Vocal nodules (singer's nodes)
Size	Larger	Smaller
Number	Usually single	Usually multiple
Shape	Spherical, may have a pedicle	Small elevation
Color	Dark hemorrhagic	Pearly white

Treatment It includes microlaryngeal surgical excision and speech therapy.

Intubation granuloma

It is the formation of a granuloma at posterior one-third of vocal cords following overenthusiastic endolaryngeal surgery, endotracheal intubation, and rigid bronchoscopy. It causes hoarseness of voice. It is treated by voice rest and microlaryngeal surgical excision.

Epiglottitis

Epiglottitis is a rapidly progressive acute inflammation of supraglottic larynx which may result in sudden complete airway obstruction.

Etiology It is more common in diabetic patients and may be viral or bacterial (*H. influenzae*) in origin.

Pathology It is characterized by acute inflammation of epiglottis, pharyngoepiglottic fold, aryepiglottic fold, arytenoids, and ventricular folds. There is heavy infiltration of neutrophils with the formation of small abscesses in mucosa and submucosa. Hyperemia and edema of supraglottic larynx may cause airway obstruction.

Clinical Features

- The patient presents with rapidly developing sore throat and odynophagia with minimal oropharyngeal findings on examination.
- The patient looks ill and has fever and malaise. He/she prefers to sit and has drooling of saliva. On protrusion of tongue, the cherry red tip of swollen epiglottis may be seen.
- The examination with a tongue depressor should be avoided.

Investigations

- Blood shows polymorphonuclear leukocytosis.
- Indirect laryngoscopy in an adult reveals a swollen and cherry red epiglottis.
- Lateral plain radiography of neck may show the swollen epiglottis ("thumb sign").
- CT scan may be done which may reveal an endolaryngeal abscess.

Complications The complications include airway obstruction, spread of infection, and abscess formation.

Treatment

- It includes hospitalization, intravenous antibiotics (e.g., ceftizoxime 1–2 g intravenously every 8–12 hours or cefuroxime 750–1500 mg intravenously every 8 hours), dexamethasone (4–10 mg initial bolus, and then 4 mg intravenously every 6 hours), and observation of airway.
- As the symptoms abate, the parenteral antibiotics are substituted with oral antibiotics to complete a 10-day course and the corticosteroids are tapered.
- The indications for endotracheal intubation include dyspnea, rapid pace of sore throat, and endolaryngeal abscess. Less than 10% of patients require intubation.
- If the patient is not intubated, monitoring of oxygen saturation and pulse oximetry must be done.

3. TUMORS OF LARYNX

Recurrent respiratory papillomatosis

It was previously known as laryngeal papilloma; its present name is given as it may involve the entire upper respiratory tract and has a tendency to recur.

Etiology It is the most common benign laryngeal tumor caused by human papillomavirus (HPV) types 6 and 11.

Types

- **Juvenile papillomatosis**: It occurs from infancy to childhood (up to 12 years). It occasionally regresses spontaneously. A history of maternal condylomas is present in 50% of these patients.

- **Adult-onset papillomatosis**: It has the peak onset of disease in the third and fourth decades of life and affects the anterior half of true vocal cords or anterior commissure. It is probably related to sexual exposure.

Clinical Features

- Hoarseness of voice is the primary symptom.
- It is always associated with some degree of respiratory obstruction (stridor).
- In juvenile-onset disease, the patient may present with sudden airway obstruction which may occur during an intercurrent upper respiratory tract infection.

Diagnosis Diagnosis is confirmed by laryngoscopy and biopsy.

Complications Complications include laryngeal obstruction, spread to adjacent areas, and recurrence.

Treatment

- The mainstay of treatment is repeated laser vaporization or cold knife resection via operative laryngoscope. Repeat treatment may be required at 6-week intervals to maintain a patent airway.
- Tracheostomy must be avoided as far as possible as it provides an additional squamociliary junction for recurrence.
- Interferon has been used but should be used in severe cases with pulmonary involvement. Cidofovir has been used intralesionally in recurrent disease. Quadrivalent recombinant human HPV vaccine (Gardasil) may be used for eventual eradication of this disease.

Carcinoma of larynx

It is the most common malignancy of larynx. About 13,000 new cases of this cancer are seen in the USA each year.

Etiology

It is an epithelial malignant tumor of larynx of unknown etiology. The main risk factors include smoking and alcohol drinking. Other risk factors are radiation exposure, nickel workers, and HPV type 16 or 18 infection.

Pathology

Almost 90–95% of all laryngeal cancers are squamous cell carcinoma. Verrucous carcinoma is a variant of squamous cell carcinoma that is locally invasive but almost never metastasizes. Adenocarcinoma and lymphoepithelioma are other cancers of larynx.

Mode of Spread

It spreads by local infiltration and by lymphatics. The vocal cords do not have lymphatics; hence, a carcinoma of vocal cords does not spread by lymphatics till it is confined to vocal cords. The lymphatic metastasis occurs in neck nodes. Hematogenous metastases are rare.

Clinical Features

- It is usually seen in men aged 50–70 years.
- A change in the voice quality or hoarseness of voice is the most often presenting complaint. Stridor, cough, hemoptysis, dysphagia, odynophagia, and aspiration are other symptoms. Presentation with a swelling in the neck is uncommon.
- Neck metastases are not common in early glottis cancers. Supraglottic carcinoma, on the other hand, often metastasizes on both sides of the neck early in the disease.

Investigations

Endoscopy Direct laryngoscopy shows the site, size and extent of the lesion, and mobility of the cords (Figs 22.4–22.6). Biopsy can be taken at the same time with a special forceps.

Radiology

- CT scan and MRI are helpful in assessing the extent and volume of tumor, neck nodes, and sclerosis or destruction of laryngeal cartilages. Chest X-ray is indicated if there are level VI enlarged lymph nodes or there is a suspicion of a second primary lesion.

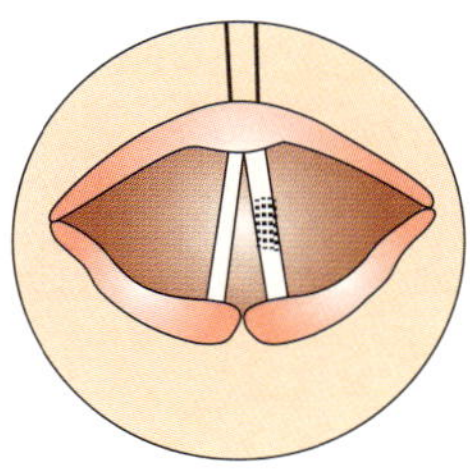

Figure 22.4 Early carcinoma of larynx involving left vocal cord.

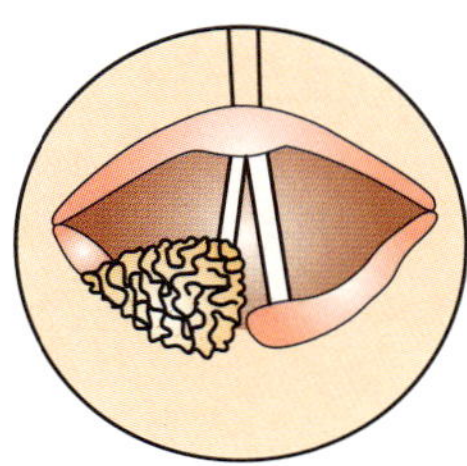

Figure 22.5 Carcinoma of larynx, right side, involving posterior half of right vocal cord, aryepiglottic fold, arytenoid, and false vocal cord.

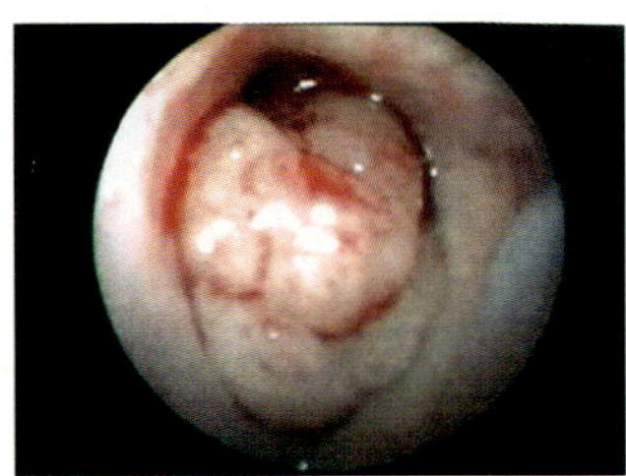

Figure 22.6 Laryngoscopic view of carcinoma of larynx. (Courtesy: Professor S.P. Agarwal)

- Positron emission tomography (PET) or CT-PET may be done to assess distant spread of disease.

TNM Staging

The TNM staging of this tumor is done to plan the treatment and to tell the prognosis.

Tumor Size "T" denotes the tumor size. Tis is carcinoma in situ. The four stages of tumor size in laryngeal carcinoma are described in Table 22.4.

Nodal Involvement and Distant Metastasis It is described in Table 22.5.

Stage Grouping

It is a combination of TNM stages into four clinical stages for the purpose of simplification of staging, planning the treatment, and predicting the results of treatment.

- **Stage I**: T1 N0 M0
- **Stage II**: T2 N0 M0
- **Stage III**: T3 N0 M0, T1–T3 N1 M0
- **Stage IV**: T4 or N2, N3 or M1

Treatment

The treatment depends on the stage of disease. The aims of treatment include:

- Cure of cancer
- Preservation of voice

Table 22.4 Staging of tumor size in laryngeal carcinoma

T stage	Supraglottic carcinoma	Glottic carcinoma	Subglottic carcinoma
T1	Confined to site of origin with normal mobility	Confined to one vocal cord or both vocal cords with normal mobility	Localized subglottic lesion
T2	Supraglottic lesion extending into glottis with normal cord mobility	Supraglottic and/or subglottic extension with normal cord mobility	Subglottic lesion extending into vocal cords with normal or impaired mobility
T3	Tumor limited to larynx with fixation, and/or extension to cricoid area, medial wall of pyriform sinus, or pre-epiglottic space	Tumor limited to larynx with vocal cord fixation	Tumor limited to larynx with vocal cord fixation
T4	Large tumor extending outside larynx involving oropharynx, tissues of neck, or destruction of thyroid cartilage	Large tumor with thyroid cartilage destruction and/or extension beyond larynx	Large tumor with cartilage destruction and/or extension beyond larynx

Table 22.5 Nodal involvement and distant metastasis in laryngeal carcinoma

Nodes	Description
N1	Single homolateral lymph node less than 3 cm
N2	Homolateral node or nodes, none of them more than 6 cm • N2a: Single node 3–6 cm • N2b: Multiple nodes
N3	Massive nodes, bilateral nodes, or contralateral nodes • N3a: Homolateral nodes >6 cm • N3b: Bilateral nodes • N3c: Contralateral nodes
Distant metastasis	• M0: No distant metastasis • M1: Presence of distant metastasis

- Preservation of safe and effective swallowing
- Avoidance of permanent tracheostomy as far as possible

Treatment of Tis It involves excision of involved vocal cord mucosa and then regular monitoring.

Treatment of T1 and T2 Glottic and Supraglottic Cancers and Selected Advanced Cancers (T3 and T4) T1 and T2 glottic and supraglottic cancers are treated by radiotherapy with cure rates >95% and 80%, respectively. But it carries substantial morbidity. Hence, T1 and T2 cancers and selected advanced cancers (T3 and T4) may be treated with partial laryngectomy if at least one cricoarytenoid unit can be preserved. In supraglottic tumors, even with N0 nodes, elective limited neck dissection with excision of tumor should be done because of high risk of neck node involvement.

Treatment of Advanced Stage III and IV Tumors They are treated with cisplatin-based chemotherapy concomitant with radiation. The same results are obtained with the epidermal growth factor receptor blocker cetuximab with lower toxicity and better tolerance. But these treatments are associated with prolonged gastrostomy-dependent dysphagia. Hence, instead of this extended treatment, less than total laryngectomy may be done in which one cricoarytenoid unit is preserved (organ preservation surgery). The patient's choice after thorough discussion plays an important role in selecting between chemoradiation and surgery.

Treatment of Neck Nodes They can be treated by surgery or chemoradiation or both. The choice of treatment depends on the treatment chosen for primary and extent of neck involvement.

The treatment of carcinoma of larynx is described in Table 24.6.

Table 22.6 Treatment of laryngeal carcinoma

TNM stages	Treatment
Tis	• Excision of involved vocal cord mucosa • Regular monitoring
T1 and T2 glottic and supraglottic cancers	• Radiotherapy with cure rates >95% and 80%, respectively (or) • Partial laryngectomy if at least one cricoarytenoid unit can be preserved • Supraglottic tumors (including no nodes): Elective limited neck dissection with excision of tumor
T3 and T4	• Partial laryngectomy if at least one cricoarytenoid unit can be preserved
Advanced stage III and IV tumors	• Cisplatin-based chemotherapy concomitant with radiation (or) • Less than total laryngectomy may be done in which one cricoarytenoid unit is preserved (organ preservation surgery)
Neck nodes	• Surgery or chemoradiation or both

Total laryngectomy

It includes resection of whole of the larynx up to below the true vocal cords, resection of a part of anterior wall of pharynx, repair of pharynx, and tracheostomy (Fig. 22.7).

Indications It is a major procedure, the indications of which are as follows:

- Advanced resectable cancer with extralaryngeal spread or cartilage involvement
- Persistent tumor following chemoradiation
- Recurrent or second primary tumor following radiotherapy

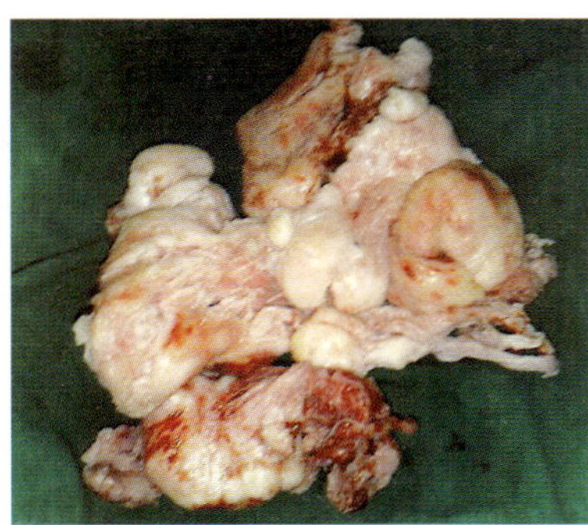

Figure 22.7 Excised specimen of carcinoma of larynx. (Courtesy: Professor S.P. Agarwal)

Complications The main complications of laryngectomy are loss of speech, pharyngeal fistula, and permanent tracheostomy.

Voice Rehabilitation Total laryngectomy patients undergo voice rehabilitation. Although a primary or at times secondary tracheoesophageal puncture provides intelligible and serviceable speech in 75–85% of patients, indwelling prostheses are a common alternative but they have to be changed every 3–6 months. The patient-inserted prostheses are also available but they need to be changed more frequently.

Prognosis

About 65% of patients of carcinoma of larynx are cured; most have useful speech and many resume their prior livelihoods with adaptations. The survival rates of glottic carcinoma are more than those of supraglottic and infraglottic cancers.

4. OTHER DISEASES OF LARYNX

Laryngocele

It is dilatation or herniation of laryngeal ventricle.

Types It is of two types:

1. **Internal**: It is confined within the larynx and presents as a bulge of false vocal cords and aryepiglottic folds.
2. **External**: It is herniation of the ventricle through the thyrohyoid membrane and presents as a swelling in the neck on one side of midline.

Etiology

- A persistent increase in transglottic air pressure such as in trumpet players and glass blowers leads to increase in the size of ventricle and formation of laryngocele. Another theory suggests that laryngocele is an atavistic problem as cervical air containing pouches are present in many mammals, for example, howling pouches in monkeys (atavism is the inheritance of a characteristic from remote rather than from immediate ancestor due to chance recombination of genes).

Pathology It is a narrow necked sac made up of herniated mucous membrane of larynx which contains seromucinous glands. Hence, it contains a variable amount of mucoid fluid.

Clinical Features It is commonly seen in men older than 50 years of age. It may be asymptomatic.

- A symptomatic laryngocele presents with hoarseness of voice, intermittent swelling in the neck, dyspnea, stridor, sore throat, cough, and sometimes snoring.

- On examination, there is a smooth, soft paramedian swelling in the neck which increases in size on Valsalva maneuver (Fig. 22.8) which is increase in intrathoracic pressure by forcible exhalation effort against closed glottis (nose).
- If the neck of the sac gets obstructed due to recrudescence of infection, the swelling does not abate completely for hours and days. Then the attack terminates with gurgling noise in the neck and discharge of mucus into the pharynx.

Investigations

- Radiography of the neck may show an air-filled cavity by the side of larynx (Fig. 22.9). It may have a fluid level.
- CT scan reveals the origin of the lesion from ventricle of larynx.

Complications The complications include infection, rupture with cellulitis of neck and subcutaneous emphysema, and laryngeal obstruction.

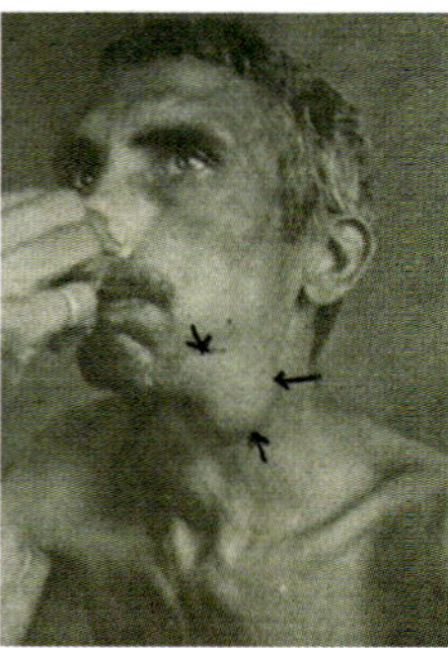

Figure 22.8 Swelling of laryngocele in the upper neck which has become more prominent during Valsalva maneuver.

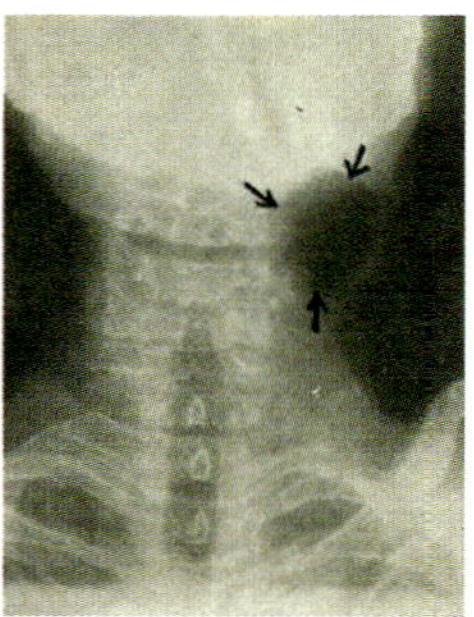

Figure 22.9 Anteroposterior radiograph of neck showing air shadow of laryngocele in the upper neck on the left side.

Treatment

- An asymptomatic laryngocele needs no treatment.
- An external laryngocele is excised by an external neck incision.
- An internal laryngocele is treated by endolaryngeal endoscopic marsupialization.

Airway obstruction

The airway extends from the nose down to the terminal bronchi, and the upper airway from the nose to the level of vocal cords. The upper airway is the common site of airway obstruction and requires urgent attention.

Etiology

The causes of upper airway obstruction are described in Box 22.5.

Box 22.5 Causes of upper airway obstruction

- **Obstruction above the larynx**
  - Choanal atresia
  - Micrognathia (Pierre Robin syndrome)
  - Accumulation of secretions, blood, and vomitus in oropharynx
- **Laryngeal obstruction**
  - Congenital
    - Laryngomalacia
    - Laryngeal web
    - Subglottic stenosis
  - Edema of larynx (glottis)
  - Infections
    - Acute epiglottitis
    - Laryngotracheobronchitis (croup)
  - Trauma
    - Injuries of larynx
    - Laryngeal foreign body
  - Tumors
    - Recurrent respiratory papillomatosis
    - Carcinoma of larynx

Clinical Features

The signs of airway obstruction include urgent dyspnea of sudden onset, inspiratory stridor, labored breathing, air hunger, active accessory muscles of respiration and alae nasi, and intercostal retraction.

Airway Management

The investigation includes laryngoscopy and treatment is removal of the cause and management of airway. The airway management needs mention here as airway obstruction is a common life-threatening emergency. All the medical personnel must be well trained to provide immediate treatment to save life. The management procedures include endotracheal intubation, cricothyrotomy, and tracheostomy.

Endotracheal intubation

In this procedure, a tube is passed in the upper airway to keep the passage clear for breathing. The larynx is visualized by using a laryngoscope and an endotracheal tube is passed up to subglottic region which is connected to Ambu bag, Boyle's machine, or ventilator. Initially, the respiratory failure is managed by endotracheal intubation but there is danger of subglottic stenosis with extended intubation. Hence, as soon as it is clear that the patient will require protracted ventilator support, tracheostomy should replace endotracheal tube.

Cricothyrotomy

In acute emergency, cricothyrotomy secures an airway more rapidly than tracheostomy with fewer immediate complications such as pneumothorax and hemorrhage. But one should change it to tracheostomy as soon as possible.

Technique

It is done by making an opening in cricothyroid membrane just below the notch of thyroid cartilage and above the cricoid cartilage, and inserting a small endotracheal or tracheostomy tube.

Tracheostomy

It is a surgical procedure in which an opening is made in the anterior wall of trachea to bypass the larynx. It is done in acute upper airway obstruction when the larynx cannot be intubated.

Indications of tracheostomy

- Airway obstruction at or above the level of larynx
- Respiratory failure requiring respiratory support
- Life-threatening aspiration pneumonia, need to improve pulmonary toilet to correct problems related to insufficient clearing of tracheobronchial secretions, and sleep apnea, which are less frequent indications

Technique

- **Anesthesia**: It is usually done under local anesthesia infiltrated along the line of incision.
- **Preparation and position**: A child patient is wrapped in a towel to prevent movements. An adult patient lies supine with head extended by putting a pillow behind the shoulders. The chin and suprasternal notch must be in the same straight line.
- **Skin incision**: A midline vertical incision is given from the upper border of cricoid to suprasternal notch dividing the skin, subcutaneous tissue, and investing and pretracheal fascia. For cosmetic reasons, tracheostomy may be done by a transverse incision between the thyroid cartilage and the suprasternal notch.
- **Identification of trachea**: The isthmus of thyroid is either retracted up or divided. The trachea is now exposed and recognized by its corrugated appearance due to tracheal rings.
- **Tracheostomy incision**: The cricoid is steadied by cricoid hook and an incision is made through the third and fourth rings of trachea with the scalpel directed upwards to avoid injury to left innominate vein. Too deep a cut into trachea may injure its posterior wall; hence, care is required.
- **Insertion of tracheal dilator**: The tracheal dilator is inserted into the opening to dilate

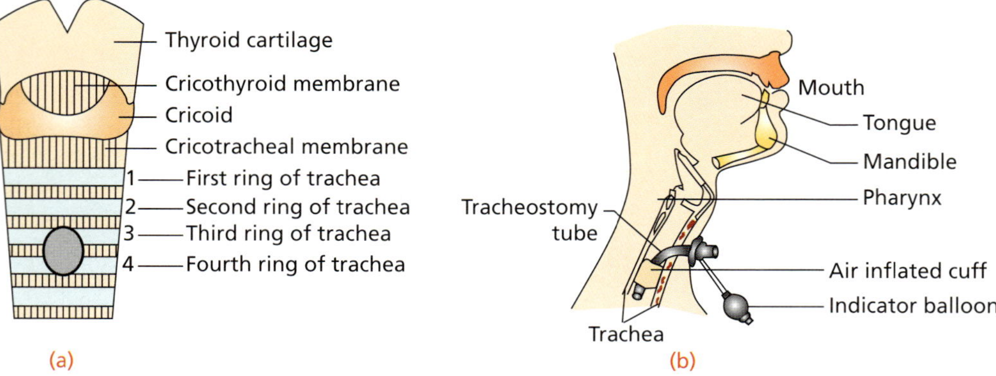

Figure 22.10 Tracheostomy. (a) Site of tracheostoma (third and fourth rings of trachea) and (b) tracheostomy tube.

the tracheal wound. Air gushes immediately in and out of the tracheal wound. In adults, the edges of tracheal wound are slightly trimmed to make an oval hole to prevent pressure necrosis of cartilage and for easy insertion of tracheostomy tube.

- **Insertion of the tracheostomy tube**: Now the tracheostomy tube (no. 5 or 6 in adults and 00 or 0 in a newborn) is inserted in the tracheal wound and tapes are tied around the neck to fix the tube. The wound is closed (Fig. 22.10a and b).

Complications

The complications of tracheostomy are described in Box 22.6. One of the common postoperative complications includes dislodgement of tracheostomy tube which may be difficult to reinsert. The surgical creation of an inferiorly based tracheal flap sutured to the inferior neck skin wound (Bjork flap) may make reinsertion of a dislodged tube easier.

Postoperative care

- Humidification of inspired air to prevent crusting and obstruction of inner tube
- Cleaning of tube several times daily
- Frequent tracheobronchial suction

Percutaneous dilatational tracheostomy (Ciaglia)

It is a quick bedside method of tracheostomy which is being practiced more and more. It is now the primary choice for elective surgical airway management in critically ill adults expected to require mechanical ventilation for more than 1–2 weeks. Here the skin is punctured and the puncture is dilated for passing a tube in the trachea; hence, it gives better cosmetic results.

Stridor

Stridor denotes a symptom of partial airway obstruction characterized by a harsh vibrating

Box 22.6 Complications of tracheostomy

Intraoperative complications

- Hemorrhage, mostly venous ooze
- Difficulty in exposure of trachea, especially in children
- Injury to posterior wall of trachea and structures in vicinity
- Difficulty in introduction of tube

Postoperative complications

- Obstruction of inner tube
- Dislodgement of tracheostomy tube
- Tracheal stricture or stenosis
- Tracheoesophageal fistula
- Tracheomalacia

noise produced as the air passes in and out of partially obstructed air passage.

Types It is of three types:

- Inspiratory stridor which is due to laryngeal obstruction above vocal cords
- Expiratory stridor which is thoracic tracheal and bronchial obstruction below vocal cords
- Biphasic stridor which is due to subglottic and cervical tracheal obstruction

Etiology The causes of stridor are described in Box 22.7.

Management

The cause of stridor is found by clinical features and investigations, and treated by removal of the cause.

Box 22.7 Etiology of stridor

- **Congenital causes**
  - Laryngomalacia
  - Laryngeal web
  - Micrognathia
  - Laryngeal cleft
- **Traumatic lesions**
  - Birth trauma
  - Postnatal intubation injury
  - Tracheal stenosis following tracheostomy or endotracheal intubation
  - Foreign body
- **Extrinsic pressure**
  - Thyromegaly
  - Enlarged lymph nodes, for example, lymphoma
  - Aortic aneurysm
- **Infections and inflammations**
  - Acute laryngitis
  - Acute laryngotracheobronchitis
  - Laryngeal diphtheria
  - Whooping cough
  - Laryngeal tuberculosis
- **Neurological problems**
  - Bilateral abductor paralysis of vocal cords
  - Vocal cord spasm, for example, tetany, hysteria
- **Tumors of larynx**
  - Papilloma
  - Carcinoma

Hoarseness of voice

It is the main symptom of laryngeal disease characterized by roughness of voice resulting from variations of periodicity and/or intensity of consecutive sound waves. Laryngeal overuse is the commonest cause of hoarseness. The causes of hoarseness of voice are described in Box 22.8.

The cause of hoarseness of voice is found by clinical and investigative assessment and the treatment is removal of the cause.

Box 22.8 Etiology of hoarseness of voice

- **Congenital causes**
  - Laryngeal web
  - Laryngeal cyst
- **Trauma**
  - Laryngeal overuse
  - Blunt injury, sharp injury
  - Foreign body
  - Intubation
- **Tumors of airway**
  - *Benign*: Papilloma, hemangioma, chondroma
  - *Malignant*: Carcinoma
- **Tumor-like lesions**
  - Vocal cord nodules
  - Vocal cord polyp
- **Infections and inflammations of larynx**
  - Acute
    - Acute laryngitis
    - Laryngotracheobronchitis
    - Diphtheria
  - Chronic
    - Tuberculosis
    - Syphilis
    - Fungal infection
    - Chronic laryngitis
    - Atrophic laryngitis
- **Other causes**
  - Vocal cord paralysis
  - Arthritis of cricoarytenoid joint
  - Laryngeal leukoplakia
  - Functional dysphonia or aphonia

KEY POINTS

- The most important structure inside the larynx is vocal cords. The cricoid is the only complete cartilaginous ring in the airway. Hence, its integrity is critical in maintaining a patent airway.
- The most common cause of laryngeal trauma is an automobile accident. The most common injury is vertical fracture of thyroid cartilage with or without fracture of cricoid cartilage. An unreduced fracture of cricoid may result in subglottic stenosis. Escape of air into tissues around larynx may cause subcutaneous emphysema, pneumomediastinum, and pneumothorax.
- Vocal cord paralysis may occur from a lesion or damage to the vagus nerve or recurrent laryngeal nerve but in most cases it results from injury to the laryngeal nerves during thyroid surgery. The paralysis of vocal cords manifests as vocal cord immobility. The vocal cords may become immobile due to causes other than palsy.
- Unilateral vocal cord paralysis is treated by medialization of paralyzed cord by using injectable materials. Acute-onset bilateral palsy causes airway obstruction that requires emergency tracheostomy.
- If a foreign body is lodged in larynx, there is immediate pain in the neck, laryngospasm, dyspnea, and inspiratory stridor. Heimlich maneuver or endoscopic removal of the foreign body is the treatment of choice.
- Acute laryngitis is caused mainly by viruses. It is usually a self-limiting problem. If the hoarseness of voice persists for more than a few days, the possibility of secondary bacterial invasion must be considered.
- Chronic inflammation of larynx is related to many causative factors such as voice misuse, chronic smoking, inhalation of vocal irritants, gastroesophageal reflux (GOR), and alcoholism. Hoarseness of voice of a long duration is the presenting symptom.
- GOR into the larynx (laryngopharyngeal reflux) can cause chronic hoarseness even without heartburn and regurgitation. It is treated by omeprazole.
- Intubation granuloma is the formation of a reparative granuloma at posterior one-third of vocal cords following overenthusiastic endolaryngeal surgery, endotracheal intubation, and rigid bronchoscopy.
- Epiglottitis is a rapidly progressive acute inflammation of supraglottic larynx characterized by cherry red tip of swollen epiglottis and "thumb sign" on radiography. Airway management and antibiotics are the treatment of choice.
- Recurrent respiratory papillomatosis is caused by human papillomavirus (HPV) types 6 and 11. Hoarseness of voice is the primary symptom. It is treated by repeated laser vaporization or cold knife resection via operative laryngoscope.
- Carcinoma of larynx is etiologically related to smoking and alcoholism and characterized by hoarseness of voice. The diagnosis is confirmed by endoscopic biopsy. Early cancer is treated by radiation and late by surgical excision including laryngectomy and chemoradiation or both.
- Laryngocele is dilatation or herniation of laryngeal ventricle due to a persistent increase in transglottic air pressure as in trumpet players. The treatment of symptomatic laryngocele is excision.
- In acute emergency, cricothyrotomy secures an airway more rapidly than tracheostomy with fewer immediate complications. But one should change it to tracheostomy as soon as possible.
- Tracheostomy is done in acute upper airway obstruction when the larynx cannot be intubated by inserting a tracheostomy tube through third and fourth rings of trachea.
- Percutaneous dilatational tracheostomy is now the primary choice for elective surgical airway management in critically ill adults expected to require mechanical ventilation for more than 1–2 weeks.
- Stridor is characterized by a harsh vibrating noise produced as the air passes in and out of partially obstructed air passage. Inspiratory stridor is laryngeal and the obstruction is above vocal cords. Expiratory stridor is thoracic tracheal and bronchial with obstruction below the vocal cords. Treatment is removal of cause and endotracheal intubation or tracheostomy.
- Hoarseness of voice is the main symptom of laryngeal diseases. Treatment is removal of the cause.

SELF-ASSESSMENT

Long answer questions

1. What is laryngitis? Discuss the etiology, clinical features, and treatment of tuberculous laryngitis.
2. What are the causes of upper airway obstruction? Describe the clinical signs of airway obstruction and discuss its treatment.
3. Discuss the indications, technique, and complications of tracheostomy.

Short answer questions

1. Vocal cord palsy
2. Tuberculosis of larynx
3. Recurrent respiratory papillomatosis
4. Laryngocele
5. Cricothyrotomy
6. Tracheostomy

Multiple choice questions

1. The most important structure in the anatomy of larynx is
   (a) Thyroid cartilage
   (b) Vocal cords
   (c) Cricoid cartilage
   (d) Aryepiglottic fold
2. Which of the following is the only complete cartilaginous ring in the respiratory passage?
   (a) Thyroid cartilage
   (b) Cricoid cartilage
   (c) First tracheal ring
   (d) Second tracheal ring
3. What is the commonest cause of vocal cord paralysis?
   (a) Carcinoma of thyroid
   (b) Injuries of neck
   (c) Thyroid surgery
   (d) Skull base tumors
4. Which is the most common foreign body aspirated into the larynx in adults?
   (a) Coins
   (b) Pins
   (c) Poorly chewed pieces of food
   (d) Beans
5. The most common cause of acute laryngitis is
   (a) Staphylococcal infection
   (b) Streptococcal infection
   (c) Viral infection
   (d) Chlamydial infection
6. Chronic laryngitis is related to all of the following factors, except
   (a) Voice misuse
   (b) Diabetes mellitus
   (c) Gastroesophageal reflux
   (d) Chronic allergies
7. Stage II tuberculous laryngitis is characterized by all of the following, except
   (a) Mouse-nibbled appearance of vocal cords
   (b) Pallid mucosa due to edema
   (c) Perichondritis
   (d) Necrosis of laryngeal cartilages
8. All of the following are true about recurrent respiratory papillomatosis, except
   (a) It is caused by human papillomavirus 6 and 11
   (b) It may involve the entire respiratory tract
   (c) The first site of occurrence in the larynx is subglottic region
   (d) Hoarseness of voice is the primary symptom
9. What is the first treatment of choice in recurrent respiratory papillomatosis?
   (a) Interferon alfacon
   (b) Aerosolized 5-fluorouracil
   (c) Microscopic CO_2 laser excision
   (d) Podophyllum
10. Which of the following is the most common benign tumor of larynx?
   (a) Lipoma
   (b) Chondroma
   (c) Recurrent respiratory papillomatosis
   (d) Neurofibroma
11. Which of the following is the most important etiological factor in laryngeal carcinoma?
   (a) Tobacco chewing
   (b) Smoking
   (c) Syphilis
   (d) Alcoholism

(CONTD...)

SELF-ASSESSMENT *(...CONTD)*

12. Which of the following is the most common cancer type of larynx?
    (a) Adenocarcinoma
    (b) Squamous cell carcinoma
    (c) Basal cell carcinoma
    (d) Transitional cell carcinoma
13. Which of the following is the most common symptom of carcinoma of larynx?
    (a) Odynophagia
    (b) Inspiratory stridor
    (c) Hemoptysis
    (d) Hoarseness of voice
14. The most common site of metastases in carcinoma of larynx is
    (a) Cervical lymph nodes
    (b) Lungs
    (c) Brain
    (d) Bones
15. The most important diagnostic investigation of carcinoma of larynx is
    (a) Laryngoscopy
    (b) Laryngoscopy and biopsy
    (c) CT scan
    (d) Barium swallow
16. What is a T3 tumor in carcinoma of larynx?
    (a) Carcinoma in situ
    (b) Tumor confined to site of origin
    (c) Tumor which has spread to an adjacent laryngeal site with tumor or impaired vocal cord mobility
    (d) Tumor confined to larynx with fixation of hemilarynx
17. All of the following are true about laryngocele, except
    (a) It occurs in trumpet players and glass blowers
    (b) It is due to chronically raised intralaryngeal pressure
    (c) It is herniation of mucous membrane of larynx through cricothyroid membrane
    (d) The patient may have an intermittent swelling in the neck near the midline
18. How do you treat a laryngocele?
    (a) By complete excision of sac
    (b) By partial excision of sac
    (c) By inversion of sac
    (d) Does not need any treatment
19. Stridor is a sign of
    (a) Nasopharyngeal obstruction
    (b) Oropharyngeal obstruction
    (c) Obstruction in the hypopharynx
    (d) Laryngeal obstruction
20. What do you mean by laser?
    (a) Light amplification by stimulated emission of radiation
    (b) Light amplification by stimulated electronic radiation
    (c) Limited augmentation by stimulated electronic radiation
    (d) Light augmentation by stimulated emission of radiation

Answers

1. (b) 2. (b) 3. (c) 4. (c) 5. (c) 6. (b) 7. (a) 8. (c) 9. (c) 10. (c) 11. (b) 12. (b) 13. (d) 14. (a) 15. (b) 16. (d) 17. (c) 18. (a) 19. (d) 20. (a)

Diseases of Thyroid

23

Surgical anatomy

The thyroid gland is a shield-shaped structure lying in the lower part of front of neck in close relationship to larynx and trachea in the visceral compartment of neck. It is a bilobed structure and the lobes are joined together by an isthmus which is situated in front of second, third, and fourth rings of trachea (Fig. 23.1). It weighs about 20–25 g. Posteriorly, it has two structures of surgical importance, that is, recurrent laryngeal nerve and parathyroids (Fig. 23.2).

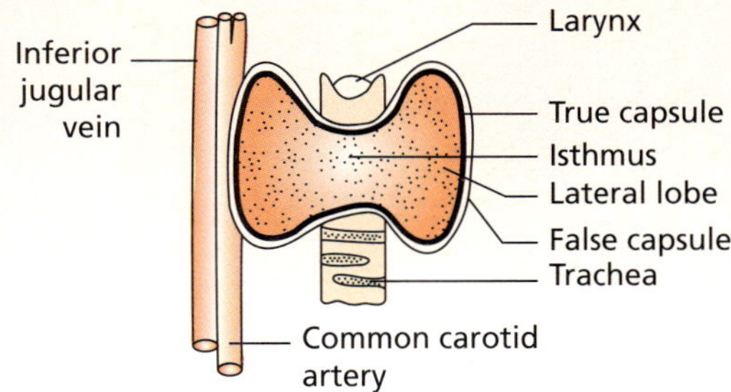

Figure 23.1 Anatomy of thyroid as seen from the front.

Embryology It develops mainly from the thyroglossal tract which passes from the foramen cecum at the base of tongue to the isthmus.

Arterial Supply

- Superior thyroid artery is a branch of external carotid artery which enters the upper pole of the lateral lobe.
- Inferior thyroid artery is a branch of thyrocervical trunk that enters the posterior aspect of gland and crosses the recurrent laryngeal nerve.
- Thyroidea ima artery is a branch of brachiocephalic trunk or direct branch of aortic arch and enters the lower part of thyroid.

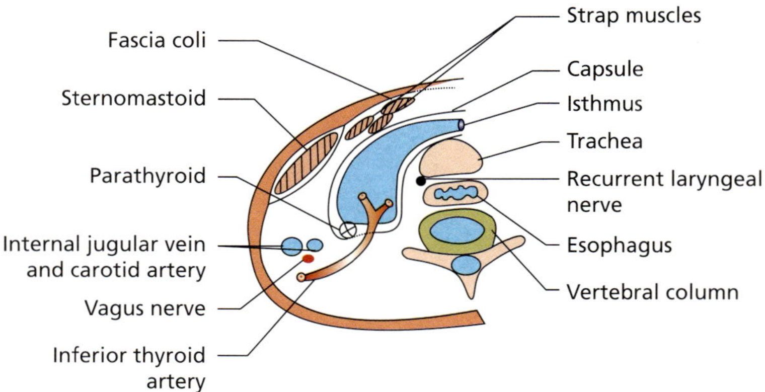

Figure 23.2 Anatomy of thyroid as seen in a transverse section of right half of neck.

Venous Drainage

- Superior thyroid vein at upper pole that enters the internal jugular vein
- Middle thyroid vein that drains into internal jugular vein
- Inferior thyroid veins which drain into innominate vein

Lymphatic Drainage From subcapsular lymphatic plexus, it occurs into pretracheal nodes (Delphic nodes) and prelaryngeal nodes which finally drain into lower deep cervical and mediastinal nodes.

Nerves Related to Thyroid

- External laryngeal nerve is a branch of superior laryngeal nerve that runs close to superior thyroid vessels and supplies cricothyroid muscle. This nerve is close to the artery near its origin and away at the upper pole of thyroid. Hence, during thyroidectomy, the upper pedicle is ligated as close to thyroid as possible.
- Recurrent laryngeal nerve runs in the tracheoesophageal groove and runs in the branches of inferior thyroid artery. Hence, this artery is ligated away from the gland to prevent injury to this nerve.

Physiology

The follicles of thyroid secrete two main thyroid hormones, that is, triiodothyronine (T_3) and thyroxine (T_4), which are under the control of thyroid-stimulating hormone (TSH) of anterior pituitary, and regulates (stimulates) the body metabolism. In between the follicles, there are parafollicular or C-cells which secrete calcitonin that helps in calcium metabolism.

The steps of synthesis of T_3 and T_4 are:

- Trapping of iodine from blood into thyroid
- Oxidation of iodine to inorganic iodine with the help of peroxidase
- Formation of iodotyrosine by combination of iodine with tyrosine resulting in the formation of monoiodotyrosine and diiodotyrosine
- Coupling of two molecules of diiodotyrosine resulting in the formation of thyroxine (T_4), and that of one molecule of monoiodotyrosine and one of diiodotyrosine resulting in the formation of triiodothyronine (T_3) (these hormones combine with globulin to form a colloid called thyroglobulin stored in thyroid gland and released as and when required)

Clinical presentation of thyroid diseases

The thyroid diseases present clinically in the manner given in the subsequent text.

Swelling The normal thyroid is neither visible nor palpable. Visibility and palpability are the commonest abnormalities of thyroid. Thyroid diseases present as a swelling in front of neck which moves up with deglutition. (*Note*: A thyroglossal cyst moves up with deglutition and protrusion of tongue.)

- **Generalized thyroid swelling**: It has the shape of thyroid like a shield or butterfly. The common causes of a generalized swelling include puberty goiter, colloid goiter, nodular goiter, and thyroiditis.
- **Localized thyroid swelling**: Common causes are carcinoma, adenoma, or cyst (localized nodule).
- **Smooth swellings of thyroid**: These include puberty goiter, colloid goiter, and goiter of Graves' disease.
- **Irregular or nodular swellings of thyroid**: These include carcinoma, nodular goiter, and Hashimoto's thyroiditis.

Abnormality of Thyroid Function It presents as hypothyroidism (less than normal function) or hyperthyroidism (more than normal function).

- **Hypothyroidism**: It is characterized by weight gain, fatigue, lethargy, depression, weakness, dyspnea on exertion, arthralgia, muscle cramps, menorrhagia, constipation, dry skin, and headache.
- **Hyperthyroidism**: It is characterized by nervousness, restlessness, heat intolerance, increased sweating, pruritus, fatigue, weakness, frequent bowel movements, and loss of weight. There may be palpitation and menstrual irregularities.

As other parts or systems of the body, the thyroid is examined under the headings of inspection, palpation, percussion, and auscultation, the first two being the most important.

Inspection The inspection of thyroid is done from the front and both sides as such and when the patient swallows.

Palpation

- It is usually done by standing behind the patient and keeping both thumbs on the nape of neck and fingers of both hands on the front of neck on the thyroid. The neck is kept relaxed with a little flexion and tilt to the side that is being palpated and then the opposite side is palpated in the same manner.
- In Lahey's method, the palpation is done from the front. To palpate the right lobe, the gland is pushed to the same side with one hand and palpated with the other hand. The opposite is done to palpate the left lobe. By this method, the consistency and nodularity of the lobe and the posteromedial aspect of the gland is palpated.

Goiters

The term goiter is derived from the Latin word "guttur" which means "neck." Strictly speaking, goiter is a noninflammatory and non-neoplastic swelling of the whole thyroid, but now this term is employed for all types of swellings of thyroid. The goiters cause cosmetic problem or pressure symptoms on structures of neck, or may become toxic (functional problem).

Etiology

- A goiter usually develops due to persistent long-term stimulation of thyroid by TSH in response to long-term low levels of circulating thyroid hormone which are due to many causes, described in Table 23.1.
- It may sometimes occur due to inappropriate secretion of TSH from a microadenoma of pituitary.

Pathogenesis of Goiters

The pathogenesis of goiters is described in Flowchart 23.1.

Physiological goiter (diffuse parenchymatous goiter)

Etiology This goiter is mostly seen in females at the time of puberty, pregnancy, or lactation due to

Table 23.1 Causes of low levels of circulating thyroid hormone

Causes	Description
Iodine deficiency	• Average daily requirement of iodine: 0.1–0.15 mg • Endemic goiter occurs in areas where iodine is deficient in water and soil, thereby in the local food • Inadequate intestinal absorption may also result in iodine deficiency
Goitrogens	• Long-term use of goitrogens may produce a goiter • Examples of goitrogens include thiocyanate in cabbage, para-aminosalicylic acid (PAS), and antithyroid drugs such as methylthiouracil
Deficiency of thyroid hormone synthesis enzymes	Deficiency of thyroid hormone synthesis enzymes, for example, thyroperoxidase, may be responsible in many sporadic goiters
Estrogen receptors in thyroid tissue	All types of simple goiter are more common in females than in males due to the presence of estrogen receptors in thyroid tissue

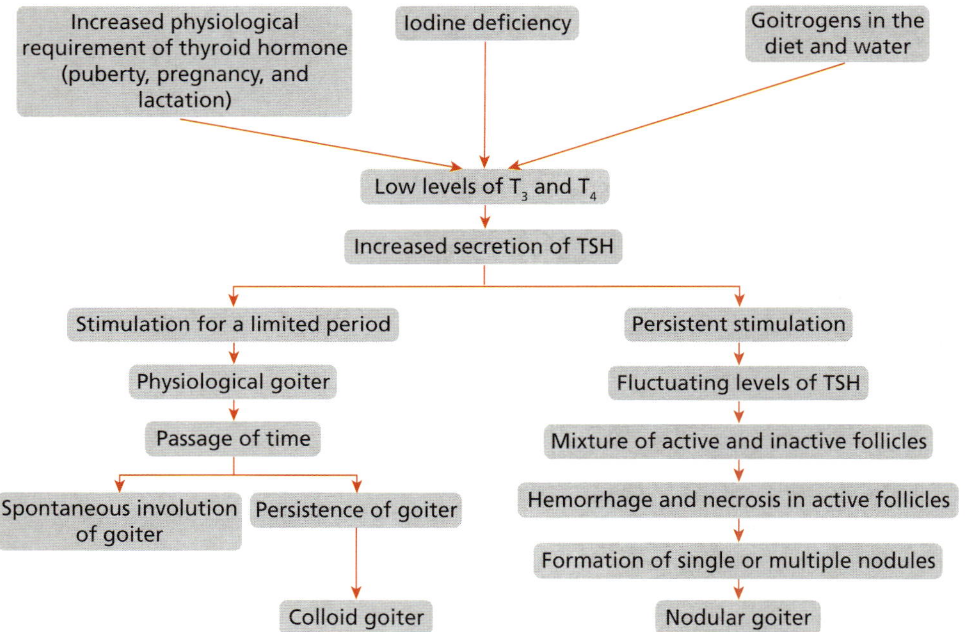

Flowchart 23.1 Pathogenesis of goiters. *TSH*, thyroid-stimulating hormone.

persistent stimulation of thyroid by elevated TSH level as a result of increased demand or stress.

Pathogenesis The stimulation causes diffuse hyperplasia of thyroid with active follicles all over and uniform iodine uptake. It usually settles down once the stress is over (reversible).

Clinical Features The patient presents with a mild, soft, smooth, uniform, and diffuse enlargement of thyroid (Fig. 23.3). There are no clinical signs of thyroid dysfunction.

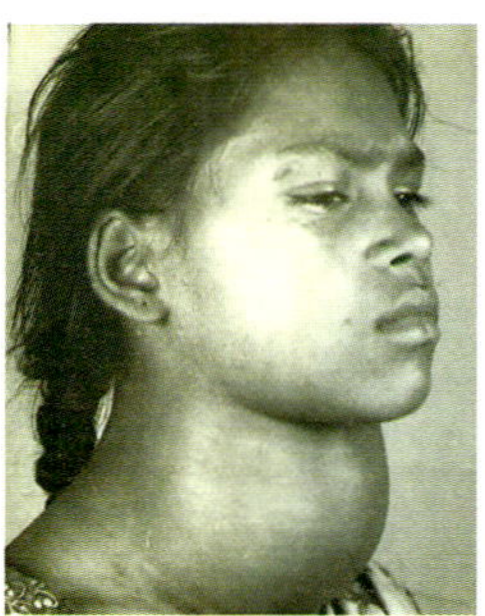

Figure 23.3 Puberty goiter in a girl aged 16 years.

Diagnosis Ultrasound shows uniform thyromegaly and thyroid function tests are within normal limits.

Treatment It is treated with thyroid hormone supplementation in doses of 0.15–0.2 mg daily.

Diffuse colloid goiter

Etiology If the stimulation of thyroid growth persists for many years or beyond puberty, the goiter continues and presents as a diffuse colloid goiter. It usually occurs due to iodine deficiency and hence commonly seen in endemic areas. It may occur sporadically in other areas where it may be due to dietary goitrogens. Microscopically the gland shows acini with flattened lining and distended with densely staining colloid.

Clinical Features The patient is usually 20–30 years of age, usually a woman who presents with a diffuse, soft, smooth, and uniform enlargement of thyroid (larger than a physiological goiter). Pressure symptoms may be present.

Diagnosis

- Serum T_3, T_4, and TSH levels are normal. ^{131}I study shows uniformly increased uptake which remains increased up to 48–72 hours.
- The 24-hour urinary excretion of ^{131}I is decreased which is indicative of iodine deficiency.
- Ultrasound shows uniform thyromegaly.

Treatment It is managed by avoidance of goitrogens, use of iodized salt, and thyroid hormone supplementation. If it fails, partial thyroidectomy or subtotal thyroidectomy with thyroid hormone supplementation should be done.

Nodular (multinodular) goiter

This goiter is characterized by enlargement of the whole thyroid having single or multiple nodules.

Pathogenesis Long-term persistent or recurrent TSH stimulation results in a mixed pattern with areas of active and inactive lobules. The active nodules are present only in the internodular tissue. Nodularity of the goiter may be due to the presence of clones particularly sensitive to TSH stimulation. The stages of development of a nodular goiter are described in Box 23.1.

Box 23.1 Stages of development of a nodular goiter

- **Stage I**: Diffuse hyperplasia due to persistent thyroid-stimulating hormone (TSH) stimulation
- **Stage II**: Overstimulation of some areas due to fluctuating levels of TSH leading to active follicles with increased vascularity
- **Stage III**: Hemorrhage and necrosis in some follicles which join together to form nodules

Clinical Features

- It is common in women in their late thirties and forties who present with a swelling in the front of the neck of long duration.
- The patient may present with dyspnea and dysphagia.
- It is a euthyroid goiter where the gland is enlarged as a whole, is firm, and has a single or multiple nodules (Fig. 23.4). The nodules may be colloid or cellular.
- The most common site of nodule is at the junction of isthmus with one lateral lobe.
- Pressure symptoms may be present.

Investigations The investigations done in a multinodular goiter are described in Table 23.2.

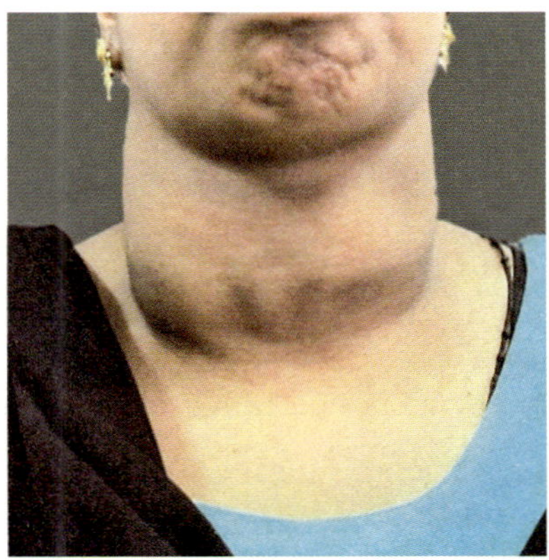

Figure 23.4 Multinodular goiter in a middle-aged woman. (Courtesy: Dr. A.C. Dwivedi)

Table 23.2 Investigations in a multinodular goiter

Investigations	Findings
Thyroid functions	Normal
Isotope study	Thyromegaly with areas of increased and decreased uptake
Radiography of neck	• Soft-tissue shadow • Retrosternal extension if present • Tracheal compression or shift, and ring or rim calcification
High-resolution ultrasound	• Identifies impalpable nodules and their vascularity • Nodules less than 0.3 cm are identifiable
FNAC	Ultrasound-guided FNAC is done from the most dominant and suspicious nodule
Indirect laryngoscopy	Done before operation to see the vocal cords as there may be asymptomatic vocal cord palsy of one cord
Blood	• Serum calcium • Thyroid antibodies to differentiate multinodular goiter from autoimmune thyroiditis

Complications The complications include compression of trachea, hemorrhage causing pain and rapid increase in the size of swelling, secondary thyrotoxicosis, calcification, and malignant change (usually into a follicular carcinoma).

Treatment

- Total thyroidectomy: It is a disease of the whole thyroid; hence, total thyroidectomy is the appropriate treatment, but it is associated with a significant risk of injury to parathyroids and recurrent laryngeal nerves.
- Subtotal thyroidectomy: The deeper or posterior part of thyroid is not much diseased. Hence, it can be left and not removed. Thus, subtotal thyroidectomy is the most popular operation in which nearly the whole thyroid is removed (Fig. 23.5). About 8 g of relatively normal thyroid tissue is left in each tracheoesophageal groove which is likely to protect the parathyroids and recurrent laryngeal nerves.
- Hartley-Dunhill operation: It includes removal of one complete lateral lobe (more diseased one), isthmus, and subtotal or partial removal of other lobe. After this treatment, it is easy to reoperate (one side only) in case of recurrence.
- Postoperatively, levothyroxine is given to meet the thyroid hormone requirement and to prevent recurrence.

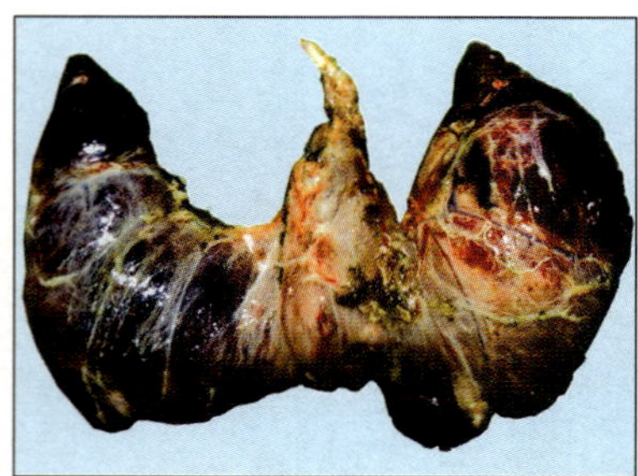

Figure 23.5 Subtotal thyroidectomy for multinodular goiter. (Courtesy: Professor Sandeep Tewari)

Retrosternal goiter

It is a goiter that extends more than 50% below the suprasternal notch behind the sternum.

Etiology Etiologically it may be primary type or secondary type.

- **Primary**: The primary type is very rare. It arises from ectopic thyroid tissue in the mediastinum. It is not related to the normal thyroid in the neck.
- **Secondary**: The secondary type is common. It is the extension of enlarged thyroid from the neck. It is usually a nodular goiter that usually arises from the lower pole. It goes into the mediastinum due to negative intrathoracic pressure, strong pretracheal muscles, short neck, and obesity.

Types Clinically it is of three types:

- **Substernal type**: It is the most common type in which the lower part of thyroid is behind the sternum.
- **Plunging type**: It is an intrathoracic goiter which comes out in the neck during coughing.
- **Intrathoracic type**: It is all the time present in the thorax and never in the neck.

Clinical Features

- The patient is usually a middle-aged, short-necked male who presents with dyspnea on lying down, cough and stridor, dysphagia, and engorged neck veins.
- Pemberton's sign: The patient is asked to raise the arms above the head. It results in visible dilated veins over the neck and upper part of the chest wall. Dull note is present on the sternum on percussion.

Investigations

- Chest X-ray shows the soft-tissue shadow behind the sternum.
- The diagnosis is confirmed by radioactive iodine (RAI) study and CT scan. The nature of goiter can be nodular, toxic, or malignant.

Treatment

- The goiter is usually excised by a neck incision as the blood supply of this goiter is from the neck.
- In a large retrosternal goiter or a malignant one, the mediastinum is opened by median sternotomy.

Thyrotoxicosis

Thyrotoxicosis is the symptom complex due to elevated levels of thyroid hormones. Hyperthyroidism is overproduction of thyroid hormones by the thyroid. Thyrotoxicosis can occur due to causes other than hyperthyroidism.

Etiology

Thyrotoxicosis can occur due to the diseases of thyroid and other causes listed in Box 23.2.

Box 23.2 Causes of thyrotoxicosis

- **Diseases of thyroid (Fig. 23.6)**
  - Graves' disease
  - Toxic nodular goiter
  - Toxic adenoma
- **Other less common causes**
  - Excessive intake of thyroid hormone
  - Administration of large doses of iodides in hyperplastic endemic goiter and autoimmune thyroiditis

Graves' Disease

It is a common form of hyperthyroidism.

Etiology

Graves' disease is caused by a wide variety of specific antibodies resulting in a thyroid-stimulating process. There is hyperplasia and hypertrophy of the whole thyroid due to prolonged action by binding of thyroid-stimulating antibodies to TSH receptor sites.

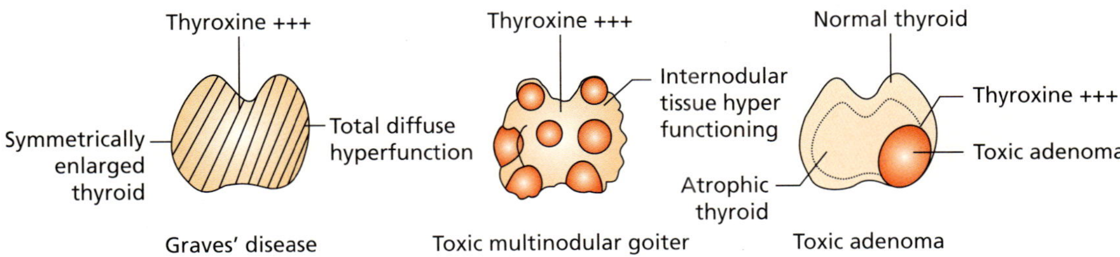

Figure 23.6 Three main causes of hyperthyroidism.

Pathology

The whole thyroid is uniformly and mildly or moderately enlarged with increased vascularity. Microscopically there is acinar cell hypertrophy and hyperplasia with absence of colloid in the acini lined by tall columnar epithelium. The epithelial cells are empty and look vacuolated.

Clinical features

- Most patients are women between 20 and 40 years of age.
- It is characterized by excessive sweating, weight loss, heat intolerance, and increased thirst.
- The thyroid is diffusely and uniformly enlarged, mild to moderate in size, soft, and smooth, and has a bruit (Fig. 23.7).

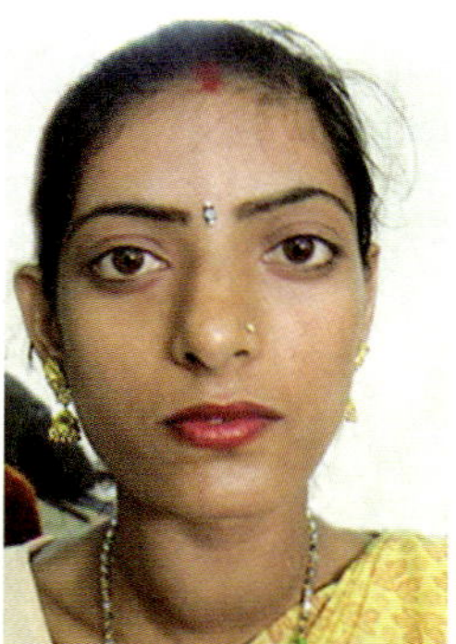

Figure 23.7 Young female with Graves' disease controlled on drugs.

The systemic signs of Graves' disease are described in Table 23.3.

Scoring system

The severity of toxicity is assessed by the presence and severity of some symptoms and signs, and is called Wayne's clinical diagnostic index. If the score is less than 11, the patient is nontoxic; if it is above 19, it is indicative of hyperfunction. Values between 11 and 19 are equivocal.

Investigations

- **Blood**: Serum T_4 and FT_4 (free thyroxine), and T_3 and FT_3 are usually elevated. Serum TSH (or TSHrAb) is usually detectable (65%). Antithyroglobulin or antithyroperoxidase antibodies are usually elevated but are nonspecific.

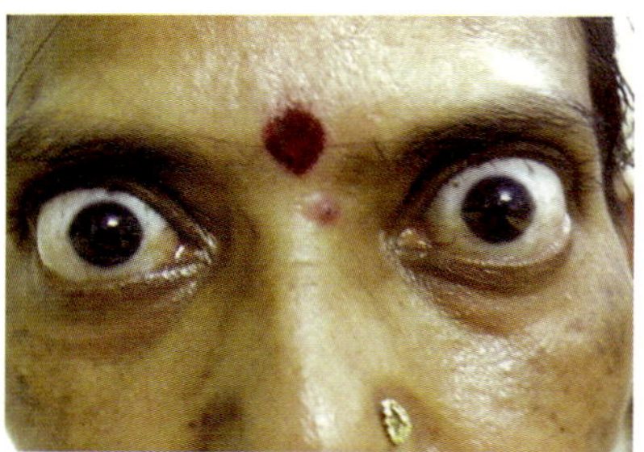

Figure 23.8 Graves' ophthalmopathy. (Courtesy: Professor Anand Misra)

Table 23.3 Systemic signs of Graves' disease

System involved	Signs and symptoms
Central nervous system	• Sleeplessness with altered sleep pattern • Emotional mood swings • Fatigue, excitability, agitation • Fine tremors
Gastrointestinal system	• Increased appetite • Increased bowel frequency to the point of diarrhea
Cardiovascular system	• Arrhythmias including ventricular tachycardia or atrial fibrillation • High-output cardiac failure or congestive cardiac failure
Graves' ophthalmopathy	The eyeballs have moved (pushed) forwards with exposure of upper part of cornea with a staring look (Fig. 23.8), lid lag, lack of convergence, and ophthalmoplegia (Graves' ophthalmopathy). These changes are related to the production of exophthalmos-producing substance (EPS)
Graves' dermopathy (pretibial myxedema)	It occurs in 3% of patients in whom the pretibial skin becomes erythematous with a thickened rough texture due to accumulation of glycosaminoglycans and lymphoid infiltration

- **RAI scanning and uptake**: It may be helpful in determining the cause of hyperthyroidism. In Graves' disease, it shows increased uptake throughout the gland (Fig. 23.9a and b).
- **MRI and CT scan**: MRI and CT scan of orbits are done to visualize Graves' ophthalmopathy affecting the extraocular muscles.

Treatment

It is treated by three methods: drug therapy, radioiodine (^{131}I), and surgery.

Drug Therapy It is the initial treatment given to all patients with the aim of symptomatic control. It includes:

- **Propranolol**: It is a β-blocker and relieves symptoms by reducing tachycardia. The dose is 10–20 mg two or three times daily orally depending on the pulse rate.
- **Thiourea compounds**: Carbimazole is given 10–15 mg 6 hourly orally followed by a maintenance dose of 10 mg two or three times daily. It may control hyperthyroidism. Then the patient is kept on a maintenance dose. The side effects include bone marrow depression, characterized by sore throat, and thiouracil goiter.
- **Lugol's iodine**: 10 to 12 drops 3 times a day is given for 14 days before thyroidectomy to reduce vascularity of the thyroid.

Radioiodine (^{131}I)

- The administration of radioiodine is an excellent method of destroying overactive thyroid tissue.
- The dose is 160 mCi/g of thyroid tissue.
- Indications: These include Graves' disease after 45 years of age, recurrent thyrotoxicosis after surgery, and autonomous toxic nodule.
- Contraindications: It should not be given to pregnant and lactating women as it is harmful to the fetus and suckling child.
- Advantages: The advantages are avoidance of surgery and its potential complications.
- Disadvantages: The disadvantages are hypothyroidism requiring hormone replacement and the ^{131}I facility not being available everywhere.

The toxicity of RAI (^{131}I) is described in Box 23.3.

Box 23.3 Toxicity of radioactive iodine (^{131}I)

- Worsening of ophthalmopathy and dermopathy
- May cause genetic damage resulting in leukemia
- May induce hyperparathyroidism
- Risk of malignant transformation of thyroid

Surgery

- It is the most rapid and effective method of treatment.
- Indications: Failure of medical and radioiodine treatment, younger patients, pregnant women, and patients with suspicious masses contained in a large thyroid are the indications of surgery in thyrotoxicosis.

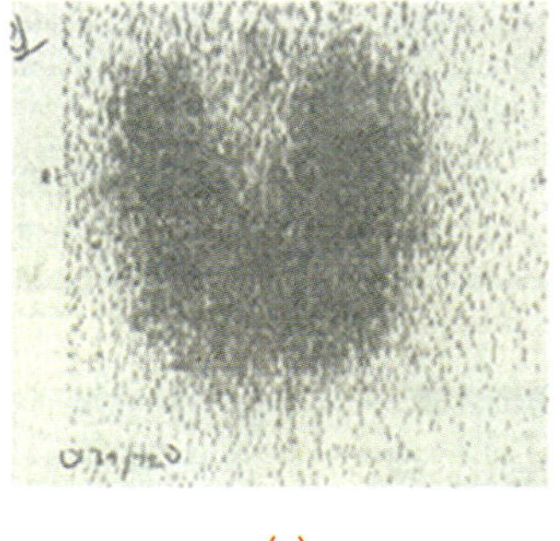

(a)

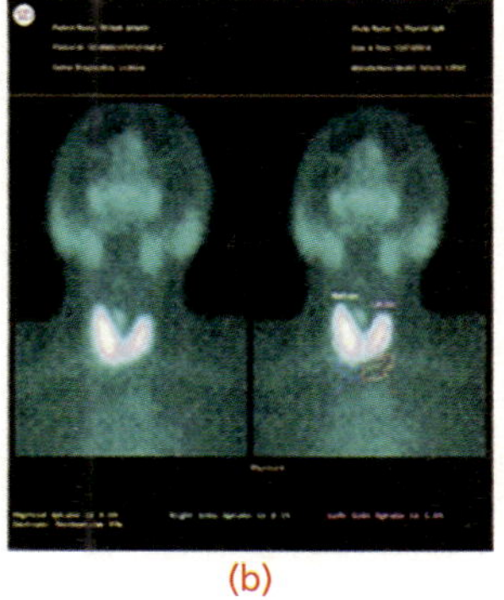

(b)

Figure 23.9 Radioactive iodine (RAI) scanning and uptake. (a) Isotope (^{123}I) scan of thyroid in Graves' disease showing uniform increased uptake of isotope and (b) ^{99m}Tc thyroid uptake and scan showing Graves' disease. (Courtesy: Dr. Himanshu, Sarkar Diagnostics)

- Types: These include total thyroidectomy, near-total thyroidectomy, and subtotal thyroidectomy.
- Preoperative preparation: The patient is rendered euthyroid before operation by the use of antithyroid drugs and β-blockers to control tachycardia. Preoperative use of Lugol's iodine for a few days reduces the vascularity of thyroid.
- Complications: The complications include hemorrhage, compression of trachea, and recurrent laryngeal nerve and parathyroid injury. They are described in Box 23.4. The thyrotoxic crisis (storm) is a specific complication of thyroidectomy in thyrotoxicosis which is now extremely rare (Box 23.5).

Box 23.4 Complications of thyroidectomy

- Immediate complications
  - Hemorrhage
  - Compression of trachea
  - Recurrent laryngeal nerve palsy
  - Hypoparathyroid tetany
  - Thyrotoxic crisis (storm)
- Delayed complications
  - Hypoparathyroidism
  - Recurrence of disease for which operation was done

Box 23.5 Thyrotoxic crisis (storm)

- It is acute exacerbation of hyperthyroidism
- It occurs in a thyrotoxic patient inadequately prepared for thyroidectomy
- It may follow an unrelated operation in a thyrotoxic patient very rarely
- It is characterized by hyperpyrexia, dehydration, restlessness, and uncontrolled atrial fibrillation
- Treatment includes intravenous fluids, cooling with ice packs, oxygen, diuretics, digoxin, sedation, and hydrocortisone
- Specific treatment includes carbimazole 10–20 mg 6 hourly, Lugol's iodine 10 drops 8 hourly orally or sodium iodine 1 g intravenously, and propranolol 1–2 mg IV or 60 mg 6 hourly orally to block α-adrenergic effects of thyroid hormone
- It has a very high mortality

Toxic Multinodular Goiter (Plummer's Disease)

- It is a multinodular goiter with secondary hyperthyroidism.
- Clinical features: It occurs in middle-aged and elderly people and has a milder course than Graves' disease. In this type, the cardiovascular manifestations are predominant while the central nervous system signs including tremors and eye signs are frequently absent.
- Investigations: The diagnosis is usually confirmed by ultrasonography which shows the nodules and radioiodine study which shows irregular increased uptake.
- Complications: The complications of a toxic goiter include hemorrhage with compression of trachea and high-output cardiac failure.
- Treatment: Antithyroid drugs such as methimazole and propranolol ER can control the symptoms but relapse is very common. Hence, it is usually treated by near-total or total thyroidectomy. The radioiodine treatment is not as effective as it is in Graves' disease.

Toxic Adenoma

Sometimes a solitary nodule in the thyroid may cause hyperfunction and produce clinical thyrotoxicosis.

- **Diagnosis**: On isotope scan, such a nodule is "hot" that causes suppression of iodine uptake by rest of the thyroid. This nodule is usually a follicular adenoma but malignancy must be excluded by biopsy as a follicular adenoma cannot be differentiated by FNAC from follicular carcinoma.
- **Treatment**: It is treated by hemithyroidectomy or lobectomy. Patients older than age 40 years or in poor health may be treated with ^{131}I therapy.

Hot and Cold Nodules

Based on radioiodine study, the solitary thyroid nodules can be functionally classified into two types as described in Box 23.6.

Box 23.6 Hot and cold thyroid nodules

- Hot and cold thyroid nodules are seen in radioactive isotope uptake study
- Hot nodule takes up more isotope than rest of thyroid. It is usually benign, for example, a toxic adenoma
- Cold nodule takes up less or no isotope than rest of thyroid. It may be a malignant nodule, hence needs further study

Primary and Secondary Thyrotoxicosis

Primary Thyrotoxicosis It starts with symptoms of both hyperthyroidism and a goiter at the same time, that is, the whole disease comes in one installment. Graves' disease comes under this category.

Secondary Thyrotoxicosis It occurs in a patient who has a preexisting nontoxic goiter for many years, usually a multinodular goiter and sometimes a solitary nodule (adenoma), and the toxicity appears after some time. Here the total disease comes in two installments.

The differences between the two types of thyrotoxicosis are described in Table 23.4.

The treatment of thyrotoxicosis is schematically described in Flowchart 23.2.

Hypothyroidism

Deficient thyroid function is called hypothyroidism. It may be due to primary disease of thyroid itself or due to deficiency of TSH of pituitary. It is of two types: hypothyroidism with goiter and hypothyroidism without goiter.

Etiology

The causes of hypothyroidism are described in Box 23.7.

Clinical Types of Hypothyroidism

Types of hypothyroidism include cretinism, juvenile myxedema, and adult hypothyroidism.

Cretinism

It is congenital lack of thyroid hormone.

Types

- **Sporadic cretinism**: It is due to complete or near-complete failure of development of thyroid. The parents and other children may be normal. It is a nongoitrous hypothyroidism.
- **Endemic cretinism**: It is due to maternal and fetal iodine deficiency. It is a type of goitrous hypothyroidism. A mother taking antithyroid drugs during pregnancy gives birth to a cretin.

Table 23.4 Differences between primary and secondary thyrotoxicosis

Features	Primary thyrotoxicosis	Secondary thyrotoxicosis
Age	15–25 years	30–50 years
Onset	Total disease appears in one step and in a short time period	Total disease comes in two steps, hence takes a long time period
Symptoms and signs	• Appears simultaneously • Duration is short	• Long duration of goiter • Short duration of symptoms of thyrotoxicosis
Goiter	Mild, diffuse, soft, smooth, and vascular	Multinodular or a solitary nodule
Predominant symptoms and signs	Pertains to CNS (e.g., tremors) and eyes (e.g., exophthalmos)	Pertains to CVS, for example, tachycardia and atrial fibrillation
Auscultation of goiter	Bruit may be present	Silent
Pretibial myxedema	May be present	Absent

CNS, central nervous system; *CVS*, cardiovascular system.

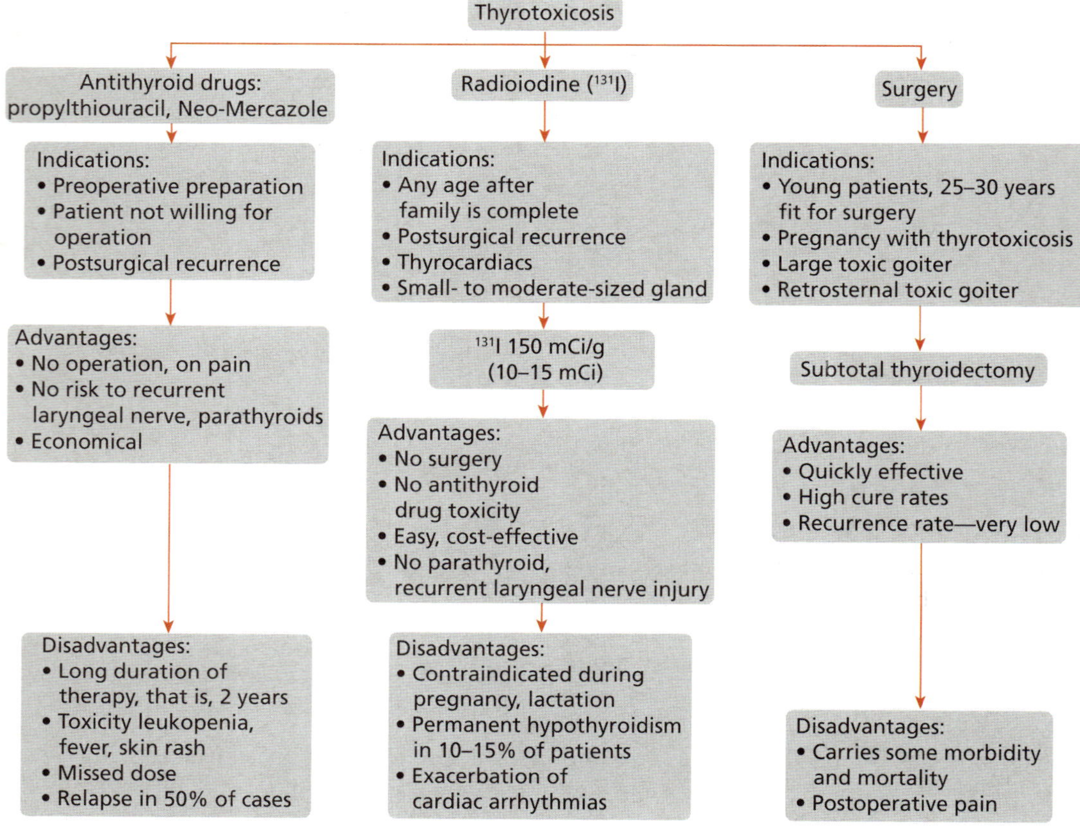

Flowchart 23.2 Treatment of thyrotoxicosis.

Box 23.7 Etiology of hypothyroidism

- **Hypothyroidism with goiter**
  - Hashimoto's disease
  - Iodine deficiency
  - Genetic thyroid enzyme defects
  - Drug goitrogens, for example, lithium, iodine, propylthiouracil, sulfonamides
  - Food goitrogens in iodine-deficient areas, for example, turnips, cassava
  - Increased peripheral resistance to thyroid hormone
  - de Quervain's thyroiditis following initial hyperthyroidism
- **Hypothyroidism without a goiter**
  - Deficient TSH secretion of pituitary
  - Destruction of thyroid by surgery or ^{131}I

TSH, thyroid-stimulating hormone.

Clinical Features The patient often presents with a pot belly, umbilical hernia, protruding tongue, and a pale and puffy face.

Diagnosis It should be diagnosed as early as possible in subclinical phase. To detect subclinical deficiency in neonates, biochemical screening of heel pad blood sample should be done for TSH and T_4.

Treatment It is treated with oral thyroid hormone for normal physical and mental development.

Juvenile myxedema

It occurs in adolescent children due to partial failure of development of thyroid.

Adult hypothyroidism

Types

- **Subclinical hypothyroidism**: It is more common.

- **Myxedema**: It is a severe form of hypothyroidism. Full-blown myxedema is rare.

Clinical Features

- **Early symptoms of hypothyroidism**: Fatigue, lethargy, weakness, arthralgia or myalgia, muscle cramps, cold intolerance, constipation, dry skin, headache, and menorrhagia
- **Early signs**: Thin brittle nails, thinning of hair, pallor, poor turgor of mucosa, and delayed response to deep tendon reflexes
- **Late symptoms**: Low speech, absence of sweating, constipation, peripheral edema, hoarseness of voice, decreased sense of taste and smell, muscle cramps, aches and pains, dyspnea, weight gain, and diminished auditory acuity
- **Late signs**: Goiter, puffiness of face and eyelids, carotenemic skin color, thinning of outer half of eyebrows, thickening of tongue, hard pitting edema, and effusions into pleural, peritoneal, and pericardial cavities as well as into joints; possibility of presence of hypotension

Investigations

- FT_4 may be low or low normal.
- TSH is increased in primary hypothyroidism, and low or normal in pituitary insufficiency. T_3 assay is not a good test.
- Serum cholesterol, liver enzymes, creatine kinase, and prolactin are increased.
- There occur hyponatremia, hypoglycemia, and anemia.
- There is a high titer of antibodies against thyroperoxidase and thyroglobulin in Hashimoto's disease.

Complications They include advanced coronary artery disease and congestive heart failure, increased susceptibility to infection, megacolon, carpal tunnel syndrome, organic psychosis, and myxedema coma.

Treatment Levothyroxine (T_4) is the treatment of choice. It is partially converted in the body into T_3. It is taken early in the morning, 25–70 μg daily with water. The dosage can be changed according to the clinical response and serum TSH which is kept between 0.4 and 2.0 μm/mL. Once the patient is put on thyroid hormone, it has to be taken for the rest of the life. Nevertheless, the dose has to be tailored from time to time.

Prognosis With early treatment, striking transformation takes place with return to normal state in most of the cases.

Myxedema Coma

- It is a rare complication of severe hypothyroidism.
- Etiology: It is often induced by infection; cardiac, respiratory, or central nervous system illness; and cold exposure or drugs. It is often seen in elderly women with hypothyroidism who have missed to take thyroid hormone.
- Clinical features: It is characterized by deep stupor (coma) with severe hypothermia, hypoventilation, hyponatremia, hypoxia, hypercapnia, and hypotension. Convulsions may occur. It has a high mortality.
- Treatment: Liothyronine (T_3, Triostat) 5–10 μg is given intravenously every 8 hours for the first 48 hours. The hypothermia is corrected by the use of blankets, as faster warming may precipitate cardiovascular collapse. Hypercarbia requires intubation and assisted mechanical ventilation. Infections are treated aggressively.

Tumors of thyroid

Tumors of thyroid are not uncommon and include adenoma, carcinoma, and lymphoma which are described in the subsequent text.

Adenoma

- It is a benign tumor of thyroid which is not uncommon.
- Clinical features: It presents as a painless solitary nodule of insidious onset (Figs 23.10 and 23.11). It is commonly situated at the junction of isthmus with one of the lateral lobes or in a lateral lobe. It is hemioval or hemispherical, smooth, and firm but elastic. The rest of the thyroid is normal.
- Diagnosis: It is usually a follicular adenoma. It cannot be differentiated from a follicular carcinoma by FNAC; hence, biopsy should be

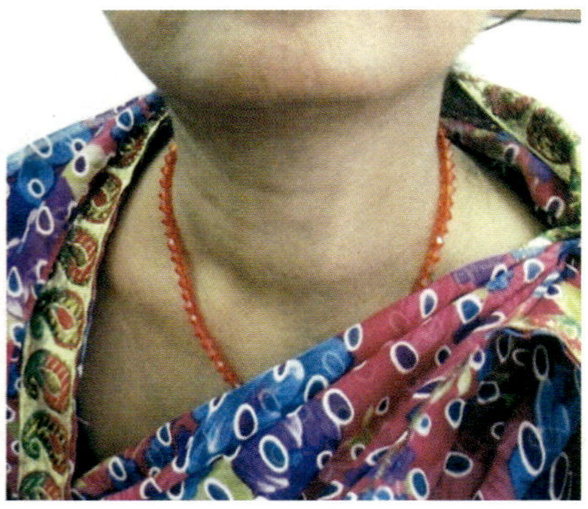

Figure 23.10 Adenoma of thyroid.

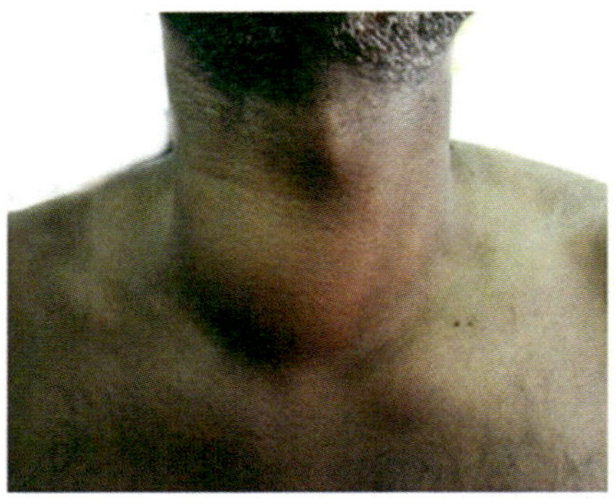

Figure 23.11 Adenoma of right lobe of thyroid without signs of thyrotoxicosis.

done to make an accurate diagnosis. X-ray of neck may show a soft-tissue shadow, maybe with shift of trachea.

- Complications: It may become toxic and cause secondary thyrotoxicosis.
- Treatment: It is treated by lobectomy or hemithyroidectomy.

Carcinoma of Thyroid

The carcinoma of thyroid is not a common form of malignancy as about 37,000 cases of this carcinoma are diagnosed every year in the USA (Fig. 23.12).

Early Disease

- The patient has a solitary nodule or localized swelling of thyroid of recent onset. A nodule is more likely to be malignant if it is present in a child or young adult or in a male.
- The diagnosis of carcinoma is made by investigations, that is, ultrasonography which shows a solid or complex nodule, radioisotope scan which shows a cold nodule, and ultrasound-guided FNAC or frozen section.

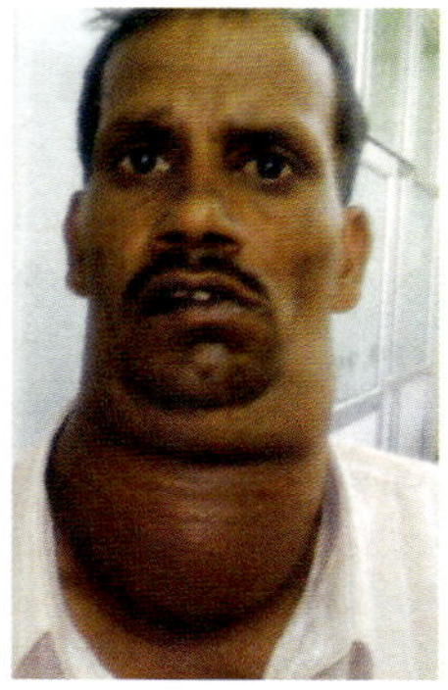

Figure 23.12 Carcinoma of thyroid in a male with a relatively fixed thyroid swelling with proximal edema of neck. (Courtesy: Professor Sandeep Tiwari)

Late Disease

- The patient has a large, irregular, and nodular swelling of hard or variable consistency. It may be mobile or fixed.
- The carotid artery on the side of the lesion may not be palpable (Berry's sign).
- Local pressure symptoms and/or signs of spread of disease, for example, pulsating scalp metastasis, may be present.

Etiology

Carcinoma of thyroid is idiopathic in most of the cases but the persons who have received a low dose of therapeutic radiation to thymus, tonsils, scalp, and skin during infancy, childhood, and adolescence have an increased risk of developing thyroid cancer (papillary carcinoma). It may run in families, especially the medullary carcinoma.

Types of Carcinoma

This cancer shows a wide range of variation. At one end of the spectrum is papillary carcinoma which occurs in young adults, grows very slowly, spreads through the lymphatics, and is compatible with a long life even in the presence of secondaries. At the other end is undifferentiated carcinoma which occurs late in life and is unencapsulated and invasive producing a large infiltrating mass leading to an early death due to local recurrence, pulmonary metastases, or both. Between these two extremes are follicular and medullary carcinomas.

Papillary carcinoma

Etiology The main etiological factor is irradiation given to the neck during early childhood.

Pathology Pathologically it is made up of colloid-filled follicles with papillary projections. In some cases, calcified lesions are found which are called psammoma bodies which are diagnostic of this cancer. Characteristic pale, empty nuclei are present in some cases which are described as orphan Annie eye nuclei.

Mode of Spread It spreads by intraglandular lymphatics within the thyroid and then the subcapsular and pericapsular lymph nodes. That is why 80% of children and 20% of adult patients present with lymph node metastasis. It may metastasize to lungs and bones.

Clinical Features It accounts for 80–85% of thyroid carcinoma and occurs usually in early adult life, more commonly in females, and presents as a solitary nodule with or without deep cervical lymph node enlargement.

Diagnosis The diagnosis can be confirmed by FNAC. Serum thyroglobulin is elevated in most metastatic papillary carcinomas.

Follicular carcinoma

Etiology It arises in a multinodular goiter especially in cases of endemic goiter. It should be suspected when the goiter starts growing rapidly.

Pathology It is an encapsulated lesion and contains follicles which make it difficult to differentiate from normal thyroid tissue. Capsular invasion and vascular invasion help in the diagnosis and differentiate it from a follicular adenoma.

Mode of Spread It usually spreads by hematogenous route to lungs, bones, and liver, and occasionally by lymphatic route to regional lymph nodes. The osseous metastases commonly involve the flat bones, for example, ribs and sternum, and vertebral column. They are vascular and pulsatile.

Clinical Features It accounts for 14% of thyroid cancers and occurs later in life than papillary carcinoma and presents as a solitary nodule or nodular enlargement of the whole thyroid. It may be hard or soft in consistency.

Diagnosis FNAC can be done but it cannot differentiate a follicular adenoma from carcinoma; hence, biopsy should be done. Serum thyroglobulin is elevated in most follicular tumors.

Hurthle Cell Carcinoma It is a variant of follicular carcinoma which is more likely to be multifocal and involves lymph nodes more than a follicular carcinoma. It makes thyroglobulin but does not have much avidity to radioiodine.

Anaplastic carcinoma (undifferentiated carcinoma)

Etiology It sometimes evolves from a papillary or follicular carcinoma.

Pathology Microscopically it is of three major types: giant cell, spindle cell, and small cell.

Mode of Spread It spreads to cervical lymph nodes and by bloodstream into the lungs.

Clinical Features It accounts for 2% of thyroid cancers and occurs in elderly persons. It grows rapidly producing a solid, hard, and irregular lump, diffusely involving the gland and invading trachea, muscles, and neurovascular structures early, causing laryngeal or esophageal obstruction. It may be painful and slightly tender.

Diagnosis Diagnosis is confirmed by FNAC or biopsy. The tumor can be imaged by CT scan or MRI.

Medullary carcinoma

Etiology About one-third of cancers are sporadic, one-third familial, and one-third are associated with MEN type 2. Medullary carcinoma is often caused by an activating mutation of the RET oncogene on chromosome 10.

Pathology It arises from parafollicular thyroid cells and can secrete calcitonin, prostaglandins, serotonin, ACTH, corticotropin-releasing hormone, and other peptides. It contains amyloid and is solid, hard, and nodular.

Mode of Spread It spreads by lymphatic and hematogenous route.

Clinical Features It accounts for about 3% of thyroid cancers and occurs at 50–70 years of age or in a young person with familial occurrence. It may be associated with diarrhea, episodic flushing, Cushing's syndrome, and cervical lymphadenopathy. The thyroid may have a single or multiple nodules.

Diagnosis All the patients should be screened for RET proto-oncogene point mutation on chromosome 10. Serum calcitonin is elevated in this cancer.

Investigations

Blood

- Thyroid function tests are generally normal in all thyroid carcinomas.
- Follicular carcinoma may secrete enough T_4 to suppress TSH and produce clinical hyperthyroidism.
- Serum thyroglobulin is elevated in most metastatic papillary and follicular tumors.
- Serum calcitonin is elevated in medullary carcinoma.

Ultrasonography It images the tumor and cervical metastases. It determines the site and extent of the tumor.

FNAC It can be done under ultrasound guidance. It gives the cytological diagnosis in most of the cases but in a follicular carcinoma biopsy should be done as FNAC cannot differentiate between a follicular adenoma and carcinoma.

CT Scan and MRI CT scan shows the primary tumor, its extent, and its metastases, especially pulmonary metastases, but it is less sensitive than ultrasound for detecting neck metastases.

^{18}FDG-PET Whole-Body Scanning It is useful in detecting metastases that do not take sufficient iodine to be visible on radioiodine scanning.

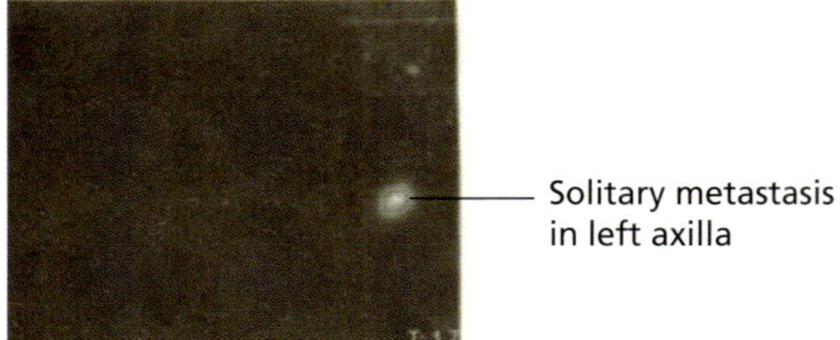

Figure 23.13 Transaxial SPECT image showing a focal area of increased radioiodine (^{131}I) uptake (round, small, white area) in the left axilla in a case of follicular carcinoma of thyroid—solitary metastasis in left axilla.

Radioiodine (^{131}I or ^{123}I) Scanning Neck and whole-body radioiodine scanning after thyroidectomy in a differentiated carcinoma is done to find local recurrence and distant metastases (Fig. 23.13).

Treatment

Differentiated Carcinoma These are papillary and follicular.

- **Thyroid lobectomy**: An indeterminate follicular lesion ≤4 cm in diameter is treated by thyroid lobectomy. If it turns out to be a carcinoma, a completion thyroidectomy is done. A lesion more than 4 cm in size is treated with total thyroidectomy.
- **Near-total thyroidectomy**: Instead of total thyroidectomy, near-total thyroidectomy can be done with nearly the same result but lesser chances of damage to recurrent laryngeal nerve and parathyroids.
- **Neck dissection**: In papillary and follicular carcinomas, limited removal of cervical lymph nodes is done.
- **Thyroid supplementation**: Postoperatively, oral levothyroxine 0.5–1.0 mg is given to do TSH suppression without causing clinical thyrotoxicosis. The serum TSH should be suppressed below 0.1 milliunit/L in patients with stage I and II disease, and below 0.5 milliunit/L in patients with stage III and IV disease.
- **Radioiodine**: After 2–4 months of surgery, the patient should be re-evaluated with radioiodine to find local and metastatic recurrence which is treated with radioiodine.

Medullary Carcinoma It is treated by total thyroidectomy with repeated neck dissection. It does not respond to ^{131}I therapy and is relatively resistant to chemotherapy.

Anaplastic Carcinoma

- It is treated with local resection (if possible) and radiation.
- Lovastatin may be given as it causes differentiation and apoptosis of cancer cells, but clinical studies have not been performed.
- It does not respond to radioiodine.

The differences between various types of carcinoma of thyroid are described in Table 23.5.

Lymphoma of thyroid

They are more common in elderly women and are most commonly B-cell lymphomas (50%), or mucosa-associated lymphoid tissue (MALT, 23%). They are treated with external radiotherapy and with chemotherapy in extensive lymphomas. MALT lymphoma is treated with simple thyroidectomy.

Thyroiditis

It is a rare disease of thyroid which is characterized by inflammation of thyroid.

Table 23.5 Differences between various types of carcinoma of thyroid

Features	Papillary	Follicular	Medullary	Anaplastic
Incidence	80%	14%	2%	3%
Main etiological factor	Irradiation of neck	Endemic goiter	Sporadic or familial	Unknown
Sex incidence	70% in females	72% in females	56% in females	56% in females
Microscopy	• Orphan Annie nuclei • Psammoma bodies	• Angioinvasion • Capsular invasion	Amyloid stroma like carcinoid	Poorly differentiated cells
Resemblance to normal thyroid	Very slight	Marked	Very slight	Very slight or not at all
Spread	Mainly by lymphatics	Mainly by bloodstream	By both lymphatics and bloodstream	Local infiltration
Clinical features	Nodular thyroid swelling with enlarged cervical lymph nodes	Nodular thyroid swelling with bony metastases	Thyroid swelling (difficult to diagnose clinically)	Irregular, rapidly growing thyroid swelling with local fixity and stridor
Diagnosis	FNAC	Frozen section	FNAC, calcitonin	FNAC, biopsy
^{123}I uptake	Minimal	Significant	Nil	Nil
Treatment of primary	Near-total thyroidectomy	Near-total thyroidectomy	Total thyroidectomy	Total thyroidectomy; if not possible, isthmusectomy and EBRT
Treatment of secondary	Excision or functional lymph node dissection of neck	Radioiodine or EBRT	Radical excision	Palliative EBRT
TSH dependence	Yes	Yes	No	No
Hormone production	Thyroxine rarely	Thyroxine rarely	Calcitonin, 5-HT, ACTH	Nil
Prognosis	Excellent	Good	Bad	Worst

ACTH, adrenocorticotropic hormone; *EBRT*, external beam radiotherapy; *TSH*, thyroid-stimulating hormone.

Acute Suppurative Thyroiditis

- **Etiology**: It is acute inflammation of thyroid with pus formation caused by streptococci, staphylococci, and pneumococci.
- **Clinical features**: The symptoms and signs include high fever, chills, severe pain in the neck, and a diffuse, very tender swelling of thyroid.
- **Diagnosis**: Ultrasound shows swollen thyroid with localized collection of pus. The diagnosis can be further confirmed by needle aspiration and culture of pus.
- **Complications**: The complications include formation of a thyroid abscess with spread of infection, that is, cellulitis, bacteremia, septicemia, and rupture on the local skin with sinus formation.
- **Treatment**: It is treated with antibiotics, pain relief, and drainage of pus.

Subacute (De Quervain's) Thyroiditis

- **Etiology**: It is probably viral infection of thyroid.
- **Clinical features**: The patient presents with neck pain, fever, malaise, and mild, uniform, and tender enlargement of thyroid. It may be associated with odynophagia and transient hyperthyroidism with mild tremor and tachycardia.
- **Diagnosis**: Erythrocyte sedimentation rate (ESR) is raised, T_4 is moderately increased, and TSH is low or normal. Radioiodine scan shows very low uptake.
- **Treatment**: Nonsteroidal anti-inflammatory drugs (NSAIDs) such as aspirin are given for relief of pain and inflammation. For symptomatic control of hyperthyroidism, propranolol 40–60 mg is given thrice daily for 4–6 weeks. If there is no relief of symptoms, prednisone 10–20 mg is given daily till symptoms are relieved. It is then tapered off in the next 3–4 weeks.

Autoimmune Thyroiditis (Hashimoto's)

It is more common than other types of thyroiditis. It is an autoimmunity-mediated destruction of thyrocytes.

- **Clinical features**: The patient is usually a premenopausal woman who presents with moderate diffuse enlargement of thyroid which is gently bosselated, very firm, and with or without pain and tenderness. It may present like a nodular goiter. There may be mild hyperthyroidism at the onset of illness followed by slowly progressive hypothyroidism.
- **Diagnosis**: It is characterized by low T_3 and T_4 levels and elevated TSH. Serum levels of antithyroperoxidase (90%) and antithyroglobulin antibodies (40%) are elevated. Ultrasound shows diffuse heterogenous density and hypoechogenicity. FNAC helps further in the diagnosis.
- **Treatment**: If hypothyroidism is present, levothyroxine is given in replacement doses, that is, 0.05–0.2 mg orally daily. If the goiter is large with normal or elevated TSH, it may shrink following levothyroxine therapy in doses to reduce serum TSH below normal while maintaining clinical euthyroidism. A large goiter not responding to thyroxine treatment may be treated with subtotal thyroidectomy.

Riedel's Struma (Riedel's Thyroiditis)

- **Etiology**: The cause of this condition is not known. It may be associated with retroperitoneal fibrosis, fibrosing mediastinitis, sclerosing cervicitis, subretinal fibrosis, and sclerosing cholangitis.
- **Pathology**: It is characterized by replacement of thyroid tissue with fibrous tissue which may extend to extrathyroidal structures.
- **Clinical features**: The thyroid is mildly enlarged, often asymmetric, stony hard, and often adherent to neck structures causing compression and invasion. Most of the patients have subclinical hypothyroidism.
- **Diagnosis**: It can be confirmed by CT scan which shows the abnormal thyroid and involvement of organs in the vicinity. FNAC may be done at the same time.
- **Treatment**: It is treated with tamoxifen 20 mg orally twice daily for years. It causes partial to complete remission in most patients within 3–6 months. Short-term corticosteroids may

be given. Surgical decompression is difficult and usually fails to permanently alleviate compression symptoms.

Solitary thyroid nodule

A solitary thyroid nodule is a common mode of presentation of thyroid disease. Apart from this, there is no other abnormality in the thyroid.

Etiology

The causes of a solitary thyroid nodule are described in Box 23.8.

Box 23.8 Etiology of a solitary thyroid nodule

- **Common causes**
  - Solitary dominant nodule of multinodular goiter where no other nodules are clinically evident
  - Follicular adenoma
- **Uncommon causes**
  - Differentiated thyroid carcinoma
  - Cyst of thyroid
- **Rare causes**
  - Thyroiditis
  - Lymphoma
  - Metastases

Clinical Features

A thyroid nodule is a very important clinical entity as 10–20% of them are malignant, without clinical signs of malignancy, that is, hardness, irregularity, and fixity. 30–40% of these are follicular adenomas. Hence, a solitary thyroid nodule must be carefully assessed.

The clinical features associated with a higher incidence of malignancy are described in Box 23.9.

Box 23.9 Features associated with higher incidence of malignancy in a solitary thyroid nodule

- Age: A solitary thyroid nodule in a patient younger than 25 or older than 60 years of age is more likely to be malignant. Between these two ages, it is usually a nodule of multinodular goiter
- Sex: A solitary nodule in a male is more likely to be malignant than in a female
- Family history: If there is a family history of a follicular or medullary carcinoma, the nodule is more likely to be carcinomatous
- History: A history of radiation to the neck during childhood is suggestive more of a carcinoma than of a benign nodule
- A nodule of recent onset, rapid increase in size, and associated with hoarseness of voice and/or cervical lymphadenopathy is more likely to be malignant

Investigations

Radiology

- **Thyroid scan**: Serum TSH level is determined. If it is subnormal, a radionuclide (^{123}I or ^{99m}Tc-pertechnetate) thyroid scan is done to find if the nodule is hyperfunctioning as the hyperfunctioning nodules are rarely malignant. Hypofunctioning (cold) nodules have an increased risk of being malignant but most are benign.
- **Ultrasonography**: It segregates the nodules into completely cystic, completely solid, and complex lesions. The first type is usually benign. The third type is likely to be malignant. This investigation has reduced the importance of thyroid scan.
- **Radiography of neck**: It shows shell-like calcification in a benign nodule, and punctate calcification in a malignant nodule. CT scan and MRI are not required

Biopsy

- FNAC: It is an investigation of choice in discrete nodule as it diagnoses a papillary carcinoma with great accuracy. It cannot differentiate a follicular adenoma from a follicular carcinoma where biopsy should be done. It helps in the diagnosis of the nodule of a multinodular goiter due to the presence of colloid.
- All benign thyroid nodules may be monitored by regular periodic palpation and ultrasound at every 6 months. If it enlarges, rebiopsy should be done.

Treatment

The treatment depends on the nature of the nodule. A nodule of one lobe may be treated by hemithyroidectomy.

Thyroid cysts

A cyst of thyroid is one of the common causes of a solitary thyroid nodule.

Etiology About 50% of cysts are due to colloid degeneration and most of the remainder are due to involution of a follicular adenoma. 10–15% of cysts are follicular carcinomas. A papillary carcinoma may also present as a cyst.

Clinical Features Bleeding may occur into a cyst when it presents as a painful swelling of sudden onset of the thyroid.

Diagnosis

- A tense cyst may feel hard and may mimic carcinoma. Hence, it should be confirmed by ultrasound (Fig. 23.14).
- Needle aspiration: The cyst is emptied by needle aspiration under ultrasound control, if possible, and the aspirate is sent for cytology. It may yield altered blood which is removed completely, but reaccumulation is quite common.

Treatment

- If the cytology is negative and the cyst does not refill, no further treatment is required.

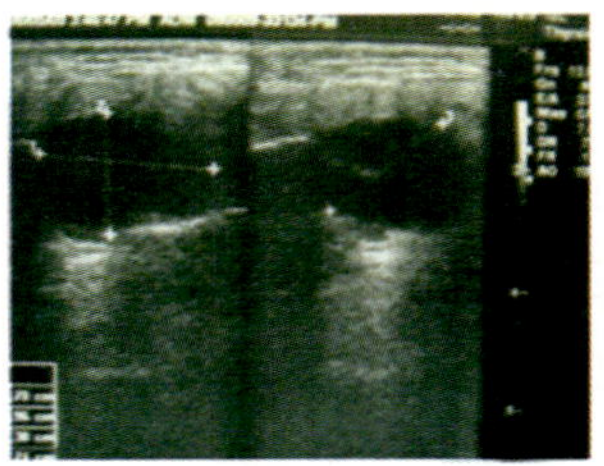

Figure 23.14 Ultrasonography of neck showing a cyst of thyroid. (Courtesy: Professor Surajit Bhattacharya)

- If it refills, ethanol injection may be given into the cyst. It has a success rate of 80%. Repeat injection may be required.
- Failures are treated by lobectomy.
- Malignant cysts are treated like a carcinoma.

Swellings of thyroid

A swelling of the thyroid is a very common clinical presentation. The differential diagnosis of thyroid swellings is being described here. It depends on two things:

1. What is the functional status of thyroid, that is, euthyroid or hyperthyroid?
2. Is it a swelling of whole gland or a localized swelling?

Depending on these two things, the swellings of thyroid are classified as described in Box 23.10. The patterns of thyroid swellings are given in Figure 23.15.

Box 23.10 Classification of swellings of thyroid

- **Euthyroid swellings**
  - *Swellings of the whole gland*
    - Puberty or physiological goiter
    - Colloid goiter
    - Nodular (or multinodular) goiter
  - *Localized swellings or a solitary nodule*
    - Adenoma
    - Carcinoma
    - Cyst
- **Hyperthyroid (toxic) swellings**
  - Graves' disease or primary thyrotoxicosis
  - Toxic multinodular goiter (Plummer's disease)
  - Toxic adenoma
- **Uncommon swellings**
  - Acute suppurative thyroiditis
  - Subacute (de Quervain's) thyroiditis
  - Hashimoto's thyroiditis
  - Riedel's struma

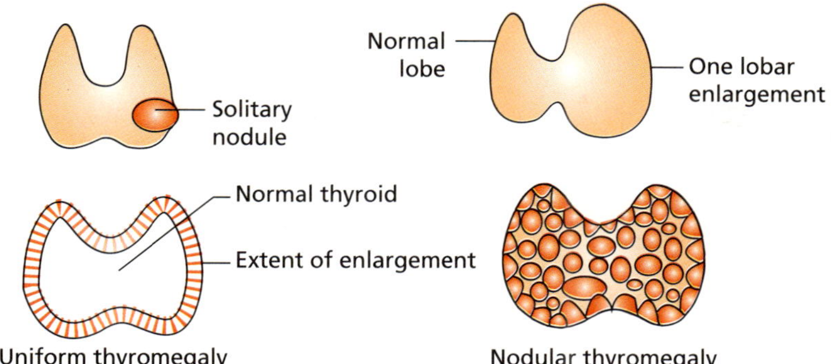

Figure 23.15 Patterns of swellings of thyroid.

Clinical Features of a Thyroid Swelling

The signs of a thyroid swelling include swelling in front of the neck which moves up with deglutition and may have the shape of thyroid. The symptoms and signs of hyperthyroidism are really the manifestations of stimulated body metabolism, that is, excessive sweating, weight loss, heat intolerance, sleeplessness, excitability, tremors, increased appetite and bowel frequency, and tachycardia.

Euthyroid Swellings

Nodular/Multinodular Goiter

- The patient is usually an adolescent girl or a young pregnant or lactating woman who comes with painless, mild enlargement of the whole thyroid of insidious onset.
- The swelling is uniform, smooth, and soft. There are no clinical signs of thyroid dysfunction.
- Ultrasound shows uniform thyromegaly and thyroid function tests are within normal limits.
- It is treated with thyroid hormone supplementation.

Colloid Goiter

- The patient is usually more than 20 years of age, commonly a female who presents with a painless, slow-growing swelling of thyroid. The whole gland is moderately and uniformly enlarged. It is smooth and soft or firm. Pressure symptoms may be present.
- Ultrasound shows uniform thyromegaly. Thyroid function tests may show mild hypothyroidism.
- It is treated by avoidance of goitrogens, use of iodized salt, and thyroid hormone supplementation. If it fails, partial thyroidectomy or subtotal thyroidectomy with thyroid hormone supplementation should be done.

Nodular/Multinodular Goiter

- The patient is usually a female 25–40 years of age who presents with a painless, slow-growing swelling of thyroid of insidious onset and long duration. The whole of the thyroid is enlarged and has a single (solitary nodular goiter) or multiple (multinodular goiter) nodules which may be felt as elevations on the surface. Pressure symptoms may be present.
- The lesion can be imaged by ultrasonography.
- A large multinodular goiter is treated with subtotal thyroidectomy or Hartley–Dunhill operation, and thyroid hormone supplementation to prevent recurrence.

Adenoma

- It presents as a solitary nodule of thyroid that is painless and slow growing. It is commonly situated at the junction of isthmus with one of the lateral lobes or in a lateral lobe. It is hemioval or hemispherical, smooth, and firm but elastic. The rest of the thyroid is normal.
- The diagnosis can be confirmed by ultrasound and FNAC but the latter cannot differentiate between a follicular adenoma and carcinoma. Hence, a biopsy is required to confirm the diagnosis.

- It is treated with lobectomy or hemithyroidectomy.

Papillary Carcinoma

- It is usually seen in a child or young adult who comes with a solitary nodule in the thyroid, or cervical lymphadenopathy mainly involving the lower deep cervical lymph nodes, or both.
- It is treated with total or near-total thyroidectomy with limited removal of cervical lymph nodes (functional dissection) followed by levothyroxine for TSH suppression.

Follicular Carcinoma

- It is usually seen between 20 and 50 years of age and presents as a solitary nodule or as a recent change in a long-standing goiter. It metastasizes in the bones and lungs.
- Follicular carcinomas are treated with total or near-total thyroidectomy with limited removal of cervical lymph nodes (functional dissection) followed by levothyroxine for TSH suppression. A metastatic follicular carcinoma is treated with RAI.

Anaplastic Carcinoma

- It is usually seen in a woman 60–80 years of age who presents with a rapidly growing, irregular, and hard thyroid swelling which produces early pressure symptoms.
- It should be treated by total thyroidectomy which is usually not possible in most of the cases. In such scenarios, it is treated by isthmusectomy and radiotherapy.

Medullary Carcinoma

- It usually occurs at 50–70 years, or in a young person with familial occurrence of this lesion. The thyroid has single or multiple nodules. The patient may have diarrhea, episodic flushing, Cushing's syndrome, and cervical lymphadenopathy.
- The diagnosis can be confirmed by FNAC and estimation of serum calcitonin which is elevated.
- This cancer is treated with total thyroidectomy with radical excision of cervical lymph nodes.

Cyst of Thyroid

- It has symptoms and signs similar to those of an adenoma of thyroid from which it cannot be differentiated.
- It is diagnosed by ultrasonography and ultrasound-guided needle aspiration.
- It is aspirated dry under ultrasound guidance. If it refills, it is treated with local ethanol injection.

Hyperthyroid (Toxic) Swellings

Graves' Disease (Primary Thyrotoxicosis)

- The patient is usually a young woman who presents with nervousness, irritability, insomnia, weight loss, increased appetite and bowel activity, heat intolerance, excessive sweating, muscle weakness, and menstrual irregularity. There are tremors in the hands (and tongue).
- Exophthalmos, retraction of upper eyelid, lid lag, lack of wrinkling of forehead when the patient looks up, and other eye signs may be present. Tachycardia, irregularity of pulse, and pretibial myxedema may be present.
- The thyroid is uniformly enlarged, mild to moderate in size, smooth, and vascular frequently with a thrill and bruit.
- The diagnosis is confirmed by estimation of T_3 and T_4 which are elevated, and TSH which is suppressed. The radioiodine uptake is increased uniformly all over the thyroid.
- It is treated with antithyroid drugs, radioiodine, or subtotal thyroidectomy depending on the age and physiological status of the patient, for example, radioiodine after 45 years of age and subtotal thyroidectomy or Hartley–Dunhill operation during pregnancy.

Toxic Multinodular Goiter (Plummer's Disease)

- The patient is usually a middle-aged person, more commonly a female, who presents with palpitation, exertional dyspnea, tachycardia, water hammer pulse, and missed and irregular heartbeat. The signs of central nervous system and eye involvement are absent. The thyroid is enlarged as a whole and has a single or multiple nodules.
- Serum T_3 and T_4 are elevated and TSH is suppressed. Radioisotope uptake shows patches of increased uptake all over the thyroid.
- It can be treated by antithyroid drugs, radioiodine, or subtotal thyroidectomy but subtotal

or near-total thyroidectomy is the treatment of choice.

Toxic Adenoma

- The patient has a solitary overactive nodule in the thyroid with atrophy of rest of the thyroid. It has clinical manifestations similar to Plummer's disease.
- Ultrasound shows a solitary nodule which shows overactivity on radioisotope scan ("hot" nodule). The rest of the thyroid is atrophic.
- It is ablated by radioiodine or surgery.

Uncommon Swellings

Acute Suppurative Thyroiditis

- The symptoms and signs include high fever, chills, severe local pain, and very tender swelling of thyroid.
- Blood shows polymorphonuclear leukocytosis, and ultrasound shows pus in swollen thyroid which can be aspirated at the same time and sent for culture.
- It is treated with broad-spectrum antibiotics and ultrasound-guided needle aspiration if pus has formed.

Subacute (de Quervain's) Thyroiditis

- The patient is usually a young man who has pain in the neck, sore throat, malaise, anxiety, fever, headache, and weakness, and may be associated with odynophagia and transient hyperthyroidism. The thyroid is slightly enlarged, smooth, tender, and firm.
- It is treated by giving aspirin to the patient.

Hashimoto's Disease (or Thyroiditis)

- The patient is usually a middle-aged woman who has a swelling of the whole thyroid or one lobe. The thyroid may be firm or hard, and sometimes rubbery and smooth or irregular.
- Elevated serum levels of antithyroid antibodies (antithyroperoxidase or antithyroglobulin antibodies or both) are often found.
- A patient with minimal enlargement of thyroid with euthyroidism should be kept under regular checkup. If hypothyroidism is present, levothyroxine 0.05–0.2 mg is given orally daily. It reduces the size of goiter an average of 30% over 6 months.

Riedel's Struma (or Thyroiditis)

- The patient is usually an elderly person who presents with mild enlargement of thyroid of insidious onset and long duration. The thyroid is irregular, hard, fixed, and nontender. It may be associated with mild hypothyroidism, and retroperitoneal and mediastinal fibrosis.
- The treatment of choice is tamoxifen 20 mg orally twice daily for many years. It may cause partial or complete remission within 3–6 months in most patients. Corticosteroids may also be given for a short period. Surgical decompression may be done to relieve pressure symptoms but it is difficult and associated with some complications.

KEY POINTS

- Thyroid gland is a bilobed structure joined together by an isthmus which is situated in front of second, third, and fourth rings of trachea. It is related to external and recurrent laryngeal nerves.
- The thyroid diseases may be disorders of structure (thyroid swelling or goiter) or function (hyperthyroidism or hypothyroidism).
- Goiter is a noninflammatory and non-neoplastic swelling of the whole thyroid. Goiters cause cosmetic problem and pressure symptoms on structures of neck, or may become toxic (functional problem). They include physiological goiter, colloid goiter, nodular goiter, and a retrosternal goiter. They are treated by dietary modification, thyroid hormone supplementation, and partial or subtotal thyroidectomy.
- Hyperfunction of thyroid is characterized by symptoms of stimulation of metabolism, that is, nervousness, irritability, insomnia, tachycardia, etc. It is of two types: Graves' disease (primary thyrotoxicosis) and secondary thyrotoxicosis.

(CONTD...)

KEY POINTS (...CONTD)

- Graves' disease presents mainly with symptoms of stimulation of nervous system, gastrointestinal tract, and exophthalmos. It is treated with antithyroid drugs, radioactive iodine, or thyroidectomy.
- Secondary thyrotoxicosis is due to toxic multinodular goiter or adenoma. It mainly produces cardiovascular symptoms and is treated by surgery. Adenoma may be treated by radioiodine.
- Hypothyroidism is due to low levels of thyroid hormones resulting in lowered metabolism. It may be congenital (cretinism) or that occurring later in life (myxedema).
- Cretinism is characterized by pot belly, umbilical hernia, protruding tongue, and a pale and puffy face. It is treated with thyroid hormone supplementation.
- The symptoms of myxedema include symptoms of hypometabolism, that is, fatigue, lethargy, weakness, constipation, dry skin, etc. Levothyroxine (T_4) is the treatment of choice.
- Adenoma is a benign tumor which presents as a solitary nodule of thyroid that is painless and slow growing. It is treated with lobectomy or hemithyroidectomy.
- Carcinoma of thyroid is characterized by solitary nodule, localized swelling, or total enlargement of thyroid of recent onset. It is of four types: papillary, follicular, medullary, and anaplastic.
- Papillary carcinoma occurs usually in early adult life and presents as a solitary nodule with or without deep cervical lymph node enlargement. Follicular carcinoma arises in a multinodular goiter. Capsular invasion and vascular invasion are the characteristic features. It usually spreads by hematogenous route to lungs, bones, and liver.
- Medullary carcinoma arises from parafollicular thyroid cells and can secrete calcitonin and other hormones.
- Papillary, follicular, and medullary carcinomas are treated by near-total thyroidectomy or total thyroidectomy followed by thyroid supplementation.
- Anaplastic carcinoma grows rapidly and causes early invasion of trachea, muscles, and neurovascular structures leading to laryngeal or esophageal obstruction. It is treated with local resection (if possible) and radiation.
- Inflammations of thyroid (thyroiditis) are uncommon and are of four types: acute suppurative thyroiditis, subacute (de Quervain's thyroiditis), autoimmune thyroiditis (Hashimoto's), and Riedel's thyroiditis. The first one is treated with antibiotics; the others are given symptomatic treatment.
- A solitary thyroid nodule may be seen in 10–20% of patients without clinical signs of malignancy. The features associated with a higher incidence of malignancy include a nodule of recent onset, rapid increase in size and associated with hoarseness of voice and/or cervical lymphadenopathy, solitary nodule in a male, family history of follicular or papillary carcinoma, history of radiation to the neck in childhood, and age (patient younger than 25 or older than 60 years of age).
- A cyst of thyroid is one of the common causes of a solitary thyroid nodule. Needle aspiration and cytology is done for diagnosis. If the cyst refills, ethanol injection may be given into the cyst or it is excised.

SELF-ASSESSMENT

Long answer questions

1. What do you understand by a goiter? Describe the etiology, pathology, clinical features, and treatment of a multinodular goiter.
2. Describe the etiology, pathology, clinical features, and treatment of Graves' disease.
3. Discuss the differential diagnosis of swellings of thyroid.
4. Describe the etiology, pathology, and clinical features of various types of carcinoma of thyroid. How will you treat a papillary carcinoma?

Short answer questions

1. Puberty goiter
2. Toxic adenoma
3. Adenoma of thyroid
4. de Quervain's disease
5. Riedel's thyroiditis

(CONTD...)

SELF-ASSESSMENT *(...CONTD)*

Multiple choice questions

1. Normal thyroid secretes which of the following hormones?
   (a) Thyroxine
   (b) TSH
   (c) Parathormone
   (d) ACTH
2. Calcitonin is secreted by
   (a) Parathyroid
   (b) Pituitary
   (c) Hypothalamus
   (d) Parafollicular cells of thyroid
3. Isthmus of thyroid lies in front of
   (a) Thyroid cartilage
   (b) Cricothyroid membrane
   (c) First, second, and third rings of trachea
   (d) Second, third, and fourth rings of trachea
4. Which of the following is the main function of calcitonin?
   (a) Increasing the calcium levels in serum
   (b) Decreasing the calcium levels in serum
   (c) Stimulation of thyroid function
   (d) Inhibition of thyroid function
5. A goiter is defined as
   (a) Any swelling in neck
   (b) Any swelling of thyroid
   (c) A swelling of lymph nodes of neck
   (d) A noninflammatory and non-neoplastic swelling of thyroid
6. Which one of the following is not a causative factor of a goiter?
   (a) Low levels of TSH in blood
   (b) Iodine deficiency
   (c) Para-aminosalicylic acid
   (d) Thiocyanate in cabbage
7. Which of the following swellings of the neck moves up with deglutition?
   (a) Suprasternal dermoid cyst
   (b) Sebaceous cyst
   (c) Pharyngeal pouch
   (d) Adenoma of thyroid
8. Which of the following swellings moves up with protrusion of tongue?
   (a) Thyroid carcinoma
   (b) Adenoma thyroid
   (c) Laryngocele
   (d) Thyroglossal cyst
9. What is the dose of thyroxine used for treating a physiological goiter?
   (a) 0.15–0.2 mg daily
   (b) 1–2 mg daily
   (c) 2–3 mg daily
   (d) 3–4 mg daily
10. Which of the following is not a complication of a multinodular goiter?
    (a) Compression of trachea
    (b) Hyperthyroidism
    (c) Hypoparathyroidism
    (d) Hemorrhage
11. Which of the following is not a radiographic finding in a multinodular goiter?
    (a) Soft-tissue shadow in neck
    (b) Calcification
    (c) Fluid level
    (d) Compression or shift of trachea
12. Which of the following is not a complication of subtotal thyroidectomy?
    (a) Hypoparathyroidism
    (b) Hyperparathyroidism
    (c) Hemorrhage
    (d) Recurrent laryngeal nerve injury
13. Graves' disease is
    (a) A type of hypothyroidism
    (b) A type of hyperthyroidism
    (c) A type of hyperparathyroidism
    (d) A type of thyroid carcinoma
14. Exophthalmos is a sign of
    (a) Hypothyroidism
    (b) Toxic adenoma
    (c) Plummer's disease
    (d) Graves' disease
15. Pretibial myxedema is a sign of
    (a) Graves' disease
    (b) Plummer's disease
    (c) Myxedema
    (d) Hyperparathyroidism
16. Graves' disease during pregnancy is treated by
    (a) Antithyroid drugs
    (b) Radioiodine
    (c) Subtotal thyroidectomy
    (d) None of the above

(CONTD...)

SELF-ASSESSMENT *(...CONTD)*

17. Plummer's disease is
    - (a) A type of hypothyroidism
    - (b) Toxic multinodular goiter
    - (c) Toxic adenoma
    - (d) Same as Graves' disease
18. All of the following are true about cretinism, except
    - (a) It is of two types: sporadic and endemic
    - (b) In sporadic type, the thyroid is not palpable
    - (c) The patient presents with pot belly, umbilical hernia, and protruding tongue
    - (d) It is an acquired lack of thyroid hormone
19. Cretinism is treated by
    - (a) Partial thyroidectomy
    - (b) Subtotal thyroidectomy
    - (c) Hemithyroidectomy
    - (d) Thyroid hormone replacement
20. All of the following are the features of myxedema, except
    - (a) There is fatigue, lethargy, and cold intolerance
    - (b) The skin is rough, dry, and cold
    - (c) Exophthalmos is present
    - (d) There is puffiness and weight gain
21. All of the following are the investigative findings in myxedema, except
    - (a) Low FT_4
    - (b) High titers of thyroid antibodies
    - (c) Increased TSH in primary type
    - (d) Lower serum cholesterol level
22. Which of the following is not a complication of myxedema?
    - (a) Megacolon
    - (b) Increased susceptibility to infection
    - (c) Carpal tunnel syndrome
    - (d) Thyroid crisis
23. Myxedema is treated by
    - (a) Levothyroxine
    - (b) Partial thyroidectomy
    - (c) Subtotal thyroidectomy
    - (d) Hemithyroidectomy
24. The dose of levothyroxine in myxedema is
    - (a) 25–100 μg daily
    - (b) 10–50 μg daily
    - (c) 1–2 μg daily
    - (d) 5 μg daily
25. The most common mode of spread of a papillary carcinoma is by
    - (a) Local infiltration
    - (b) Bloodstream
    - (c) Lymphatic route
    - (d) Both local infiltration and hematogenous route
26. The metastases of a follicular carcinoma commonly go to
    - (a) Cervical lymph nodes
    - (b) Mediastinal lymph nodes
    - (c) Bones
    - (d) Ovary
27. All of the following are true about anaplastic carcinoma of thyroid, except
    - (a) It commonly occurs in women beyond midlife
    - (b) It produces a hard and irregular lump of the whole thyroid
    - (c) It invades trachea
    - (d) It is usually a slow-growing cancer
28. All of the following are true about medullary carcinoma, except
    - (a) It arises from acinar cells of thyroid
    - (b) It is a solid, hard tumor
    - (c) It secretes calcitonin
    - (d) It is a familial tumor in 25% of cases
29. Metastatic follicular carcinoma is treated by
    - (a) Total thyroidectomy with chemotherapy
    - (b) Total thyroidectomy followed by radioiodine therapy
    - (c) Total thyroidectomy with radiotherapy
    - (d) Radioiodine only
30. Which of the following radioiodine uptake findings is suggestive of a carcinoma of thyroid?
    - (a) Hot nodule
    - (b) Cold nodule
    - (c) Higher uptake by the rest of thyroid
    - (d) Lower uptake by the rest of thyroid
31. Which of the following solitary nodules of the thyroid is least likely to be malignant?
    - (a) A solitary nodule of recent onset
    - (b) A solitary nodule in a male
    - (c) A solitary nodule in a female of 25–60 years of age of long duration
    - (d) A solitary nodule in a patient who received radiation to the neck during childhood

(CONTD...)

SELF-ASSESSMENT *(...CONTD)*

32. The initial treatment of a solitary thyroid nodule is
    - (a) Partial thyroidectomy
    - (b) Hemithyroidectomy
    - (c) Subtotal thyroidectomy
    - (d) Enucleation of nodule
33. The initial treatment of a thyroid cyst is
    - (a) Emptying by needle aspiration
    - (b) Enucleation of cyst
    - (c) Partial thyroidectomy
    - (d) Hemithyroidectomy
34. All of the following statements are true about de Quervain's thyroiditis, except
    - (a) The patient is usually a young man who has sore throat, malaise, anxiety, fever, headache, and weakness
    - (b) One lobe of thyroid is significantly enlarged and tender
    - (c) There may be signs of mild hyperthyroidism
    - (d) It is treated symptomatically mainly by aspirin
35. Which of the following statements is false about Hashimoto's disease?
    - (a) The patient is usually a premenopausal woman
    - (b) Thyroid is diffusely enlarged and gently bosselated
    - (c) It has initial hypothyroidism followed by hyperthyroidism
    - (d) Antibodies against thyroglobulin are present in serum
36. Which of the following statements is false about Riedel's struma?
    - (a) The thyroid is markedly enlarged, smooth, soft, and mobile
    - (b) It may compress the trachea producing difficulty in breathing
    - (c) It may compress the esophagus causing dysphagia
    - (d) It may be associated with retroperitoneal fibrosis

Answers

1. (a) 2. (d) 3. (d) 4. (b) 5. (d) 6. (a) 7. (d) 8. (d) 9. (a) 10. (c) 11. (c) 12. (b) 13. (b) 14. (d) 15. (a) 16. (c) 17. (b) 18. (d) 19. (d) 20. (c) 21. (d) 22. (d) 23. (a) 24. (a) 25. (c) 26. (c) 27. (d) 28. (a) 29. (b) 30. (b) 31. (c) 32. (b) 33. (a) 34. (b) 35. (c) 36. (a)

Diseases of Parathyroids

24

Surgical anatomy

Parathyroid glands are two pairs of yellowish brown ovoid glands lying between the posterior border of the lateral lobes of thyroid and its capsule. The anastomosing vessels joining the superior and inferior thyroid arteries run very close to parathyroids and form a good guide to locate them.

The superior parathyroids are more constant in their position at the level of the middle of the posterior border of the lateral lobe of thyroid (Fig. 24.1). The inferior parathyroids are variable in their position. They may even lie in the thyroid, superior mediastinum, or behind the esophagus in the posterior mediastinum.

The parathyroids may sometimes vary in number. They secrete the parathormone which controls the calcium metabolism and increases its levels in blood by mobilization of calcium from bones. It is not under the control of pituitary but balanced by calcitonin secreted by C-cells of thyroid.

Hypoparathyroidism

Hypoparathyroidism is defined as less than normal function of parathyroids and characterized by hypocalcemia due to deficiency of parathormone.

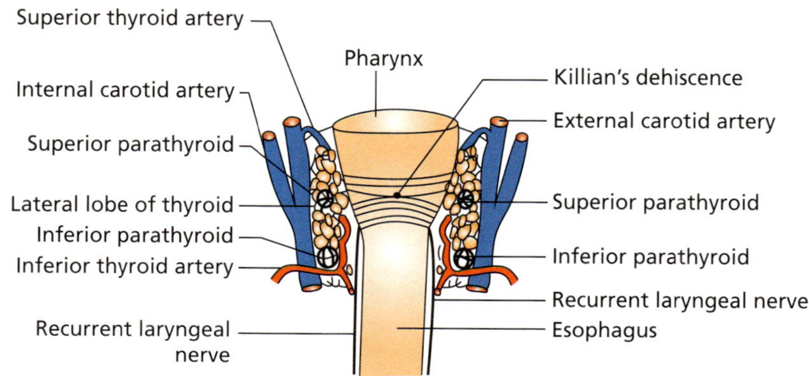

Figure 24.1 Pharynx and thyroid from behind showing the parathyroids.

Etiology

The most common cause is damage to parathyroids during thyroidectomy. Other causes include lymph node dissection of neck, Wilson's disease, hemochromatosis, autoimmune hypoparathyroidism, and granulomas.

Clinical Features

Clinical features of hypoparathyroidism are those of hypocalcemia which include tetany, muscle cramps, carpopedal spasm (Fig. 24.2), irritability, altered mental status, convulsions, and stridor. Tingling of circumoral area, hands, and feet is common. The symptoms of chronic disease include lethargy, personality changes, anxiety state, and blurring of vision. Tetany can be demonstrated by two clinical tests: Chvostek's sign and Trousseau's sign described in Box 24.1.

Investigations

Laboratory Findings The serum calcium is low, serum phosphate is high, and PTH levels and urinary calcium are low. The serum calcium level can be corrected from serum albumin level as follows:

Corrected serum calcium = serum calcium (mg/dL) + [0.8 × (4.0 – albumin [g/dL])]

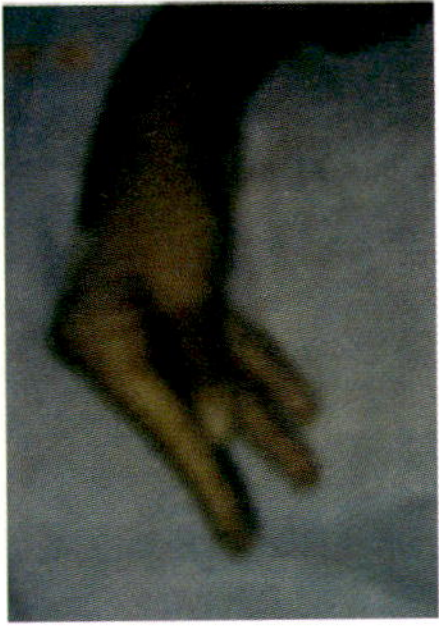

Figure 24.2 Carpopedal spasm (accoucheur's hand) of tetany.

Box 24.1 Clinical tests to demonstrate tetany of hypoparathyroidism

- **Chvostek's sign**: Contraction of facial muscles elicited by tapping the facial nerve in front of pinna
- **Trousseau's sign**: Occurrence of carpal spasm after application of sphygmomanometer cuff and inflating it to occlude the blood flow of the forearm (Fig. 24.3)

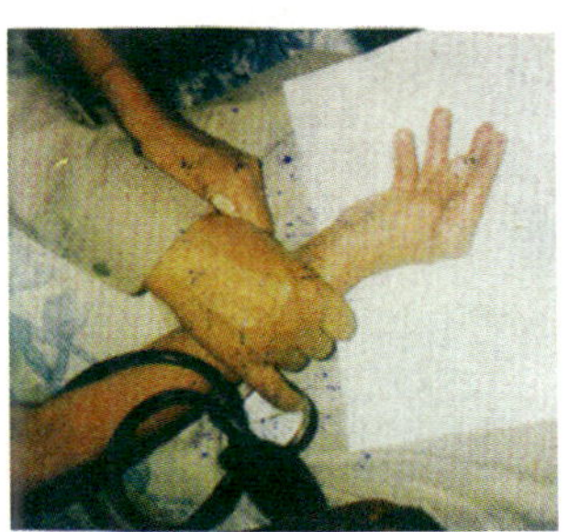

Figure 24.3 Trousseau's sign of tetany.

Imaging X-ray or CT scan of skull may show calcification of basal ganglia, and the bones may be denser than normal. In chronic disease, there may be increased bone mineral density, especially in lumbar spine.

Other Investigations Slit lamp examination may show early posterior lenticular cataract. ECG shows prolonged QT interval and abnormal T wave.

Treatment

Treatment of acute attack (hypoparathyroid tetany)

- Maintenance of airway is the first step.
- Intravenous calcium: Intravenous calcium gluconate 10–20 mL of 10% solution is given till tetany comes under control followed by slow intravenous drip of 10–50 mL of 10% calcium gluconate added to 1 L of 5% glucose. The aim should be to maintain serum calcium level in the range of 8–9 mg/dL.
- Oral calcium: As soon as possible, the patient is shifted to oral calcium, that is, calcium carbonate 500 mg/5 mL in a dose of 1–3 g calcium daily. Calcium citrate is associated with better gastrointestinal tolerance.
- Vitamin D: With oral calcium, the active metabolite of vitamin D, 1,25-dihydroxycholecalciferol (calcitriol), is started in the dose of 0.25 μg orally each morning with upward dosage titration to near normocalcemia.

- If hypomagnesemia is also present, magnesium is given.
- Transplantation of cryopreserved parathyroid tissue accidentally removed during thyroid surgery may be done. It restores normocalcemia in 23% of patients.

Maintenance therapy

- Patients with mild asymptomatic hypocalcemia require no treatment.
- Others are given calcium supplementation 1 g daily along with vitamin D with the aim of maintaining serum calcium level a slightly low but at an asymptomatic range of 8–8.6 mg/dL. The commonly used agents are calcitriol 0.25–2.9 μg/day orally and ergocalciferol.
- Another drug is teriparatide, a recombinant preparation of human PTH 1-34. The disadvantages of this drug include its very high cost and the necessity for injections.

Hyperparathyroidism

Hyperparathyroidism is defined as hyperfunction of parathyroids leading to hypercalcemia.

Types of Hyperparathyroidism

Primary Hyperparathyroidism It is characterized by hypercalcemia, elevated or inappropriately raised PTH levels, and parathyroid gland enlargement which may be due to adenoma (85%), hyperplasia (14%), or carcinoma (1%).

Secondary Hyperparathyroidism It is due to compensatory hyperplasia of parathyroids caused by persistent hypocalcemia as occurs in chronic renal failure, rickets, osteomalacia, malabsorption, and pseudohypoparathyroidism. Out of these causes, the chronic renal failure is the main cause. Hence, this type of secondary hyperfunction is called renal hyperparathyroidism.

Tertiary Hyperparathyroidism It occurs following renal transplantation when the hyperfunctioning parathyroid tissue becomes autonomous.

Clinical Features

- It occurs at all ages but most commonly in the seventh decade and in women (74%). Before age 45, the occurrence is similar in both the sexes. It is a familial disease in about 10% of patients. It may be entirely asymptomatic.
- The symptomatic disease presents with renal pain, polyuria (renal calculi), hypertension, constipation, fatigue, mental changes, bone pain, and rarely cystic lesions in bones associated with fibrosis (osteitis fibrosa cystica) and pathological fractures as described in Box 24.2.
- It may present as a "brown tumor" of lower jaw which is a multiloculated giant cell lesion associated with hypercalcemia and elevated serum levels of PTH.
- The examination of neck is normal; when a mass is palpable, it usually turns out to be an incidental thyroid nodule.

Box 24.2 Clinical features of hyperparathyroidism

A disease of bones, stones, abdominal groans, psychic moans with fatigue overtones

- Bone pain
- Renal calculi
- Constipation
- Mental changes
- Fatigue

Investigations

Laboratory Findings

- The most important finding is hypercalcemia with serum-adjusted total calcium >10.5 mg/dL.
- The urinary calcium excretion may be high or normal.
- The serum phosphate is often low (< 2.5 mg/dL).
- Elevated serum levels of intact PTH (IRMA assay) confirm the diagnosis.

The laboratory findings in hypoparathyroidism and hyperparathyroidism are described in Table 24.1.

Table 24.1 Laboratory values in hypoparathyroidism and hyperparathyroidism

Laboratory tests	Hypoparathyroidism	Hyperparathyroidism
Serum calcium	Low	High
Serum phosphate	High	Low
PTH levels	Low	Elevated
Urinary calcium levels	Low	High/normal

Imaging Studies

- Sestamibi–iodine subtraction imaging (Fig. 24.4) and ultrasound of neck may locate a parathyroid adenoma.
- CT scan and MRI are usually not required but MRI offers better soft-tissue contrast than CT scan. CT scan is useful to see the kidneys for calcium-containing stones.
- Bone density measurements by dual-energy X-ray absorptiometry (DXA) determine the extent of bone loss. It occurs mostly in long bones. DXA should include lumbar spine, hip, and distal radius. Radiography of bones is usually normal in early stages of the disease. Radiographic features of advanced disease are described in Box 24.3.

Box 24.3 Radiographic features of hyperparathyroidism

- Early disease: Hardly any change
- As the disease advances:
  - Demineralization of bones
  - Subperiosteal resorption especially in the radial aspect of fingers
  - Loss of lamina dura of the teeth
  - Cysts in all bones (osteitis fibrosa cystica)
  - Mottling of skull ("salt and pepper appearance")
  - Pathological fractures
  - Chondrocalcinosis—calcification of articular cartilages

Treatment

Mild Asymptomatic Hyperparathyroidism It needs no active treatment. These patients should avoid immobilization and thiazide diuretics, and drink adequate fluids. Indications of surgery are described in Box 24.4.

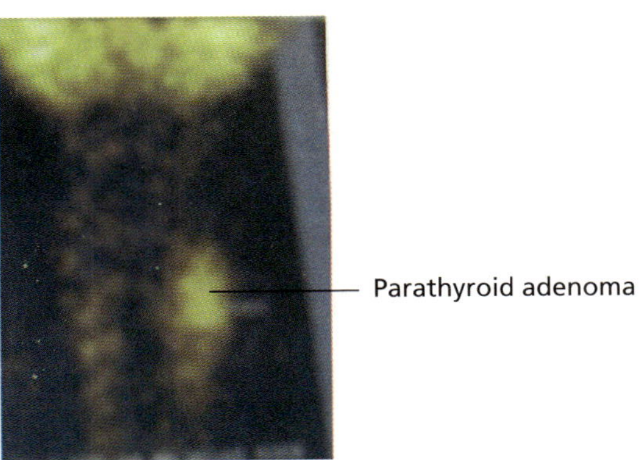

Figure 24.4 ^{99m}Technetium-labeled sestamibi isotope scan showing a parathyroid adenoma of left side of neck.

Box 24.4 Indications of surgery in asymptomatic hyperparathyroidism

- Serum calcium 1 mg/dL above upper limit of normal, that is, 10.5 mg/dL
- Urine calcium excretion more than 400 mg/24 hours
- Creatinine clearance <60 mL/minute

Symptomatic Hyperparathyroidism It is treated with parathyroidectomy. The neck is explored and the adenoma or parathyroids are located. The different treatment options are enumerated in Box 24.5.

The complications of parathyroidectomy include injury to recurrent laryngeal nerve and neck vessels, persistent hypocalcemia, and wound infection.

Medical Measures Medical measures to control hypercalcemia are enumerated in Box 24.6.

Box 24.5 Treatment of symptomatic hyperparathyroidism

- **Parathyroid adenoma**: Excision
- **Parathyroid hyperplasia**: Excision of 3.5 parathyroid with a metal clip left in residual parathyroid to locate it in future
- **Parathyroid carcinoma**: En bloc resection with ipsilateral thyroid lobe
  - Reoperation for neck recurrence with adjuvant radiation

Box 24.6 Medical measures to control hypercalcemia

- Large fluid intake
- Intensive hydration with intravenous saline
- Bisphosphonates (e.g., pamidronate or zoledronic acid intravenously)
- Vitamin D, vitamin D analogs, and cinacalcet

Tetany

It is a syndrome characterized by sharp flexion of wrist and ankle joints (carpopedal spasm), muscle twitchings, cramps, and convulsions, sometimes with attacks of stridor. It is due to abnormal calcium metabolism (hypocalcemia) and occurs in hypoparathyroidism, hypovitaminosis D, alkalosis, and ingestion of alkaline salts. Treatment is removal of the cause.

MEN syndrome

Multiple endocrine neoplasia (MEN) syndromes are inherited as autosomal dominant traits that predispose to occurrence of tumors of two or more different endocrine glands. They are caused by different germline mutations and are of four types as described in Box 24.7. These patients should be examined and investigated accordingly and should have genetic testing of their first-degree relatives.

Box 24.7 Types of MEN syndrome

- MEN 1 includes tumors of parathyroids, endocrine pancreas and duodenum, anterior pituitary, adrenal gland, thyroid, carcinoid, lipomas, and facial angiofibromas
- MEN 2 includes medullary carcinoma of thyroid, pheochromocytoma, and Hirschsprung's disease
- MEN 3 includes medullary carcinoma of thyroid, pheochromocytoma, Marfan-like habitus, mucosal neuromas, intestinal ganglioneuroma, and delayed puberty
- MEN 4 includes tumors of parathyroids, anterior pituitary, adrenal glands, ovary, testis, and kidney

Dental aspects of parathyroid dysfunction

The dental aspects of parathyroid dysfunction are described in Box 24.8. The dental problems of parathyroid disease are managed by removal of the cause and treatment of the dental problem on its merits.

Box 24.8 Dental aspects of parathyroid dysfunction

- **Hyperparathyroidism**
  - Defective teeth if the parathyroid disease occurs during childhood
  - Weak jaws, especially mandible due to mobilization of calcium
  - May be weak and loose teeth
  - Brown tumor of lower jaw (it is a multiloculated giant cell lesion associated with hypercalcemia and elevated serum levels of PTH)
- **Hypoparathyroidism**
  - Hardly any effect on jaws and teeth

KEY POINTS

- Parathyroid glands are two pairs of yellowish brown ovoid glands lying between the posterior border of the lateral lobes of thyroid and its capsule. They secrete parathormone.
- Hypoparathyroidism is defined as less than normal function of parathyroids and characterized by hypocalcemia. It is usually due to damage of parathyroids during thyroidectomy. It is characterized by tetany, carpopedal spasm, irritability, altered mental status, stridor, and Chvostek's and Trousseau's signs. Its treatment includes maintenance of airway and intravenous calcium followed by oral calcium and vitamin D.
- Primary hyperparathyroidism is mainly due to adenoma of parathyroid glands and is characterized by hypercalcemia and elevated or inappropriately raised PTH levels.
- Secondary hyperparathyroidism is due to compensatory hyperplasia of parathyroids caused by persistent hypocalcemia mainly due to chronic renal failure, hence called renal hyperparathyroidism.
- Hyperparathyroidism is "a disease of bones, stones, abdominal groans, psychic moans with fatigue overtones" with bone pain, renal calculi, constipation, and mental changes. Laboratory findings include hypercalcemia, low levels of serum phosphate, elevated PTH levels, and high or normal urinary calcium levels.
- In the lower jaw, hyperparathyroidism may present as "brown tumor" which is a multiloculated giant cell lesion. Other dental manifestations of parathyroid dysfunction include defective teeth and decreased density of jaw bones due to calcium mobilization.
- Parathyroid adenoma is detected by sestamibi–iodine subtraction imaging and ultrasound of neck. It is treated by excision which gives the best results.
- Parathyroid hyperplasia is treated by resection of 3.5 parathyroids and parathyroid carcinoma by en bloc resection of tumor and ipsilateral thyroid lobe.
- Tetany is a syndrome that occurs in hypoparathyroidism and is characterized by sharp flexion of wrist and ankle joints (carpopedal spasm), muscle twitchings, cramps, and convulsions, sometimes with attacks of stridor.
- Multiple endocrine neoplasia (MEN) syndromes are inherited as autosomal dominant traits that predispose to occurrence of tumors of two or more different endocrine glands.

SELF-ASSESSMENT

Long answer question

1. What are the dental manifestations of parathyroid disorders? Describe the clinical features and treatment of hyperparathyroidism.

Short answer questions

1. Hypoparathyroidism
2. Brown tumor
3. Osteitis fibrosa cystica
4. Tetany

Multiple choice questions

1. Commonly the parathyroids are ____ in number.
   (a) 3
   (b) 4
   (c) 5
   (d) 6
2. Parathyroids are usually situated
   (a) Behind the posterior border of lateral lobe of thyroid
   (b) Near the upper pole of lateral lobe of thyroid
   (c) Along the upper border of thyroid
   (d) Along the lateral border
3. The parathyroids secrete
   (a) Thyroxine
   (b) Parathormone
   (c) ACTH
   (d) Calcitonin

(CONTD...)

SELF-ASSESSMENT *(...CONTD)*

4. All of the following are the effects of parathormone, except
   (a) Increased mobilization of calcium from bones
   (b) Hypercalcemia
   (c) Hyperphosphatemia
   (d) Hypercalciuria
5. The most common cause of hypoparathyroidism is
   (a) Damage or removal of parathyroids during thyroidectomy
   (b) Lymph node dissection of neck
   (c) Wilson's disease
   (d) DiGeorge's syndrome
6. All of the following are the manifestations of hypoparathyroidism, except
   (a) Tetany
   (b) Tetanus
   (c) Circumoral tingling and numbness
   (d) Carpopedal spasm
7. Hypoparathyroidism is characterized by all of the following features, except
   (a) Low serum calcium
   (b) Low serum phosphate
   (c) Hypocalciuria
   (d) Prolonged QT interval on ECG
8. The commonest cause of hyperparathyroidism is
   (a) Parathyroid adenoma
   (b) Carcinoma
   (c) Parathyroid hyperplasia
   (d) Wilson's disease
9. All of the following are features of hyperparathyroidism, except
   (a) Hypercalcemia
   (b) Hypophosphatemia
   (c) Hypocalciuria
   (d) Increased PTH levels in serum
10. All of the following are features of hyperparathyroidism, except
   (a) Bone pain due to osteitis fibrosa cystica
   (b) Renal pain due to renal calculi
   (c) Psychiatric symptoms
   (d) Carpopedal spasm
11. Tertiary hyperparathyroidism is caused
   (a) By parathyroid adenoma
   (b) By carcinoma of parathyroid
   (c) By rickets
   (d) Following renal transplantation when the hyperfunctioning parathyroid tissue becomes autonomous

Answers

1. (b) 2. (a) 3. (b) 4. (c) 5. (a) 6. (b) 7. (b) 8. (a) 9. (c) 10. (d) 11. (d)

Diseases of Lymph Nodes

25

Introduction

There are about 800 lymph nodes in the body, out of which 300 are present in the neck.

Normal lymph nodes are neither visible nor palpable. If they are diseased, they get enlarged and then they become visible and palpable. The enlargement of lymph node is called lymphadenopathy and is a sign of disease. Any (localized lymphadenopathy) or many lymph nodes together (regional or generalized lymphadenopathy) may enlarge.

Causes of lymph node enlargement

Infection is the commonest cause of lymph node enlargement, especially the presence of a focus of infection in the drainage area. For example, cervical lymph nodes may get infected (and enlarged) in infective lesions in their drainage area, that is, oral and nasal cavities, tonsils, pharynx, larynx, ears, face, and scalp. The causes of lymph node enlargement are described in Box 25.1.

Box 25.1 Causes of lymph node enlargement

Infections

- Acute lymphadenitis
- Chronic lymphadenitis
  - Chronic nonspecific infection
  - Tuberculosis
  - Syphilis
  - Filariasis
  - Lymphogranuloma inguinale
  - Infectious mononucleosis (glandular fever)
  - AIDS

Tumors

- **Benign**: Very rare
- **Malignant**: Common
  - *Primary*: Hodgkin's lymphoma, non-Hodgkin's lymphoma, chronic lymphatic leukemia
  - *Secondary*: Metastasis from carcinoma, melanoma, and synoviosarcoma

Acute lymphadenitis

- **Etiology**: The lymph node or nodes draining an area or organ having acute infection usually get enlarged due to spread of infection into the lymph nodes through the draining lymphatics.
- **Clinical features**: The node/nodes are tender. Systemic response symptoms such as pyrexia, anorexia, and malaise may be present. If the inflammation continues, it may result in an abscess formation (lymphadenitic abscess) when the overlying skin becomes red and hot (Fig. 25.1).
- **Diagnosis**: Diagnosis is clinical and usually no investigations are done but blood counts show leukocytosis.
- **Treatment**: Appropriate antibiotic treatment of the primary infection usually leads to resolution of inflammation. If an abscess has formed, drainage of pus is required.

Chronic nonspecific lymphadenitis (reactive lymphadenopathy)

- **Etiology**: It is a common condition in which the lymph nodes of the neck, oral cavity, nasal cavity (caused by chronic or recurrent infection of pharynx), salivary glands, and scalp are enlarged.
- **Clinical features**: In the neck it usually affects the upper cervical lymph nodes. The nodes are enlarged, mild to moderate in size, and firm but elastic, discrete, mobile, and mildly tender. There is no matting.

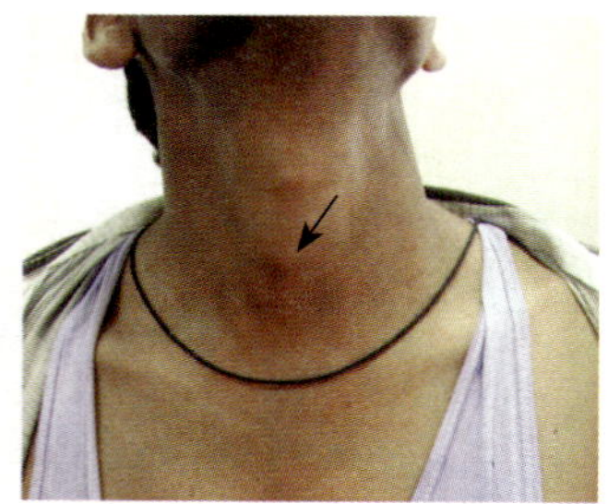

Figure 25.1 Acute nonspecific lymphadenitis of lower midline lymph nodes of neck.

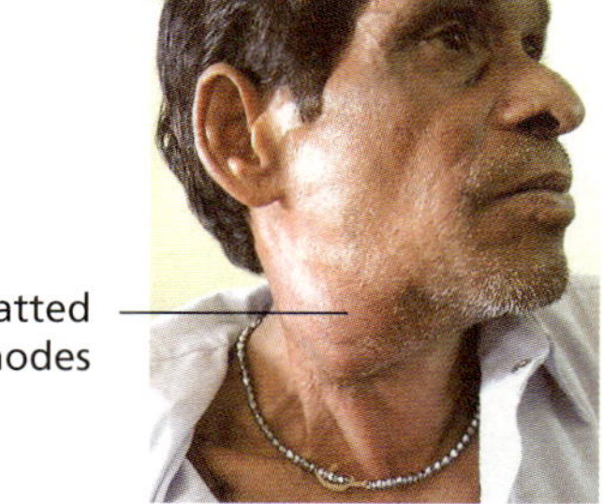

Figure 25.2 Matted upper cervical lymph nodes due to tuberculosis. In the lower part they are pointing on the skin and preparing to rupture.

- **Diagnosis**: FNAC or biopsy may be done to confirm the diagnosis.
- **Treatment**: The treatment includes removal of cause, that is, eradicating the primary focus of infection, and giving relief in symptoms.

Tuberculous lymphadenitis

Etiology It is a common disease of lymph nodes caused by *Mycobacterium tuberculosis.*

Clinical Features It usually affects young people, more commonly the females. Generally the deep cervical, mesenteric, and axillary lymph nodes are involved. They are enlarged mild to moderate in size, firm but elastic, nontender, and matted (Figs 25.2 and 25.3). The patient may have general symptoms of tuberculosis, for example, low-grade fever, night sweats, anorexia, and loss of weight. Apart from lymph node enlargement, the disease has two more presentations described as follows:

1. **Cold abscess and "collar-stud" abscess**: As the disease advances, a cold abscess (Fig. 25.4)

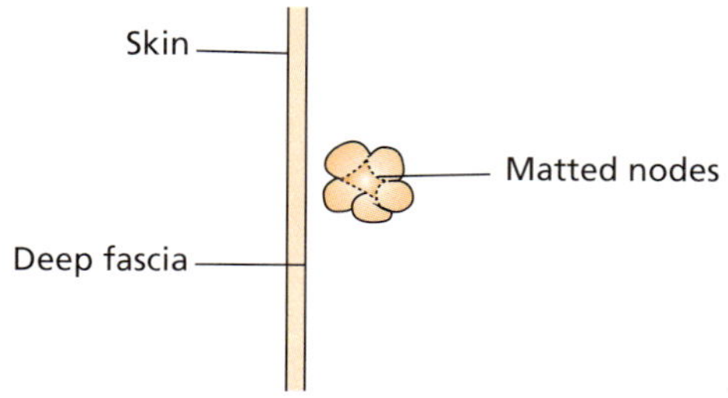

Figure 25.3 Matted nodes of tuberculous lymphadenitis.

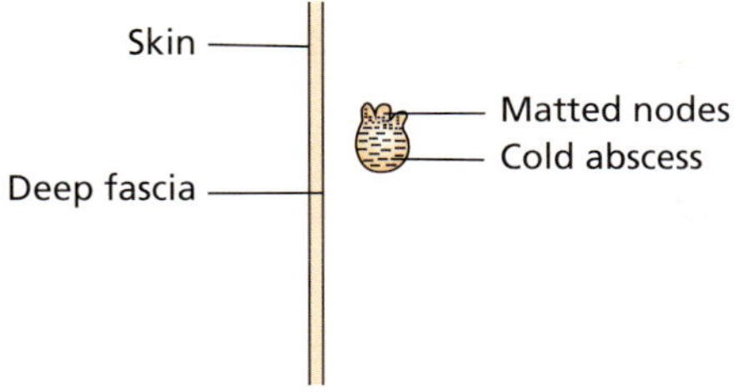

Figure 25.4 Matted nodes with cold abscess formation in tuberculous lymphadenitis.

may form deep to deep fascia which may be eroded at one point and the pus flows out through the hole thus created into the subcutaneous space forming a "collar-stud" abscess having a large subcutaneous pocket and a small subfascial pocket joined together by a narrow track (Fig. 25.5) and having cross-fluctuation.

2. **Tuberculous sinus/sinuses and ulcer**: After some time, a cold abscess may rupture on the skin producing a single or multiple sinuses or ulcers which has/have a bluish undermined edge (Fig. 25.6). They discharge thin syrup-like pus with curdy flakes.

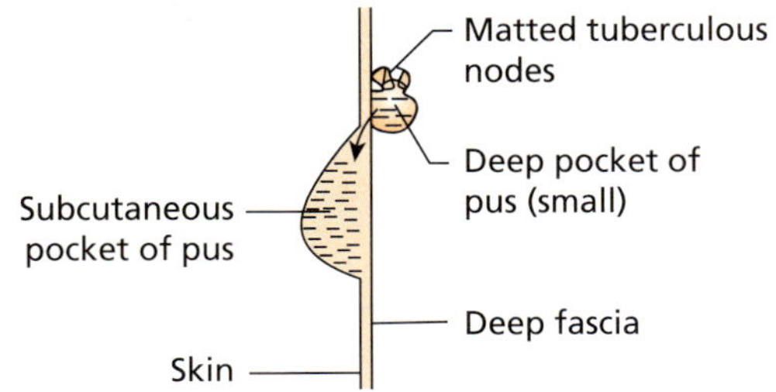

Figure 25.5 Collar-stud abscess of neck due to tuberculous lymphadenitis.

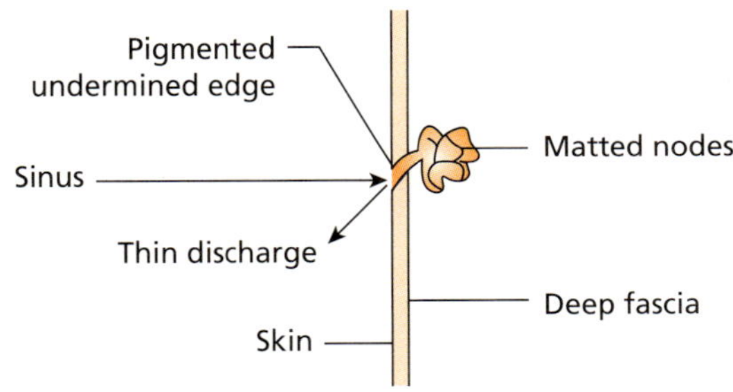

Figure 25.6 Tuberculous lymphadenitis with sinus.

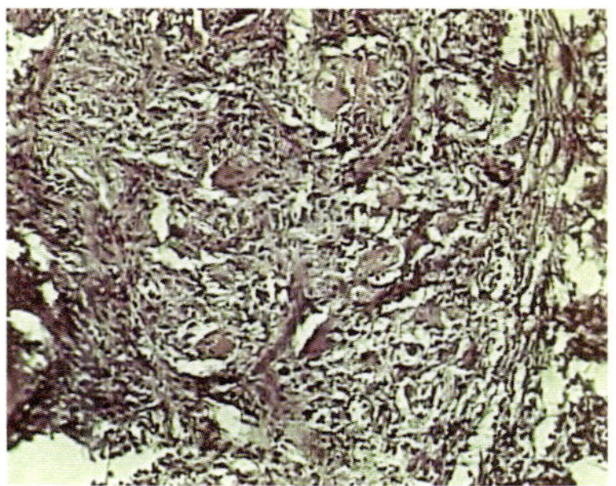

Figure 25.7 Tuberculosis of lymph node showing multiple caseous granulomata composed of central area of caseation surrounded by epithelioid cells, lymphocytes, and Langhans giant cells. (Courtesy: Professor P.K. Agarwal)

Diagnosis The diagnosis may be confirmed by FNAC or lymph node biopsy (Fig. 25.7). Culture or DNA–RNA amplification for tuberculosis of the discharge may be done. Deep node disease can be imaged by CT scan.

Treatment

- A full course of antituberculous chemotherapy cures most of the patients.
- Persistently enlarged nodes, cold abscess, and sinus or sinuses may require surgical intervention. The excision of the lesion may be difficult due to fibrosis, presence of many nerves (accessory, hypoglossal, and vagus), and the internal jugular vein in the vicinity. The excised tissue is examined microscopically and bacteriologically.

Cervical lymphadenopathy

The cervical lymph node enlargement is one of the commonest presentations of lymph node disease. The causes of cervical lymphadenopathy are described in Box 25.2.

Hard, enlarged lymph node/nodes in the neck in an elderly patient are most likely due to metastatic carcinoma which may be locoregional (e.g., carcinoma of oral cavity or a paranasal sinus) or distal (e.g., carcinoma of stomach, pancreas, or testis). Hence, one should workup the patient accordingly.

Box 25.2 Causes of cervical lymph node enlargement

- Nonspecific lymphadenitis (reactive lymph nodes)
- Tuberculous lymphadenitis
- Metastatic disease
- HIV infection
- Lymphomas
- Chronic lymphatic leukemia
- Infectious mononucleosis
- Sarcoidosis

Syphilitic lymphadenitis

- **Etiology**: Coital transmission of *Treponema pallidum* is the main cause of this disease. Sometimes the infection is transmitted by kissing an infected person.
- **Clinical features**: In primary syphilis, there is a primary chancre and mild enlargement of regional lymph nodes. Sometimes the infection is transmitted by kissing an infected person which produces a primary chancre on the lip or tongue and markedly enlarged upper cervical lymph nodes. In secondary syphilis, there is generalized lymphadenopathy. The clinical features of syphilitic lymphadenitis in relation to head and neck are described in Table 25.1.
- **Diagnosis**: The diagnosis is confirmed by finding *T. pallidum* in dark-field microscopy of fresh aspirate from the lymph nodes and serological tests for syphilis, for example, VDRL and FTA-Abs.
- **Treatment**: It is treated by giving benzathine penicillin G or aqueous penicillin G parenterally.

Filarial lymphadenitis

- **Etiology**: It is caused by *Wuchereria bancrofti* or *Brugia malayi* which enters the body by mosquito bite.
- **Clinical features**: The patient presents with fever with rigor and inguinal lymphadenopathy. There may be pain in the inguinal region, scrotum, or foot. The lymph nodes are firm and tender.
- **Diagnosis**: The diagnosis can be confirmed by the presence of microfilaria in the blood (thick smears prepared with blood collected at night) in the acute phase. In chronic disease, enzyme-linked immunosorbent assay (ELISA) and immunochromatographic card tests are done.
- **Treatment**: It is treated by diethylcarbamazine 3–5 mg/kg body weight per day in three divided doses for 3–4 weeks.

Lymphogranuloma venereum (LGV)

- **Etiology**: LGV is an acute and chronic sexually transmitted disease caused by *Chlamydia trachomatis* types L1–L3.
- **Pathogenesis**: LGV is acquired during intercourse or through contact with contaminated exudate from active lesions. Its incubation period is 5–21 days.
- **Clinical features**: LGV presents as genital vesicular or ulcerative lesions and the infection spreads to inguinal lymph nodes and rectal areas. The inguinal lymph nodes enlarge often on both sides, and fuse, soften, and break down to form multiple draining sinuses. Rectum is affected in females. It may lead to extensive scarring.

Table 25.1 Features of syphilitic lymphadenitis

Type of syphilis	Lymph nodes
• Primary syphilis involving oral cavity	• Significant enlargement of upper cervical lymph nodes which are nontender, discrete, and mobile
• Secondary syphilis	• Generalized lymphadenopathy involving epitrochlear and occipital lymph nodes
• Tertiary and congenital syphilis	• Nothing specific about the lymph nodes

- **Diagnosis**: Positive compliment fixation test helps in diagnosis.
- **Treatment**: The drug of choice is doxycycline 100 mg orally twice daily for 21 days. It is contraindicated during pregnancy. Other effective drugs are erythromycin (500 mg orally four times daily for 21 days) and azithromycin 1 g orally once weekly for 3 weeks.

Infectious mononucleosis (glandular fever)

- **Etiology**: It is an acute infective disease caused by Epstein–Barr virus.
- **Clinical features**: The patient presents with generalized lymphadenopathy associated with irregular fever, sore throat, toxemia, rash, and splenic enlargement. The lymph nodes are discrete, nonsuppurative, and slightly painful, especially those of posterior cervical chain.
- **Diagnosis**: The diagnosis is confirmed by heterophile agglutination test (monospot).
- **Treatment**: Most of the patients recover with symptomatic treatment, for example, acetaminophen for pain with throat irrigations or gargles. Acyclovir decreases viral shedding but is of no use clinically. Corticosteroids may be used in complicated cases, for example, impending airway obstruction.

Acquired immune deficiency syndrome (AIDS)

Etiology It is a serious disease caused by human immunodeficiency virus (HIV).

Risk Factors The risk factors include sexual contact with an infected person, infected blood transfusion, needle sharing, and perinatal exposure.

Clinical Features

- The patient may present with fever, sore throat, and lymphadenopathy such as infectious mononucleosis. There may be signs of transient meningitis, encephalitis, or neuropathy.
- The patient may have chronic disease with persistent generalized lymphadenopathy for 3 months or more. The lymph nodes are more than 1 cm in size at two or more extragenital sites.
- There may be prominent systemic complaints such as sweating, diarrhea, weight loss, and wasting. Opportunistic infections (cytomegalovirus, *Candida albicans*) and aggressive cancers (Kaposi's sarcoma, lymphoma) may occur.

Diagnosis The diagnosis is confirmed by HIV ELISA and Western blot.

Treatment The treatment includes prophylaxis and treatment of opportunistic infections, malignancies, and other complications; and treatment of HIV infection with combination of antiretroviral drugs (HAART).

Hodgkin's lymphoma

Etiology It is one the commonest primary malignant tumors of lymphoid tissue the cause of which is not known. It may be related to certain human leukocyte antigen (HLA), immune deficiency, and an oncogenic virus. It originates from lymphocytes of germinal center origin.

Histopathology Microscopically it is characterized by presence of Reed–Sternberg cells which are multinucleated giant cells (Fig. 25.8). They are malignant cells which are surrounded by an inflammatory lymphocytic infiltrate, the pattern of

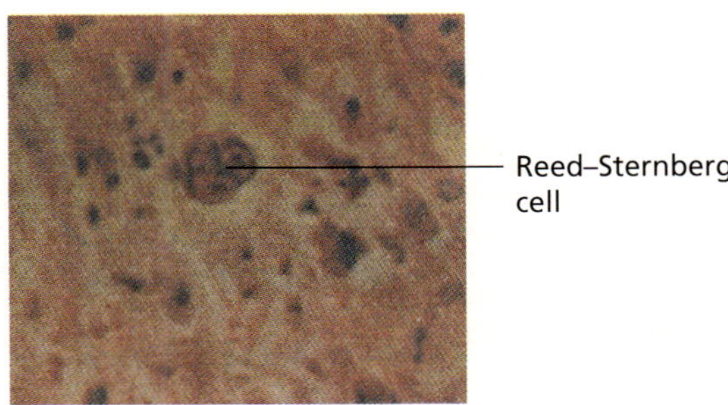

Figure 25.8 Microscopic appearance of Hodgkin's lymphoma showing a large Reed–Sternberg cell in the center. (Courtesy: Professor P.K. Agarwal)

which determines the subtypes given below (Rye's classification):

- Lymphocyte predominant
- Lymphocyte depletion
- Mixed cellularity
- Nodular sclerosis

Mode of Spread It usually arises within single lymph node areas and spreads in an orderly manner to contiguous areas of lymph nodes. Late in the course of disease, vascular invasion occurs resulting in widespread hematogenous dissemination.

Clinical Features

- There is bimodal age distribution with one peak in twenties and another above 50 years of age.
- The patient usually presents with a painless mass in the neck which may have pain following alcohol ingestion.
- Later on, other lymph nodes are involved which are mobile, discrete, and rubbery with little tendency toward matting.
- There may be irregular fever, weight loss, pruritus, and night sweats. Spleen is usually enlarged; liver may also be enlarged.

Clinical Staging (Ann Arbor) The aims of clinical staging are to decide the line of treatment and to tell the prognosis (Fig. 25.9). The Ann Arbor clinical staging is described in Box 25.3.

Box 25.3 Ann Arbor clinical staging of Hodgkin's lymphoma

- **Stage I**: Single lymph node site involved
- **Stage II**: Involvement of two or more lymphatic sites on one side of diaphragm
- **Stage III**: Lymph node regions involved on both sides of diaphragm
- **Stage IV**: Disseminated disease with extranodal involvement

It is further categorized as A if there are no constitutional symptoms and B if constitutional symptoms are present, for example, fever, weight loss, pruritus, and night sweats

Investigations The diagnosis is confirmed by lymph node biopsy in which one entire lymph node is removed to see its architecture. The staging evaluation is done by whole-body PET/CT scan and bone marrow biopsy.

Treatment The mainstay of treatment is chemotherapy and ABVD (adriamycin or doxorubicin, bleomycin, vinblastine, dacarbazine) is the standard first-line regimen. Others such as Stanford V (doxorubicin, vinblastine, bleomycin, vincristine, nitrogen mustard, prednisone, and etoposide) or escalated BEACOPP (bleomycin, etoposide, adriamycin, cyclophosphamide, Oncovin, procarbazine, and prednisone) may improve the response rates but have increased toxicity. The treatment of Hodgkin's lymphoma is described in Table 25.2.

Prognosis

- **Stages IA and IIA**: 10-Year survival more than 90%

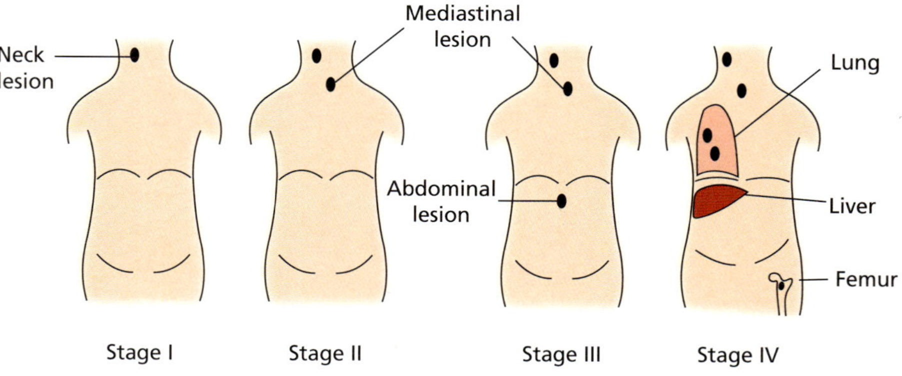

Figure 25.9 Stages of Hodgkin's lymphoma (Ann Arbor).

Table 25.2 Treatment of Hodgkin's lymphoma

Stage of disease	Treatment
Stages I and II	• Short course of chemotherapy with involved field radiotherapy (or) • Full course of chemotherapy alone
Stage II and bulky mass	• Full course of ABVD for six cycles with involved field radiotherapy
Stages III and IV	• Full course of chemotherapy and no radiotherapy • Pulmonary toxicity if occurs should be treated aggressively
Relapsing disease	High-dose chemotherapy and autologous hematopoietic stem cell transplantation. Disease relapsing after autologous stem cell transplantation may be treated with antibody–drug conjugate brentuximab

ABVD, adriamycin or doxorubicin, bleomycin, vinblastine, dacarbazine.

- **Advanced disease (stages III and IV)**: 10-Year survival rates 50–60%

Non-Hodgkin's lymphoma

It is a heterogenous group of malignant tumors of lymphocytes usually presenting as enlarged lymph nodes (Figs 25.10 and 25.11). It is of two types: nodular and diffuse (Rappaport classification).

Types of Non-Hodgkin's Lymphoma

- Eighty-five percent of these tumors are B-cell and 15% are T-cell or NK-cell in origin.
- In one-third of patients, the disease occurs outside lymph nodes, that is, extranodal in organs that normally have nests of lymphoid tissue (mucosal surfaces, bone marrow, and skin).
- They are divided into two groups depending on clinical behavior and pathology: the indolent (low-grade) and the aggressive (intermediate or high-grade).

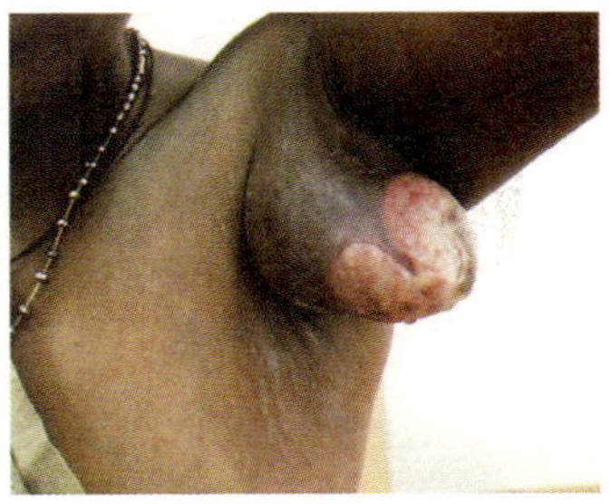

Figure 25.10 Ulcerated non-Hodgkin's lymphoma of left axilla in a person aged 54 years.

The differences between indolent and aggressive non-Hodgkin's lymphoma are described in Table 25.3.

Extranodal Lymphoma

Extranodal lymphoma occurs outside the lymph nodes in organs and tissues having lymphoid tissue most commonly in oropharynx, paranasal sinuses, thyroid, gastrointestinal tract, liver, testes, skin, and bone marrow. Of all extranodal sites, the stomach is most commonly involved.

Clinical Features of Non-Hodgkin's Lymphoma

- The patient presents with painless lymphadenopathy which may be isolated or widespread and peripheral or central (retroperitoneal, mesenteric, and pelvic).
- The indolent lymphomas are mostly disseminated, and the bone marrow involvement is common.

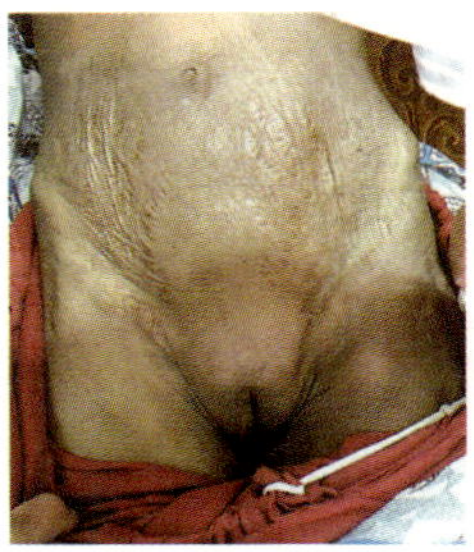

Figure 25.11 Massive enlargement of left inguinal lymph nodes with involvement of overlying skin in an elderly female due to non-Hodgkin's lymphoma.

Table 25.3 Differences between indolent and aggressive non-Hodgkin's lymphoma

Features	Indolent	Aggressive
Cell pattern	Smaller differentiated cells	Larger less differentiated cells
Architecture	Follicular	Diffuse involvement of whole lymph node
Age	Older patients	All age groups
Extent of disease	Presents as localized disease but mostly widely disseminated as found on investigations	One-third of patients present with localized disease
Course	Not very aggressive but may progress to aggressive disease	Very aggressive
Prognosis	Very difficult to cure. Most of the patients die. Median survival 6–12 years	Often curable, those not curable often die early

- The patient may have constitutional symptoms, for example, fever, drenching night sweats, and >10% loss of body weight. Extranodal involvement may be found.

Burkitt's Lymphoma

This lymphoma is common is South Africa (endemic) and New Guinea, but it occurs in our country also (sporadic). It may be etiologically related to Epstein–Barr virus. Burkitt's lymphoma is common in malaria endemic areas. It commonly occurs in children and involves abdomen with abdominal pain mainly affecting kidneys. It may affect the jaws producing a rapidly growing fleshy growth.

Staging and Diagnosis

Staging of the disease is done with whole-body PET/CT scan and bone marrow biopsy. In a lymphoma with high-risk features, a lumbar puncture is performed. The diagnosis is confirmed by lymph node biopsy or biopsy of involved extranodal site.

Treatment

Indolent lymphomas

- Localized disease may be treated with curative radiotherapy.
- Some patients have spontaneous remission.
- Most of the patients have disseminated disease which is not curable. Hence, treatment is given when symptoms develop or there is high tumor bulk. The treatment includes:
  - Anti-CD 20 monoclonal antibody rituximab 375 mg/m^2 intravenously weekly for 4 weeks alone or in combination with other drugs and the drugs include bendamustine, cyclophosphamide, doxorubicin, and vincristine.
  - Two radioimmunoconjugates, that is, yttrium-90 ibritumomab tiuxetan and iodine-131 tositumomab, are also available and give higher response rates.
- Some patients may be treated with allogenic stem cell transplantation. Mucosa-associated lymphoid tumors (MALT) of stomach are treated with a combination of anticancer antibiotics and acid blockage with endoscopic monitoring. Disease confined to stomach may be treated with radiotherapy.

Aggressive lymphomas

- **Diffuse large B-cell lymphoma**: Localized disease is treated with a short course of immunochemotherapy plus localized involved field radiation, or six cycles of immunochemotherapy without radiation. Advanced disease is treated with six cycles of immunochemotherapy such as R-CHOP which includes rituximab, cyclophosphamide, adriamycin, Oncovin, and prednisolone. Recurrent disease is managed with autologous hematopoietic stem cell transplantation.

Table 25.4 Differences between Hodgkin's and non-Hodgkin's lymphoma

Features	Hodgkin's lymphoma	Non-Hodgkin's lymphoma
Age	Bimodal age	Mostly around 50 years
Lymph node: visceral involvement	• Mostly lymph nodes are involved • Visceral involvement rare	60%:40%
Commonest presentation	Lower cervical lymph node enlargement	Upper cervical lymph node enlargement
Systemic symptoms	Common	Uncommon, late
Tonsils	Not enlarged	May be enlarged
Epitrochlear lymph node	Not enlarged	May be enlarged
Hepatomegaly	Uncommon	Common in low grade
Bone marrow involvement	Uncommon (10%)	Common (40%)
Alcohol-induced pain	Characteristic feature	Absent
Prognosis	Better	Poor

- **Mantle cell lymphoma**: It is treated with intensive initial immunochemotherapy including autologous hematopoietic stem cell transplantation.
- **High-grade lymphoma (Burkitt's or lymphoblastic lymphoma)**: It is treated with intensive cyclic chemotherapy just like acute lymphoblastic leukemia (ALL).
- **Peripheral T-cell lymphoma**: It is treated with autologous stem cell transplantation.

The differences between Hodgkin's and non-Hodgkin's lymphoma are described in Table 25.4.

Chronic lymphatic leukemia

The essentials of this disease are described in Box 25.4.

Box 25.4 Chronic lymphatic leukemia

- Clonal malignancy of B lymphocytes
- Slowly progressive accumulation of long-lived immunoincompetent small lymphocytes which causes tissue destruction by infiltration
- Isolated lymphocytosis with 75–98% lymphocytes shown in blood
- Early disease: Kept under observation
- Symptomatic and stage II disease: Fludarabine with cyclophosphamide and rituximab

Metastatic lymph nodes

- The regional lymph nodes may be involved in carcinoma, malignant melanoma, and synoviosarcoma due to lymphatic spread of cancer cells.
- Initially the lymph nodes may not be clinically palpable when their involvement can be detected by sentinel lymph node biopsy identified by injection of isosulfan blue and a radioisotope near the tumor and detection of sentinel node by color and handheld gamma camera.
- Later when the lymph nodes become palpable (Fig. 25.12), they are hard-like stone (stony hard) or like wood (wooden hard), nontender, and ill-defined when the diagnosis can be confirmed by FNAC or biopsy (Fig. 25.13).
- If the disease is not treated, the overlying skin ulcerates and the tumor fungates when the disease becomes untreatable.
- The treatment depends on the primary. The palpable and mobile lymph nodes are usually removed by block dissection, for example, suprahyoid or radical neck dissection in head and neck cancers. Fixed and nonresectable nodes are treated with palliative radiotherapy. It may be combined with chemotherapy.

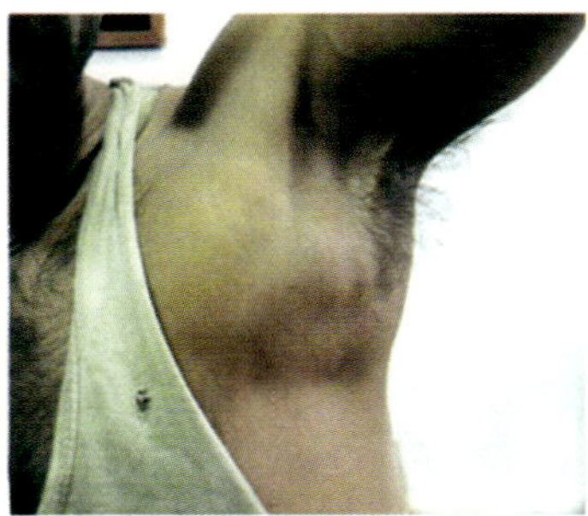

Figure 25.12 Lymph node metastasis in the axilla with a sarcoma of forearm (synoviosarcoma). (Courtesy: Dr. A.C. Dwivedi)

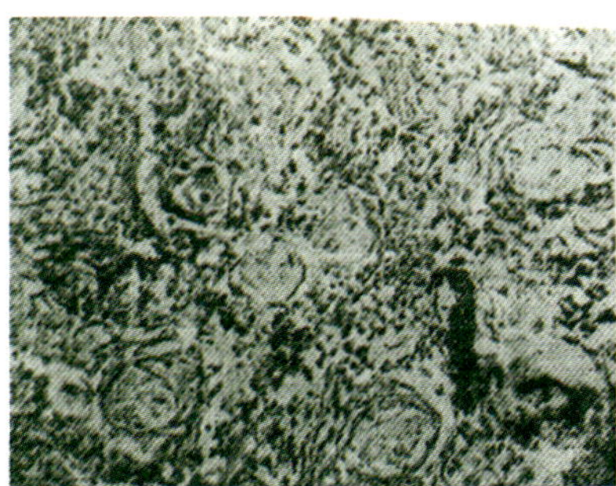

Figure 25.13 Microphotograph of lymph node metastasis from a well-differentiated squamous cell carcinoma.

KEY POINTS

- Normal lymph nodes are neither visible nor palpable. The enlargement of lymph node is called lymphadenopathy and is a sign of disease.
- Infection is the commonest cause of lymph node enlargement, especially the presence of a focus of chronic or recurrent infection in the drainage area. Tumors, both primary and secondary malignant tumors, can cause lymph node enlargement.
- Acute lymphadenitis is due to spread of infection from an area having acute infection into the lymph nodes draining that area and characterized by tender node/nodes. It may result in a lymphadenitic abscess.
- Chronic nonspecific lymphadenitis (reactive lymphadenopathy) is a common condition caused by chronic or recurrent infection.
- Tuberculous lymphadenitis affects the deep cervical lymph nodes which are nontender and matted. As the disease advances, cold abscess may form deep to deep fascia. Erosion of deep fascia leads to "collar-stud" abscess having a large subcutaneous pocket and a small subfascial pocket with cross-fluctuation joined together by a narrow track. It may rupture to produce a single or multiple sinuses which discharge thin syrup-like pus with curdy flakes.
- Infectious mononucleosis is an acute infective disease caused by Epstein–Barr virus and presents with systemic symptoms and generalized lymphadenopathy.
- In acquired immune deficiency syndrome, the patient may have chronic disease with persistent generalized lymphadenopathy. The lymph nodes are more than 1 cm in size at two or more extragenital sites.
- Hodgkin's lymphoma is one of the commonest primary malignant tumors of lymphoid tissue characterized by the presence of Reed–Sternberg cells which are multinucleated giant cells.
- It is treated by chemotherapy, for example, ABVD (adriamycin or doxorubicin, bleomycin, vinblastine, dacarbazine) is the standard first-line regimen.
- Non-Hodgkin's lymphoma is a heterogenous group of malignant tumors of lymphocytes usually presenting as enlarged lymph nodes. In one-third of patients, the disease is extranodal; the most common site is the stomach. Indolent (low grade) and aggressive (intermediate and high grade) are the types of non-Hodgkin's lymphoma based on clinical behavior and pathology. They are treated by chemotherapy.
- Regional lymph nodes may be involved in carcinoma, malignant melanoma, and synoviosarcoma due to lymphatic spread of cancer cells, that is, metastatic lymph nodes.
- The palpable and mobile malignant lymph nodes are usually removed by block dissection. Fixed and nonresectable nodes are treated with palliative radiotherapy which may be combined with chemotherapy.

SELF-ASSESSMENT

Long answer questions

1. Discuss the etiology, management,[1] and complications of tuberculous cervical lymphadenitis.
2. Describe the etiology, pathology, clinical features, and treatment[2] of tuberculous cervical lymphadenitis.
3. Discuss the differential diagnosis of cervical lymphadenopathy. How will you investigate such a case?
4. Describe the clinical features, diagnosis, and treatment of Hodgkin's lymphoma.

Short answer questions

1. Cold abscess
2. Collar-stud abscess
3. Hard lymph node in the neck in an elderly patient
4. Reed–Sternberg cells
5. Indolent lymphoma
6. Lymphadenitic abscess

Multiple choice questions

1. How many lymph nodes are present in the body?
   (a) 200
   (b) 400
   (c) 600
   (d) 800
2. How many lymph nodes are present in the neck?
   (a) 100
   (b) 200
   (c) 300
   (d) 400
3. Which of the following is the commonest cause of lymphadenopathy?
   (a) Infections
   (b) Hodgkin's lymphoma
   (c) Non-Hodgkin's lymphoma
   (d) Metastatic disease
4. The most diagnostic feature of tuberculous lymphadenitis is
   (a) Low-grade evening pyrexia
   (b) Night sweats
   (c) Hemoptysis
   (d) Enlarged matted nodes
5. Collar-stud abscess is a specific manifestation of
   (a) Acute septic lymphadenitis
   (b) Chronic nonspecific lymphadenitis
   (c) Tuberculous cervical lymphadenitis
   (d) Infectious mononucleosis
6. Infectious mononucleosis is a
   (a) Viral infection
   (b) Chlamydial infection
   (c) Bacterial infection
   (d) Fungal infection
7. All of the following are true about Hodgkin's lymphoma, except
   (a) It is the commonest primary malignant tumor of lymphoid tissue
   (b) It originates from T-cells
   (c) Reed–Sternberg cell is a characteristic histological feature
   (d) The patient may have fever, weight loss, pruritus, and night sweats
8. Hodgkin's lymphoma stage IA is treated by
   (a) Short course of chemotherapy with involved field radiotherapy
   (b) MOPP
   (c) ABVD
   (d) Combined radiotherapy and chemotherapy
9. What are 10-year survival rates of stage IA Hodgkin's lymphoma?
   (a) 40%
   (b) 50%
   (c) 70%
   (d) More than 90%
10. All of the following facts are true about non-Hodgkin's lymphoma, except
    (a) It consists of a wide variety of lymphoid tumors
    (b) They originate from B-cells, T-cells, and histiocytes
    (c) They are divided into two groups: indolent and aggressive
    (d) Asymptomatic indolent lymphoma is treated by alkylating agents

Answers

1. (d) 2. (c) 3. (a) 4. (d) 5. (c) 6. (a) 7. (b) 8. (a) 9. (d) 10. (d)

[1] *Note*: Management means diagnosis and treatment.
[2] *Note*: Treatment means treatment only.

Diseases of Bones and Joints

26

Introduction

Diseases of the bones and joints can be due to injuries, infections, and tumors. The fracture of bones and dislocation of joints are common injuries. Infections of the bones and joints include osteomyelitis, septic arthritis, and tuberculosis. Tumors can be benign, malignant, and metastatic. Apart from this, there can be osteonecrosis of the bones due to irradiation (osteoradionecrosis), chemical, and electrical injury.

1. TRAUMA

Fractures

A fracture is a linear deformation or breach in the continuity of a bone which may range from a mere dissolution of a few trabeculae with an intact periosteum to frank disruption of osteoperiosteal continuity.

Etiology

- **Direct trauma**: The bone fractures at the site of impact.
- **Indirect trauma**: The bone breaks away from the site of impact.
- **Tractional force**: Avulsion fracture is caused by sudden powerful pull of a muscle at a localized area of bone where it is attached.
- **Compressional force**: It causes impacted fracture of vertebral bodies following vertical fall from a height.
- **Diseases of the bone**: Normal bones are strong structures and do not break easily with trauma. Sometimes the bones become weak and friable due to diseases such as osteoporosis, tumors, and cysts, and these bones break due to trivial force or trauma. Such fractures are called pathological fractures.

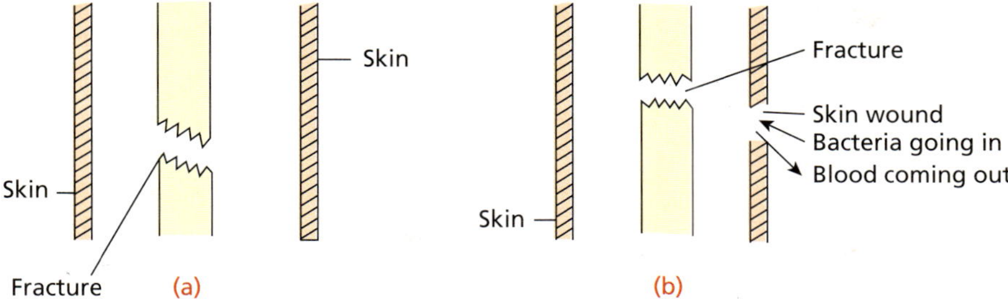

Figure 26.1 Common types of fractures: (a) simple fracture and (b) compound fracture.

Types of Fractures

- **Closed or simple fracture**: Here the fracture does not communicate with the exterior, as the skin or mucoperiosteum (on jaws) covering the fractured bone is intact (Fig. 26.1a). Hence, there is no contamination of fracture by the bacteria from the surrounding environment.
- **Open or compound fracture**: In this type, the fracture communicates with the exterior through a breach in the covering skin or mucoperiosteum (Fig. 26.1b). It is a serious injury as the infection may enter and produce the complications of delayed healing and traumatic osteomyelitis.
- **Transverse fracture**: A transverse fracture occurs at the site of impact due to direct trauma.
- **Oblique or spiral fracture**: It occurs away from the site of application of force due to indirect trauma or torsion.
- **Greenstick fracture**: It occurs in children who have softer and less brittle bones like a greenstick, not like the hard bones of an adult. Here only one cortex of the bone is broken with intact periosteum. This fracture is characterized by an angular deformity with bending of bone without displacement of bone fragments (Fig. 26.2).
- **Comminuted fracture**: Here the bone breaks into more than two fragments. It is usually produced by direct trauma. It is different from a multiple fracture where more than one bone is broken.
- **Stellate fracture**: In this fracture, the fracture lines are multiple and radiate like the rays of the sun in many directions around starting from a central point of impact. It occurs in flat bones of skull and patella.
- **Stress fracture**: It occurs when a bone is subjected to repeated or continued stress at one point or site over a period of time as in athletes and military recruits on a long march.

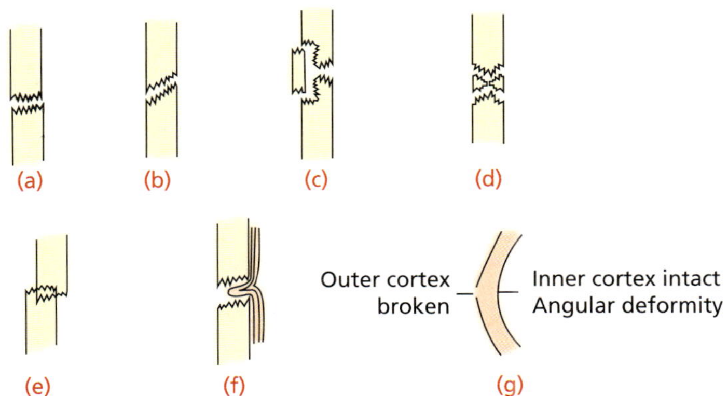

Figure 26.2 Other types of fractures: (a) transverse; (b) oblique; (c) oblique with butterfly segment; (d) comminuted; (e) impacted; (f) muscle between fragments (complicated); and (g) greenstick fracture.

- **Depressed fracture**: Here a broken segment of bone is depressed from the surface level due to direct localized impact. It usually occurs in the vault of skull. **Pond fracture** is a type of depressed fracture where the bone is indented like a ping-pong ball. It is seen in skull of small children.
- **Impacted fracture**: Here the injuring force causing the fracture (usually end on type) drives one fragment of bone into the other. It commonly occurs in vertebral bodies following a vertical fall from the height.
- **Avulsion fracture**: It occurs due to sudden contraction of a powerful muscle pulling up a small piece of bone to which it is attached, for example, sudden pull of temporalis tendon causing avulsion fracture of coronoid process of mandible.
- **Complicated fracture**: In this fracture, the neighboring soft tissues, for example, muscles, intervene in between the fractured ends and structures such as nerves or blood vessels injured.

Healing of a Fracture

Healing of a fracture is of two types: healing of fracture reduced by closed reduction and healing of a fracture reduced by open reduction.

Fracture reduced by closed reduction

This method of healing of bone is just like healing of a wound by secondary intention. The various stages in fracture healing by closed reduction are given as follows:

- **Fracture hematoma**: When a bone breaks, bleeding occurs from the broken ends of bone and other injured tissues. It accumulates around the broken ends producing a fracture hematoma which plays an important role in fracture healing.
- **Cellular proliferation**: The fracture hematoma is invaded by osteogenic cells from the periosteum and endosteum of both fractured ends which differentiate into osteoblasts and chondroblasts. In addition, there is growth of capillaries and mesenchymal tissue from the marrow and surrounding tissues.
- **Callus formation**: As time passes, osteoblasts and chondroblasts lay down irregular bone and cartilage into mesenchymal tissue. It is called callus or procallus and is present 4–6 weeks after trauma. Later on, the osteoblasts produce mature bone which bridges the broken ends. It is known as bony callus and is present 8–12 weeks following trauma.
- **Remodeling**: Remodeling is the final stage of healing wherein the bony callus between the bone ends gets organized into proper lamellar bone and the excess callus around is slowly resorbed to give the broken area normal bony architecture and shape.

Fracture fixed by open method

Here there is no fracture hematoma as it drains out during the operation. Hence, there is no callus formation. The broken tissues unite as they come and remain in close contact with each other. Hence, healing occurs by continuity such as healing of a sutured wound with primary intention. As there is no callus formation, there is no need of remodeling.

Clinical Features

- **History**: The patient presents with a history of trauma, local pain and tenderness, deformity, and loss of function. Usually the trauma is quite severe, but a pathological fracture occurs with trivial trauma.
- **Signs**: The most important sign is local bony tenderness. Other signs of a fracture include swelling, ecchymosis, abnormal mobility, palpable step deformity, and crepitus. The abnormal mobility and crepitus are the conclusive signs of fracture. However, these signs must not be elicited as they cause pain and may add to local tissue injury.

Investigations

- **Plain radiography**: It is the usual and reliable method of confirming the diagnosis (Fig. 26.3). The radiographs are taken in two planes but special views may be required in many fractures.

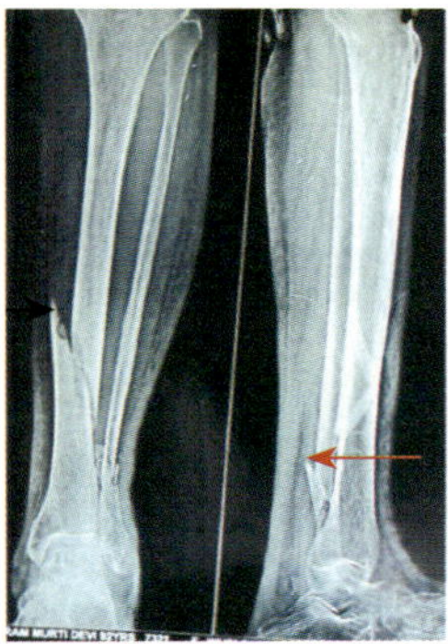

Figure 26.3 Fracture of lower third of tibia and lower fibula with oblique fracture line.

- **CT scan**: It may be required to see the finer details of the fracture (may be by 3D reconstruction) and injuries of the related structures.

Complications

The complications of fracture are of two types: early and late. They are described in Box 26.1.

Box 26.1 Complications of a fracture

Early complications
- Blood vessel injury
- Nerve injury
- Injury to other neighboring soft tissues and organs, for example, pneumothorax in fracture of ribs
- Volkmann's ischemia
- Infection, especially in a compound fracture
- Fat embolism

Late complications
- Delayed union
- Nonunion
- Malunion
- Growth disturbance
- Avascular necrosis
- Traumatic arthritis
- Osteoporosis

Treatment

First aid

Apart from ABC (airway, breathing, circulation), the fracture is immobilized by a splint or whatever is locally available, for example, ruler, stick, and umbrella.

Definitive treatment

The principles of treatment of fractures include reduction to correct displacement, immobilization to retain the broken fragments stable for healing, and rehabilitation to restore function.

Reduction

It is required if there is displacement of fracture fragments. It is of two types: closed reduction and open reduction.

Closed Reduction It is required for most of the displaced simple fractures which can be reduced by closed manipulation (may be under general anesthesia) followed by immobilization usually in a plaster cast, for example, Colles' fracture. The main disadvantage of this method is that a lot of time is required to come to normal. Some fractures are reduced by continuous traction, for example, fracture of shaft of femur which may be of two types—skin traction and skeletal traction.

Open Reduction
- **Indications**: If the closed reduction fails or is not possible and the fracture is compound type, it is treated by open reduction, for example, fracture of shaft of femur.
- **Procedure**: The fracture site is opened; the fragments are accurately reduced and fixed by wire sutures, screws, stainless steel or titanium plate, pin, nail or rod, or arch bars (Figs 26.4 and 26.5).
- **Advantages**: The open method is more accurate and the means employed to fix the fracture may dispense the need for an external cast and permit early mobilization.

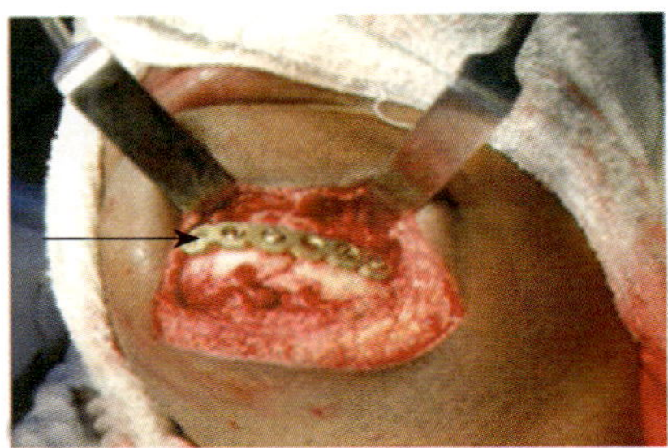

Figure 26.4 Fracture of lower jaw fixed by onlay plate and screws. (Courtesy: Professor Divya Mehrotra)

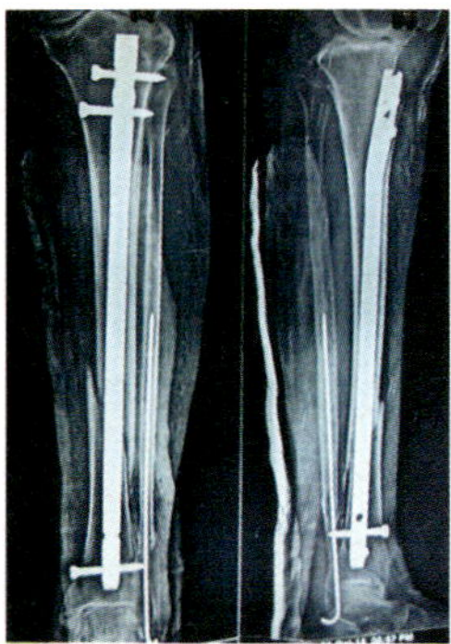

Figure 26.5 Fracture of lower end of tibia treated with intramedullary nail with screws.

- **Disadvantage**: The risk of open reduction is wound infection.

Now some of the fractures are treated with percutaneous method with minimal invasion under C-arm control, for example, fracture of shaft of femur.

Fixation or immobilization

Reduction is followed by suitable immobilization to prevent movement and displacement and pain till the fracture heals.

- Traditionally it is done by the use of a plaster cast. More recently plaster of Paris is being replaced by glass fiber casts.
- Other methods of immobilization include strapping (fracture of phalanx) and sling (fracture of clavicle).
- In open reduction, the fracture is internally fixed by steel wire, Kirschner wire, intramedullary nail, plates and screws (fracture of lower jaw), and special implants.
- Now biodegradable implants made of polyglycolic acid are also available but the fixation attained is not rigid, hence cannot be used in all fractures. Therefore, the external immobilization is also required.

Following immobilization, a check X-ray is done to see that the bone fragments are in correct or reduced position. The duration of immobilization varies from 6 weeks to 3 months. The treatment of common fractures is described in Box 26.2.

Box 26.2 Treatment of common fractures

- **Simple fracture**: Closed or open reduction with external immobilization or internal fixation
- **Compound fracture**: Debridement of wound, reduction, and immobilization by an external fixator with broad-spectrum antibiotics
- **Pathological fracture**: Open reduction and internal fixation, may be with bone grafting followed by treatment of the cause
- **Comminuted fracture**: Open reduction, removal of dead pieces of bone, and internal fixation, may be with bone grafting
- **Greenstick fracture**: External immobilization for a short period

Rehabilitation

It is done by physiotherapy by active and gentle passive movements of the affected joints to restore normal function.

Treatment of compound fractures

Under antibiotic cover, the wound is opened and washed clean, debrided, and the fracture is reduced and fixed with an external fixator. In this method, the wound can be examined and dressed daily. The vascular, nerve, or visceral injury associated with a fracture requires repair at the same time. In a contaminated wound, the cut ends of the nerve are marked to be repaired after some time when the wound becomes clean.

The details of fractures of lower jaw and maxilla are present in Chapter 12, *Maxillofacial (Faciomaxillary) Injuries*. The recent advances in fracture treatment are described in Box 26.3.

Box 26.3 Recent advances in fracture treatment

- Association for osteosynthesis (AO) method of fracture treatment which includes interfragmentary splinting (a combination of compression and splinting)
- Changing AO concepts, for example, use of locking compression plate (LCP)
- Functional bracing: A nonoperative method of treatment of fractures of long bones
- Ilizarov technique: Use of ring fixator to treat difficult nonunions, malunions, and limb length discrepancies

Pathological Fractures

It is a fracture that occurs in a bone made weak by some disease of bone. Hence, it breaks following trivial trauma or even spontaneously. The etiology of pathological fractures is given in Box 26.4.

Box 26.4 Etiology of pathological fractures

- **Local causes**
  - *Infections*: Pyogenic osteomyelitis, tuberculosis of bone
  - *Tumors*
    - Secondary cancer from carcinoma of lung, prostate, and kidney in a male; and breast, lung, and genitals in a female
    - Primary tumors of bone: Osteosarcoma, Ewing's tumor
  - *Cysts*: Simple cyst, aneurysmal bone cyst
  - *Others*: Eosinophilic granuloma, atrophic bone
- **General causes**
  - Osteoporosis
  - Hyperparathyroidism
  - Paget's disease of bones
  - Osteogenesis imperfecta
  - Rickets and scurvy
  - Multiple myeloma
  - Fibrous dysplasia

Clinical features and diagnosis

- A fracture that is sustained without significant trauma is likely to be a pathological fracture. Osteoporosis is the commonest cause of a pathological fracture and the bones most often affected include bodies of thoracic and lumbar vertebrae, neck of femur, and lower end of radius.
- In children it is commonly due to chronic osteomyelitis or a bone cyst, in adults due to bone cyst or giant cell tumor, and in elderly due to metastatic disease.
- Apart from the signs of fracture, usually there are signs of the causative lesion.
- Radiography shows the fracture and the signs of the predisposing factor. Biopsy confirms the diagnosis.

Treatment

- Fractures occurring in benign bone diseases may unite with conventional treatment but it takes more than usual time and even may not unite.
- Open reduction with bone grafting is the modern method of treatment which is the treatment of choice. In a fracture due to malignancy, postoperative chemotherapy or radiotherapy is given to complete the treatment.

Dislocation of joints

The injuries of the joints are not uncommon. The most common result of a joint injury is a dislocation.

Types of Dislocation

Joint dislocations are of two types (Fig. 26.6):

1. **Subluxation or partial dislocation**: In this injury, the joint surfaces are partially displaced, retaining some contact between them.
2. **Luxation or complete dislocation**: In this type of injury, the articular surfaces are markedly displaced, resulting in loss of all contact between them.

Etiology

It includes trauma (traumatic dislocation) and a disease of the joint, damaging its ligaments and supports, for example, tuberculosis of hip causing posterior dislocation (pathological dislocation).

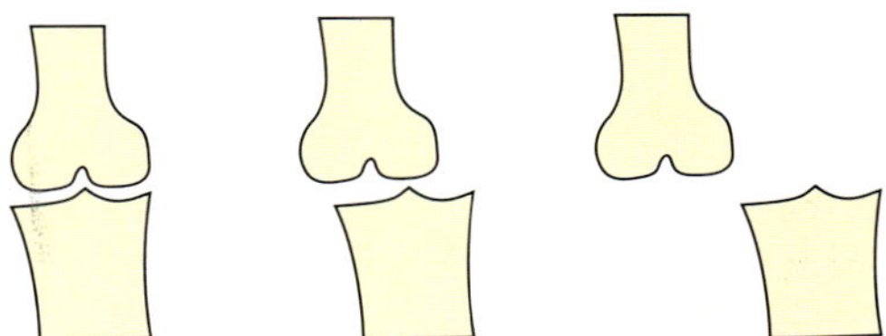

Figure 26.6 Subluxation and luxation.

Clinical Features

The patient presents with pain, swelling, and deformity of the joint with restriction of some movements and presence of some abnormal movements. Deformity is the distinguishing feature of dislocation.

Investigations

The diagnosis can be confirmed by radiography. MRI may be done to image the related ligaments.

Complications of Dislocation of a Joint

Complications include deformity, loss of function, ankylosis of the joint, and secondary osteoarthritis.

Treatment

Treatment includes reduction and immobilization for 1–3 weeks. Recurrence may occur which is treated by operative repair of stretched or injured ligaments and capsule.

2. INFECTIONS

Osteomyelitis

Infections of the bones are quite common. They may involve one component of bone or all the components together. Infection of periosteum is called periostitis, of cortical bone is called osteitis, and of endosteum or marrow cavity is called endosteitis or myelitis. Total inflammation of bone is called osteomyelitis. It is of two types: acute and chronic.

Acute Osteomyelitis

Etiology

It is acute inflammation of a bone of rapid onset and progression caused by pyogenic bacteria, the most common being *Staphylococcus aureus*. Other causative organisms include *Streptococcus pyogenes*, *Salmonella*, *Haemophilus influenzae*, and *Streptococcus pneumoniae*.

Portal of entry

- **Hematogenous spread**: The bacteria usually reach the bone by the bloodstream (hematogenous osteomyelitis) from a focus of infection anywhere in the body, for example, a boil.
- **Local spread**: Bacteria may also enter a bone wound from outside as occurs in a compound fracture (traumatic osteomyelitis). This type of osteomyelitis is uncommon.

Pathogenesis

The pathogenesis of acute hematogenous osteomyelitis is described in Box 26.5 and the pathology is shown in Figure 26.7.

Clinical features

- Most of the patients are children, more commonly male children, who present with fever, chill, toxemia, local pain, and mild swelling.
- The swelling is diffuse, red, hot, and tender like that of cellulitis.
- Hence, if a child presents with signs of cellulitis near a joint, it should be suspected as acute osteomyelitis unless proved otherwise (Rutherford Morison aphorism).

Investigations

- **Laboratory studies**: The blood shows polymorphonuclear leukocytosis with markedly elevated erythrocyte sedimentation rate (ESR) more than 100 mm. The blood must be sent for culture and sensitivity.
- **Plain radiographs**: Radiography does not reveal anything in the first 2 weeks except

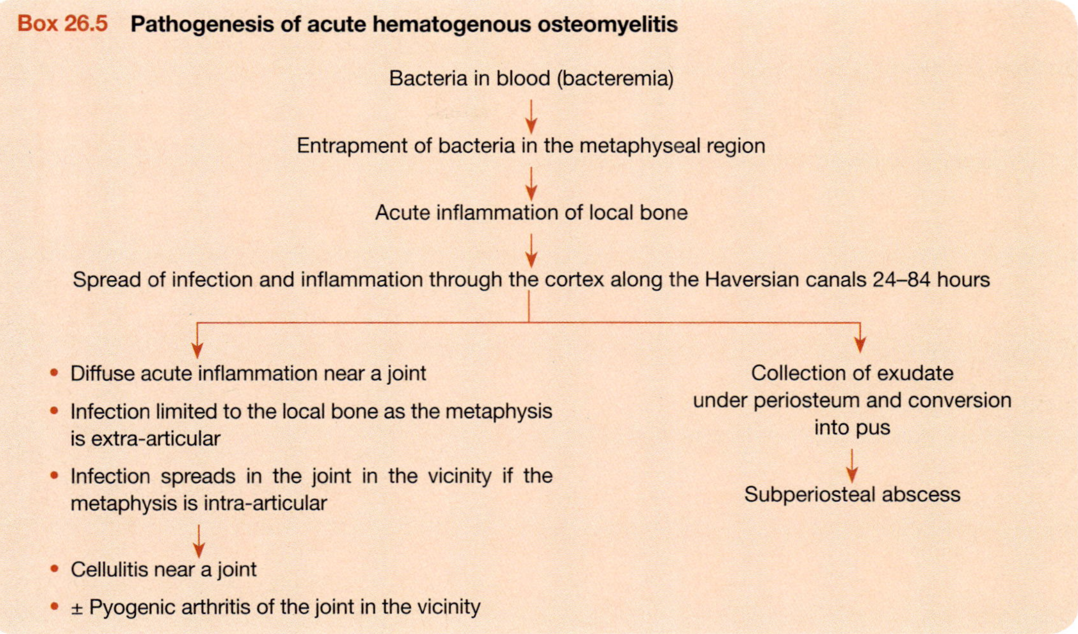

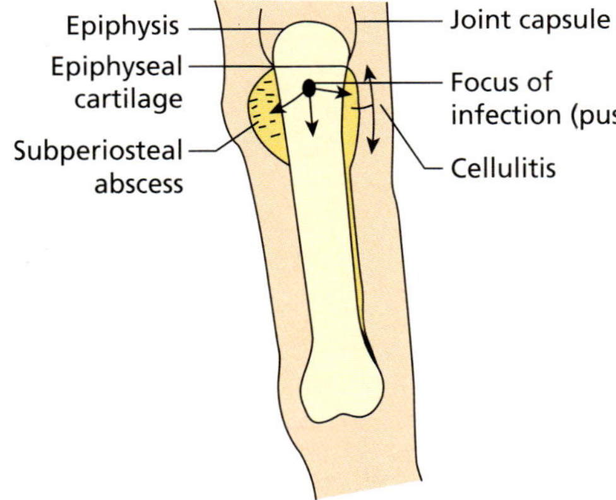

Figure 26.7 Pathology of acute osteomyelitis.

some soft-tissue swelling. Later on, it may show haziness and some decalcification of the involved bone.

- **Ultrasonography**: It is used to identify collection of fluid in the tissues and under the periosteum which may be aspirated at the same time under its guidance and sent for culture and sensitivity.
- **CT scan, MRI, and nuclear bone scan**: They are more sensitive than conventional radiography especially to detect early disease. MRI is most sensitive in detecting edema, soft-tissue collections, and sinus tracts. The bone scan shows increased uptake at the site of disease.
- **Biopsy**: It is sometimes required to differentiate the swelling from an Ewing's tumor which looks like acute osteomyelitis.

Complications

The complications of osteomyelitis are described in Box 26.6.

Box 26.6 Complications of acute osteomyelitis

Systemic complications

- Septicemia
- Pyemia
- Pyemic abscess

Local complications

- Chronic osteomyelitis
- Involvement of adjacent joint when the metaphysis is intra-articular
- Diminished bone growth due to damage to epiphyseal cartilage
- Increased bone growth due to hyperemia of epiphyseal cartilage

Treatment

Medical Treatment

- The patient is admitted and given supportive treatment.
- Intravenous antibiotics, for example, a combination of ceftriaxone and vancomycin or ceftriaxone and cloxacillin, are started.
- When the culture report comes, suitable changes are made in the antibiotic therapy. If this treatment is given within 48 hours of onset, complete resolution may occur.

Surgical Treatment In late cases or if there is collection of pus, exploration is done by making a drill hole in the region of metaphysis. If the pus wells up from the hole, the hole is enlarged for free drainage of pus. Following this, the antibiotics are continued for 6 weeks.

Acute Traumatic Osteomyelitis

- **Etiology**: It is due to infection of a fracture hematoma in open fractures.
- **Clinical features**: It can occur at any age and can affect any bone depending on the site of injury. It is less severe than acute hematogenous osteomyelitis as the open wound provides some measure of drainage of exudate and it is not a part of systemic infection.
- **Prevention**: It is more or less preventable by early and adequate treatment of a compound fracture and doing operations on the bones under strict aseptic conditions.
- **Treatment**: Apart from antibiotics, the wound is provided with effective drainage. The implants may require removal. Stabilization of the affected bone is done to prevent deformity and to help in healing.

Chronic Osteomyelitis

Acute osteomyelitis may become chronic due to either delay in treatment or inadequate treatment. Hence, a part of bone dies to form a sequestrum in this disease.

Pathology

The subperiosteal abscess of acute osteomyelitis ruptures in the soft tissues around and then on the skin to discharge pus through one or more openings called sinuses. At this stage, the fever and toxemia disappear and the patient passes into a chronic phase of disease as described in Box 26.7.

- **Sequestrum**: Due to persistent infection, a part of bone dies and a rim of granulation tissue forms around the dead bone which gradually separates the dead from the healthy bone. The separated dead piece of bone is called sequestrum (Fig. 26.8). It is smooth, shiny, and variable in size.
- **Involucrum**: The elevated and irritated periosteum gradually lays down new bone around the dead bone which is called involucrum. In chronic and long-standing disease, it may be quite thick and strong.

Box 26.7 Pathology of chronic osteomyelitis

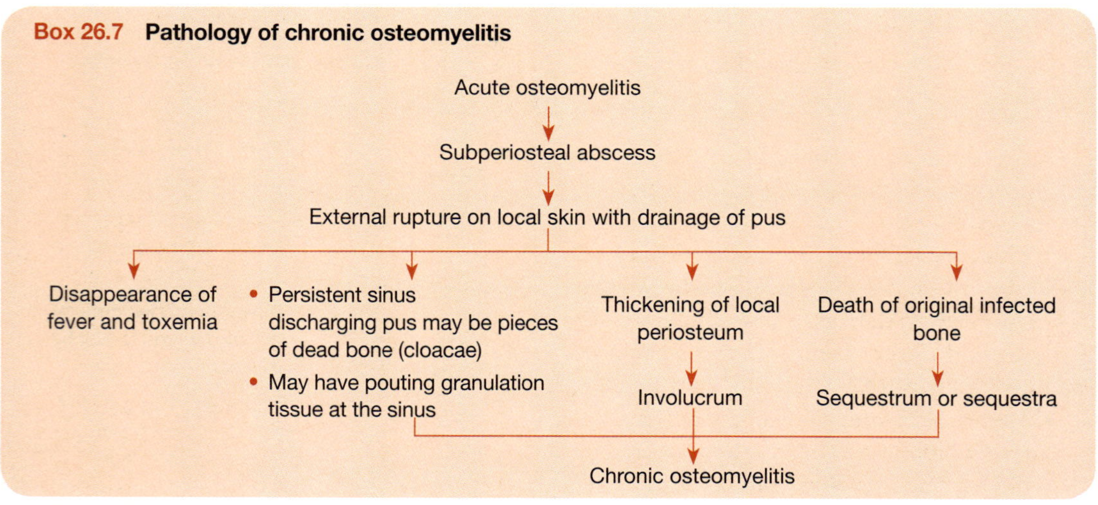

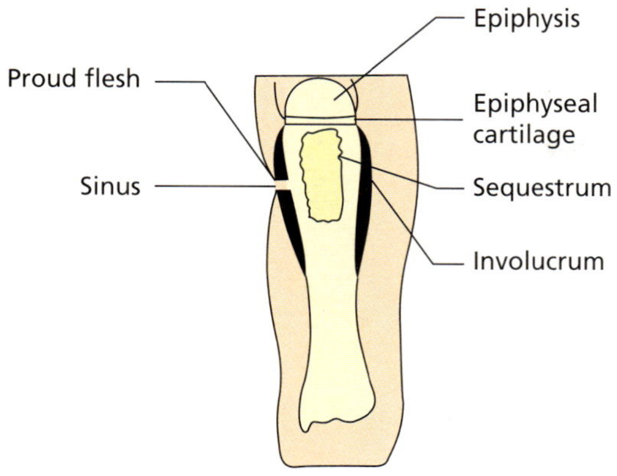

Figure 26.8 Pathology of chronic osteomyelitis.

- **Cloacae**: The involucrum has many holes which discharge pus (liquid) and chips of dead bone (solid) outside. These holes in the involucrum are called cloacae (cloaca is the anus of frog which discharges both urine and feces).

Clinical features

The patient presents with a discharging sinus or sinuses, usually near the ends of a bone which is thickened and tender on deep pressure. The sinus is fixed to the underlying bone. It may have excessive granulation tissue protruding out from its mouth. It is called "proud flesh." It is a sign of presence of sequestrum (or a foreign body) inside the bone.

Investigations

- **Laboratory**: The blood is examined for hemoglobin and counts. The pus is sent for culture and sensitivity. Repeat culture may be done from time to time.
- **Radiology**: It reveals the whole pathology of this disease.
  - The involucrum is thick, irregular, and sclerotic newly formed bone which covers the diseased bone. It has small area or areas of lesser density indicating the sites of cloacae. The sequestrum appears denser than the rest of bone which has undergone some resorption due to inflammatory hyperemia while the sequestrum does not have blood supply, hence retains its minerals. It is separated from the involucrum and the normal bone by a rim of radiolucency which indicates the presence of granulation tissue.
  - CT scan may be done to see further details.
- **Biopsy**: Biopsy from the mouth of sinus and needle biopsy of thickened bone may be done but is not always required.
- **Sinography**: Sinography may be done to delineate the size and extent of osteomyelitic cavity.

Complications

The complications of chronic osteomyelitis include pathological fracture if the involucrum is weak, recurrent attacks of acute inflammation, and amyloidosis in long-standing suppuration.

Treatment

- The treatment is basically surgical. Antibiotics are given during exacerbations and during surgical treatment, and the choice depends on culture and sensitivity report of pus.
- The surgical treatment includes removal of dead bone, granulation tissue and sinus, and elimination of dead space which means sequestrectomy and saucerization. During the latter step, one must be careful not to produce a fracture. After the operation, the wound is closed over a catheter connected to continuous suction–irrigation system.
- Hyperbaric oxygen therapy is also used but its usefulness is not yet proved. Rarely amputation is required in extensive infection.

Acute Osteomyelitis of Jaws

Jaws are special bones as they have so many teeth embedded in their sockets. In spite of the fact that dental infections are very common, the osteomyelitis of jaws is not so common. It may occur at any age but more than half of the cases comprise adults. It is twice more common in males.

Etiology

- **Causative organisms**: The causative bacteria are the resident bacteria of the oral cavity. Ninety percent of instances of osteomyelitis of jaws are the result of local spread of infection. *Streptococcus* is the commonest causative organism. It spreads from a local focus directly into the bone during periodontal inflammation and extraction of tooth during acute pulp or periodontal inflammation.

- **Failure to adequately treat an apical abscess related to lower molar tooth**: It can lead to involvement of the mandibular neurovascular bundle interfering with the blood supply of medullary bone leading to osteomyelitis. Hence, the osteomyelitis of mandible is characterized by anesthesia of lower lip.
- **Fracture of mandible**: A fracture of horizontal ramus of mandible is compound into the mouth. If it is not treated early and properly, the infected saliva is sucked into the wound when the fractured ends move in relation to each other.
- **Gunshot injury in the mandibular region**: It produces many devitalized fragments of bone which if not removed and the adjacent viable ones not covered with soft tissues are infected soon.
- **Hematogenous spread**: Infection may sometimes reach from a distal focus of infection, for example, boil or abscess elsewhere in the body, by bloodstream. In such cases, the causative organism is *S. aureus*. In children, staphylococci may be implanted from nipple to tooth germ. Poor nourishment tips the balance in favor of disease.

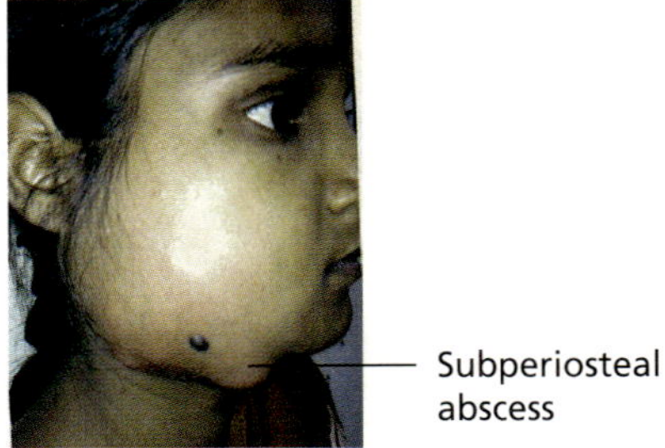

Figure 26.9 Acute osteomyelitis of mandible (right) with subperiosteal abscess. (Courtesy: Professor Divya Mehrotra)

Pathology

The pathological changes are more or less the same as occur in osteomyelitis of long bones. Although the disease is acute, the whole tempo is slower than that of acute osteomyelitis of long bones.

Clinical features

The symptoms are just like those of acute osteomyelitis of other bones.

- There is swelling of overlying soft tissues, pain (boring or throbbing), malaise, and pyrexia. The gums over the affected segment are swollen and the related teeth may become loose and tender.
- When the pus forms, it may present as a localized swelling on the skin outside (Fig. 26.9) or on the alveolus inside. It may subsequently rupture, discharging pus with relief of pain, pyrexia, and toxemia. It may present as a sinus along the lower border of mandible including its angle when the disease becomes chronic.
- From lower jaw disease, the pus may burrow into submandibular region, upper deep neck, anterior pillar of fauces, and muscles of mastication (which causes trismus) or temporomandibular joint.
- From upper jaw, the infection may spread into orbit, ethmoid, and even cavernous sinus of brain.

Investigations

- **Laboratory studies**: The blood shows polymorphonuclear leukocytosis.
- **Radiography**: The diagnosis can be confirmed by orthopantomogram, CT scan, or MRI which shows the bony changes, that is, rarefaction, bone destruction, and new bone formation (Fig. 26.10).

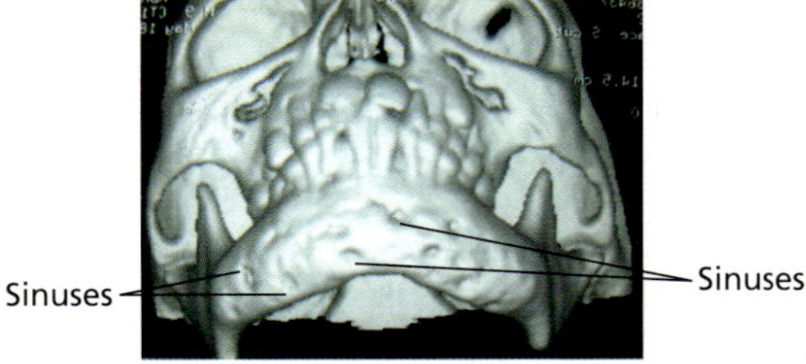

Figure 26.10 3D CT reconstruction of skeleton of lower face showing multiple sinuses in the thickened periosteum due to chronic osteomyelitis of mandible. (Courtesy: Professor Divya Mehrotra)

- **Aspiration**: The pus may be aspirated from related abscess and examined bacteriologically.

Complications

Complications include bacteremia, loss of related teeth, and local spread of infection causing submandibular cellulitis.

Treatment

Medical Therapy If effective antibiotic therapy is started rather early (at the onset of mental anesthesia), frank osteomyelitis involving large parts of mandible does not occur. The antibiotics of choice include ceftriaxone (1 g parenterally daily) or ciprofloxacin (750 mg twice daily) given for 4–6 weeks.

Surgical Therapy The subperiosteal abscess is drained and loose teeth surrounded by pus and grossly carious teeth are extracted as they are a source of persistent infection.

Acute Osteomyelitis of Maxilla

It usually occurs during infancy in the first few weeks of life.

- **Clinical features**: It produces swelling and redness of midface with gross swelling leading to closure of the eye. Hence, it may be mistaken as orbital cellulitis. The palate is edematous. Very soon suppuration occurs and the pus may point below the medial corner of the eye or over as yet unerupted second deciduous molar tooth germ.
- **Investigations**: The diagnosis can be confirmed by CT scan and/or MRI.
- **Complications**: The long-term sequelae of this disease are hypoplasia of enamel of related primary teeth and retardation of growth of maxilla.
- **Treatment**: It is treated with broad-spectrum antibiotics; the pus is aspirated or drained and the necrotic tissue is excised.

Chronic Osteomyelitis of Jaws

Etiology

- It usually affects the sclerosed bone which may develop at the periphery of a segment of mandible involved in acute osteomyelitis. It results in local ischemia which adds to the disease process.
- Some diseases such as Paget's disease of bone may have patches of sclerosed bone which is exposed at the bottom of tooth socket and gets infected.
- Incurable osteomyelitis of mandible occurs following tooth extraction in marble bone disease.

Pathology

The discharge of pus results in the formation of a single or multiple sinuses. Following infection, there is sequestration and regeneration. The erupted and nonerupted teeth may die and then act as a foreign body. A sequestrum or sequestra may form. In the disease of maxilla, the premaxilla separates and acts as a sequestrum. The mandible produces a large sequestrum. Maxilla being a membrane bone does not produce much of a sequestrum. Under the periosteum, there is formation of new bone (not much in maxilla) which forms the involucrum.

Clinical features

- The patient usually presents with a discharging sinus on the face, maybe near the angle of mouth (or in the mouth). It may point via the periodontal membrane of teeth.
- The patient has mild discomfort which increases when flare-up of infection occurs intermittently.
- The involved bone is thickened and tender and the sinus is fixed to the underlying bone. Sequestra may form from the cortical bone and may be discharged from time to time.

Investigations

Investigations include examination of pus and local radiography may be CT scan.

Complications

Complications include spread of infection locally and systemically, damage to local teeth, and very rarely amyloidosis.

Treatment

The sequestra are removed and the cavity is saucerized up to healthy bleeding medulla. Sclerotic bone masses are removed if they are demarcated by bone resorption.

Sinus near the angle of mandible

A sinus near the angle of the mandible is a common clinical presentation of local diseases. Its causes are described in Box 26.8.

Box 26.8 Causes of sinus near the angle of the mandible

- Tuberculosis of local structures and tissues, for example, mandible, submandibular lymph nodes, and rarely parotid and submandibular salivary glands
- Rupture or drainage of infected sebaceous cyst
- Rupture or drainage of infected branchial cyst
- Chronic osteomyelitis of mandible
- Cervicofacial actinomycosis
- The sinuses may be multiple in tuberculosis and actinomycosis

Diagnosis is confirmed by examination of discharge including culture, radiography including sinography, and biopsy from the mouth of sinus. The treatment is removal of the cause.

Septic arthritis (pyogenic arthritis)

It is acute inflammation of a joint caused by pyogenic organisms and characterized by pain, swelling, loss of function, and local redness and tenderness.

Etiology

The commonest causative organism is *S. aureus*. Other organisms include *S. pyogenes*, *S. pneumoniae*, and *Neisseria gonorrhoeae*.

Pathology

The organisms reach the joint by two routes:

1. Hematogenous route
2. Local spread from nearby osteomyelitis, penetrating injury, and intra-articular steroid injection

The pathology of septic arthritis is described in Box 26.9.

Clinical Features

- The patient is usually a child who presents with severe throbbing pain, loss of function, swelling, and redness of the affected joint.
- Any large joint may be involved but the knee joint is most commonly involved.

Box 26.9 Pathology of septic arthritis

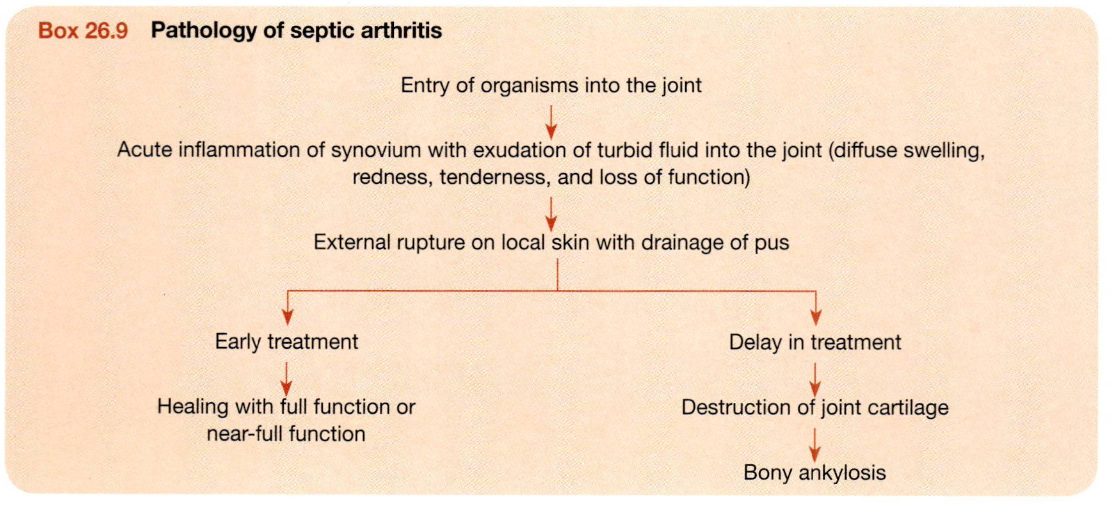

- It is associated with high-grade fever, malaise, and toxemia.
- The child does not move the limb and does not let anybody move it or even touch it. The joint is kept in the position of ease as described in Box 26.10 for different joints.

Box 26.10 Position of ease of the different joints in acute arthritis

- **Shoulder joint**: Adduction and internal rotation
- **Elbow joint**: Flexion and midpronation
- **Wrist joint**: Slight flexion
- **Hip joint**: Flexion, abduction, and external rotation
- **Knee joint**: Mild flexion
- **Ankle joint**: Plantar flexion

Investigations

- **Laboratory studies**: The blood shows polymorphonuclear leukocytosis and elevated ESR. Blood culture may also reveal the causative organism.
- **Radiography**: In the early stage, radiography may be normal or may show increased joint space and enlarged soft-tissue shadow. Later on, the joint space is reduced and joint surface becomes irregular. The joint may be subluxated or luxated.
- **Ultrasonography and needle aspiration**: It may be done to see the fluid in the joint which may be aspirated under its guidance and sent for culture. Gram staining may give a clue to bacteriological diagnosis. Other features of the aspirate are: it is opaque and contains white cells more than 50,000/μL and often >1,00,000/μL with 90% or more polymorphs. It has low glucose.

Complications

Complications of this disease include stiffness or ankylosis, deformity, pathological dislocation, and secondary osteoarthritis.

Treatment

Medical Treatment The patient is admitted, and given supportive treatment and intravenous broad-spectrum antibiotics, for example, a combination of ceftriaxone and cloxacillin. It may require change when culture and sensitivity report of the aspirate is received.

Surgical Treatment If pus is found on aspiration, the joint is opened (arthrotomy), pus and necrotic tissue are removed, and joint cavity irrigated and closed with a suction drain. Now this procedure can be done arthroscopically. The antibiotics are continued for 6 weeks. After arthrotomy and debridement, the joint is immobilized in the position of optimum function because the disease will heal with fibrosis (ankylosis), may be with some function.

Tuberculosis of bones and joints

Tuberculosis is a common infective disease of our country. After the lungs and lymph nodes, bones and joints are the next common site of this disease.

Etiology

- **Causative organism**: The causative organism is *Mycobacterium tuberculosis*. This disease is always secondary to a primary focus in the lungs, lymph nodes, and other sites.
- **Mode of spread**: The diseases may spread from the primary focus may be either by hematogenous or by direct spread from a focus of disease in the vicinity.

Pathology

As the bacteria enter the bone or joint, they cause chronic granulomatous inflammation with caseous necrosis and pus formation (cold abscess) in the affected tissues as described in Box 26.11.

Box 26.11 **Pathogenesis of tuberculosis of bones and joints**

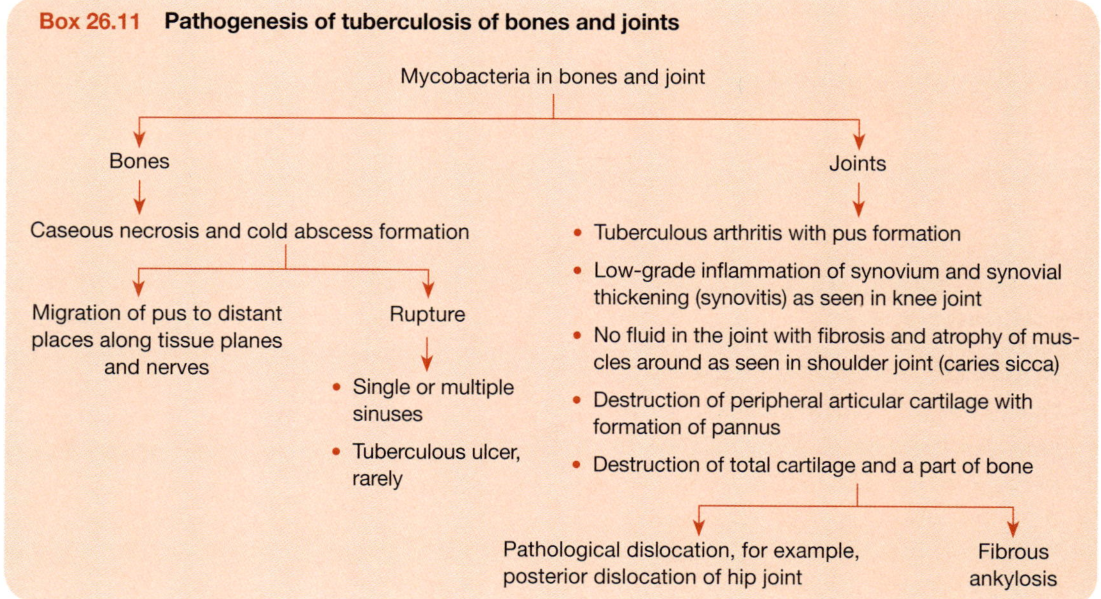

Clinical Features

This disease can occur at any age and in both sexes but is a little more common in young females. The patient presents with local pain, swelling, and loss of function of the affected part of gradual onset. The swelling may be due to collection of pus or synovial thickening which becomes more prominent because of atrophy of muscles in the vicinity. The constitutional symptoms are present in only 20% of patients.

Investigations

- **Laboratory studies**: The blood shows lymphocytosis and elevated ESR. It may be examined for mycobacterial antibodies which are likely to be present.
- **Aspiration**: Aspirate of the cold abscess or synovial fluid in joint disease may be cultured for tuberculosis or may be tested by DNA/RNA amplification for tuberculosis.
- **Radiography**
  - In early disease, there are hardly any signs.
  - In bone disease, there is rarefaction and destruction with minimal reactive new bone formation.
  - The joint disease is characterized by reduction of joint space, erosion of articular surfaces, and marked periarticular rarefaction. The joint may be totally destroyed followed by fibrous (Fig. 26.11) or osseous ankylosis.
  - CT scan or MRI may be required.
- **Biopsy**: Biopsy may be taken from granulation tissue by curettage and sent for histopathology.

Complications

Complications include spread of infection, sinus/sinuses formation, ulceration, and pathological fracture and dislocation.

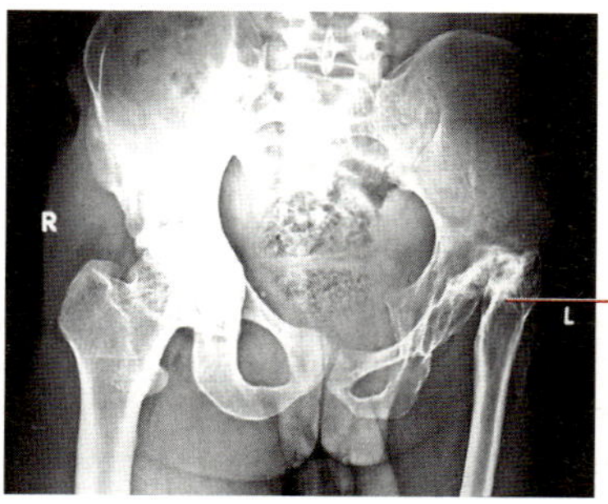

Figure 26.11 Radiography of the pelvis showing destruction of left hip joint including the head of femur with posterior dislocation and atrophy of lower half of left hip bone and femur due to tuberculosis.

Treatment

Antituberculous Drugs The drugs include rifampicin, isoniazid, pyrazinamide, and ethambutol for the first 2 months, and then the last two drugs are withdrawn and the other two drugs are continued for 7 months or more depending on the response.

Supportive Measures The patient is given nourishing diet and exposed to fresh air and sunlight. The affected part is given rest till the pain is relieved. In the upper extremity, it is done with a plaster slab and in the lower by traction. In spinal disease, bed rest may be sufficient, sometimes a spinal brace is required.

Surgical Treatment A cold abscess is aspirated or evacuated, excessive granulation tissue is curetted, and hypertrophied synovium is excised. Later on, salvage operations are done to save whatever useful function is possible, for example, Girdlestone arthroplasty for tuberculosis of hip.

Tuberculosis of Jaws

The tuberculosis of the jaws is rare. It may constitute 5% of all osteoarticular tuberculoses.

Etiology

- It mostly occurs secondary to pulmonary tuberculosis with infection reaching the jaws by hematogenous route.
- It may spread to the jaws from a surface lesion in the mouth.
- Rarely the infection may enter the alveolar process from tuberculous periodontitis.

Clinical Features

- **Maxilla**: The infection usually occurs first at the infraorbital margin of maxilla. The severity of infection in maxillary disease varies inversely with the distance of the lesion from the orbit.
- **Mandible**: Tuberculous infection of the mandible is more common than that of maxilla. The patient presents with a single or multiple sinuses in the mouth or face. In mandible, the infection may spread into the muscles of mastication causing trismus.
- There is necrosis of bone with crumbling sequestration. Secondary infection may make the condition indistinguishable from pyogenic osteomyelitis.

Investigations The diagnosis can be confirmed by X-ray, CT scan, bacteriological examination of discharge for tuberculosis, and biopsy including FNAC of lymph nodes, if enlarged.

Treatment Apart from a full course of antituberculous drugs, the pus is drained and the necrotic tissue excised.

3. TUMORS

Introduction

Bone tumors are not uncommon. They are of two types: primary and secondary.

- **Primary tumors**: They are the tumors of bone that arise from osseous tissue, for example, osteoma and osteosarcoma.
- **Secondary tumors**: They are metastatic tumors of bone due to spread from a primary malignant tumor usually situated at a distant site, for example, carcinoma prostate spreading into bones.

Of the primary malignancies, multiple myeloma is the commonest, and of the benign tumors osteochondroma is the commonest.

Classification

The bone tumors are of many types. Their classification is described in Box 26.12.

Box 26.12 Classification of bone tumors

- Bone-forming tumors
  - *Benign*: Osteoma
  - *Malignant*: Osteosarcoma
- Cartilage-forming tumors
  - *Benign*: Osteochondroma (exostosis), enchondroma (chondroma)
  - *Malignant*: Chondrosarcoma
- Giant cell tumor
- Bone marrow tumors: Ewing's sarcoma, multiple myeloma
- Metastatic tumors from a primary malignant tumor somewhere else in the body, for example, carcinoma of breast and prostate

Osteoma

It is a very slow-growing benign tumor that is composed of sclerotic well-formed bone protruding from the cortical surface of a bone.

- **Clinical features**: The most commonly affected bones are skull and facial bones. It is usually asymptomatic. Sometimes it may bulge into one of the air sinuses and may produce pain.
- **Radiography** shows a smooth bony projection.
- **Treatment**: Asymptomatic tumor does not require any treatment; a symptomatic tumor is excised.

Osteosarcoma

It is a highly malignant primary bone tumor characterized by formation of osteoid tissue or bone by tumor cells.

- **Site of occurrence**: It usually affects the following sites of bone in decreasing order of frequency: lower end of femur, upper end of tibia, and upper end of humerus. However, any bone of the body may be affected including both the jaws.
- **Clinical features**: The patient is usually 15–25 years of age and presents with pain followed by swelling which is shiny with prominent veins. It is warm, tender, and ill-defined. The movements of the adjacent joint may be restricted.

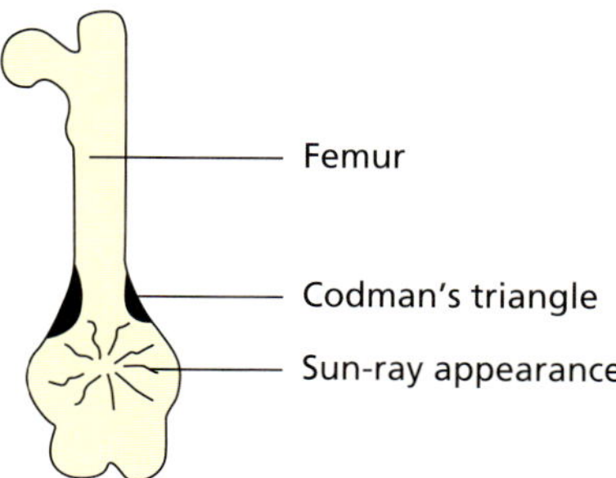

Figure 26.12 Osteosarcoma of lower metaphysis of femur.

- **Investigations**: Radiography shows irregular destruction with new bone formation giving sun-ray appearance (Fig. 26.12). Codman's triangle is a triangular area of subperiosteal new bone formation at the periphery of tumor. The diagnosis is confirmed by biopsy.
- **Treatment**: Amputation of the affected limb well above the tumor is the mainstay of treatment. The systemic macrometastases or micrometastases are controlled by chemotherapy which includes high-dose methotrexate with citrovorum factor, cyclophosphamide, and sometimes cisplatin.

Osteochondroma (exostosis)

It is the commonest benign bone tumor, but is not a true neoplasm as its growth stops with the fusion of epiphysis. It is a mushroom-like tumor with a stalk and a head made up of mature bone with its top covered with cartilage.

- **Clinical features**: The patient is usually an adolescent person who has a painless swelling around a joint, commonly the knee (Fig. 26.13). It is hard, smooth, and nontender, and may be sessile or pedunculated.
- **Radiography**: X-ray shows bony growth with translucent cartilaginous cap (Fig. 26.14).
- **Complications**: The complications include bursitis at the top of swelling, fracture of exostosis, compression of neurovascular bundle in the vicinity, and limitation of movement of adjacent joint.
- **Treatment**: A symptomatic lesion is excised.

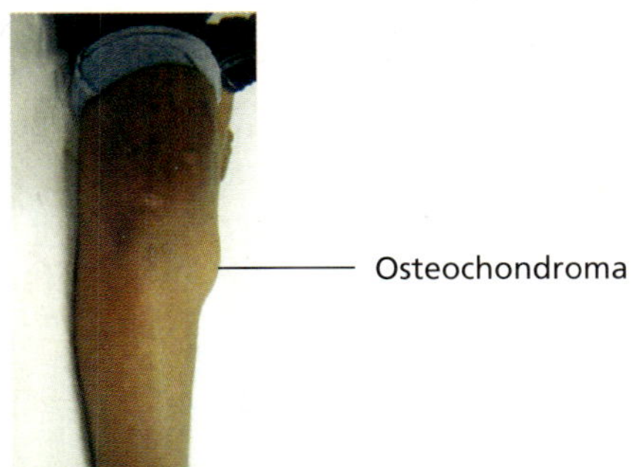

Figure 26.13 Knee region of a boy of 15 years having a bony swelling from medial side of upper end of tibia—osteochondroma (exostosis).

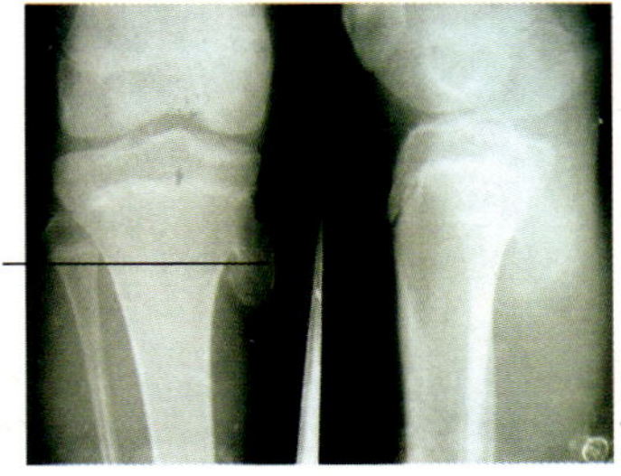

Figure 26.14 Radiograph of knee, anteroposterior and lateral views, showing an osteochondroma (exostosis) of upper metaphysis of tibia. The lesion is pointing downwards and outwards and has a terminal expansion.

Enchondroma (chondroma)

It is a benign tumor consisting of a lobulated mass of cartilage covered by fibrous capsule.

- **Clinical features**: It is usually seen at 20–30 years of age and presents as a long-standing swelling of one or more small bones of hands and feet, that is, phalanges, metacarpals, or metatarsals. The swelling increases in size very slowly, often totally replacing the bone.
- **Radiography**: Radiography shows an expanding lytic lesion with stippled calcification.
- **Treatment**: The lesion is thoroughly curetted and the cavity, if big, filled with bone graft chips.

Chondrosarcoma

It is a malignant tumor of cartilage cells which may arise from any bone but commonly from flat bones such as pelvis, scapula, and ribs.

- **Clinical features**: It usually occurs at 30–60 years of age and presents with pain and swelling. It is firm or hard, smooth or lobulated, and ill-defined.
- **Radiography**: X-ray shows shadow of tumor with mottled calcification, erosion of cortex, and irregular bone destruction.
- **Treatment**: It is usually treated with amputation well above the tumor. In some low-grade tumors, wide resection may be done. Chemotherapy and radiotherapy have hardly any role.

Giant cell tumor (osteoclastoma)

It is a common bone tumor the origin of which is uncertain. Microscopically it consists of undifferentiated spindle cells profusely interspersed with multinucleated giant cells.

- **Clinical features**: The patient is of 20–40 years of age, that is, after epiphyseal fusion, who presents with a swelling of insidious onset of lower end of femur, upper end of tibia, or lower end of radius and lower jaw and maybe with vague pain (Fig. 26.15). The swelling is eccentrically located and may reach up to the joint surface. It is smooth and may have egg-shell crackling on deep pressure.
- **Radiography**: Radiography shows a homogeneously lytic area with trabeculae of remnants of bone traversing it giving soap-bubble appearance, or a lytic lesion.

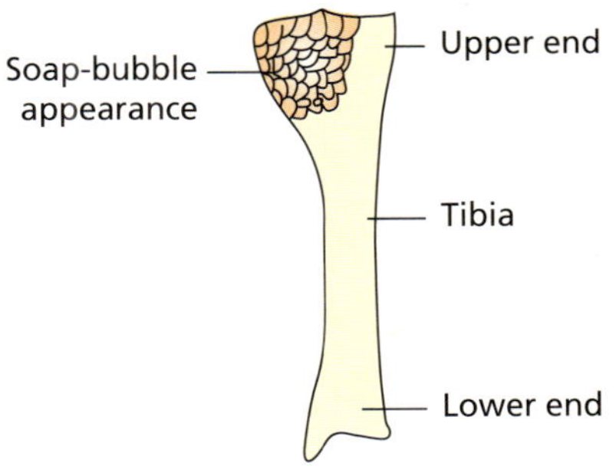

Figure 26.15 Osteoclastoma (giant cell tumor) of upper end of tibia.

- **Treatment**: The treatment is complete excision of the tumor with reconstruction of joint if required and possible, for example, turn-o-plasty of knee joint. For sites such as spine where excision is not possible, radiotherapy is given.

Ewing's sarcoma

It is a highly malignant tumor occurring at 10–20 years of age consisting of sheets of quite uniform small cells resembling lymphocytes.

- **Site of occurrence**: It can occur anywhere but commonly affects the diaphysis of long bones, mainly that of femur and tibia.
- **Clinical features**: The patient presents with pain and swelling often associated with fever. Hence, it may be confused with acute osteomyelitis.
- **Radiography**: Radiography shows an irregular lytic lesion in the medullary zone of mid-shaft and new bone formation in layers giving it an onion-peel appearance (Fig. 26.16).
- **Treatment**: It consists of local control of tumor by radiotherapy (it melts away with radiotherapy, 6000 rad) and control of systemic disease by chemotherapy consisting of vincristine, cyclophosphamide, and adriamycin.

Multiple myeloma

- **Site of occurrence**: It usually affects flat bones, that is, pelvis, vertebrae, skull, and ribs.
- **Types**: It may occur as a solitary lesion (plasmacytoma) or multiple lesions (multiple myeloma).
- **Pathology**: The lesions are mostly small and circumscribed replacing the bone. There is no

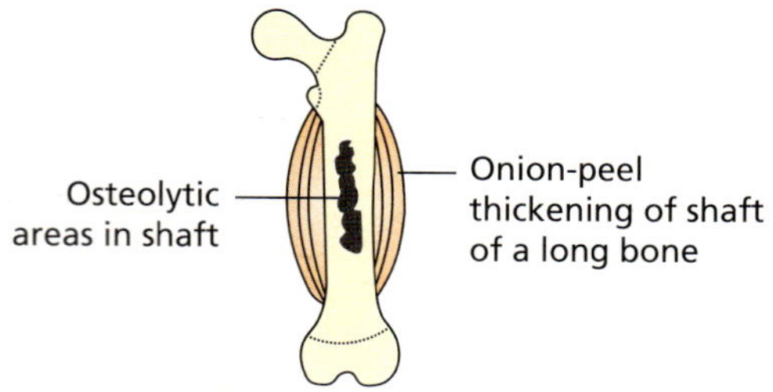

Figure 26.16 Onion-peel appearance of an Ewing's sarcoma.

reactive new bone formation. Microscopically it consists of sheets of closely packed plasma cells with eccentric nucleus with clumped chromatin.

- **Clinical features**: The patient is usually above 40 years of age, more commonly a male who presents with increasingly severe pain in the lumbar and thoracic spine. Pathological fractures, especially of vertebrae and ribs, may occur. Local tenderness may be present on the affected bone.
- **Investigations**
  - The diagnosis is confirmed by finding a paraprotein in serum or urine on protein electrophoresis (PEP) or immunofixation electrophoresis (IFE).
  - The bone marrow biopsy shows infiltration by monoclonal plasma cells.
  - Radiography shows punched-out lytic lesions in skull, spine, proximal long bones, and ribs. These lesions are better seen by MRI and positron emission tomography (PET).
- **Treatment**
  - The initial treatment includes thalidomide or lenalidomide combined with high-dose dexamethasone. Bortezomib is also given.
  - It is consolidated in patients under age 76 years with autologous hematopoietic stem cell transplantation.
  - Localized radiotherapy may be useful for palliation of bone pain or for eradicating tumor at the site of a pathological fracture.

The differences between common malignant bone tumors are described in Table 26.1.

Metastatic bone tumors

The metastatic tumors of the bone are more common than primary bone tumors. Any malignant tumor can metastasize in the bones but the commonly metastasizing tumors include bronchogenic carcinoma, carcinoma of breast, carcinoma of prostate, cancer of thyroid, renal cell carcinoma, and carcinoma of urinary bladder.

- **Clinical features**: The patient presents with bone pain at the site of metastasis, that is, in the spine, ribs, or extremities, and a pathological fracture commonly in the spine or any other bone. The primary may not be obvious.

Table 26.1 Differences between common malignant bone tumors

Features	Osteosarcoma	Chondrosarcoma	Giant cell tumor	Ewing's tumor	Multiple myeloma
Age	15–25	30–60	20–40	5–15	Adults over 40
Common sites of occurrence	Lower end of femur, upper end of tibia, jaws	Flat bones, upper end of femur	Lower end of femur, upper end of tibia, lower end of radius, horizontal ramus of mandible	Femur, tibia, flat bones	Pelvis, vertebrae, skull, ribs
Clinical features	Pain and swelling of weeks' or months' duration	Swelling, may be pain of months' duration	Pain and swelling of months' duration	Pain, swelling, and fever of weeks' or months' duration	Increasingly serve pain in lumbar and thoracic spine of weeks' or months' duration
Radiography	Sun-ray appearance, Codman's triangle, osteolysis, and new bone formation	Mottled calcification or popcorn-like appearance	Soap-bubble appearance, no new bone formation	Onion-peel appearance	Multiple punched-out areas in skull and other flat bones
Pathology	Tumor cells with osteoid or bone formation	Chondroblasts and cartilaginous matrix	Multinucleated giant cells in fibrous stroma	Layers of round cells	Sheets of closely packed cells
Treatment	Local surgical ablation and chemotherapy	Local ablation and radiotherapy	Excision of tumor with reconstruction	Radiotherapy with chemotherapy	• Thalidomide with high-dose dexamethasone • Autologous hematopoietic stem cell transplantation

- **Investigations**
  - X-ray shows a lytic lesion (Fig. 26.17) in most of the cancers and osteosclerosis in carcinoma of prostate but in 20–25% of cases there are no signs on radiography. Hence, a bone scan should be done.
  - PET scan may also be used for early detection.
  - Biopsy confirms the diagnosis.
  - In a case of secondary cancer without known primary, the common investigations include X-ray of chest, abdominal ultrasound, intravenous or CT urography, and thyroid scan.
- **Treatment**
  - Palliative measures including relief of pain
  - Treatment of a pathological fracture by open reduction and radiotherapy
  - Control of causative cancer by chemotherapy and/or radiotherapy

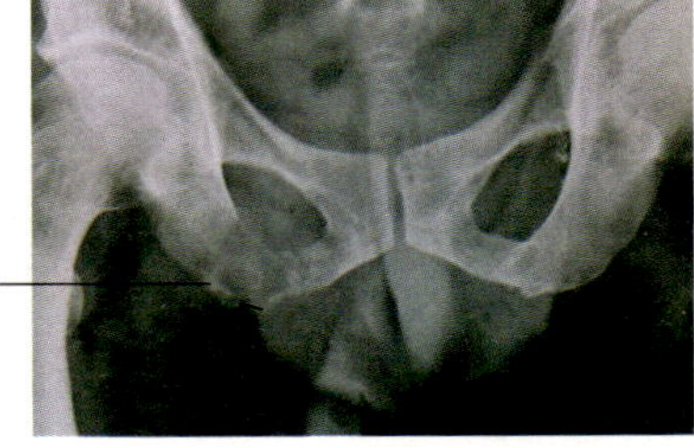

Figure 26.17 Anteroposterior view of lower part of pelvis showing osteolytic metastasis, especially in the right ischium.

4. OTHER DISEASES OF THE BONES AND JOINTS

Osteonecrosis of the jaw

It is the death of osteoid tissue of jaw bones and may be caused by irradiation, use of certain chemicals, and electric current. It is of many types which are described in the subsequent text.

Chemical Osteonecrosis

At one time it was quite common, but now it is rare. It can be caused by the use of phosphorus, arsenic, or mercury.

- In phosphoric necrosis, the involucrum surrounds the necrotic bone completely.
- Arsenic was used in bygone years to devitalize the pulp of teeth wherefrom it diffuses into the neighboring tissues causing extensive necrosis of soft tissues and bone.
- In mercurialism, the oral changes are due to the metal being secreted in saliva. A necrotizing stomatitis occurs in the first 24 hours. Later on, ulcers develop on the alveolar border exposing it to secondary infection. Subsequently, osteonecrosis is converted into osteomyelitis followed by sequestration of alveolar process.
- Use of bisphosphonates in the treatment of osteoporosis may rarely cause osteonecrosis of jaw.

Electrical Osteonecrosis

When an oral carcinoma, especially that adjacent to the jaw, is treated by electrocoagulation, it may result in extensive bone necrosis. To destroy the tumor completely, coagulation is done up to the periosteum, thus exposing the bone to secondary infection. Sequestrum forms and separates early but the continuity of the jaw is maintained.

Osteoradionecrosis

It is a complication of radiotherapy which is given to treat local squamous cell carcinomas. It was very common when these cancers were treated by conventional deep X-ray therapy. Now with the use of Co-60 therapy or linear accelerator, its incidence is markedly reduced (3%).

Etiopathogenesis

The full-blown disease is the combined effect of irradiation, trauma, and infection.

- The irradiation may lead to aseptic necrosis as the regenerative power of the bone is depressed, and the vessels are occluded by thrombosis or fibrosis. Osteonecrosis occurs irrespective of the fact whether the cancer is controlled or not controlled.
- In children, it interferes with normal growth and development of the jaw and causes irregularities in the formation and eruption of teeth.
- In adults, postirradiation crumbling and demineralization of teeth occur, called irradiation caries.
- Osteoradionecrosis is usually associated with extraction of teeth that were not removed before the start of radiotherapy, which subsequently become carious.
- Pressure of an artificial denture may cause ulceration which may not heal exposing the bone to infection. Thus, even an edentulous patient may have serious radionecrosis ending in slow and massive sequestration.
- Radiotherapy causes mucositis and secondary candidiasis preventing the patient from taking proper care of mouth and teeth leading to secondary infection. It may result in ulceration of mucosa covering the jaws.
- Reduced salivary flow and pH are contributory factors.
- This condition is also called radiation osteomyelitis.

Clinical features

- In early stages, the patient has severe burning pain in the jaw which may continue for weeks or months.

- When infection occurs, fever, swelling, and trismus are additional symptoms. One or more abscesses may occur.
- After some time, the abscess/abscesses may rupture resulting in relief of pain, fever, and swelling. One or more sinuses may form. The jaw mucosa may slough out.

Investigations

Investigations include radiography and bacteriological examination of discharge. To see the finer details of the lesion, CT scan is required.

Treatment

- Maintenance of orodental hygiene by irrigation and scaling of teeth, extraction of bad teeth
- Antibiotic therapy
- Drainage of pus
- Debridement and sequestrectomy

Prophylaxis of osteoradionecrosis

Before the start of radiotherapy in orofacial cancers, the following things are done:

- Oral hygiene is made perfect by frequent irrigation, scaling and extraction of bad teeth, and controlling infection.
- All teeth in the area of irradiation should be extracted.
- Radiotherapy is given 7–10 days after extraction to permit wound healing.
- Fluoride therapy helps in preventing irradiation caries.

KEY POINTS

- A fracture is a linear deformation or breach in the continuity of a bone which may range from a mere dissolution of a few trabeculae with an intact periosteum to frank disruption of osteoperiosteal continuity.
- The most important sign in fracture is local bony tenderness. The abnormal mobility and crepitus are the conclusive signs of fracture, but they should be avoided to elicit. The diagnosis is confirmed by radiography.
- The types of fractures include simple fracture, compound fracture, greenstick fracture, comminuted fracture, complicated fracture, and pathological fracture.
- Healing of fracture resembles healing with secondary intention in surgical wounds and occurs through the following stages: fracture hematoma, cellular proliferation, callus formation, and remodeling, but when a fracture is fixed by open method, the healing occurs without callus formation similar to primary healing of surgical wounds.
- The complications in fracture include infection, injury to nerves, vessels and surrounding tissues, fat embolism, delayed union, malunion, nonunion, growth disturbances, traumatic arthritis, and osteoporosis.
- The treatment includes reduction, fixation or immobilization, and rehabilitation. Reduction of fractures can be closed or open type. The latter type includes accurate reduction and fixation of fracture with plates and screws, wires, pins, nails, or rods. The risk of open reduction is wound infection.
- Treatment of compound fracture includes debridement of wound under antibiotic cover, reduction, and fixation with an external fixator.
- In subluxation of the joint, the joint surfaces are partially displaced but retain some contact between them. In luxation, the articular surfaces lose all contact between them. Deformity is the distinguishing clinical feature of a dislocation.
- Acute osteomyelitis is characterized by fever, local pain, redness, and swelling. Early disease can be detected by bone or CT scan. Combination of ceftriaxone and vancomycin or ceftriaxone and cloxacillin is the line of treatment. It may become chronic due to delay or improper treatment.
- Chronic osteomyelitis is characterized by sinus formation, local thickening of bone, and tenderness. Radiography shows sequestrum, involucrum, and cloacae. It is treated by sequestrectomy and saucerization.
- Acute osteomyelitis of the jaws is more or less the same as occurs in osteomyelitis of long bones but the whole tempo is slower.
- Chronic osteomyelitis of the jaw is characterized by discharging sinus on the face (or in the mouth),

(CONTD...)

KEY POINTS (...CONTD)

tender and thickened bone, and the sinus being fixed to the underlying bone. Sequestra may form from the cortical bone and may be discharged from time to time.

- Septic arthritis (pyogenic arthritis) is an acute inflammation of a joint caused by pyogenic organisms and characterized by pain, swelling, loss of function, and redness of the joint. If left untreated, it may lead to bony ankylosis.
- Tuberculosis of bones and joints is characterized by swelling which may be due to collection of pus or synovial thickening. The treatment includes antituberculous drugs, drainage of abscess, and salvage surgery when necessary.
- Tuberculosis of jaws occurs secondary to pulmonary tuberculosis with infection reaching the jaws by hematogenous route. Tuberculous infection of the mandible is more common than that of maxilla.
- The commonest benign tumor of the bone is osteochondroma, and the commonest malignant tumor is multiple myeloma.
- Osteoclastoma is a locally malignant tumor of epiphysis of long bones which can occur in the jaws also. X-ray shows a multiloculated shadow.
- Osteosarcoma is a highly malignant primary bone tumor characterized by a tender, ill-defined vascular swelling. X-ray shows bone destruction and new bone formation giving sun-ray appearance and Codman's triangle. Amputation well above the tumor is the mainstay of treatment followed by chemotherapy.
- Ewing's sarcoma commonly affects the diaphysis of long bones, mainly that of femur and tibia. Radiography shows an onion-peel appearance. Treatment consists of local control of tumor by radiotherapy and systemic control by chemotherapy.
- Multiple myeloma is a malignant tumor consisting of plasma cells that usually affects flat bones. Treatment is chemotherapy, autologous hematopoietic stem cell transplantation, and palliative radiotherapy.
- The metastatic tumors of the bone are more common than primary bone tumors. The most commonly metastasizing tumors include carcinoma of lung, breast, prostate, thyroid, kidney, and urinary bladder.
- Osteonecrosis of the jaws is the death of osteoid tissue of jaw bones and may be caused by irradiation, use of certain chemicals, and electric current.
- Osteoradionecrosis of the jaw is prevented by extraction of the teeth in the area of irradiation 7–10 days prior to radiotherapy.

SELF-ASSESSMENT

Long answer questions

1. Describe the types, clinical features, investigations, and treatment of a fracture.
2. Discuss the etiology, pathology, clinical features, investigations, and treatment of acute osteomyelitis.
3. Discuss the causes and management of a sinus situated near the angle of mandible.

Short answer questions

1. Pathological fracture
2. Dislocation of a joint
3. Osteomyelitis of mandible
4. Pyogenic arthritis
5. Tuberculosis of joints
6. Osteoradionecrosis

Multiple choice questions

1. The last step in healing of a fracture is
   (a) Hematoma formation
   (b) Consolidation
   (c) Remodeling
   (d) Callus formation
2. Which of the following is the most important clinical sign of fracture?
   (a) Local pain
   (b) Swelling
   (c) Crepitus
   (d) Restriction or loss of movement

(CONTD...)

SELF-ASSESSMENT *(...CONTD)*

3. Compound fracture is defined as
   (a) Fracture with an open skin wound
   (b) Fracture with nerve injury
   (c) Fracture of many bones
   (d) Fracture of a bone at multiple sites
4. All of the following are the principles of treatment of a compound fracture, except
   (a) Wound debridement
   (b) Immediate closure of wound
   (c) Immobilization with external fixator
   (d) Aggressive antibiotic therapy
5. The ideal method of treatment of a compound fracture is
   (a) Internal fixation
   (b) External fixation
   (c) Skeletal traction
   (d) Plaster immobilization
6. A compound fracture is treated by antibiotics, wound debridement, and
   (a) Closure of the wound
   (b) External fixation
   (c) Internal fixation
   (d) Prosthesis
7. The most serious complication of an open (compound) fracture is
   (a) Bleeding
   (b) Infection
   (c) Shortening
   (d) Muscle contracture
8. Osteomyelitis is defined as
   (a) Infection of periosteum of bone
   (b) Infection of cortical bone
   (c) Infection of endosteum
   (d) Infection of all components of bone
9. The commonest causative organism of acute osteomyelitis is
   (a) *Staphylococcus aureus*
   (b) *Streptococcus pyogenes*
   (c) *Salmonella*
   (d) *Streptococcus pneumoniae*
10. The bacteria usually reach the bone by
    (a) Lymphatic route
    (b) Open injury
    (c) Hematogenous route
    (d) Direct spread from the neighboring joint
11. Subperiosteal abscess is collection of pus
    (a) Under the periosteum of bone
    (b) Superficial to periosteum
    (c) In the marrow cavity
    (d) Inside the neighboring joint
12. All of the following facts are true about acute osteomyelitis of maxilla, except
    (a) It is usually seen during infancy
    (b) The midface of one side is swollen and red
    (c) The ipsilateral palate is edematous
    (d) The eyes are normal
13. The antibiotic of choice in the treatment of acute osteomyelitis is
    (a) Ceftriaxone + cloxacillin
    (b) Penicillin
    (c) Streptomycin
    (d) Tetracycline
14. Sequestrum is defined as
    (a) Sheath of new bone formed around the dead bone
    (b) Separated dead piece of bone in osteomyelitis
    (c) Holes in the newly formed bone discharging pus and chips of bone
    (d) Excessive granulation tissue projecting out from the sinus
15. Involucrum is defined as
    (a) Sheath of new bone formed around the dead bone
    (b) Separated dead piece of bone in osteomyelitis
    (c) Holes in the sheath of newly formed bone discharging pus and bone chips
    (d) Cavity inside the bone having sequestrum
16. All of the following statements are correct about "proud flesh," except
    (a) It is pouting granulation tissue situated at mouth of a sinus
    (b) It is a sign of sequestrum lying inside the related bone
    (c) It is also seen if there is a foreign body present in the depth of a sinus
    (d) It is indicative of malignant transformation
17. All of the following are signs of chronic osteomyelitis, except
    (a) The patient presents with a chronic sinus discharging pus
    (b) It is fixed to the underlying bone

(CONTD...)

SELF-ASSESSMENT *(...CONTD)*

(c) The related bone is tender and thickened
(d) X-ray shows a localized area of osteolysis without periosteal reaction

18. What is the treatment of choice of chronic osteomyelitis with sequestrum?
    (a) Long-term antibiotic therapy
    (b) Sequestrectomy and saucerization
    (c) Sequestrectomy
    (d) Laying open the sinus
19. The most common diagnostic investigation for chronic osteomyelitis is
    (a) Plain radiography
    (b) Sinography
    (c) CT scan
    (d) MRI
20. All of the following are true about chronic osteomyelitis of jaws, except
    (a) The causative bacteria are the local bacteria of oral cavity
    (b) The commonest organism is pyogenic *Streptococcus*
    (c) The infection may occur by hematogenous route
    (d) Maxilla produces considerable involucrum

Answers

1. (c) 2. (c) 3. (a) 4. (b) 5. (b) 6. (b) 7. (b) 8. (d) 9. (a) 10. (c) 11. (a) 12. (d) 13. (a) 14. (b) 15. (a) 16. (d) 17. (d) 18. (b) 19. (a) 20. (d)

Diseases of Vessels

27

1. DISEASES OF ARTERIES

Definitions

- **Infarction**: It is sterile necrosis of tissues following sudden complete arterial obstruction.
- **Gangrene**: It is defined as massive death of tissues with putrefaction. It occurs following arterial obstruction and infection.

There are many types of arterial diseases, for example, atherosclerosis, arterial embolism and thrombosis, arterial trauma, aneurysm, thromboangiitis obliterans, and Raynaud's disease.

Effects of arterial diseases

The main effect of arterial diseases is reduced or absent blood supply in the area supplied by that particular artery, described in Table 27.1.

Table 27.1 Effects of arterial diseases

Effects of arterial diseases	Causes	Features	Examples
Reduced blood supply	• Atherosclerosis • Thromboangiitis obliterans	• Causes intermittent pain at the time of stress or exertion • Arterial pulses are usually weak	• Angina pectoris in coronary artery disease • Intestinal angina in mesenteric arterial obstruction • Claudication (cramp-like pain) in lower limbs
Absent blood supply	• Embolism • Thrombosis	• 5 Ps—pain, pallor, puffiness, pulselessness, and paralysis • Affected part feels cold	• Infarction in sterile areas, for example, myocardial infarction and cerebral infarction • Gangrene in infected areas such as in intestine, lower limbs, and lungs

Clinical features of arterial obstruction

The clinical features of acute arterial obstruction (5 Ps) are described in Box 27.1.

Box 27.1 Clinical features of arterial obstruction (5 Ps)

- Pain
- Pallor
- Puffiness
- Pulselessness
- Paralysis, that is, loss of sensory and motor function (the part feels cold and numb to touch)

Claudication

Claudication is cramp-like pain that occurs in the lower limbs due to chronic ischemia characterized by pain after some walking which is relieved by standing still or taking some rest. It occurs again if the patient starts walking after rest. It is called intermittent claudication.

Atherosclerosis

It is a very common disease characterized by subintimal deposition of cholesterol, lipoid material, and lipophages in large and medium-sized arteries (atheroma) resulting in narrowing (stenosis) of the artery. It commonly occurs at branching or bifurcation sites, of large and medium-sized arteries.

Etiopathogenesis

The predisposing factors include smoking, fat-rich diet, diabetes mellitus, obesity, lack of exercise, and hypercholesterolemia. The etiopathogenesis and effects of atherosclerosis are described in Box 27.2.

Clinical Features

- The patient is usually above 50 years of age, more commonly a male. It is more common in diabetics, obese, and tobacco users.
- It is asymptomatic in two-thirds of patients. In symptomatic patients, its main symptom is pain on exertion when the demands for blood increase, for example, claudication in lower limbs and angina pectoris in the heart.

Box 27.2 Etiopathogenesis and effects of atherosclerosis

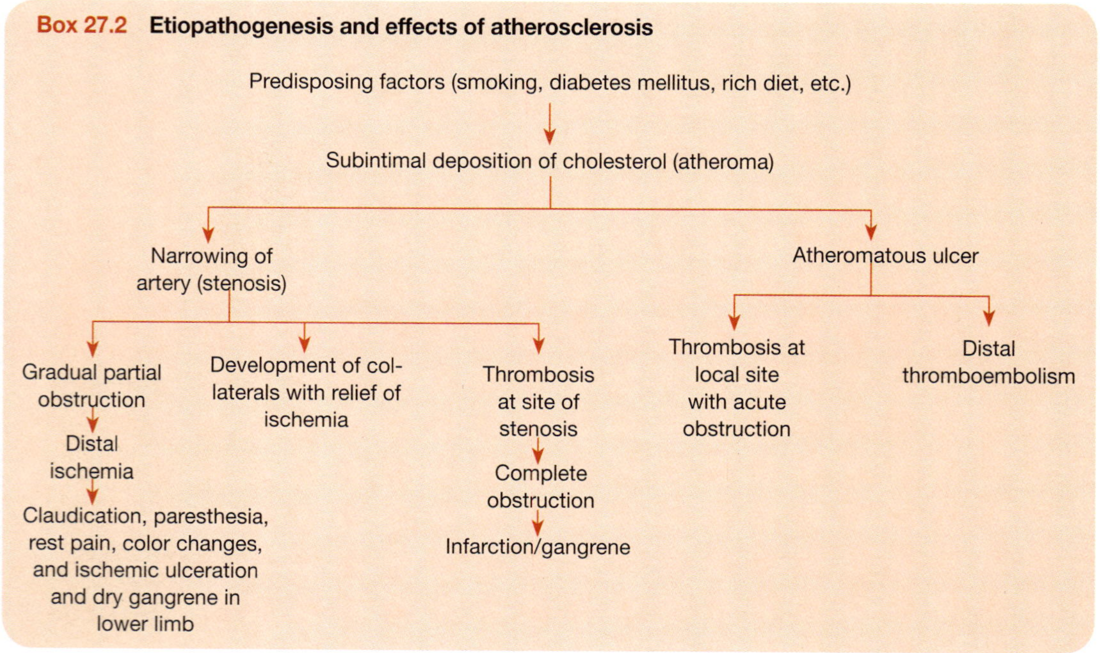

- The arterial wall may be palpably thickened and a systolic bruit may be heard on large arteries.

Investigations

The blood is sent for hemoglobin, blood sugar, and lipid profile. The disease can be imaged by CT angiography or MR angiography (Figs 27.1 and 27.2). The arteries can also be seen by Doppler, color duplex, and arteriography; the latter investigation is required if surgery is being planned on the arteries.

Arteriography is radiographic visualization of arteries after injecting a radio-opaque contrast medium into lumen of targeted artery.

Treatment

Removal of Risk Factors These include smoking cessation, risk factor reduction such as control of hypertension and blood sugar, dietary modification, and moderate exercise.

Drug Therapy It includes cilostazol 100 mg twice daily orally and antiplatelet agents. There is hardly any drug to relieve the pain of ischemia but vasodilators may be used. The pain of coronary atherosclerosis (coronary angina) is relieved by long-acting nitrates, for example, isosorbide nitrate, and/or β-blockers.

Surgical Methods Segmental atheromatous narrowing (known as arterial stenosis) is treated with percutaneous balloon dilatation and stenting. It is the commonest method of treatment which is done percutaneously. Another method is bypass grafting using a prosthetic graft or a segment of vein.

Arterial embolism

Etiology It is due to sudden arterial obstruction caused by impaction of some particulate material in the arterial lumen, for example, thrombus, air, fat, and tumor tissue.

Site The arteries of lower limb and heart, and pulmonary artery are the most common sites of embolism.

Clinical Features The patient presents with pain of sudden onset (like bolt from blue) at the site of impaction radiating along the course of that artery and signs of severe arterial insufficiency.

Investigations The diagnosis is confirmed by urgent arteriography. Doppler is a better investigation during emergency as it saves time.

Complication The main complication of arterial embolism is acute ischemic loss of the affected organ.

Treatment

- The thromboembolism is treated with unfractionated heparin and catheter-directed chemical thrombolysis with the use of tissue plasminogen activator (TPA).
- The surgical treatment is urgent embolectomy which is done by interventional Fogarty balloon catheter method or an open operation.

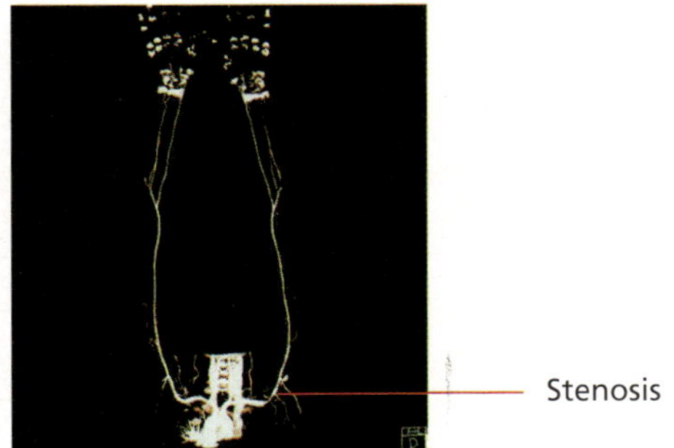

Figure 27.1 CT angiography showing left subclavian arterial stenosis (the upper limbs are abducted above head). (Courtesy: Dr. S.S. Sarkar, Sarkar Diagnostics)

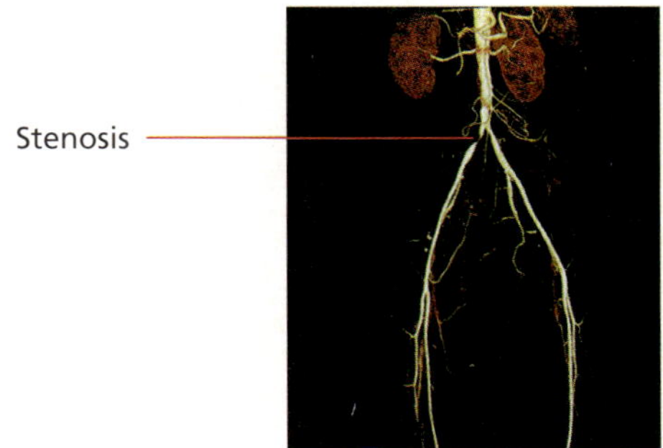

Figure 27.2 CT angiography showing arterial stenosis of right common iliac artery at its origin and absent internal iliac artery. (Courtesy: Dr. S.S. Sarkar, Sarkar Diagnostics)

It is mostly required to remove other types of emboli than a thrombus.

Arterial thrombosis

- It usually occurs on an atheromatous plaque and causes acute arterial obstruction but is of slow onset as compared to embolism.
- It does not cause acute ischemia as collaterals are likely to have developed due to preexisting chronic atheromatous obstruction making the effect of eventual acute occlusion less dramatic. The arterial thrombosis must be differentiated from arterial embolism as described in Table 27.2.
- Treatment: The patient is given 5000–10,000 units of heparin by intravenous infusion and arrangement is made for intra-arterial thrombolysis using urokinase. Percutaneous mechanical thrombectomy may be required. Later on, the stenosis (localized narrowing) is treated by balloon dilatation.

Arterial trauma

Etiology The arteries can be injured in any type of trauma, that is, blunt, sharp, or firearm injury. It is usually associated with injury to other structures around.

Clinical Features An artery may be contused, punctured, cut partially or completely, or lacerated. It is characterized by arterial hemorrhage (external in open wounds and internal in closed wounds) and distal ischemia, that is, pallor and pulselessness.

Investigations The diagnosis can be confirmed by Doppler ultrasound. For seeing full details of injury and planning treatment, arteriography is done.

Treatment Apart from emergency general care, the contused and thrombosed segment of the artery is excised followed by end-to-end repair or repair with a segment of vein. Puncture is suture repaired or repaired with a venous patch. Cut ends are suture repaired (anastomosed).

Arterial aneurysm

Etiology It is a localized dilatation of an artery which is caused by weakness of arterial wall due to atherosclerosis, syphilis, and other causes.

Types An arterial aneurysm is of two types—true and false. A true aneurysm is of two morphological types—saccular (spherical in shape) and fusiform (like a spindle). They are shown in Figure 27.3. Pseudoaneurysm has a fibrous wall and usually follows arterial punctures. Its features are described in Box 27.3.

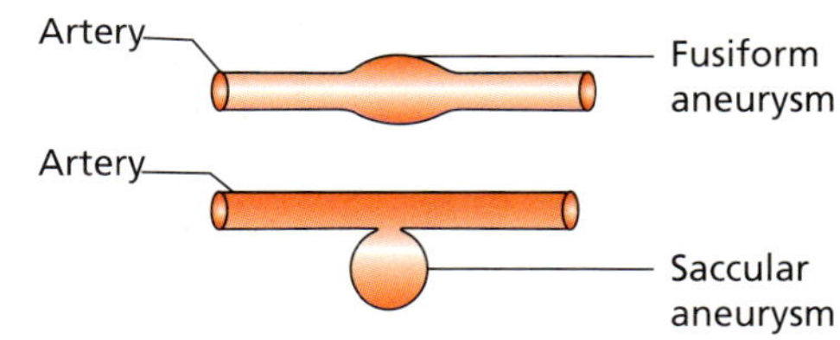

Figure 27.3 Two main types of true arterial aneurysm.

Table 27.2 Differences between arterial embolism and arterial thrombosis

Features	Arterial embolism	Arterial thrombosis
Onset	Sudden like bolt from blue	Acute but a little slow (few minutes to an hour)
Pulse	Proximal pulse and opposite-side pulses are normal	Same-side pulse and opposite-side pulses may be normal or weak with thickened arterial wall
Temperature	Severely cold	Cold or normal
Arteriography	• Sharp cutoff sign • No or very few collaterals	• Gradual tapering of artery (stenosis) to complete obstruction • Well-developed collaterals
Distal ischemia	Likely to be significant—5 Ps	Usually mild

Box 27.3 Features of a pseudoaneurysm

- It has a fibrous wall and not true arterial wall
- It usually follows arterial puncture for arteriography and cardiac catheterization. Hence, it commonly affects the femoral artery. It may rupture or cause thromboembolism, hence should be repaired when it is more than 2 cm in size

Clinical Features

- It may be asymptomatic when it is detected by investigations.
- Symptomatic aneurysm is characterized by a pulsatile mass, pressure symptoms on local veins and nerves, and symptoms of recurrent distal embolism.
- On examination there is a tense pulsatile swelling along the course of a large artery.

Investigations The diagnosis can be confirmed by Doppler color ultrasound. MR angiography or CT angiography is required to define local arterial anatomy for its reconstruction.

Complications It may rupture leading to sudden massive hemorrhage, or may contain a thrombus which may cause repeated distal thromboembolism.

Treatment Operation is indicated when an aneurysm is associated with distal embolism, has attained a certain size (different in different-site aneurysms), and has a mural thrombus. The treatment methods include bypass, endovascular repair, and open operation with prosthetic interposition.

Thromboangiitis obliterans (Buerger's disease)

It is a segmental inflammatory and thrombotic process of distal-most arteries and sometimes of neighboring veins.

Etiology Its cause is not known but it is mostly seen in heavy smokers.

Clinical Features The patient is usually a male younger than 40 years of age who presents with rest pain in lower limbs, especially in the toes. If the patient continues to smoke, the pain progresses to dry gangrene. The distal arterial pulses are weak or absent.

Diagnosis Angiography shows obliteration of distal arterial tree.

Complications The complications include loss of a digit or limb, mostly the lower limb.

Treatment Smoking cessation is the mainstay of treatment which gives relief in symptoms but it should be total and forever. As the distal small arteries are occluded, revascularization is not possible.

Raynaud's phenomenon (RP) and Raynaud's disease

RP is a syndrome of paroxysmal digital ischemia usually caused by an exaggerated response of digital arteries to exposure to cold or emotional stress.

Etiology It may occur without a known cause (primary RP or Raynaud's disease), or due to a variety of rheumatic diseases, especially scleroderma (secondary RP).

Clinical Features

- It mainly affects fingers but may affect toes, nose, and ears.
- It is clinically characterized by pallor due to excessive vasoconstriction followed by cyanosis and subsequent recovery with vasodilatation leading to rubor (RP).
- Primary RP is more common, mostly occurs in young women, and poses more as a nuisance than a serious disease.
- The secondary RP is less common and may cause digital ulceration or gangrene.

Investigations These depend on the clinical suspicion about the cause.

Complications The complications include digital ulceration, dry gangrene, and loss of a digit.

Treatment

- The patient should avoid cold exposure and sympathomimetic agents, and stop smoking.
- Calcium channel blockers, for example, nifedipine, are useful.
- Finally cervicodorsal sympathectomy may be required.

2. DISEASES OF VEINS

The veins are thin-walled tubes which carry deoxygenated blood to the right side of the heart. The veins of the lower half of body drain blood into the heart against gravity which is helped by provision of valves in them and the muscle pump present in the calf muscles. Because of this factor, the diseases of veins commonly affect the lower limbs.

Varicose veins

They are dilated, tortuous, and lengthened superficial veins. They commonly occur in the lower extremities in about 15% of adults (Fig. 27.4).

Etiology They are etiologically related to prolonged standing, heavy weight lifting, and pregnancy. The great saphenous vein and its tributaries are commonly involved. Dilatation of vein prevents the valves from coapting causing incompetence and venous stasis.

Types The varicose veins are of two types:

1. **Primary**: They occur without a definite cause. Most of the varicose veins belong to this group.
2. **Secondary**: They are less common and are due to extrinsic pressure in the pelvis due to a large tumor or cyst, ascites, pregnancy, and acquired arteriovenous fistula.

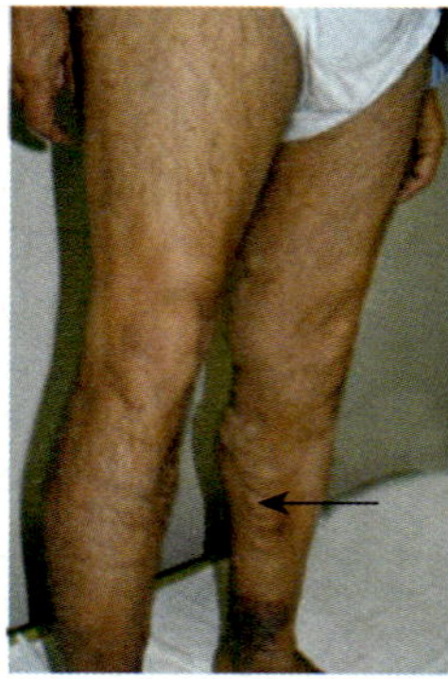

Figure 27.4 Varicose veins of lower limbs as seen from the front, more marked in the left leg. (Courtesy: Professor Sandeep Tewari)

Clinical Features It may be asymptomatic or may produce dull pain and fatigue in the leg. The dilated tortuous veins are visible at the site of affected vein, for example, long saphenous vein, short saphenous vein, or communicating veins. The valvular incompetence is detected by Trendelenburg's and Schwartz test and deep vein thrombosis (DVT) by bandage test.

Investigations Duplex ultrasonography helps in diagnosis and finds the site of venous reflux. Rarely, venography may be done.

Complications The complications of varicose veins include hemorrhage, thrombosis, lipodermatosclerosis, and ulceration.

Treatment

- Early disease is treated by use of elastic graduated compression stocking, elevation of limb at night, and gentle massage from bottom up.
- Advanced or unresponsive disease is treated with endovenous ablation using radiofrequency waves or laser, or stripping of diseased vein.
- The complications of stripping of the vein include injury to the accompanying nerve and formation of a local hematoma which may be at multiple sites.
- Small varicose veins less than 4 mm diameter are treated with injection sclerotherapy when the sclerosant is injected into the lumen of empty vein.
- Foam sclerotherapy can be employed to treat larger veins.

Deep vein thrombosis

It is clotting of blood in the deep veins which is a dangerous problem as it can cause pulmonary embolism (impaction of thromboembolus in pulmonary artery which kills a large number of victims).

Etiology The main etiological factors include stasis, hypercoagulability, and vein wall injury (Virchow's triad). Hence, it occurs in bed-ridden patients due to disease, operation, or childbirth, especially in obese and elderly people. It commonly affects calf veins (soleus muscle) and pelvic veins.

Clinical Features

- It is asymptomatic in most of the patients (60%). An asymptomatic patient may present suddenly with pulmonary embolism characterized by chest pain, breathlessness, and hemoptysis.
- In symptomatic patients, the symptoms include fever, pain and swelling in the calf and thigh, and positive Homans' and Moses' signs. The pain may be so severe that it may be difficult to flex or move the limb.
- The clinical features of DVT are described in Box 27.4.

Box 27.4 Clinical features of deep vein thrombosis

- The leg involvement may be asymptomatic
- In a symptomatic case, there is fever, pain, and swelling in the calf and thighs
- Positive Homans' sign is characterized by pain in the calf when the foot is dorsiflexed forcefully with extended knee
- Positive Moses' sign is characterized by pain when the calf is gently squeezed and moved from side to side

- Iliofemoral venous thrombosis: It may occur during confinement in late pregnancy and after delivery. It is of two types as described in Box 27.5.

Box 27.5 Two types of iliofemoral vein thrombosis

- **Phlegmasia alba dolens**: Massively swollen leg with pitting edema, pain, and blanching (pale whitish)
- **Phlegmasia cerulea dolens**: Result of further progression with arterial compromise characterized by painful massively swollen blue leg

Box 27.6 Venous ulcers

It is a chronic nonhealing ulcer of lower limb caused by chronic venous insufficiency, and occurs around medial malleolus that has bluish color with sloping edge and pigmented surrounding skin. It is of two types:

- Varicose ulcer is due to varicose veins. It is superficial and often rides a vein
- Post-thrombotic ulcer is a complication of deep vein thrombosis. It goes deep to deep fascia

- Post-thrombotic ulcers: It is a complication of DVT. General features and types of venous ulcers are described in Box 27.6.

Investigations The diagnosis can be confirmed by duplex ultrasound. Venography (radio or MR venography) may be done.

Treatment

- **Anticoagulants**: The patient is given intravenous heparin 25,000 units daily for 7 days. Warfarin is also given orally as early as possible 10 mg daily orally for the first 2 days and 5 mg daily subsequently for 3–6 months. The therapy is controlled by periodic assessment of activated partial thromboplastin time (aPTT). Anticoagulant therapy retards additional thrombus formation allowing endogenous fibrinolytic activity to lyse existing clot. It increases the risk of hemorrhage.
- **Thrombolytic therapy**: It is given within the first 24 hours to lyse the existing clots by increasing the plasmin levels. The drugs include streptokinase, urokinase, and recombinant tissue plasminogen activator (rt-PA).
- **Caval filter**: Interruption of inferior vena cava by putting a filter in it by percutaneous transjugular technique may be done in patients with a major contraindication to anticoagulants and who are at a high risk of development of pulmonary embolism.
- **Prevention**: It is prevented by avoidance or control of predisposing factors, heparin therapy, and use of pneumatic compression devices during and after major operations and long-term confinement to bed.

3. GANGRENE

Gangrene is massive or macroscopic death of tissues associated with putrefaction. It commonly affects the distal parts of body, for example, toes, foot (Fig. 27.5) or leg, finger, and intestine.

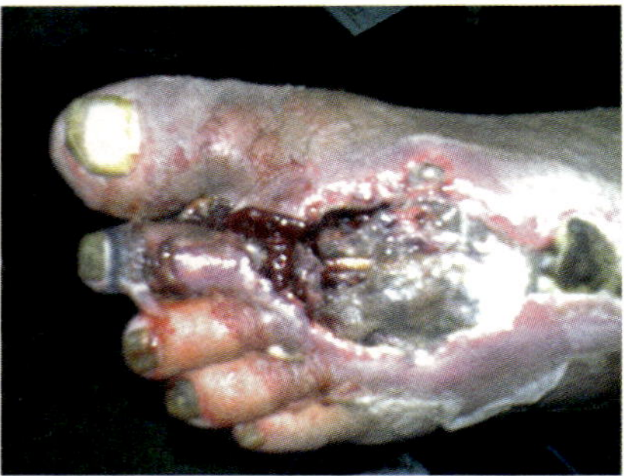

Figure 27.5 Gangrene of foot with gangrene of second toe and part of dorsum with surrounding inflammation. (Courtesy: Professor Sandeep Tewari)

Etiology

The diabetics and the people having peripheral arterial disease, peripheral neuropathy, and heart disease are more liable to suffer with this problem. The causes of gangrene are described in Box 27.7.

Clinical Diagnosis

- The problem of gangrene can occur at any age and in both sexes.
- Initially there is severe pain, except when there is peripheral neuropathy which gradually reduces when the affected part dies.
- The gangrenous part changes its color through a variety of shades—pale, dusky red, mottled, purple, and then to dark brown, greenish black, or black. The black color is due to disintegration of hemoglobin and formation of iron sulfide.
- The part loses its normal warmth and becomes cold. It becomes numb (loss of sensation). There is lack of arterial pulsation, venous return, and capillary response to pressure.

Box 27.7 Etiology of gangrene

- **Arterial diseases causing ischemia leading to massive death of tissues**
  - Thrombosis of atherosclerotic artery
  - Arterial embolism
  - Thromboangiitis obliterans (Buerger's disease)
  - Intra-arterial injection of toxic drugs
- **Infections (infective gangrenes)**
  - Gas gangrene
  - Fournier's gangrene of scrotum
  - Carbuncle
  - Cancrum oris
- **Trauma**
  - *Direct trauma*
    - Crush injury
    - Persistent pressure at one point or area causing pressure sores
  - *Indirect trauma*: Injury to vessels at some distance from the site of gangrene, for example, pressure on brachial artery by supracondylar fracture of humerus
  - *Physical and chemical agents*
    - Excessive heat, for example, burns
    - Excessive cold, for example, frostbite, trench foot
    - Chemical burns
    - Radiation injury
    - Electrical injury
- **Gangrene of multifactorial etiology:** Diabetic gangrene
- **Ergotism**
- **Venous gangrene**

Specific Types of Gangrene

Some specific types of gangrene are described in Box 27.8.

Types of Gangrene

The gangrene is of two types.

Box 27.8 Some specific types of gangrene

- **Fournier gangrene of scrotum**: It is gangrene of the scrotum of acute onset without an obvious cause and associated with mixed infection
- **Frostbite**: It is a pale and waxy tissue necrosis of pinna, external nose, fingers, and toes following exposure to cold below freezing point at a high altitude and high winds
- **Trench foot**: It is peripheral gangrene of lower limb due to prolonged exposure to moist cold as occurs in a trench
- **Ainhum**: It is a condition occurring chiefly in Negroes in tropical conditions marked by linear constriction of a toe, especially the little toe which by its contraction gradually amputates the toe
- **Cancrum oris**: It is extensive ulceration and gangrene of cheek that occurs in malnourished children suffering with some major illness such as diphtheria and typhoid

Dry Gangrene

- It occurs when the ischemic tissues are desiccated by gradual reduction of arterial supply as happens in atherosclerosis. The part becomes dry and shriveled, discolored from disintegration of hemoglobin, and greasy to touch.
- Line of demarcation: After the gangrenous process is established, a line of demarcation appears gradually between the live and gangrenous tissues. It is seen on the surface and in a slow gangrenous process and not in an acute problem.

Moist (Wet) Gangrene

- It occurs when the main artery supplying a part or limb is suddenly occluded as occurs following ligation or embolism. The part is swollen and discolored, and may have blebs with absent line of demarcation.
- The other types of wet gangrene include diabetic gangrene and gas gangrene.

The differences between dry and wet gangrenes are described in Table 27.3.

Investigations

Investigations include Doppler ultrasound and arteriography (radiography, MR, or CT angiography).

Treatment

- Removal of the cause, for example, control of diabetes, stopping smoking in Buerger's disease, calcium channel blockers in Raynaud's disease, and penicillin in gas gangrene
- Excision of the gangrenous part

Table 27.3 Differences between dry and wet gangrenes

Features	Dry gangrene	Wet gangrene
Etiology	Atherosclerosis, thromboangiitis obliterans	Arterial embolism, arterial ligation, crush injury, gas gangrene, uncontrolled diabetes
Pathogenesis	Gradual loss of arterial supply leading to gradual desiccation and death of tissues	Sudden occlusion of blood supply
Extent of involvement	Small area of gangrene due to presence of collaterals	Large area of involvement due to absence of collaterals
Onset	Gradual onset	Acute onset
Appearance	Gangrenous part is dry, shriveled, and mummified	Gangrenous part is wet, swollen, putrefied, and discolored
Line of demarcation	Usually present	Absent
Crepitus	Absent	May be present
Discharge	Nil	Significant serous or blood-stained discharge
Treatment	• Conservative amputation • Treatment of cause	• Major amputation • Treatment of cause

4. DISEASES OF LYMPHATICS

Acute lymphangitis

It is acute inflammation of cuticle along with its lymphatics caused by *Streptococcus haemolyticus* (commonly) and *Staphylococcus aureus* (uncommonly) characterized by spreading inflammation with a border or limit. It is treated by penicillin or co-amoxiclav intravenously.

Lymphedema

It is swelling of a part of body due to accumulation of lymph in its interstitial tissue. It commonly affects the lower limbs, scrotum, and penis, and may affect other areas. It is a chronic process.

Etiology

Primary Lymphedema

- It occurs due to congenital insufficiency of lymphatics the cause of which is not known.
- Lymphangiography done by injecting a radio-opaque dye in lymphatics shows abnormal lymphatics in these patients, for example, aplasia, hypoplasia, or hyperplasia.
- It is of three types depending on the age of occurrence:
  - Congenital lymphedema at birth (Milroy's disease is a type of lymphedema congenita that runs in families)
  - Lymphedema praecox at puberty
  - Lymphedema tarda later in life

Secondary Lymphedema It is the accumulation of lymph in the tissues due to the following causes:

- Lymphatic filariasis which is the commonest cause in India
- After inguinal or axillary block dissection of lymph nodes
- Radiotherapy of metastatic nodes of inguinal or axillary areas
- Advanced malignancy of inguinal or axillary lymph nodes

Filarial Lymphedema

It is the commonest type of secondary lymphedema in our country.

Etiopathogenesis It is caused by *Wuchereria bancrofti* and *Brugia malayi* which enter the body through the mosquito bite that occurs on the lower limbs. This parasite enters the lymphatics of the limb and causes recurrent attacks of adenolymphangitis (inflammation of lymphatics and lymph nodes). The pathogenesis is schematically described in Box 27.9.

Clinical Features

Primary Lymphedema

- These patients are usually young between 2 and 35 years of age. A positive family history may be present.
- It may be unilateral or bilateral and commonly involves the lower limb. The edema is pitting type and remains so throughout life. The overlying skin is normal.

Secondary Lymphedema

- The patient presents with swollen lower limb (or scrotum or penis) which starts from below up (tree-trunk pattern).
- The swelling occurs with fever with rigor that increases with each attack.
- The dorsum of the foot and toes are swollen (buffalo hump and squaring of toes) and the malleolar shape is lost due to edema.
- The skin of dorsum of toes cannot be pinched (Stemmer's sign).
- As the disease progresses, the skin gets thickened and nodulated, and may be depigmented (Fig. 27.6).

Box 27.9 Pathogenesis of filarial lymphedema (elephantiasis)

Recurrent adenolymphangitis following mosquito bite
↓
Fibrous scarring
↓
Adenolymphatic obstruction
↓
Accumulation of lymph in distal tissue spaces (lymphedema, pitting type)
↓
Recurrent attacks of adenolymphangitis
↓
Addition of protein to edema fluid
↓
Increasing fibrosis of edematous tissue
↓
Nonpitting edema and dermal thickening (elephantiasis)

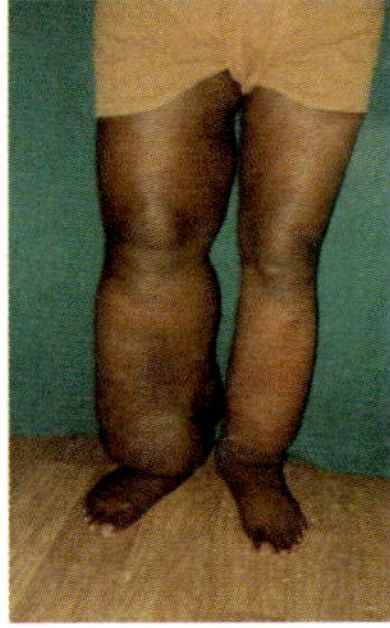

Figure 27.6 Chronic filarial lymphedema of right leg. (Courtesy: Professor Brijesh Mishra)

The differences between primary and secondary lymphedema are described in Table 27.4.

Diagnosis

It is confirmed by finding eosinophilia, microfilariae in the night blood smear, positive immunological tests, and very rarely lymphangiography.

Grading of Lymphedema

The grading is done to decide the line of treatment and may predict about the results of treatment. It is described in Box 27.10.

Complications

The complications of lymphedema include dermal fissuring, cracks, ulceration, lymphorrhea, recurrent

Table 27.4 Differences between primary and secondary lymphedema

Features	Primary lymphedema	Secondary lymphedema
Etiology	Congenital insufficiency of lymphatics the cause of which is not known	Recurrent/chronic adenolymphatic obstruction commonly due to filariasis
Age	Younger age group (2–35 years of age)	Middle ages
Sex	Females are more affected	Males are more affected
Regional lymph nodes	Absent or may have undergone fatty degeneration	Enlarged, removed, or destroyed by cancer or radiotherapy
Skin	Normal	• Thickened, may have grooves or nodules • Skin of dorsum of toes cannot be pinched (Stemmer's sign)
Edema	Present	Tree-trunk pattern (swelling from below upwards)
Pitting	Always present	Initially pits, later it does not

Box 27.10 Grades of lymphedema

- **Grade I**: Pitting edema without skin changes, completely relieved on rest and elevation of part
- **Grade II**: Pitting edema without skin changes, partly relieved on elevation
- **Grade III**: Nonpitting edema with skin thickening, slightly reduced on elevation
- **Grade IV**: Nonpitting edema with gross skin changes with nodules or warty projections, may be lymphorrhea, and no relief on elevation

cellulitis, and abscess, but they are very rare in primary lymphedema due to absence of infection.

Treatment

Supportive Measures This treatment does not cure the problem but may keep the problem under reasonable control.

- A course of diethylcarbamazine 100 mg thrice daily orally after meals for 3–4 weeks
- Prevention of further mosquito bite
- Intermittent elevation of affected limb by 6 inches
- Use of elastic crepe pressure bandage or pressure garment
- Massage of affected limb from below up
- Care of skin to prevent infection and immediate treatment if infection occurs

Surgical Treatment If the obstructed and dilated lymph vessels or lymph nodes can be identified by imaging, the following procedures can be done to improve lymphatic drainage:

- **Lymphovenous shunt**: It is anastomosis of a dilated lymphatic to the same-sized tributary of the long saphenous vein by microvascular technique (lymphovenous shunt). At least four lymphatics should be anastomosed (Fig. 27.7a).
- **Nodovenous shunt**: It is anastomosis of transected dilated lymph node to a vein (Fig. 27.7b).

These operations are technically demanding and give poor results, hence are not popular. They may be employed in primary lymphedema where it may be possible to do them but in secondary lymphedema they are difficult to perform.

- **Charles' operation**: Another approach is excisional in which the diseased tissues are excised up to the healthy tissue and the raw area is covered by split-thickness grafts obtained from healthy areas of skin of affected limb or other donor areas.
- **Thompson Swiss-roll operation**: It combines both excision and improving lymphatic drainage. By a longitudinal incision a skin flap is raised after denuding its epidermis near the edge. The underlying elephantoid tissue is excised and the denuded skin flap is buried with its edge close to the main vessels of the limb and the wound closed (Fig. 27.8). The results of this operation are not good.

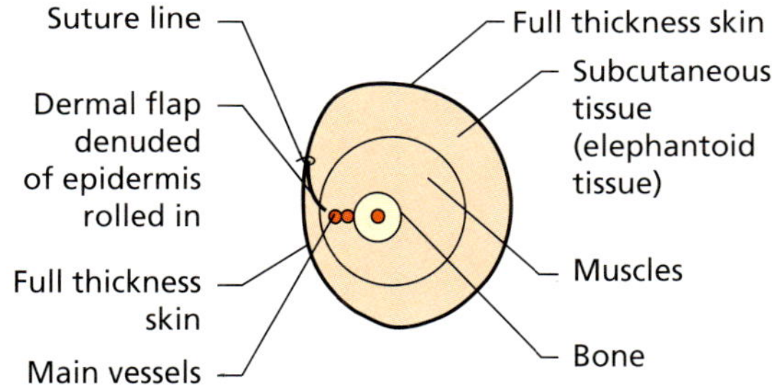

Figure 27.8 Thompson Swiss-roll operation for chronic lymphedema.

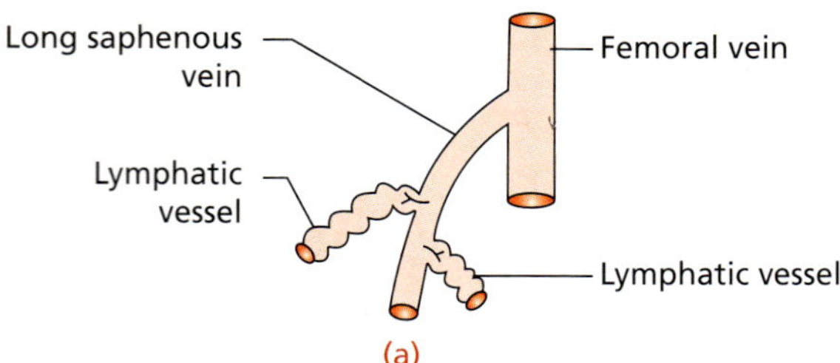

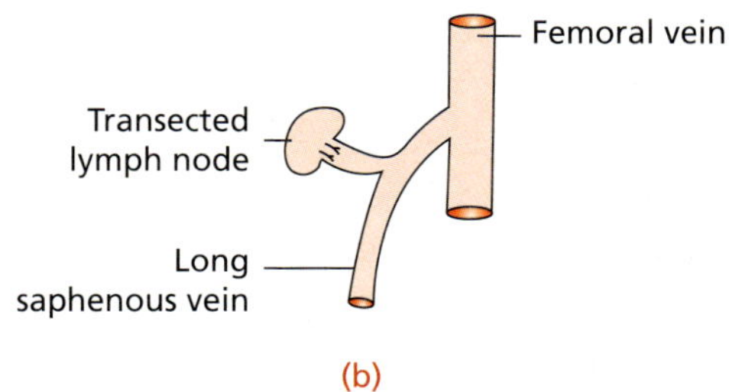

Figure 27.7 Lymphangioplasty for treating lymphedema: (a) lymphovenous shunt (O'Brien) and (b) nodovenous shunt (Neibulowitz).

KEY POINTS

- Infarction is sterile necrosis of tissues following sudden complete arterial obstruction. Gangrene is massive death of tissues with putrefaction which occurs following arterial obstruction and infection.
- Reduced arterial blood supply causes intermittent pain at the time of stress or exertion and claudication in lower limbs. Clinical features of acute arterial obstruction include pain, pallor, puffiness, pulselessness, and paralysis (5 Ps).
- Atherosclerosis is characterized by subintimal deposition of cholesterol, lipoid material, and lipophages in large and medium-sized arteries (atheroma) resulting in narrowing (stenosis) of the artery.
- Arterial embolism is sudden arterial obstruction caused by impaction of some particulate material, for example, thrombus, air, fat, and tumor tissue. The arteries of lower limb and pulmonary artery are the most common sites of embolism. The patient presents with pain of sudden onset (like bolt from blue) at the site of impaction radiating along the course of that artery and signs of severe arterial insufficiency.
- Arterial thrombosis usually occurs on an atheromatous plaque and causes acute arterial obstruction but not acute ischemia as collaterals are likely to have developed.
- Arterial trauma is caused by blunt, sharp, or firearm injury in which an artery may be contused, punctured, cut partially or completely, or lacerated. It is characterized by hemorrhage and distal ischemia.
- Arterial aneurysm is a localized dilatation of an artery which is caused by weakness of its wall characterized by a tense pulsatile swelling along the course of a large artery.
- Thromboangiitis obliterans (Buerger's disease) is a segmental inflammatory and thrombotic process of distal-most arteries and sometimes of neighboring veins. It is usually seen in males who are heavy smokers, and is characterized by rest pain which may progress to dry gangrene. The main line of treatment is complete avoidance of smoking.
- Raynaud's phenomenon (RP) is a syndrome of digital ischemia usually caused by an exaggerated response of digital arteries to exposure to cold or emotional stress.
- Varicose veins are dilated, tortuous, and lengthened superficial veins which commonly occur in the great saphenous vein and its tributaries. They are treated initially by supportive measures and sclerotherapy. Advanced or unresponsive disease is treated with endovenous ablation using radiofrequency waves or laser or stripping of diseased vein.
- Deep vein thrombosis (DVT) is clotting of blood in the deep veins (calf veins and pelvic veins) which may cause pulmonary embolism. It is treated with anticoagulants and thrombolysis, and may be by putting a filter in inferior vena cava.
- Gangrene is massive death of tissues associated with putrefaction and commonly affects the distal parts of body. The diabetics and the people having peripheral arterial disease, peripheral neuropathy, and heart disease are more liable to suffer with this problem.
- Dry gangrene occurs when the ischemic tissues are desiccated by gradual reduction of arterial supply as happens in atherosclerosis and a line of demarcation appears gradually between the live and gangrenous tissues.
- Moist (wet) gangrene occurs when the main artery supplying a part or limb is suddenly occluded as occurs following ligation or embolism. Diabetic gangrene and gas gangrene are other examples of moist gangrene.
- Acute lymphangitis is an acute inflammation of lymphatics (red streaks in the skin) caused by *Streptococcus haemolyticus*. Treatment includes antibiotics and supportive measures.
- Lymphedema is swelling of a part of body due to accumulation of lymph in the interstitial tissue. It commonly affects the lower limbs, scrotum, and penis, and may affect other areas. It is usually due to filariasis in our country.

SELF-ASSESSMENT

Long answer questions

1. Describe the etiology, pathology, clinical features, and treatment of atherosclerosis.
2. Discuss the etiology, clinical features, complications, and treatment of varicose veins.

Short answer questions

1. Aneurysm
2. Arterial stenosis
3. Stenting
4. Buerger's disease

(CONTD...)

SELF-ASSESSMENT *(...CONTD)*

5. Raynaud's disease
6. Prevention of deep vein thrombosis
7. Acute lymphangitis
8. Chronic lymphedema

Multiple choice questions

1. Arterial stenosis is commonly caused by
   (a) Atherosclerosis
   (b) Trauma
   (c) Arterial embolism
   (d) Infection
2. Effects of arterial occlusion include
   (a) Claudication
   (b) Rest pain
   (c) Ischemic ulcer
   (d) All of the above
3. All of the following are features of intermittent claudication, except
   (a) Cramp-like pain in muscles
   (b) Brought up by walking
   (c) Relieved by standing still or taking rest
   (d) Present on taking the first step
4. Ischemia of lower limb is characterized by
   (a) Pallor
   (b) Coldness
   (c) Paresthesia
   (d) All of the above
5. Arterial obstruction may cause all of the following clinical features, except
   (a) Pain on effort
   (b) Ulceration
   (c) Color changes
   (d) Increased temperature
6. The commonest cause of aneurysm is
   (a) Atherosclerosis
   (b) Syphilis
   (c) Diabetes mellitus
   (d) Old age
7. The most important etiological factor of Buerger's disease is
   (a) Smoking
   (b) Diabetes mellitus
   (c) Immobility
   (d) Obesity
8. The commonest site of varicose veins is
   (a) Upper limb
   (b) Lower limb
   (c) Abdominal wall
   (d) Scrotum
9. The treatment of varicose veins includes
   (a) Elastic compression garments
   (b) Injection sclerotherapy
   (c) Excision or stripping of varicose vein
   (d) All of the above
10. In injection sclerotherapy the sclerosant is injected into
    (a) Filled vein
    (b) Empty vein
    (c) Partially empty vein
    (d) All of the above
11. The commonest side effect of stripping of varicose vein is
    (a) Wound infection
    (b) Hemorrhage
    (c) Phlebedema
    (d) Cutaneous hypoesthesia
12. The first sign of deep vein thrombosis is
    (a) Claudication
    (b) Calf tenderness
    (c) Fever
    (d) Homans' sign
13. The treatment of deep vein thrombosis is
    (a) Intravenous heparin
    (b) Oral anticoagulants
    (c) Thrombolytic therapy
    (d) All of the above
14. The commonest causative organism of acute lymphangitis is
    (a) *Streptococcus pyogenes*
    (b) *Staphylococcus aureus*
    (c) *Salmonella typhi*
    (d) *Mycobacterium tuberculosis*
15. Milroy's disease is
    (a) Filarial lymphedema
    (b) Congenital lymphedema
    (c) Phlebedema
    (d) Congenital arteriovenous fistula

(CONTD...)

SELF-ASSESSMENT (...CONTD)

16. Which of the following parts is usually affected by elephantiasis?
    (a) Leg
    (b) Scrotum
    (c) Penis
    (d) All of the above

17. All of the following are the operative procedures used in the treatment of lymphedema, except
    (a) Microsurgery
    (b) Charles' operation
    (c) Amputation
    (d) Thompson operation

Answers

1. (a) 2. (d) 3. (d) 4. (d) 5. (d) 6. (a) 7. (a) 8. (b) 9. (d) 10. (b) 11. (d) 12. (c) 13. (d) 14. (a) 15. (b) 16. (d) 17. (c)

Diseases of Nerves

28

Nerve injuries

Nerve injuries are not uncommon and are one of the important causes of disability and deformity.

These injuries are classified into many types as described in Box 28.1.

Box 28.1 Classification of nerve injuries

- **Seddon's classification**
  - Neuropraxia
  - Axonotmesis
  - Neurotmesis
- **Sunderland's classification**
  - Conduction block, that is, temporary neuronal block
  - Axonotmesis with endoneurium preserved
  - Axonotmesis with disruption of endoneurium with perineurium preserved
  - Axonotmesis with disruption of endoneurium and perineurium but epineurium preserved
  - Neurotmesis with disruption of endoneurium, perineurium, and epineurium

Neuropraxia

Pathology It is the physiological paralysis of conduction of impulses through a nerve as a result of stretching or distortion without any anatomical discontinuity. The nerve and nerve fibers are intact within their sheaths; hence, there is no Wallerian degeneration of axons distal to the site of injury.

Clinical Features It is characterized by temporary weakness of muscles, sensory loss, and paresthesias for a variable interval followed by full recovery within a short time. There is no residual neurological deficit.

Treatment It is treated by giving rest to the part by splinting in functional position. If there is a cause, it must be removed.

Axonotmesis

Pathology In this injury the axons are disrupted within the intact nerve sheath. Hence, Wallerian degeneration occurs proximally up to next node of Ranvier and distally the total length of axon.

Clinical Features It is characterized by neurological deficit distal to the site of injury, that is, weakness or paralysis of muscles, sensory loss, and paresthesia.

It usually recovers with passage of time as the anatomy of the nerve is nearly normal, but the recovery may be complete or incomplete depending on the extent of intraneural fibrosis.

Assessment The progress of recovery (axons regenerate 1–2 mm/day) is assessed by examining the recovery of nerve function and Tinel's sign.

For eliciting the Tinel's sign, the course of the nerve is gently tapped with a hammer from below upwards to find the tingling sensation at the level of regeneration.

Treatment The paralyzed part is given rest by splinting. The nutrition of muscles is maintained by physiotherapy. Most of the injuries recover spontaneously but if the recovery is delayed, the nerve is explored and the scar tissue is excised.

Neurotmesis

Pathology It is the partial or complete division of a nerve, that is, nerve sheath and nerve fibers. Neurotmesis occurs due to open injuries, for example, cuts and penetrating wounds. Accidental division of a nerve can occur during operations, for example, facial nerve during operations on parotid, and superior and recurrent laryngeal nerves during thyroidectomy.

Clinical Features It is characterized by motor and sensory loss in the area supplied by the injured nerve. As the time passes, partial division produces a lateral neuroma at the site of injury, and a complete division a terminal neuroma at the upper cut end of the nerve.

Investigations Investigations in nerve injuries include nerve conduction studies and electromyography. Neurotmesis is characterized by absence of fibrillation on electromyography. MRI is now being used to image large nerves.

Treatment

- The nerve is repaired immediately by suturing provided the wound is clean (Fig. 28.1), for example, accidental division of facial nerve during excision of a parotid adenoma.
- If the wound is contaminated or infected, the nerve repair is delayed till the wound becomes clean (delayed repair).
- The nerve repair is done by accurate coaptation of divided ends without tension in a healthy tissue bed by suturing with very fine sutures.

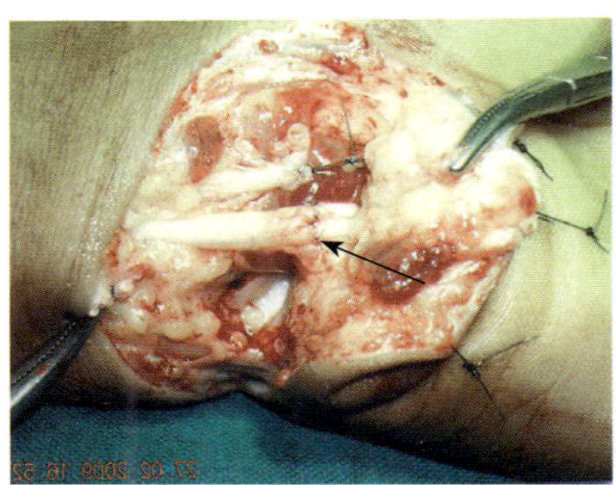

Figure 28.1 End-to-end anastomosis of divided ulnar nerve of upper limb. (Courtesy: Dr. R.K. Mishra, Sushrut Institute of Plastic Surgery Hospital, Lucknow)

- The nerve tissue deficit may be made good by nerve grafting. A microscope may be used for fine anastomosis.

The differences between the three types of nerve injury are described in Table 28.1.

Trigeminal neuralgia (tic douloureux)

It is momentary episodes of sudden lancinating facial pain that usually arises on one side of face and shoots toward the ear, or nostril on the same side.

Etiology

The cause is not known in most of the cases (primary neuralgia). In some cases ectatic vascular loops may cause compression of trigeminal nerve root. In young patients it may be related to multiple sclerosis. It may rarely be a symptom of brain tumor or intracranial arterial aneurysm (secondary neuralgia).

Clinical Features

- It is most common in middle-aged and late life and affects women more than men.
- There are attacks of severe dagger-like pain in the area supplied by one or more divisions of

Table 28.1 Differences between neuropraxia, axonotmesis, and neurotmesis

Features	Neuropraxia	Axonotmesis	Neurotmesis
Definition	Functional paralysis of nerve conduction	Division or rupture of axons	Partial or complete division of the nerve
Cause	Minor injury, for example, compression or passage of a missile near a nerve	More severe blow or stretch injury	Open injury, for example, stab wound
Motor loss	Complete	Complete	Complete
Sensory loss	Partial	Complete	Complete
Autonomic function	Spared	Lost	Lost
Nerve conduction	Present	Absent	Absent
Electromyography	Fibrillation occasionally detectable	Incomplete denervation potentials	Denervation potentials present
Recovery	Complete spontaneous recovery	Good recovery	Incomplete or no recovery
Rate of recovery	Rapid in days of weeks	1–2 mm/day	1–2 mm/day after repair
Quality of recovery	Perfect	Nearly perfect	Always imperfect
Treatment	Supportive	Supportive, sometimes exploration	Exploration and repair

the nerve (usually maxillary or mandibular division) which many be triggered by touch (trigger areas), movement, drafts, and eating. To prevent an attack, many patients try to hold the face still while talking.

- Spontaneous remissions may occur but as the disease progresses the remissions become less common and shorter.

Investigations

The neurological examination including the imaging studies of the brain is normal except when it is due to multiple sclerosis and brainstem tumor.

Treatment

Medical Therapy It is treated with oxcarbazepine (900–1800 mg) and carbamazepine (400–1600 mg ER). Other drugs are phenytoin, baclofen, and gabapentin.

Surgical Interventions

- In the past, alcohol injection into the nerve, rhizotomy, or tractotomy was being done if drug treatment failed.
- Recently posterior fossa exploration has revealed an anomalous artery or vein impinging on the trigeminal nerve root. In these patients, separation of anomalous vessel from the nerve root produces lasting relief. In elderly patients with limited life expectancy, radiofrequency rhizotomy can be done as it is easy to perform. Gamma radiosurgery is also effective.
- In infraorbital neuralgia, the avulsion of affected nerve (peripheral) is an effective treatment.

Glossopharyngeal neuralgia

- **Etiology**: It is an uncommon disorder the cause of which is not known. In some cases, it may be due to multiple sclerosis.
- **Clinical features**: It is characterized by attacks of pain in the throat about the tonsillar area, sometimes deep in the ear and back of tongue. The attack may be precipitated by swallowing, chewing, talking, or yawning and may be accompanied by syncope.
- **Investigations**: MRI may be used to visualize the whole course of glossopharyngeal nerve.
- **Treatment**: Oxcarbazepine and carbamazepine are the drugs of choice. If medical treatment fails, microvascular decompression is indicated.

Facial nerve paralysis

Out of all the cranial nerves, facial nerve paralysis is one of the commonest.

Surgical Anatomy

The facial (seventh) nerve supplies all the muscles of facial expression. Its sensory component, nerves intermedius, is small and conveys the taste sensation from anterior two-thirds of the tongue and probably skin sensation from anterior wall of external auditory meatus. Its motor nucleus lies anterior and lateral to abducens nucleus. After leaving pons, it enters the internal auditory meatus with the auditory (eighth) nerve. It continues its course in the stylomastoid foramen and enters the parotid salivary gland where it divides into five branches (pes anserina) to supply facial muscles (Fig. 28.2).

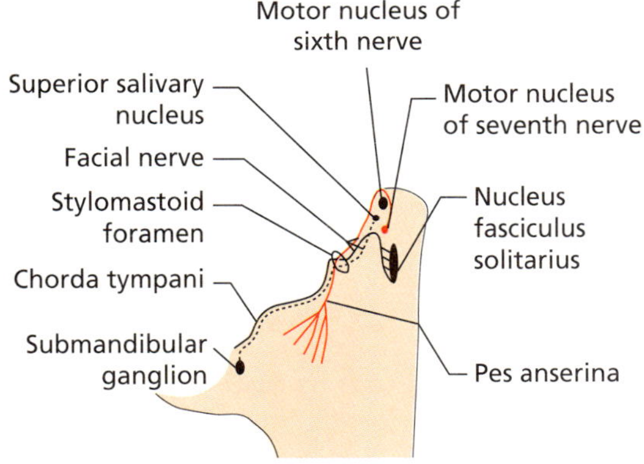

Figure 28.2 Anatomy of facial nerve.

Etiology

The causes of facial nerve paralysis are described in Box 28.2.

Clinical Features

Supranuclear Facial Paralysis (Upper Motor Neuron Paralysis)

- It is usually caused by cerebrovascular accidents and is a part of hemiplegia.

Box 28.2 Causes of facial nerve paralysis

- **Supranuclear (upper motor neuron) paralysis**
  - Cerebrovascular accidents
  - Cerebral degenerative disease
  - Intracranial tumors
- **Nuclear paralysis—lesions of pons**
- **Infranuclear (lower motor neuron) paralysis**
  - Intracranial causes
    - Bacterial and viral infections
    - Cholesteatoma
    - Cerebropontine angle tumors
    - Temporal bone trauma
  - Extracranial causes
    - Carcinoma of parotid gland
    - Maxillofacial trauma
    - Iatrogenic causes, for example, parotid gland surgery, temporomandibular joint (TMJ) surgery, and arthroscopy
  - Bell's palsy (idiopathic, may be viral mononeuritis)

- The motor supply of upper half of the face has bilateral cortical representation. Hence, this type of paralysis results in muscle weakness of lower face with preservation of eye closure and forehead movements. It is contralateral involvement. The taste sensation of anterior two-thirds of tongue is lost.

Nuclear Paralysis It is characterized by involvement of abducent nerve also, as the fibers of facial nerve loop around nucleus of abducent nerve in the pons.

Differences between upper neuron and lower neuron facial palsy are described in Table 28.2.

Infranuclear or Lower Motor Neuron Paralysis

- It is the most common type of facial palsy (palsy and paralysis are synonyms). The most frequent cause is the Bell's palsy (Fig. 28.3) which is a type of viral mononeuritis and facial nerve injury after its exit from stylomastoid foramen. Other important causes are carcinoma of parotid and parotidectomy. The signs of infranuclear facial palsy are given in Box 28.3.

Table 28.2 Differences between upper motor neuron and lower motor neuron facial palsy

Features	Upper motor neuron or supranuclear facial palsy	Lower motor neuron facial palsy
Site of lesion	Contralateral lower motor cortex	Ipsilateral facial nerve nucleus in the pons or the nerve coming out of pons up to its branches on the face
Causes	Cerebrovascular accidents, trauma, tumor	Lesions of pons and lesions of whole course of the nerve including Bell's palsy
Clinical features	Hemifacial palsy of the opposite side but forehead movements (frowning) and eye closure are not affected	• Total hemifacial paralysis of the same side • In lesions of pons, abducent nerve is also paralyzed along with facial nerve

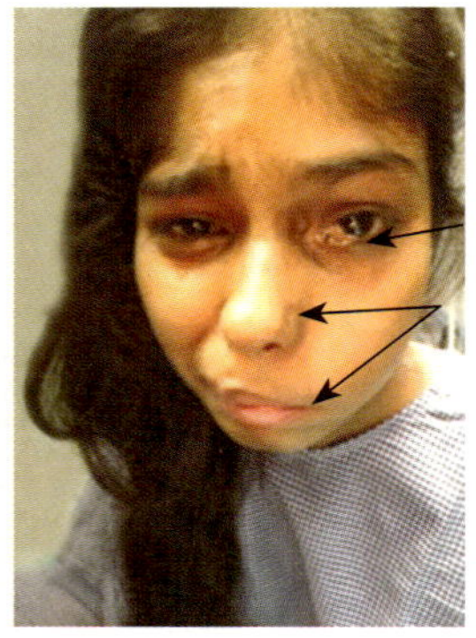

Figure 28.3 Left facial nerve palsy "with a tear in the eye that does not fall." (Courtesy: Dr. Diwakar)

Box 28.3 Signs of infranuclear facial palsy (Bell's palsy)

- The face looks expressionless and asymmetrical even at rest
- The eye cannot be closed and an attempt to close the eye results in eyeball turning upwards and outwards (Bell's phenomenon)
- The nasolabial fold is obliterated and the angle of mouth is drooped down
- Frowning of forehead and whistling is not possible
- When the patient is asked to show the teeth, the lips on the affected side do not separate
- The food accumulates inside the cheek during mastication
- The taste sensation in the anterior two-thirds of tongue is lost

Investigations

CT Scan/MRI A CT scan is done if there is history of head injury to see along the course of the nerve. MRI may be required to image the whole course of the nerve to see the soft tissue.

Other Investigations They include electromyography, evoked electromyography, and electroneurography. Magnetic transcranial and electrical stylomastoidal stimulation allows differentiation of the causative lesions, especially Bell's palsy.

Treatment

General Care

- Reassurance as the condition (Bell's palsy which is the commonest clinical type) resolves in many cases without any residual defect
- Protection of eye from exposure keratitis by a topical lubricant or ointment and pad and bandage (tarsorrhaphy may be required in which the lateral portions of upper and lower eyelids are stitched together)

Medical Therapy Bell's paralysis recovers in many cases by itself. Steroids are given if paralysis is complete and there is severe pain, for example, prednisone 60–80 mg daily for 5 days followed by tapering over next 7–10 days.

Surgical Treatment

- If possible, the cause is removed, for example, excision of acoustic neuroma to decompress the facial nerve.
- Nerve repair: The injured nerve during parotidectomy for a pleomorphic adenoma should be repaired immediately in a clean wound, or after some time when the wound becomes clean (delayed repair). If some part of the nerve is lost, the deficit is made good by put-

ting a nerve graft taken from great auricular nerve, sural nerve, or a piece of freeze-thawed skeletal muscle.

- If repair is not possible, cross-face nerve transfer may be carried out.
- Repair of facial drooping: In long-standing paralysis the facial drooping is corrected by transposition of strips taken from regional muscles, for example, temporalis, masseter or platysma to upper and lower eyelids, and lips (Fig. 28.4).

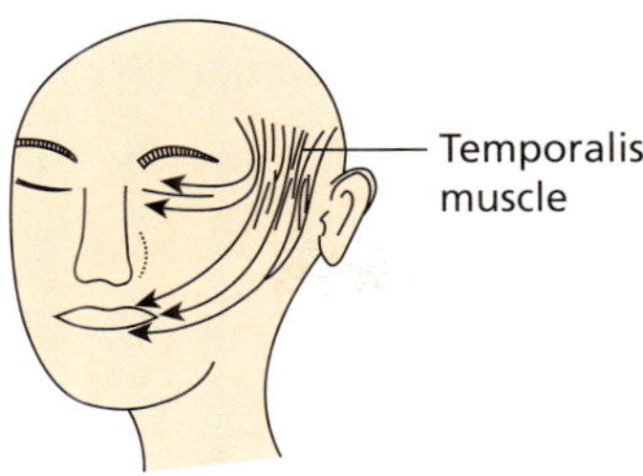

Figure 28.4 Muscle sling transposition from temporalis to upper and lower eyelids and lips to correct facial drooping following facial palsy.

KEY POINTS

- Neuropraxia is due to the physiological paralysis of conduction of impulses. It is characterized by temporary loss of nerve function followed by full recovery within a short time.
- In axonotmesis, the axons are disrupted within the intact nerve sheath resulting in Wallerian degeneration and characterized by neurological deficit distal to the site of injury, which usually recovers with passage of time.
- The progress of nerve recovery (axons regenerate 1–2 mm/day) is assessed by recovery of nerve function by Tinel's sign in which the course of the nerve is gently tapped from below up to find the tingling sensation at the level of regeneration.
- Neurotmesis is the partial or complete division of a nerve, leading to motor and sensory loss in the area supplied by the injured nerve. Nerve repair is done by suturing the cut ends. The nerve tissue deficit is treated by nerve grafting.
- Trigeminal neuralgia is characterized by momentary episodes of sudden lancinating facial pain near one side of face that shoots toward the ear, or nostril on the same side. It is treated by oxcarbazepine or carbamazepine. In case of anomalous artery or vein impinging on the trigeminal nerve root, posterior fossa exploration is done to excise them. In elderly patients with limited life expectancy, radiofrequency rhizotomy can be done.
- Supranuclear facial palsy is usually caused by cerebrovascular accidents and is a part of hemiplegia. It results in weakness of face with preservation of eye closure and forehead movements.
- Bell's palsy is characterized by inability to frown and close the eyes on the side of lesion. Bell's phenomenon is the inability to close the eye and an attempt to close the eye results in eyeball turning upwards and outwards. It recovers by itself in many cases or treated with steroids.
- The signs of facial palsy are obliteration of nasolabial fold, drooping of the angle of the mouth, inability to whistle, and loss of taste sensation in the anterior two-thirds of the tongue.

SELF-ASSESSMENT

Long answer question

1. What are the various types of nerve injuries? Describe their clinical features and treatment.

Short answer questions

1. Neuropraxia
2. Axonotmesis
3. Neurotmesis
4. Trigeminal neuralgia
5. Bell's palsy

Multiple choice questions

1. Neuropraxia is defined as
   (a) Disruption of axons within the intact nerve sheath
   (b) Physiological paralysis of nerve conduction without any organic discontinuity

(CONTD...)

SELF-ASSESSMENT *(...CONTD)*

(c) Partial division of a nerve
(d) Complete division of a nerve

2. Axonotmesis is defined as
(a) Disruption of axons within the intact nerve sheath
(b) Physiological paralysis of nerve conduction without any organic discontinuity
(c) Partial division of a nerve
(d) Complete division of a nerve

3. All of the following are the features of neurotmesis, except
(a) The nerve is divided partially or completely
(b) There are signs of neurological deficit in the area supplied by the affected nerve
(c) On EMG denervation potentials are present
(d) It is treated by surgical nerve repair

4. All of the following are the features of trigeminal neuralgia, except
(a) It is characterized by episodes of sudden lancinating facial pain in one or more divisions of trigeminal nerve
(b) The cause can be found in most of the cases
(c) It occurs mostly in middle ages and late in life
(d) It affects women more often than men

5. Which is the drug of choice for treating trigeminal neuralgia?
(a) Phenobarbitone
(b) Dilantin sodium
(c) Carbamazepine
(d) Ibuprofen

6. If drug treatment fails, which of the following is the best method of treatment of trigeminal neuralgia?
(a) Injection of absolute alcohol into the ganglion
(b) Decompression and separation of anomalous vessels from the nerve root
(c) Percutaneous thermocoagulation of trigeminal ganglion
(d) Gamma radiosurgery of the trigeminal root

7. The most common cause of upper motor neuron type of facial nerve paralysis is
(a) Brain tumor
(b) Tuberculoma
(c) Cerebrovascular accident
(d) Subdural hematoma

8. Which of the following features is not true about upper motor neuron facial palsy?
(a) It is usually caused by a cerebrovascular accident
(b) The upper half of face escapes paralysis
(c) The taste sensation of anterior two-thirds of tongue is preserved
(d) The eye closure is preserved

9. Bell's paralysis is
(a) Paralysis of mandibular nerve
(b) Paralysis of maxillary division of the trigeminal nerve
(c) Infranuclear type of facial paralysis of unknown origin
(d) Upper motor neuron facial paralysis

10. All of the following statements are true about Bell's palsy, except
(a) It may be due to viral mononeuritis
(b) It usually recovers slowly with conservative treatment
(c) Corticosteroids may be required
(d) It is a supranuclear type of facial paralysis

11. Which of the following is the commonest cause of facial palsy when the nerve is passing through the parotid salivary gland?
(a) Pleomorphic adenoma
(b) Parotid abscess
(c) Carcinoma
(d) Warthin's tumor

12. When a segment of facial nerve is excised along with the carcinoma of parotid, what is the treatment?
(a) End-to-end anastomosis of cut ends of nerve
(b) Putting a nerve graft in the defect
(c) Cross-face nerve transfer
(d) Tarsorrhaphy only

(CONTD...)

SELF-ASSESSMENT *(...CONTD)*

13. What is tarsorrhaphy?
    (a) Stitching of lateral portions of upper and lower eyelids together
    (b) Repair of a laceration of upper eyelid
    (c) Reconstruction of lower eyelid
    (d) Reconstructive surgery of tarsal bones of foot

14. During superficial parotidectomy for pleomorphic adenoma, if the facial nerve is accidentally divided, how will you treat this complication?
    (a) Nerve grafting
    (b) Nerve suture
    (c) Lateral tarsorrhaphy alone
    (d) Cross-face nerve transfer

Answers

1. (b) 2. (a) 3. (c) 4. (b) 5. (c) 6. (b) 7. (c) 8. (c)
9. (c) 10. (d) 11. (c) 12. (b) 13. (a) 14. (b)

Swellings of the Jaws

29

Introduction

A swelling is a localized enlargement, elevation, or protuberance usually associated with some disease process. As a swelling can arise from other bones, a swelling can arise from jaw bones also. Jaw bones have some structural differences from other bones. Hence, the scenario of swellings here is a little different. The peculiar features of jaw bones are:

- They have teeth, each root of which is held in a socket of its own.
- A significant part of each jaw near the row of teeth is lined by oral mucosa which is fused with local periosteum and is called mucoperiosteum.
- They have a special tissue called gingivae which are situated near the neck of teeth and in between teeth.
- The upper jaw is hollow and contains a cavity (antrum or sinus) lined by columnar epithelium. The lower jaw contains inferior dental canal which carries the inferior dental nerve and vessels (Fig. 29.1).

Classification of swellings of jaws

A large variety of swellings can affect the jaws. Their classification is described in Box 29.1.

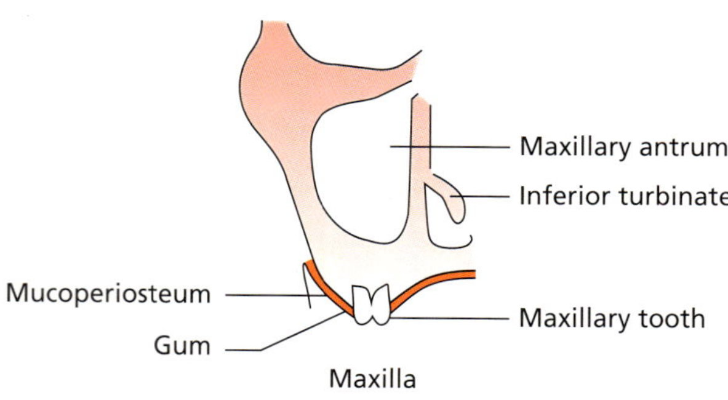

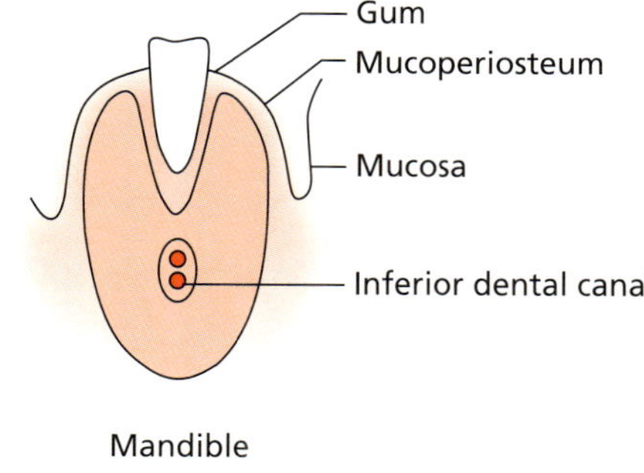

Figure 29.1 Surgical anatomy of jaws.

Box 29.1 Classification of swellings of jaws

- **Traumatic swellings**
  - Fracture hematoma
  - Displaced ends of a fracture
  - Callus
  - Malunited fracture
- **Inflammatory swellings**
  - Alveolar abscess
  - Osteomyelitis
  - Cervicofacial actinomycosis
  - Empyema of maxillary antrum
- **Epulides (epulis, on the gum)**
  - Fibrous epulis
  - Myeloid epulis
  - Granulomatous epulis
  - Congenital epulis
- **Cysts**
  - Odontogenic cysts
    - Epstein's pearls
    - Dental or radicular cyst
    - Dentigerous cysts
  - Fissural cyst
    - Nasopalatine cyst
    - Nasolabial cyst
- **Tumors**
  - Odontogenic tumors
    - Ameloblastoma
    - Cementoma
    - Myxoma
    - Odontomes
    - Keratocystic odontogenic tumor
  - Primary bone tumors
    - Fibroma
    - Ossifying fibroma
    - Osteoma
    - Chondroma
    - Osteoclastoma
    - Osteosarcoma
    - Carcinoma
    - Burkitt's lymphoma
  - Secondary tumors
- **Osteodystrophies**
  - Cherubism
  - Hyperparathyroidism
  - Paget's disease
  - Fibrous dysplasia

Clinical diagnosis of swelling of jaws

The points that are important for making a clinical diagnosis are given in the subsequent text.

Duration of Swelling

- **Short duration**: Traumatic and acute inflammatory swellings
- **Long duration**: Chronic inflammations, tumors, and cysts

Mode of Onset

- Traumatic swellings usually occur immediately after trauma or sometime after trauma.
- Acute inflammatory swellings are painful and of short duration, and chronic inflammatory swellings usually have a painless insidious onset.
- The tumors and cysts usually have an insidious onset.

Site of Start of Swelling

- A swelling of gum starts near the dental border of jaws.
- A bony swelling usually starts from inside the jaw a little away from the row of teeth.
- An osteoclastoma usually affects the chin.
- Ameloblastoma usually affects the ascending ramus near the angle of mandible.

Nature of the Swelling

- Surface swelling: The surface swellings of the jaws include epulis, ossifying fibroma, localized fibrous osteoma, ivory osteoma, carcinoma of gum, and malignant melanoma.
- An expanding lesion involving both the tables includes dentigerous cyst and osteosarcoma.

1. DIFFERENTIAL DIAGNOSIS OF SWELLINGS OF JAWS

Traumatic swellings

The trauma of the jaws can produce a variety of swellings of jaws described in the subsequent text.

Fracture Hematoma

The patient presents with a swelling following maxillofacial trauma. It is diffuse, soft, and tender, and has bruising of overlying skin.

Displaced Ends of a Fracture

Following local trauma, there is a swelling, deformity, malalignment of teeth, crepitus, and abnormal mobility. The displaced ends are palpable.

Fracture Callus

It is a diffuse, hard, and nontender fusiform, swelling around the fractured ends that forms few days after the injury. Radiography shows diffuse opacity in relation to fractured ends.

Malunited Fracture

The patient comes with a history of fracture of jaws which was not properly treated and characterized by swelling, deformity, and malalignment of teeth. Radiography confirms the diagnosis.

Inflammatory swellings

The swelling is an important sign of inflammation. Hence, inflammation is an important cause of a swelling of jaws.

Alveolar Abscess

- It occurs mostly in children and young adults and arises from the molar teeth of mandible or maxilla at the root of decaying or impacted teeth (Fig. 29.2). It usually progresses outwards eroding the lateral plate of alveolus forming a subcutaneous abscess on lower face. The patient presents with constant dull-aching or throbbing pain aggravated by hot or cold drinks. The jaw swelling is red, hot, and tender, and associated with edema of gum related to affected tooth. Trismus may be present.

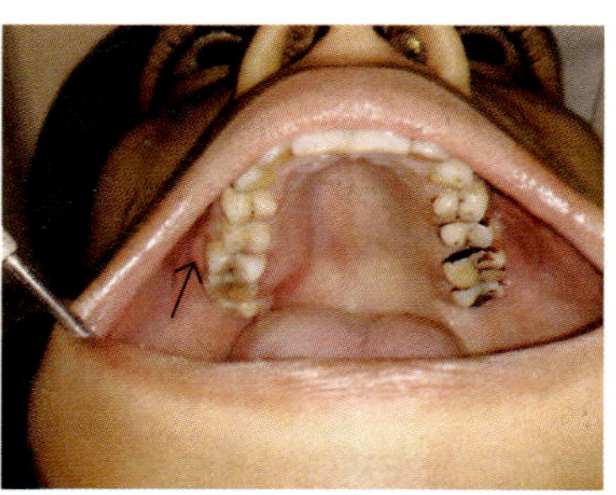

Figure 29.2 Alveolar abscess of right upper molar region. (Courtesy: Professor Divya Mehrotra)

Osteomyelitis

- **Acute osteomyelitis of mandible**: It presents with fever, pain, swelling, and tenderness of acute onset in the lower part of face. The patient is usually a child.
- **Acute osteomyelitis of maxilla**: It usually occurs in children with swelling and redness of the cheek and closure of eye of same side due to edema of lower eyelid. The hard palate is also edematous.
- **Chronic osteomyelitis**: It is characterized by a sinus fixed to underlying bone which is thickened and tender.

Cervicofacial Actinomycosis

The patient presents with a hard, diffuse, and nodular swelling of the gum or mandible near the angle. The overlying skin may be swollen, bluish, and wooden hard and there may be one or more ("sulfur granules" containing) pus-discharging sinuses near the angle of mandible.

Empyema of Maxillary Antrum

- The patient is usually a young person who has facial pain, toothache, frontal headache, and severe constitutional symptoms of recent onset. The pain is aggravated by bending the head forwards and downwards. There is diffuse swelling of midface extending into the lower eyelid and tenderness below the prominence of cheek. Speculum examination of nose may show pus under middle meatus of nose.

Epulides (epulis—upon the gum)

Epulides are the swellings of the gum due to variety of causes. Their signs are described in the subsequent text.

Fibrous Epulis

It is a fibroma that arises from periodontal membrane. Fibrous epulis is the commonest type of epulis. It is commonly seen in women in their thirties or forties. The patient presents with a painless, slow-growing swelling of the gum (Fig. 29.3). It is usually present between two incisors commonly of the lower jaw on its outer surface. It is pink, smooth, firm, nontender, and longitudinal with a narrow base.

Myeloid Giant Cell Epulis or Giant Cell Reparative Granuloma

It can occur at any age but is common between 25 and 45 years. Myeloid giant cell epulis presents as a purplish, hyperemic, smooth or lobulated, soft or firm swelling of the gum (Fig. 29.4). It may be associated with a periosteal osteoclastoma which underlies it. It affects the outer surface of upper or lower gum.

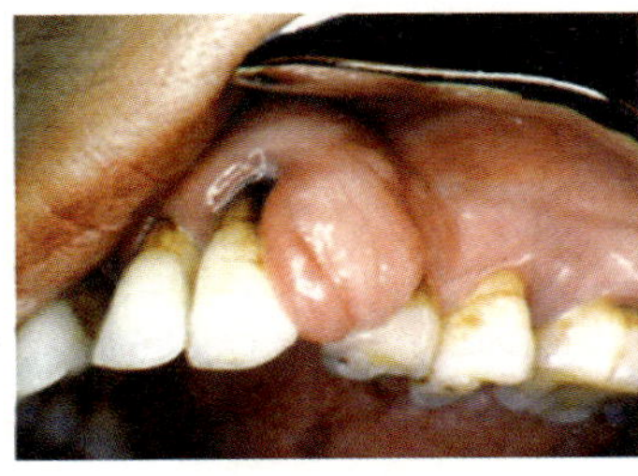

Figure 29.3 Fibrous epulis. (Courtesy: Professor Surajit Bhattacharya)

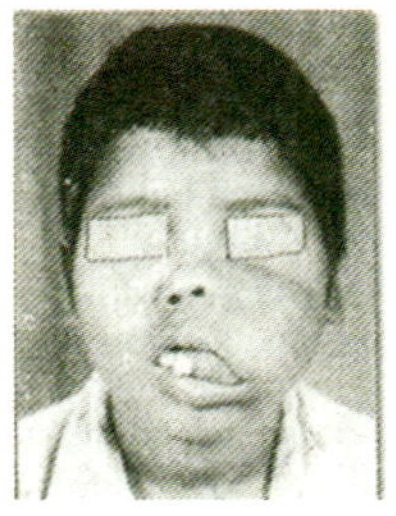

(a)

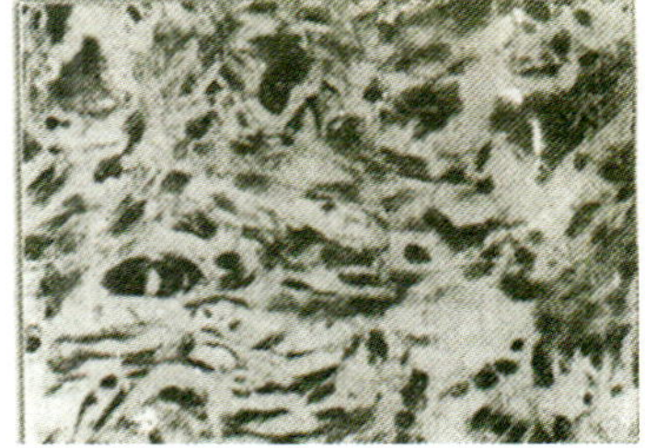

(b)

Figure 29.4 A large myeloid epulis of left maxilla. (a) Clinical photograph; (b) microscopic picture.

Granulomatous Epulis

The patient is usually a middle-aged or elderly person who presents with a small, pink, and soft swelling of the gum that bleeds on touch (pyogenic granuloma). It is a mass of reactive granulation tissue present around a carious tooth or at a pressure point of an ill-fitting denture.

Congenital Epulis

It is a small pink swelling of gum seen in small children in relation to an unerupted incisor.

Cysts

Epstein's Pearls (Bohn's Nodules)

They probably arise from the epithelial remnants of dental lamina which proliferate, keratinize, and form small cysts. They are small, white nodules

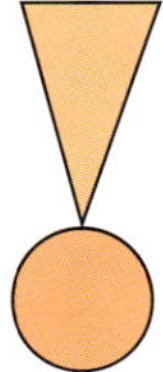

Figure 29.5 Dental cyst.

2–3 mm in diameter occurring on the crest of maxillary or mandibular ridges in a newborn. They tend to rupture or involute spontaneously and disappear before 3 months of age. Hence, no treatment is required.

Dental or Radicular Cyst

- It is the commonest odontogenic cyst (70%). The patient is usually a middle-aged person who presents with a painless and slow-growing swelling attached to the fang of a pulpless tooth which is carious (Fig. 29.5). It affects the upper jaw more commonly than the lower jaw (Fig. 29.6). It is usually small when it is not obvious clinically, but can be detected on radiography. Larger cysts occurring in the maxilla may push into the antrum.
- Radiography shows a round radiolucent area with a clearly defined outline in close relation to root of a tooth.

Dentigerous Cyst (Follicular Odontome)

- It is commonly seen in young adults at the site of an unerupted permanent tooth, usually the lower third molar (Figs 29.7 and 29.8). Other sites include upper cuspids, upper third molar, and lower bicuspids. It develops from enamel epithelium of the crown of an unerupted tooth which is displaced deeper by the cyst, thus preventing its eruption. A thin-walled cyst may have egg-shell crackling.
- Radiography shows a pear-shaped or ovoid unilocular translucency (cyst) surrounding the crown of an unerupted tooth (Fig. 29.9).

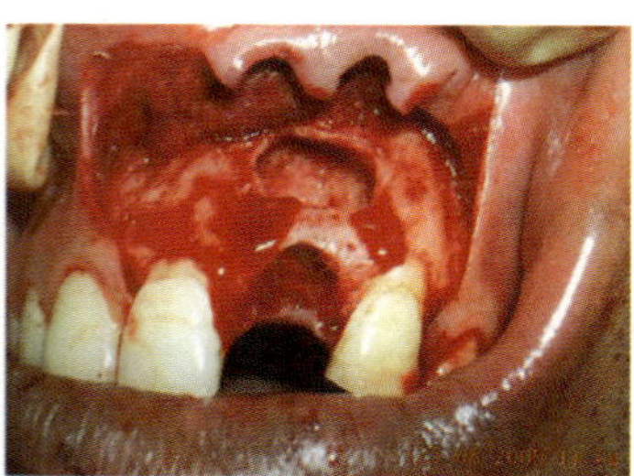

Figure 29.6 Intraoperative picture of a dental cyst of upper central incisor. (Courtesy: Professor Divya Mehrotra)

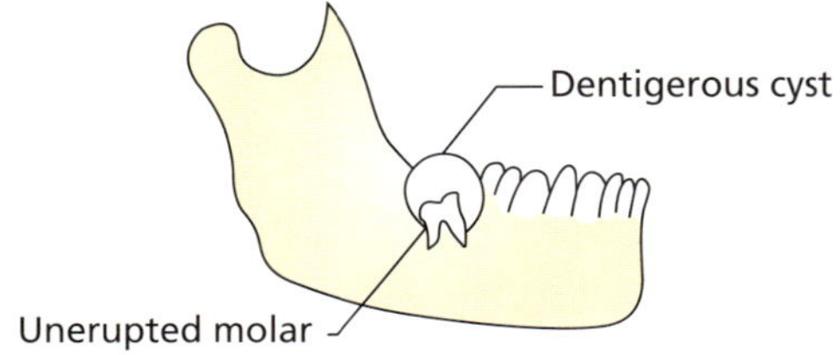

Figure 29.7 Dentigerous cyst of lower jaw.

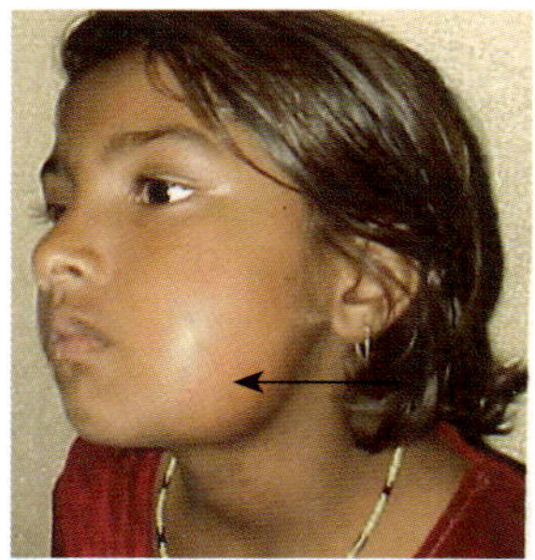

Figure 29.8 Dentigerous cyst of lower jaw on the left side in a girl of 12 years of age.

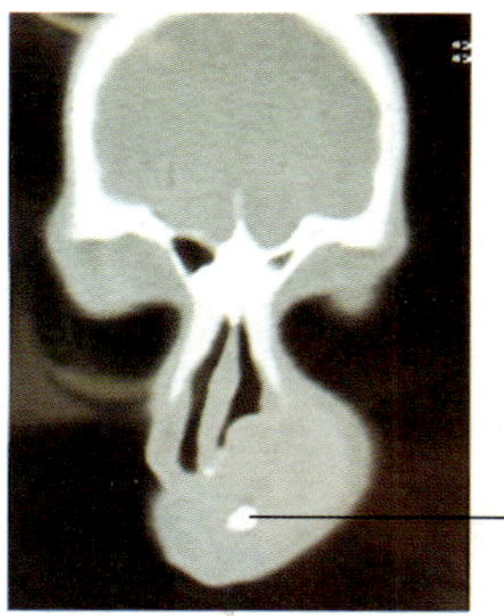

Figure 29.9 Coronal CT scan of face showing a large dentigerous cyst of left horizontal ramus of mandible. The unerupted tooth is seen within the cyst.

A dentigerous cyst must be differentiated from an ameloblastoma. Their differences are described in Table 29.1.

Nasopalatine Cyst

It is a slow-growing swelling of midline of hard palate or of the labial aspect of upper alveolus. It develops from embryonic epithelial residues in the nasopalatine canal. Radiography shows a round or heart-shaped radiolucency in the midline above or between the roots of central incisor teeth. The heart-like shape is due to notching in the middle due to nasal septum or nasal spine.

Nasolabial Cyst

It probably arises from epithelium embedded at the line of fusion of the lateral nasal and maxillary processes or from the lower end of nasolacrimal duct. It is commonly seen as a swelling in the external surface of maxilla deep to the nasolabial fold. The patient presents with a slowly enlarging fluctuant swelling of the upper lip. There may be bulge in the labial sulcus and floor of the nose with distortion of the nostril. X-ray shows a well-defined radiolucency at the site of cyst.

Tumors

Ameloblastoma (Adamantinoma)

- Most of the ameloblastomas occur in forties predominantly in the mandible and usually in the molar region or ascending ramus (Fig. 29.10). It is characterized by a painless, slow-growing swelling which may attain a huge size if left untreated. The outer table of mandible is expanded, the inner being nearly normal, and it may have egg-shell crackling. The local lymph nodes are not enlarged.
- X-ray shows a well-defined radiolucent area which is characteristically multilocular with small cysts at periphery (soap-bubble

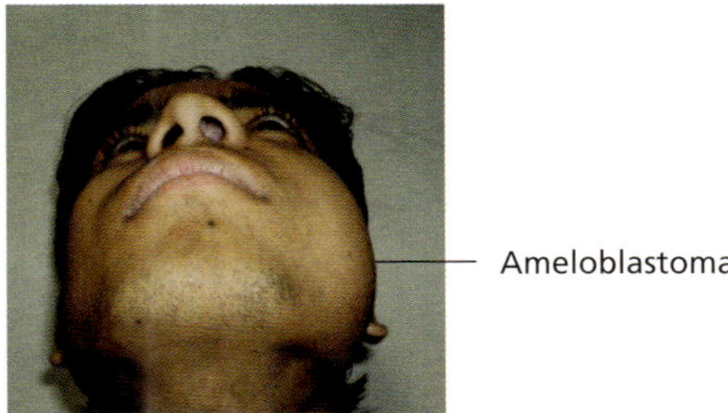

Figure 29.10 Ameloblastoma of left angle of mandible. (Courtesy: Professor Surajit Bhattacharya)

Table 29.1 Differences between a dentigerous cyst and an ameloblastoma

Features	Dentigerous cyst	Ameloblastoma
Definition	A developmental cyst developing around an unerupted permanent molar	A locally malignant tumor of ameloblasts of developing teeth
Age	20–30 years	30–60 years
Sex	More in females	Equal in both sexes
Symptoms	Painless, very slow-growing swelling near the angle of mandible	Painless swelling of insidious onset near the angle of mandible
Signs	• Expanding lesion with outer table expanded more than the inner table • Smooth surface • Egg-shell crackling may be present	• Expanding lesion with outer table expanded predominantly • Smooth or irregular, may be ulcerated • No egg-shell crackling
Spread	Does not occur	Local invasion only
Radiography	Unilocular expanding radiolucent lesion around the crown of an ill-developed unerupted molar	Usually large expanding lesion with fine honeycombing and scalloping border
Treatment	Excision of lining of cyst with push-in of the cyst wall. Normal tooth in the axis of eruption retained, otherwise removed	Wide excision which may amount to hemimandibulectomy

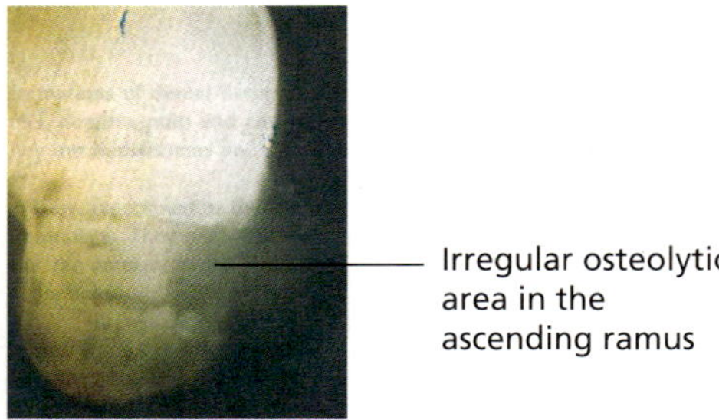

Figure 29.11 Anteroposterior radiograph of head and jaws showing an irregular osteolytic lesion of left ascending ramus of mandible—ameloblastoma.

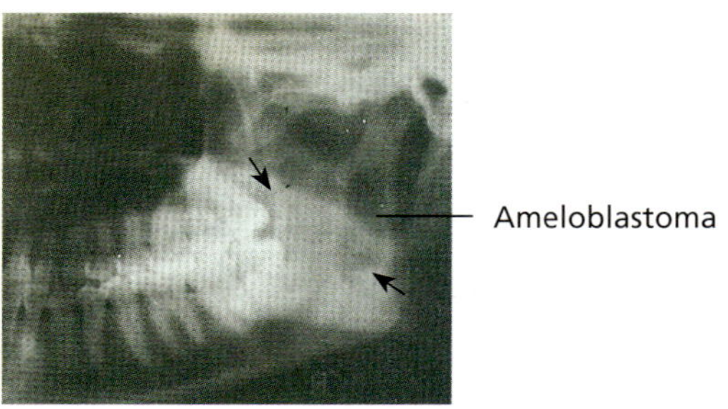

Figure 29.12 Orthopantomogram showing a multiloculated lytic lesion of the ascending ramus of mandible—ameloblastoma. (Courtesy: Professor G.N. Agrawal)

appearance) leading to scalloping (Figs 29.11 and 29.12).

Cementoma

This tumor is produced by continuing proliferation of cementum, and is of three types.

Benign Cementoblastoma It occurs in young adults and presents as an irregular or round mass of cementum attached to the root of a mandibular molar or premolar tooth.

Cementifying Fibroma The patient is a middle-aged person who has a painless, slow-growing swelling in the molar region. It consists of a mass of connective tissue in the jaw containing nodules of cementum-like material.

Gigantiform Cementoma It develops from fusion of several tumors and presents as enlargement of jaws and appears as a loculated radio-opaque mass with a radiolucent border.

Myxoma

The patient is usually young and presents with a painless, slow-growing swelling of jaws of insidious onset (Fig. 29.13). Radiography shows a finely trabeculated soap-bubble radiolucency expanding the bone. The diagnosis is confirmed by biopsy which reveals spindle-shaped cells scantily distributed in mucoid intercellular material having a resemblance to dental mesenchyme. It is an infiltrative lesion; hence, recurrence is common after excision.

Odontomes

Odontomes are malformations of dental tissue of developmental origin. They consist of enamel, dentine, pulp, and cementum in a variable relationship with one another. Thus, they are hamartomas and composite in nature. They are five in number and described in the subsequent text.

Enamel Pearls They are present at the bifurcation of roots of normal molars and premolars. Enamel pearls probably result from the displacement of ameloblasts at the amelocemental junction. They are spherical, a few millimeters in diameter, and may contain a core of dentine and pulp.

Dilated Odontomes They are severely distorted teeth due to invagination and proliferation of cells during development. The abnormality ranges from a pit into cingulum of the crown to the apparent occurrence of tooth within a tooth (dens in dente).

Germinated Odontome It occurs due to fusion of two adjacent tooth germs, or incomplete division

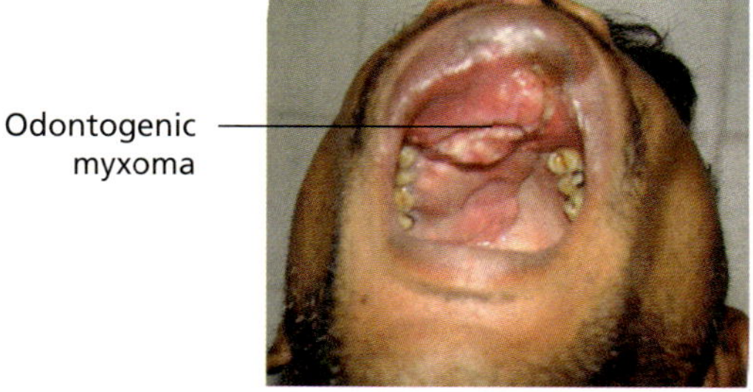

Figure 29.13 Odontogenic myxoma of upper jaw. (Courtesy: Professor Divya Mehrotra)

of a single tooth germ. Thus, fusion may be seen at either the crown or the root. This abnormality usually occurs in the incisor region.

Compound Follicular Odontome This lesion consists of many denticles surrounded by a fibrous capsule. The patient presents with a painless swelling which becomes painful when infected. This odontome develops from normal portions of dental lamina forming separate and multiple tooth germs.

Complex Composite Odontome It is composed of disordered arrangement of dental tissues and produces a mass of enamel, dentine, and cementum together with pulp and periodontal membrane in varying proportions. The patient is a young person who presents with a painless hard swelling. Radiography shows an irregular radio-opaque mass.

Keratocystic Odontogenic Tumor

It is a rare tumor that arises from the epithelium of primordial dental lamina or its remnants and contains semisolid keratin. More than 70% of tumors occur in the mandible near angle or ascending ramus. Expansion of jaw is minimal, especially of inner table; otherwise the clinical features are similar to other odontogenic swellings. In the maxilla, the inner surface is also expanded. Radiography shows a unilocular cyst. It may sometimes be multilocular which may have scalloped margins.

Fibroma

It is a rare tumor that may arise endosteally when it presents as an expanding lesion, or may originate from under the periosteum when it presents as a surface tumor. Fibroma is a painless and slow-growing swelling which is smooth and firm. It may invade the antrum when it becomes quite large.

Ossifying Fibroma

It is a painless, slow-growing swelling which mostly arises from horizontal ramus of mandible or antral wall. It is smooth, firm, and nontender. X-ray shows a circular, well-defined, translucent area with flakes or rings of calcification. Biopsy shows mature fibrous tissue with areas of calcification or ossification.

Osteoma

It is a very rare tumor which is painless and very slow-growing. It may occur as a central tumor expanding the bone and ultimately erupting on the surface as a bony excrescence. It is of two types.

Localized Fibrous Osteoma

- It is a painless, slow-growing tumor that grows chiefly into the mouth or cheek. The patient is usually a middle-aged person of any sex. It usually affects maxilla leading to obliteration of canine fossa and enlargement of alveolus. Hence, the upper lip and cheek are pushed out.
- X-ray in a child shows a shadow like rind of an orange, and a dense structureless mass in an adult. Biopsy shows trabeculae of cancellous bone separated by vascular fibrous tissue.

Ivory Osteoma

- The patient is a middle-aged or elderly person who has a very slow-growing, painless, and hard swelling of any aspect of alveolar process of mandible, outer aspect of maxilla, palate, orbital surface, or antrum. It looks like a limpet.
- X-ray shows a dome-shaped densely opaque shadow.

Chondroma

It is also a rare swelling of jaws which presents as a round hard mass which may cause asymmetry of face and a radiolucent expansion of either jaw having characteristic trabeculation.

Osteoclastoma

It may occur in the mandible as a central tumor which begins in the ramus (Fig. 29.14) or near the symphysis. In maxilla it erupts early into antrum or orbital cavity. It may rarely fungate through the

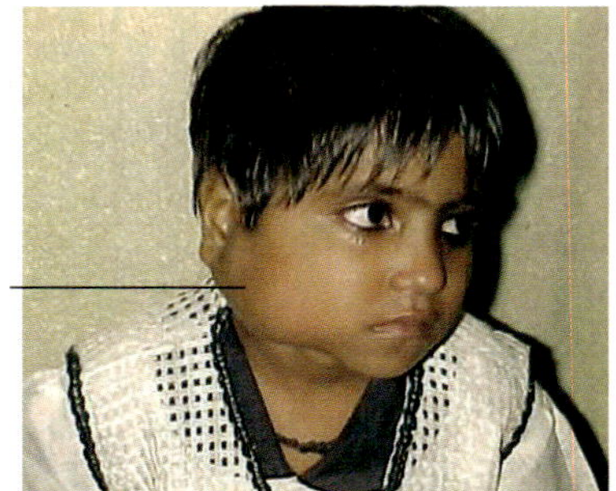

Figure 29.14 Osteoclastoma of mandible presenting as a smooth swelling near the right angle of mandible. (Courtesy: Professor Sandeep Kumar)

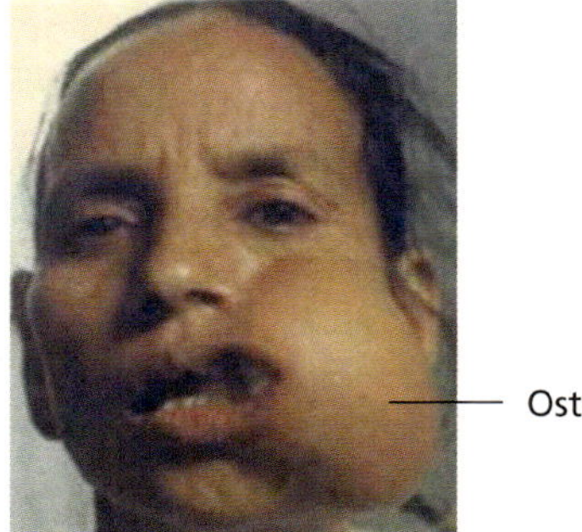

Figure 29.15 Osteosarcoma of left ascending ramus of mandible. (Courtesy: Dr. Surajit Bhattacharya)

socket of an extracted tooth. It expands the jaw and may have egg-shell crackling. X-ray shows a multiloculated lytic lesion.

An osteoclastoma of the symphysis has to be differentiated from other swellings of this region described in Box 29.2.

Box 29.2 Differential diagnoses of swellings of symphyseal region

- Osteoclastoma
- Dental cyst
- Fibrous epulis
- Osteomyelitis of symphysis
- Inframylohyoid sublingual dermoid
- Enlarged submental lymph nodes

Osteosarcoma

- It usually occurs in young adults but may occur in elderly after irradiation.
- Osteosarcoma is characterized by a swelling of jaw of recent onset which grows rapidly causing loosening and extrusion of teeth (Figs 29.15 and 29.16). Pain may be present. X-ray shows resorption of normal bone with expansion and occasional radio-opacities due to irregular new bone formation. Biopsy confirms the diagnosis.
- Fibrosarcoma and chondrosarcoma can also arise from jaws but their growth is slower than that of osteosarcoma.

Carcinoma

A squamous cell carcinoma can arise from mucoperiosteum of alveolus and presents as a swelling (carcinomatous epulis) or an ulcer. It is hard and irregular and may bleed on touch. X-ray shows erosion of the underlying bone. The diagnosis is confirmed by biopsy.

Carcinoma of Maxillary Antrum The patient is usually an elderly person who presents with a variety of symptoms depending on the site and direction of growth of the lesion as described in Table 29.2.

The patient may present with only cervical lymph node enlargement due to metastasis. It may present with recalcitrant toothache and offensive, purulent, blood-tinged nasal discharge.

Antral puncture reveals frank blood. Radiography shows soft-tissue shadow with irregular erosion of antral wall.

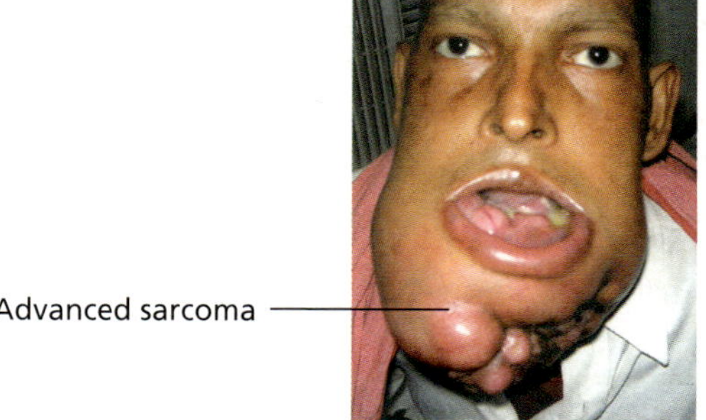

Figure 29.16 Advanced sarcoma of mandible with skin involvement.

Table 29.2 Clinical features of carcinoma of maxillary antrum

Site of involvement	Clinical features
Roof	Proptosis and diplopia
Anterolateral wall	A painless, irregular, hard swelling of insidious onset on the face
Floor	Bulging of hard palate
Medial wall	Nasal obstruction, epiphora, and epistaxis
Posterior wall and extension	Swelling in the temporal fossa with hardly any change in the contour of face

Burkitt's Lymphoma

- It is usually seen in children 3–7 years of age and presents with a swelling of maxilla. It affects the molar or premolar region which is expanded on both the sides. The teeth of affected segment become loose. As the tumor grows, it distorts the face. There is hardly any pain. It may affect the mandible. There may be multiple tumors in the abdomen. Splenic involvement is not significant.
- Radiography shows disappearance of lamina around the affected teeth. Subsequently many small foci of osteolysis appear and eventually coalesce forming a large area of bone destruction.

Secondary Tumors

Secondary deposits can occur in the jaws from carcinoma of bronchus, breast, kidney, thyroid, or prostate. The deposits tend to occur in lingula or at mental foramen. They may not produce a local swelling. X-ray shows irregular osteolysis.

Osteodystrophies

Cherubism

- It is characterized by bilateral symmetrical mandibular swelling near the angle of mandible giving winged face appearance and swelling of both cheeks. The bulging of cheek causes downward pull on lower eyelids which gives the appearance of looking toward the heaven. The lesions consist of fibrous tissue and plenty of giant cells. It is a familial disease that occurs mainly in boys during childhood.
- Radiography shows lesions to be multilocular. It regresses spontaneously with time when the normal bone replaces the abnormal tissue.

Hyperparathyroidism

The jaws may have giant cell lesions (brown tumors) in this disorder. The patient is usually an elderly female who has recurrence of a giant cell lesion of the jaw after complete excision. The serum calcium and parathormone are elevated. Radiography shows a multiloculated cyst-like lesion with loosening of teeth.

Paget's Disease of Bone (Osteitis Deformans)

The patient is usually an elderly male in whom a large number of bones are thickened and deformed including both maxillae. X-ray shows irregular patches of sclerosis and radiolucency (cotton wool appearance), enlargement of bone, and hypercementation of the roots of teeth.

Fibrous Dysplasia

- The patient is a child or adolescent person who presents with a painless bony swelling or swellings. It may involve one bone (monostotic) or many bones (polyostotic). The jaw bones are frequently affected in the former type of dysplasia. Facial asymmetry may be present due to involvement of one or more facial bones.
- X-ray shows expansion of the affected jaw, commonly of ascending ramus of mandible with a dense uniform opacity or ground glass appearance. The expansion usually affects the outer table. The teeth are normal. CT scan images the lesion more accurately (Fig. 29.17).

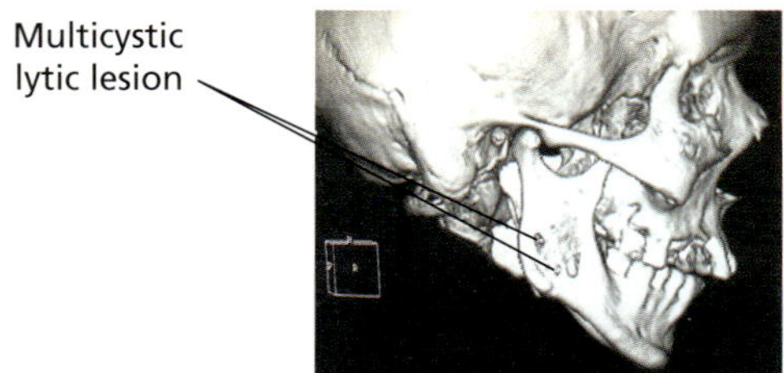

Figure 29.17 Multicystic lytic lesion of mandible near its angle seen in 3D reconstruction CT scan. (Courtesy: Dr. A.C. Dwivedi)

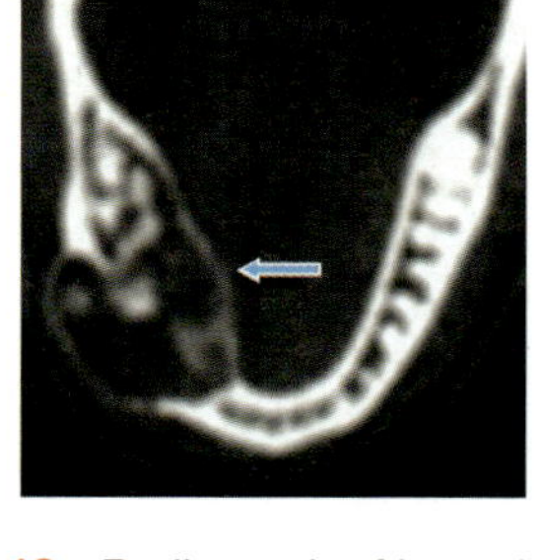

Figure 29.18 Radiograph of lower jaw showing expanding lesion near the right angle with multiloculation. (Courtesy: Professor Surajit Bhattacharya)

Investigations

The investigations include radiography including orthopantomogram (Figs 29.18 and 29.19), CT scan, biopsy, and examination of discharge, if any, for example, anaerobic culture in actinomycosis.

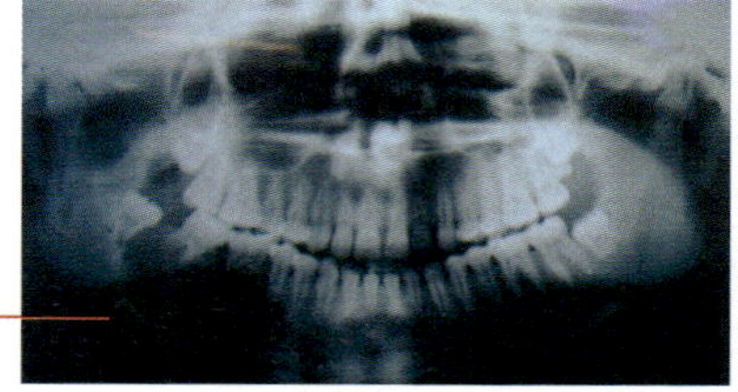

Figure 29.19 Orthopantomogram showing a dentigerous cyst at the right mandibular last molar region. (Courtesy: Professor Divya Mehrotra)

Treatment of swellings of jaws

The treatment of swellings of the jaws requires a multidisciplinary team approach, including a reconstructive and cosmetic surgeon, cancer surgeon, dental surgeon, and radiotherapist. Face is an area of the body which is most important cosmetically. Hence, a reconstructive and cosmetic surgeon is needed from the very beginning when the treatment is being planned.

Specific Swellings

- The fractures are reduced and immobilized. Malunited fracture is refractured, reduced, and immobilized.
- Inflammatory swellings are treated with appropriate antibiotics, drainage of pus, and excision of necrotic tissue.
- Epulides are excised completely and excised tissue is sent for histopathological examination.
- Cysts are excised. A dentigerous cyst is opened; its lining is excised with malformed, misplaced tooth. If the tooth is in correct alignment, it is retained. The shape to the jaw is given by gentle push into the cyst wall (Fig. 29.20).

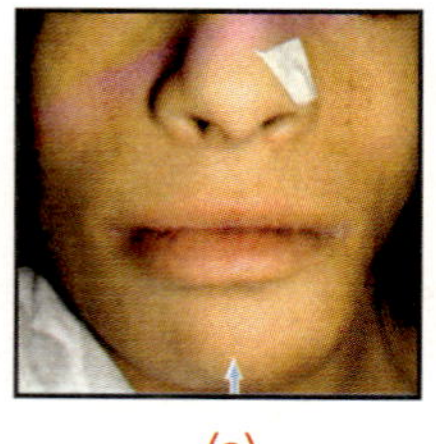
(a)

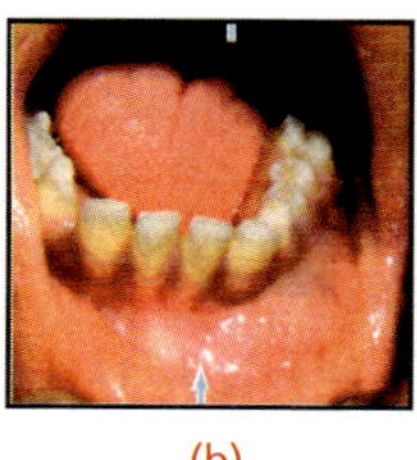
(b)

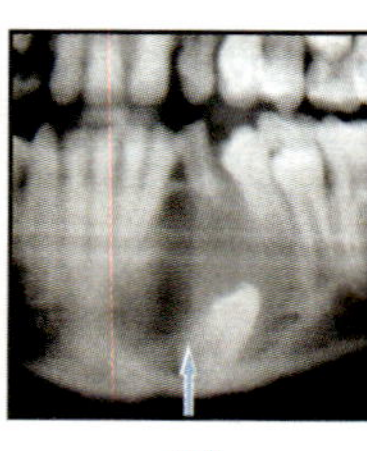
(c)

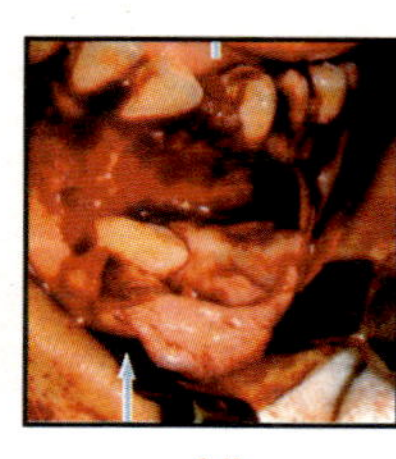
(d)

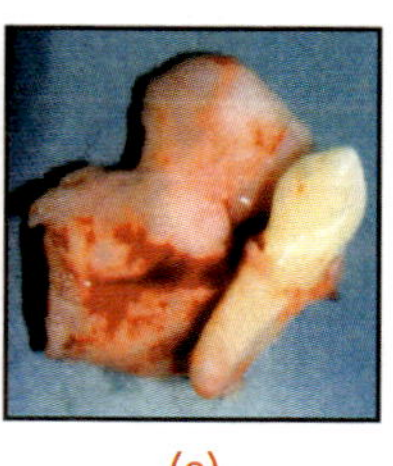
(e)

Figure 29.20 Dentigerous cyst of symphyseal region of mandible. (a) Patient with smooth swelling of chin; (b) swelling in anterior lower labiogingival sulcus; (c) radiograph showing cyst containing the missing left canine; (d) intraoperative appearance of the cyst with contained tooth; (e) excised specimen. (Courtesy: Professor Surajit Bhattacharya)

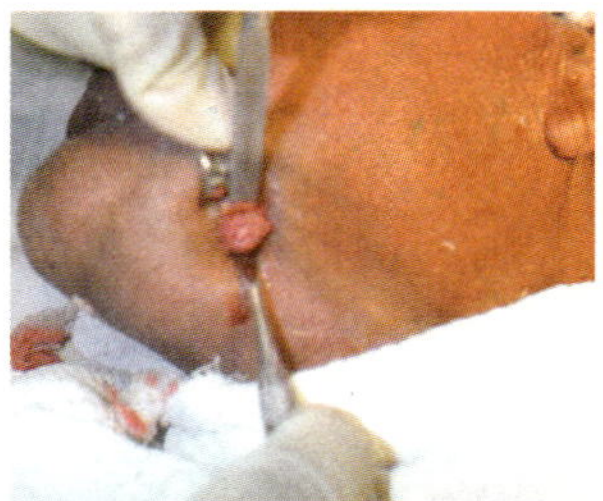

Figure 29.21 Osteoma of mandible being excised. (Courtesy: Professor Divya Mehrotra)

- The benign tumors are excised with their capsule (Fig. 29.21).
- The malignant tumors are widely excised (Figs 29.22 and 29.23). They may require chemotherapy and/or radiotherapy depending on the nature of tumor.
- Osteodystrophies: Brown tumor of the jaw is treated by control of hyperparathyroidism, for example, excision of a parathyroid adenoma. The Paget's disease of bone is treated with calcitonin and bisphosphonates.

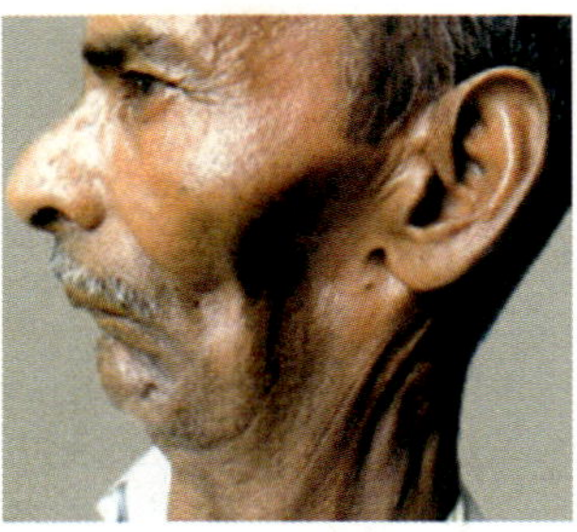

Figure 29.22 Appearance after excision of ameloblastoma of left ascending ramus of mandible without reconstruction of mandible. (Courtesy: Professor A.A. Sonkar)

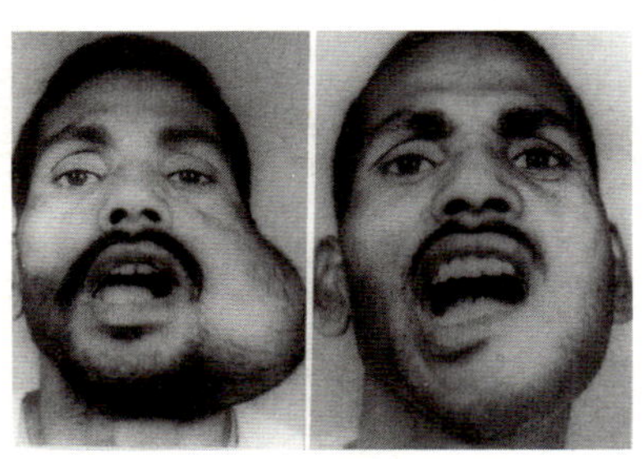

Figure 29.23 Ameloblastoma of mandible near its left angle—before and after treatment (excision and reconstruction). The left facial nerve is partially paralyzed.

- Fibrous dysplasia: The deformities are corrected and localized swellings are excised.

Swellings near the angle of mandible

It is a common clinical presentation of diseases of this region, the causes of which are described in Box 29.3.

Box 29.3 Causes of swellings near the angle of mandible

- **From mandible**
  - Chronic osteomyelitis
  - Ameloblastoma of mandible
  - Dentigerous cyst
  - Keratocystic odontogenic tumor
- **From lower part of parotid gland**
  - Pleomorphic adenoma
  - Warthin's tumor
  - Carcinoma
- **From submandibular salivary gland**
  - Pleomorphic adenoma
  - Carcinoma
  - Distended gland due to calculus obstruction of Wharton's duct
- **From submandibular lymph nodes**
  - Tuberculosis including cold abscess
  - Metastatic lymph nodes
  - Lymphoma
- **Cysts**
  - Branchial cyst
  - Cervical part of plunging ranula

Swellings near the symphysis of mandible

Sometimes a patient presents with a swelling near the symphysis of mandible the causes of which are described in Box 29.4.

The diagnosis of both the above-mentioned groups of swellings (Boxes 23.3 and 29.4) is made by clinical features and investigations. The treatment depends on the cause.

Box 29.4 Causes of swelling near the symphysis of mandible

- **From mandible**
  - Chronic osteomyelitis
  - Osteoclastoma
  - Dental cyst
- **From soft tissues related to symphysis**
  - Inframylohyoid sublingual dermoid
  - Carcinoma of alveolus of symphysis

KEY POINTS

- A swelling is a localized enlargement, elevation, or protuberance usually associated with some disease process. Traumatic swellings include fracture hematoma, fracture callus, and malunited fracture.
- Alveolar abscess occurs mostly in children and young adults and arises from the molar teeth of mandible or maxilla at the root of decaying tooth. It usually progresses outwards eroding the lateral plate of alveolus forming a subcutaneous abscess on lower face.
- Acute osteomyelitis presents with fever, pain, swelling, and tenderness at the site of infection. Chronic osteomyelitis is characterized by a sinus fixed to underlying bone which is thickened and tender. Radiography shows involucrum and sequestrum.
- Cervicofacial actinomycosis presents as hard, diffuse, and nodular swelling of the gum or mandible near the angle with pus-discharging sinuses. The pus contains "sulfur granules."
- Empyema of maxillary antrum presents with facial pain which is aggravated by bending the head forwards and downwards, toothache, and frontal headache. CT scan and CT-guided needle aspiration reveal pus.
- Fibrous epulis arises from the periodontal membrane and presents with a painless, slow-growing swelling of the gum usually between two incisors of the lower jaw.
- Myeloid or giant cell epulis may be associated with a periosteal osteoclastoma and presents as a purplish, hyperemic, smooth or lobulated, soft or firm swelling of the gum.
- Dentigerous cyst is seen in young adults at the site of an unerupted permanent tooth, usually the lower third molar. Radiography shows a pear-shaped or ovoid unilocular translucency (cyst) surrounding the crown of an unerupted tooth.
- Ameloblastomas occur predominantly in the mandible and usually in the molar region or ascending ramus characterized by a painless, slow-growing swelling with expansion of outer table of the mandible. Radiography shows a unilocular or multilocular radiolucency (soap-bubble appearance) with scalloping.
- Odontomes are hamartomatous malformations of dental tissue of developmental origin. They consist of enamel, dentine, pulp, and cementum in a variable relationship to one another.
- Osteoclastoma may occur in the mandible as a central tumor which begins in the ramus or near the symphysis. In maxilla it erupts early into antrum or orbital cavity.
- Osteosarcoma is characterized by a painful swelling of jaw of recent onset which grows rapidly causing loosening and extrusion of teeth. X-ray shows resorption of normal bone with expansion and occasional radio-opacities due to irregular bone formation.
- Squamous cell carcinoma can arise from mucoperiosteum of alveolus or jaws and presents as a swelling (carcinomatous epulis) or ulcer. It is hard and irregular and may bleed on touch. X-ray shows erosion of the underlying bone.
- Carcinoma of maxillary antrum usually occurs in an elderly person who presents with a variety of symptoms depending on the site and direction of growth of the lesion. Antral puncture reveals frank blood. Radiography shows soft-tissue shadow with erosion of antral wall. It is treated by a combination of surgery, chemotherapy, and radiotherapy.
- Burkitt's lymphoma is usually seen in children 3–7 years of age and presents with a painless swelling of maxilla in molar or premolar region. The teeth of affected segment become loose. The swelling may fungate into the mouth. It is treated by chemotherapy.
- The benign tumors are excised with their capsule. The malignant tumors are treated with wide or radical surgical excision, radiotherapy, and/

(CONTD...)

KEY POINTS (...CONTD)

or chemotherapy depending on the nature and extent of the tumor.

- A multiloculated giant cell lesion (brown tumor) may occur in hyperparathyroidism. It is treated by removal of its cause.
- Fibrous dysplasia may involve one bone (monostotic), most commonly the jaw bones, or many bones (polyostotic). Monostotic fibrous dysplasia may result in facial asymmetry. X-ray shows outer table expansion of the affected jaw, commonly of ascending ramus of mandible with a dense uniform opacity or ground glass appearance.

SELF-ASSESSMENT

Long answer questions

1. What is an epulis? Describe the clinical features and treatment of various types of epulides.
2. Classify the swellings of the jaws. Describe the diagnosis and treatment of ameloblastoma of mandible.
3. What is an odontome? Describe the types, diagnosis, and treatment of odontomes.
4. Describe the differential diagnosis of a swelling situated near the angle of mandible.

Short answer questions

1. Fibrous epulis
2. Dentigerous cyst
3. Ameloblastoma
4. Cherubism
5. Brown tumor

Multiple choice questions

1. All of the following facts are true about an alveolar abscess, except
   (a) It occurs mainly in children and adults
   (b) It arises from upper central incisors
   (c) It progresses outwards eroding the outer table of the jaws
   (d) X-ray shows lucency in relation to the root of affected tooth
2. Epulis is a
   (a) Nonspecific swelling of gum
   (b) Manifestation of chronic osteomyelitis of jaws
   (c) Type of odontome
   (d) Type of epidermoid carcinoma
3. Which of the following is the commonest epulis?
   (a) Fibrous epulis
   (b) Granulomatous epulis
   (c) Myeloid epulis
   (d) Congenital epulis
4. All of the following facts are correct about the fibrous epulis, except
   (a) It arises from the periodontal membrane
   (b) The patient is usually a middle-aged woman
   (c) The swelling is pink, smooth, firm, longitudinal and has a narrow base
   (d) It is usually present between two upper molars on the lingual surface
5. All of the following facts are true about a myeloid epulis, except
   (a) It is same as giant cell reparative granuloma (peripheral)
   (b) It is caused by hyperparathyroidism
   (c) It occurs in young people and mainly affects the mandible
   (d) It manifests as a swelling of gum that is painless, purplish, soft, lobulated, and sessile
6. All of the following facts are true about Epstein's pearls, except
   (a) They are known as Bohn's nodules
   (b) They occur in adults
   (c) They are small white nodules of 2–3 mm diameter affecting both the jaws
   (d) They disappear by themselves within 3 months

(CONTD...)

SELF-ASSESSMENT *(...CONTD)*

7. Which of the following is the commonest odontogenic cyst?
   (a) Dental cyst (radical cyst)
   (b) Dentigerous cyst
   (c) Epstein's pearls
   (d) Nasopalatine cyst
8. All of the following statements are true about a dental cyst, except
   (a) It is the commonest odontogenic cyst
   (b) The patient is usually young and presents with a painful swelling of the jaws
   (c) It occurs in relation to the root of a pulpless tooth which is carious
   (d) It is usually small and not clinically obvious
9. All of the following statements are the clinical features of a dentigerous cyst, except
   (a) It is usually seen in young adults
   (b) It is related to the root of a permanent tooth
   (c) It expands both the tables of jaw
   (d) It can occur in the maxilla of which the inner table is not expanded
10. All of the following facts are the features of a keratocystic odontogenic tumor, except
   (a) It is lined by columnar epithelium
   (b) It is filled with semisolid keratin
   (c) More than 70% of swellings occur in the mandible near its angle
   (d) It recurs in 60% of cases after excision
11. All of the following facts are true about a nasolabial cyst, except
   (a) It arises from external surface of maxilla deep to nasolabial fold
   (b) The patient presents with a slow-growing swelling of upper lip
   (c) It may bulge in the labial sulcus
   (d) The nostril is not distorted
12. All of the following facts are the clinical features of an ameloblastoma, except
   (a) It usually occurs in forties
   (b) It usually affects the mandible in the molar region or ascending ramus
   (c) It is characterized by a painless, slow-growing swelling
   (d) It expands both the tables of the jaw
13. All of the following facts are true about ameloblastoma, except
   (a) It usually occurs in forties
   (b) It mostly occurs in maxilla near canine tooth
   (c) It expands mainly the outer table
   (d) The lymph nodes are not enlarged
14. What is the radiographic appearance of an ameloblastoma?
   (a) Ill-defined radiodense area
   (b) Ill-defined radiolucent area
   (c) Well-defined multiloculated radiolucent area with scalloping edge
   (d) Areas of bone destruction and new bone formation
15. All of the following facts are the features of odontomes, except
   (a) They are tumors of dental tissue
   (b) They are hamartomatous in nature
   (c) They are developmental in origin
   (d) They consist of enamel, dentine, pulp, and cementum in different proportions
16. All of the following facts are the features of ossifying fibroma, except
   (a) It is a tumor of elderly people
   (b) It is usually a surface tumor
   (c) It is a painless, slow-growing swelling
   (d) X-ray shows a well-defined radiolucent area with speckled opacities
17. All of the following statements are true about osteosarcoma, except
   (a) The patient is usually a young adult
   (b) It is a rapidly growing swelling of jaws of recent onset
   (c) It spreads by lymphatic route to cervical lymph nodes
   (d) Radiography shows irregular destruction of bone, may be with some new bone formation
18. All of the following facts are features of a Burkitt's lymphoma, except
   (a) It mostly occurs in children 3–7 years of age
   (b) It usually affects mandible near molar or premolar region
   (c) Both the tables of jaw are expanded
   (d) There is hardly any pain

Answers

1. (b) 2. (a) 3. (a) 4. (d) 5. (b) 6. (b) 7. (a) 8. (b) 9. (b) 10. (a) 11. (d) 12. (d) 13. (b) 14. (c) 15. (a) 16. (a) 17. (c) 18. (b)

Swellings of the Neck

30

Introduction

Swellings of the neck are very common. They arise from the normal tissues and structures of the neck. The swelling may be acute such as an acute abscess and Ludwig's angina, or chronic such as a cold abscess, multinodular goiter, and branchial cyst.

Causes of swellings of neck

They can be classified into two groups:

1. **Nonspecific swellings**: These swellings arise from nonspecific tissues of the neck such as skin, subcutaneous tissue, and lymph nodes.
2. **Specific swellings**: They originate from specific structures of neck such as thyroid, larynx, pharynx, and sternomastoid.

The causes of swellings of the neck are described in Box 30.1.

Clinical diagnosis

Clinical diagnosis of most of the swellings of neck can be made by careful history taking and the physical examination of the patient. "Rule of 80" in neck masses (Box 30.2) must be kept in mind while making diagnosis.

The following points are especially helpful in making the diagnosis:

Box 30.1 Causes of swellings of neck

- **Nonspecific swellings**
  - Lymph node enlargement
  - Sebaceous cyst
  - Infections: Boil, acute abscess, cold abscess
  - Tumors: Papilloma, lipoma, neurofibroma, hemangioma
- **Specific swellings**
  - *Anterior midline swellings*
    - Enlarged submental, prelaryngeal, and pretracheal lymph nodes
    - Ludwig's angina
    - Dermoid cyst: Sublingual inframylohyoid and suprasternal
    - Thyroglossal cyst
    - Subhyoid bursal cyst
    - Solitary nodule of isthmus of thyroid
  - *Upper lateral neck swellings*
    - Enlarged level I lymph nodes
    - Periauricular dermoid
    - Swellings of cervical part of parotid and submandibular salivary glands
    - Branchial cyst
    - Plunging ranula
    - Faciocervical actinomycosis
  - *Middle lateral neck swellings*
    - Enlarged level II lymph nodes
    - Swellings of lateral lobe of thyroid
    - Carotid artery aneurysm
    - Pharyngeal pouch or Zenker's diverticulum
    - Laryngocele
    - Carotid body tumor
    - Sternomastoid tumor
  - *Lower lateral neck swellings*
    - Enlarged level III lymph nodes
    - Cystic hygroma
    - Cervical rib
    - Subclavian artery aneurysm
    - Pancoast's tumor
    - Lung hernia (pneumatocele)
  - *Swellings of nape (back) of neck*
    - Enlarged suboccipital lymph nodes
    - Carbuncle
    - Lipoma
    - Occipitocervical meningocele

Box 30.2 Rule of 80 in neck masses

- 80% of neck masses are neoplastic
- 80% of neoplastic neck masses occur in males
- 80% of neck masses are malignant
- 80% of malignant neck masses are metastatic
- 80% of metastatic neck masses are from primary sites above clavicle

- **Duration**: Most of the swellings of the neck area are of long duration except the acute inflammatory swellings such as an acute abscess and Ludwig's angina which have a short duration.
- **Pain**: Pain is a dominant symptom of acute inflammatory swellings; otherwise most of the swellings are painless.
- **Rate of growth**: Acute inflammatory and malignant swellings grow rapidly while the other swellings are usually slow-growing.
- **Site of swelling**: Most of the swellings of neck are site specific. The sites of the common swellings of neck are described in Table 30.1.
- **Shape**: Some swellings have a typical shape. Examples:
  - Generalized enlargement of thyroid has a butterfly-like shape.
  - Sternomastoid tumor is an ovoid swelling with its long axis parallel to the long axis of sternocleidomastoid.
  - Subhyoid bursal cyst is transversely oval.
- **Movements**: A swelling of thyroid moves up with deglutition, and a thyroglossal cyst moves up with protrusion of tongue.
- **Surface and consistency**:
  - Benign swellings are usually smooth, regular, and uniformly soft or firm in consistency.
  - Malignant swellings are usually irregular, nodular, hard, or variable in consistency.
  - A large number of swellings of neck are cystic in consistency (cystic consistency is the feel as if there is fluid inside the swelling). A classified list of cystic swellings of neck is described in Box 30.3.

Table 30.1 Sites of occurrence of the common swellings of neck

Swelling	Site of occurrence
Lymph node swelling	At the sites of lymph nodes
Dermoid cyst	Anterior midline of neck below the chin (sublingual inframylohyoid) and above manubrium, behind angle of mandible
Branchial cyst	Anterior and deep to upper third of sternomastoid below angle of mandible
Thyroglossal cyst	Anterior midline of neck just below body of hyoid bone, a little to the left
Cystic hygroma	Posterior triangle of neck
Sebaceous cyst	Anywhere in the neck
Lipoma	Anywhere but commonly at nape of neck and supraclavicular fossa
Cold abscess	At the site of lymph nodes, paravertebral region
Carbuncle	Nape of neck
Sternomastoid tumor	Lower sternomastoid
Cervical meningocele	Posterior midline of neck

Box 30.3 Causes of cystic swellings of neck

- **Anywhere in the neck**
  - Sebaceous cyst
  - Cold abscess
- **Anterior midline of neck**
  - Sublingual inframylohyoid dermoid cyst
  - Thyroglossal cyst
  - Subhyoid bursal cyst
  - Cyst of isthmus of thyroid
  - Suprasternal dermoid
- **Lateral neck**
  - Periauricular dermoid
  - Branchial cyst
  - Plunging ranula, cervical part
  - Laryngocele
  - Pharyngeal pouch
  - Cyst of lateral lobe of thyroid
  - Cystic hygroma
  - Lung hernia
- **Posterior midline of neck**
  - Occipitocervical meningocele

1. NONSPECIFIC SWELLINGS

Enlarged lymph nodes

The lymph node enlargement is the commonest cause of a swelling/swellings in the neck. The signs of a lymph node swelling are:

- It is situated at the site of lymph nodes.
- It is single or multiple, more commonly multiple.
- It is usually ovoid in shape.

The lymph node sites in the neck are classified into six levels as described in Box 30.4.

Causes of Cervical Lymphadenopathy

The clinically important causes of cervical lymphadenopathy are described in Box 30.5.

Reactive Lymph Nodes

- The normal lymph nodes in the neck are usually <1 cm in size. Infections involving oral and nasal cavities, throat, salivary glands, and

Box 30.4 Levels of cervical lymph node groups

- **Level I**: Submental and submandibular nodes
- **Level II**: Upper jugular chain nodes
- **Level III**: Middle jugular chain nodes—below hyoid bone, above cricoid, and deep to sternomastoid from its posterior border to strap muscles medially
- **Level IV**: Lower jugular chain nodes below cricoid, above clavicle deep to sternomastoid from its posterior border to strap muscles medially
- **Level V**: Posterior triangle nodes
- **Level VI**: Anterior compartment nodes below hyoid, above suprasternal notch medial to lateral border of strap muscles on both sides

Box 30.5 Clinically important causes of cervical lymphadenopathy

- Reactive lymph nodes of recurrent or chronic throat or scalp infection
- Tuberculosis
- Metastatic disease
- Lymphoma

scalp lead to their enlargement which is mild, smooth, and tender (Fig. 30.1).

- Pus may form in a reactive lymph node (lymphadenitic abscess). Chronic or recurrent infection results in persistent or recurrent lymphadenopathy. These lymph nodes are firm and may be slightly tender or nontender.
- The diagnosis should be confirmed by FNAC or biopsy.

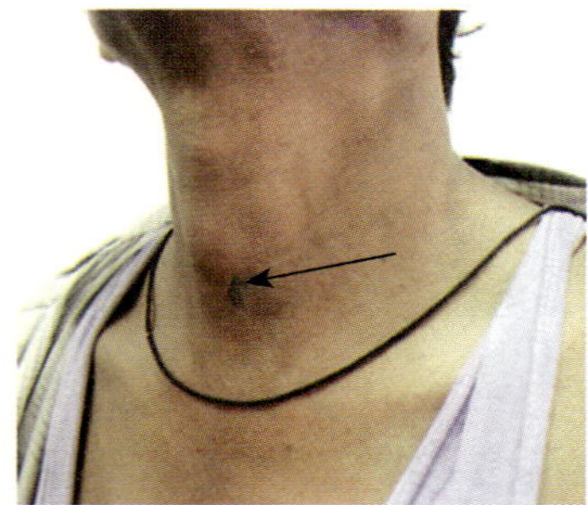

Figure 30.1 Acute nonspecific lymphadenitis of lower midline lymph nodes of neck with swelling and redness.

Tuberculous Lymphadenitis

- The patient is usually young and presents with a single or multiple enlarged neck nodes. Any group of lymph nodes may be involved.
- The lymph nodes are mild to moderate in size, firm, nontender, and matted. They may be associated with general symptoms, for example, anorexia, loss of health, low-grade evening fever, and night sweats.

Metastatic Lymph Nodes

- The patient is usually a middle-aged or elderly person, more commonly a male, who presents with a single or multiple enlarged lymph nodes.
- They are hard, nontender, and mobile or fixed. Most of these nodes are deep to anterior edge of sternomastoid.
- The patient should be carefully evaluated for the primary site in the mouth, nose, pharynx, larynx, thyroid, external auditory meatus, lungs, and in a case of left supraclavicular lymph node enlargement the abdomen and testes.

Lymphoma

- The patient presents with a single or multiple enlarged lymph nodes in neck which are nontender, firm or rubbery, and discrete without matting.
- In non-Hodgkin lymphoma, lower neck nodes are enlarged and may be associated with nonlymphatic site involvement.
- In Hodgkin lymphoma, usually upper neck nodes are involved and may be associated with splenomegaly. Apart from these features, there may be irregular fever, loss of weight, pruritus, and night sweats.

Sebaceous cyst

It is characterized by a painless and slow-growing swelling. It is smooth, soft, and hemispherical. It usually has a dark spot on the top in the center called punctum (Figs 30.2 and 30.3).

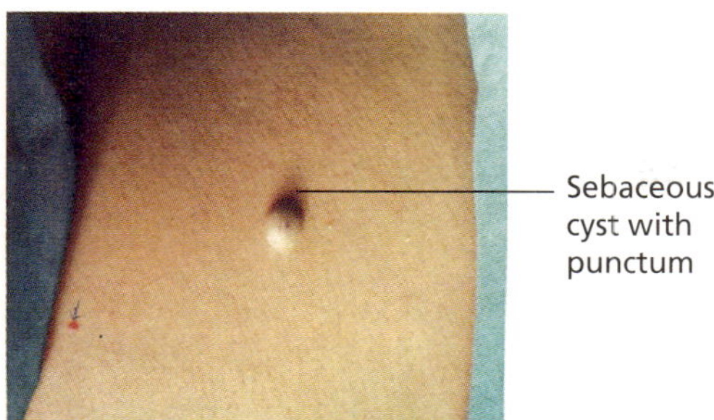

Figure 30.2 Sebaceous cyst of left side of neck with a punctum on the top. A small capillary angioma is also seen (↓).

Boil (furuncle)

It is staphylococcal infection of a hair follicle with perifolliculitis and suppuration. It can occur anywhere except in palm of hand and sole of foot. The common sites of occurrence are neck, back, scalp, thigh, and forearm. It is a small conical swelling with yellowish top (Fig. 30.4).

Acute abscess

It is a localized collection of pus in the tissues characterized by a painful swelling of short duration. It is red, hot, and tender and may be soft or boggy in the center (Fig. 30.5). The pain may be throbbing type that increases on making the part dependent.

Cold abscess

It is a manifestation of tuberculosis of cervical lymph nodes or cervical spine. The patient is usually young and has a painless, smooth, nontender, and soft cystic swelling in the neck. It is opaque to transmitted light (Fig. 30.6).

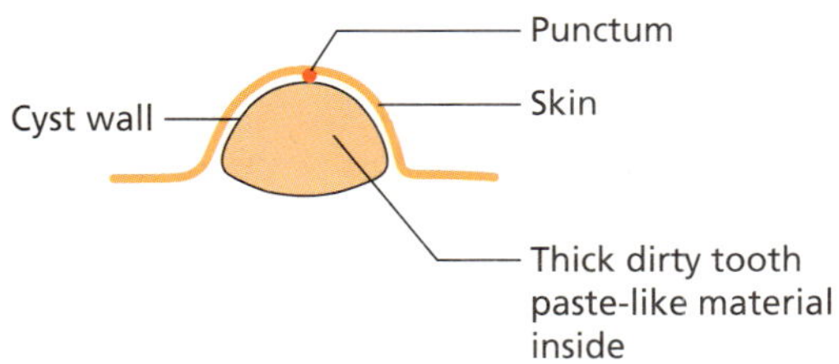

Figure 30.3 Sebaceous (epidermal) cyst.

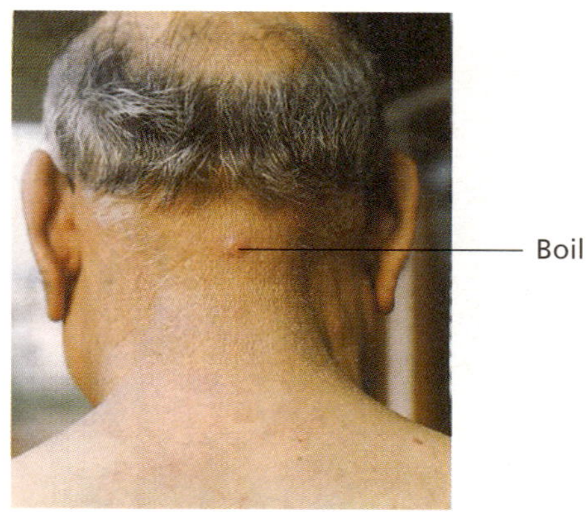

Figure 30.4 Boil or furuncle of nape of neck.

Collar-Stud Abscess

It is a presentation of cervical lymph node tuberculosis and characterized by two pockets of pus joined together by a narrow track. The upper pocket is small and a little higher up and deep to deep fascia of neck. It contains the caseating lymph node. The lower pocket is large, superficial (subcutaneous), and a little lower down. There is a cross-fluctuation between the two swellings.

Papilloma

It is a very common benign tumor of skin of neck. Papilloma may be single or multiple and may be in the form of a ring around the neck. It is firm and nontender and may look like a small tree having branches.

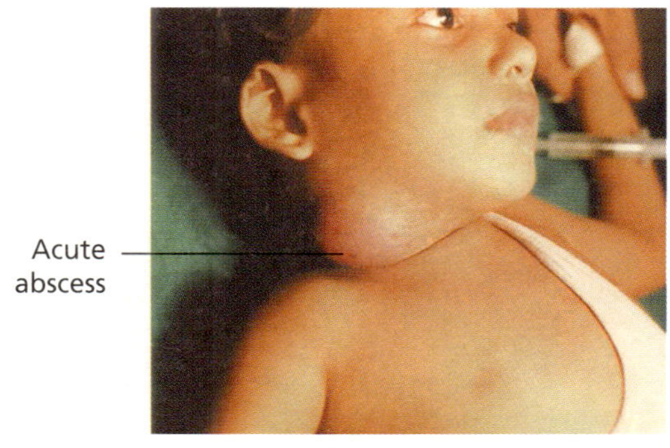

Figure 30.5 Acute abscess of neck.

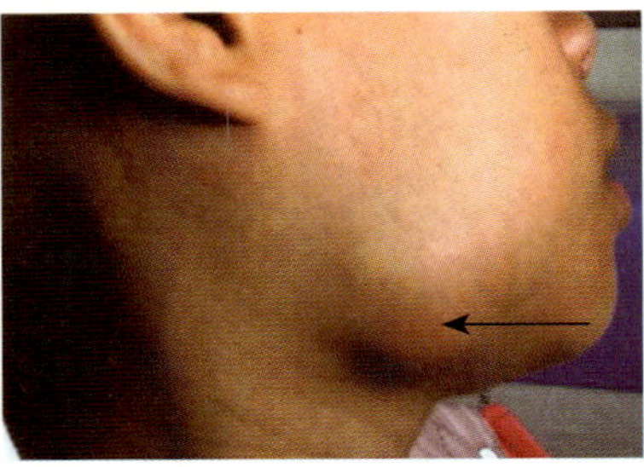

Figure 30.6 Cold abscess of right submandibular region. Note mild redness of overlying skin which is a preparation to rupture. (Courtesy: Professor Surajit Bhattacharya)

Lipoma

It is a benign tumor of fatty tissue which presents as a painless and slow-growing swelling of long duration. It can occur anywhere but is common in the supraclavicular region and nape of neck. It is soft, nontender, smooth, or lobulated and has an edge that slips under the finger.

Neurofibroma

It is a benign tumor of fibrous connective tissue of nerve sheath.

- **Solitary neurofibroma**: It is characterized by a subcutaneous nodule which is round or ovoid and firm (Fig. 30.7). It moves across the axis of nerve from which it is arising. Pressure on it may cause tingling and numbness which radiate along the course of that nerve.
- **Multiple neurofibromas**: They are present all over the body associated with coffee-brown pigmented patches on the skin (café au lait spots).
- **Pachydermatocele**: It is a plexiform lesion of small subcutaneous nerves of skin in which the skin is thickened and folds of it hang down from the neck.
- **Ganglioneuroma**: It is a tumor of ganglion cells and nerve fibers of sympathetic chain. It is a painless and slow-growing swelling of upper neck. It may present as a parapharyngeal mass that can cause dysphagia.

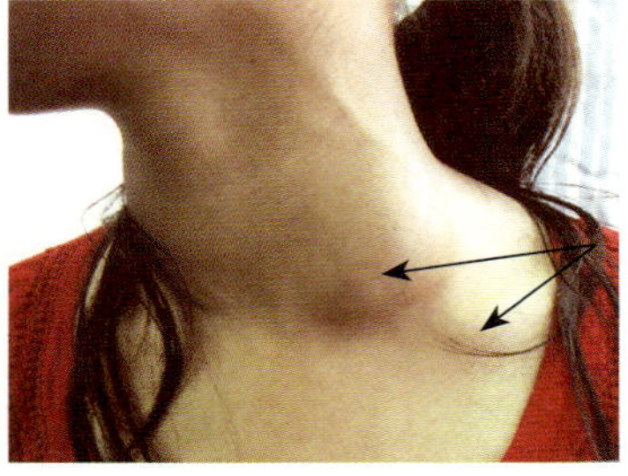

Figure 30.7 Left supraclavicular firm lobular mass—FNAC showed it to be a neurofibroma.

Hemangioma

It is a malformation of blood vessels that looks like a tumor (hamartoma). It is of three types: capillary hemangioma, venous or cavernous hemangioma, and congenital arteriovenous malformation.

Capillary Hemangioma It is of three types: salmon patch, port-wine stain, and strawberry angioma. Salmon patch occurs over the forehead and not in the neck. Port-wine stain is an extensive intradermal lesion occurring on the face, neck, shoulder, and buttocks. It is a congenital flat lesion, bluish purple in color. Strawberry angioma is a protruding skin lesion of the head–neck region which appears usually 1 month after birth. It is compressible and grows for 5–7 years when it starts regressing.

Venous or Cavernous Hemangioma It is a painless and slow-growing swelling of the neck of long duration. It usually occurs in the posterior triangle. It is bluish in color, soft, cystic, opaque, and compressible.

Congenital Arteriovenous Malformation It is characterized by congenital direct communication of arteries and veins in the neck and lack of normal capillary network. It is typically seen during adolescence initially as a quiescent lesion which progresses to an expansive mass in the carotid and subclavian region with cosmetic and functional disturbance. Schobinger (1996) has described four clinical stages of this lesion which are given in Table 30.2. The diagnosis can be confirmed by MR imaging and digital subtraction angiography.

Table 30.2 Clinical stages of congenital arteriovenous malformation

Stage	Symptoms and signs
Quiescence	Warm overlying skin, discoloration
Expansion	Pulsatile mass, bruit
Destruction	Pain, ulceration, hemorrhage
Decompensation	Congestive cardiac failure due to overload

2. ANTERIOR MIDLINE SWELLINGS OF NECK

Enlarged anterior midline lymph nodes

These lymph nodes are situated just below the chin, a little lower down in front of larynx (prelaryngeal), and still below in front of trachea (pretracheal). The common causes of their enlargement include:

- Chronic/recurrent infection of midline structures from the lower incisors to structures below when they are firm and discrete
- Tuberculosis when they are matted
- Metastasis of carcinoma of tip of tongue, floor of mouth, and central lower lip when they are hard, nontender, and mobile or fixed

Ludwig's angina

It is submandibular cellulitis characterized by swelling of submental and submandibular regions of short duration. The swelling is hot and tender on palpation. The floor of mouth is swollen with the tongue lifted upwards. Hence, the patient keeps the mouth open (Fig. 30.8).

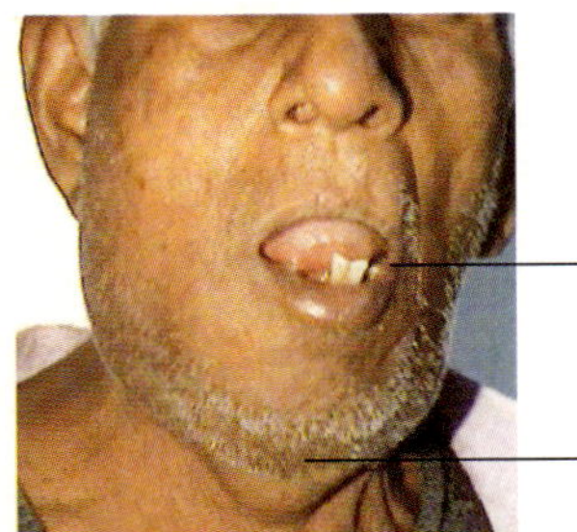

Figure 30.8 Submandibular swelling due to Ludwig's angina. (Courtesy: Professor Anupam Misra)

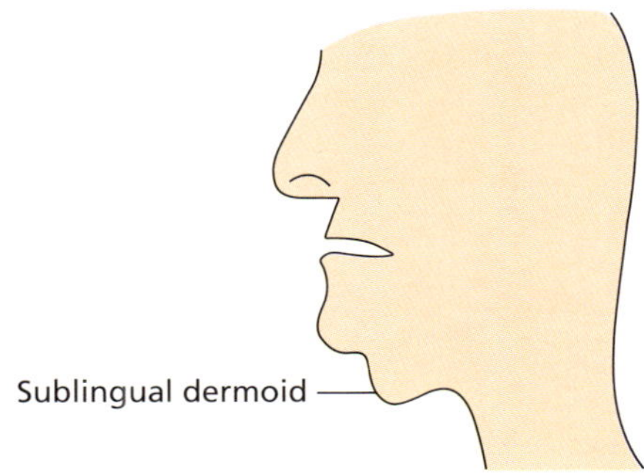

Figure 30.9 Double-chin appearance due to sublingual dermoid.

Sublingual inframylohyoid dermoid

It presents in the neck just below the chin. The patient is usually young (10–20 years) and has a painless and slow-growing swelling just below the chin giving a double-chin appearance to the patient when the patient is viewed from the side (Fig. 30.9). It is smooth, soft, cystic, nontender, and opaque. A dermoid can occur in the suprasternal space of Burns and has the signs described earlier.

Thyroglossal cyst

The patient is an adolescent person who presents with a painless swelling in the upper neck usually at the level of hyoid bone slightly to the left of midline. It moves up with swallowing and protrusion of tongue. It is smooth, cystic, and often translucent (Fig. 30.10).

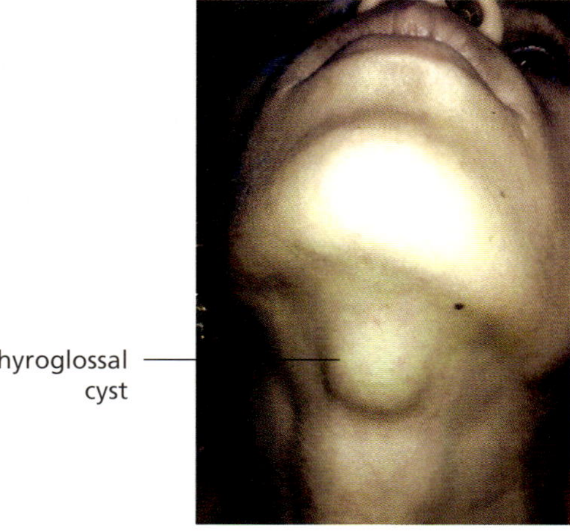

Figure 30.10 Thyroglossal cyst. (Courtesy: Dr. Ravi Mishra)

Subhyoid bursal cyst

There is a small swelling in the front of neck in midline just below the body of hyoid bone. It is soft, cystic, transversely oval, and translucent. It moves up with deglutition.

Solitary nodule of isthmus of thyroid

A solitary nodule may occur in the isthmus of thyroid, the causes of which include carcinoma, adenoma, and cyst. It moves up with deglutition. These three swellings cannot be differentiated clinically.

3. UPPER LATERAL NECK SWELLINGS

Enlarged upper lateral lymph nodes

The details of enlarged cervical lymph nodes are already described, which are same here.

Periauricular dermoid

A dermoid can occur just behind or below the pinna. It is smooth, soft, nontender, and opaque. It may be indented with digital pressure.

Swellings of cervical part of parotid and submandibular salivary glands

Swellings of Cervical Part of Parotid

The swellings limited to this part of parotid gland include pleomorphic adenoma and carcinoma. The parotid swellings are present above the submandibular swellings which are situated below the pinna.

Swellings of Submandibular Salivary Gland

- An enlarged submandibular salivary gland presents as a swelling in the submandibular triangle below the angle of mandible.
- It is transversely ovoid and palpable bidigitally (one finger in the floor of mouth on that side) as opposed to a swelling of submandibular lymph nodes.
- The common causes of submandibular salivary gland swelling are distended salivary gland due to calculus obstruction, pleomorphic adenoma, and carcinoma. Swelling due to calculus obstruction is smooth and firm and turbid fluid comes out from the opening of Wharton's duct if it is pressed. The stone may be visible in the ductal orifice or palpable in the duct in the floor of mouth.
- The swelling of pleomorphic adenoma is ovoid, lobulated, firm, and nontender.
- The swelling of carcinoma is rapidly growing and may be large, hard, irregular, and nontender.

Branchial cyst

- The patient is usually young, 15–25 years of age, who presents with a swelling of the upper neck near the angle of mandible which is partly covered by sternomastoid.
- It is smooth, cystic, and nontender, and may be translucent (Fig. 30.11). On making the sternomastoid contract, the swelling becomes less prominent.

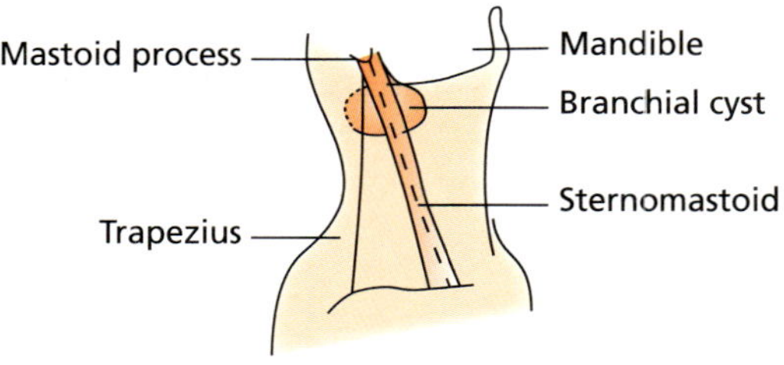

Figure 30.11 Branchial cyst.

Plunging ranula

Ranula is a bluish translucent swelling of one side of floor of mouth. Sometimes it has a cervical extension which presents as a cystic swelling in the upper neck below the angle of mandible. It is smooth, soft, and cystic with cross-fluctuation between the cervical and oral swellings.

Faciocervical actinomycosis

It is the most common type of actinomycosis. The infection spreads from adjacent infected teeth or tonsil. Initially local induration occurs followed by nodules at the junction of face and neck near the angle of mandible. They soften and burst on the skin to produce sinuses which discharge pus-containing sulfur granules. The regional lymph nodes are not enlarged.

4. MIDDLE LATERAL NECK SWELLINGS

Enlarged lymph nodes

These lymph nodes are commonly enlarged due to tuberculosis, metastatic cancer, and lymphoma.

Thyroid swellings

A thyroid swelling moves up with deglutition. Any swelling of the thyroid can present as a lateral neck swelling. They are of two types: generalized swellings and localized swellings.

Generalized Thyroid Swellings

The generalized swellings are characterized by enlargement of whole thyroid which presents as a butterfly-like swelling of anterior neck and both sides, the causes of which include physiological goiter, colloid goiter, Graves' disease, multinodular goiter, and advanced carcinoma.

- In physiological goiter, colloid goiter, and Graves' disease, the swelling is smooth, regular, and uniform. Graves' disease has signs of hyperfunction of thyroid.
- In multinodular goiter (Fig. 30.12) and advanced carcinoma, the swellings are nodular and irregular.

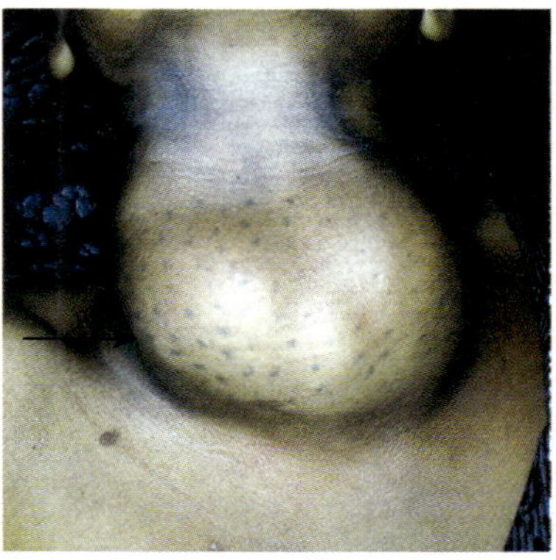

Figure 30.12 Multinodular goiter.

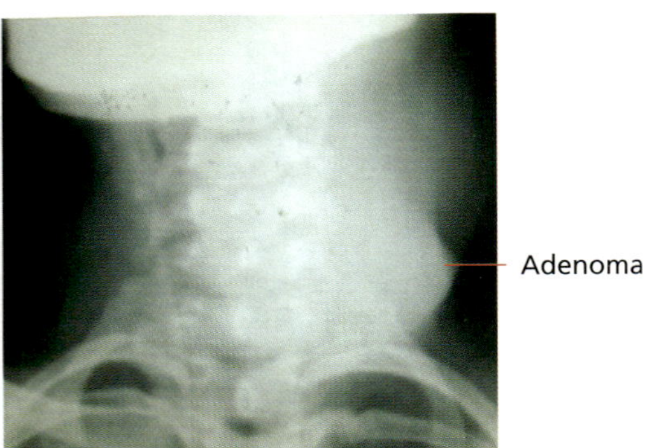

Figure 30.13 Left oblique view radiograph of the neck showing soft-tissue shadow of a large adenoma of left lobe of thyroid that has shifted tracheal gas shadow.

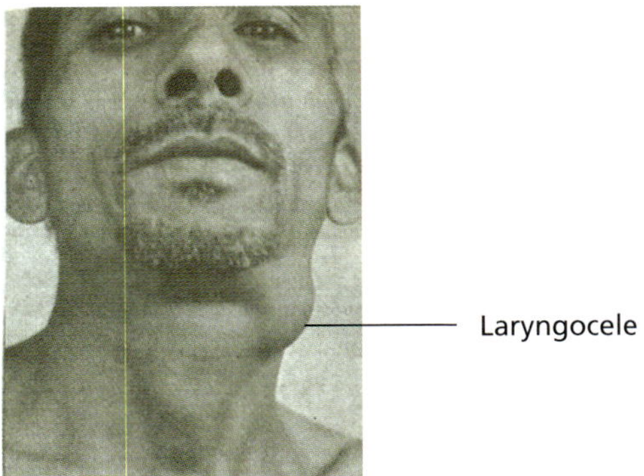

Figure 30.14 Laryngocele of left side.

Localized Thyroid Swellings

The common causes of localized enlargement are solitary nodule of a nodular goiter, adenoma (Fig. 30.13), cyst, and early carcinoma of thyroid. These swellings of thyroid may present as a lateral neck swelling.

Carotid artery aneurysm

The patient is usually a middle-aged or elderly person who presents with a pulsatile swelling which is smooth, tensely cystic, and opaque. It has expansile pulsation and a bruit on auscultation.

Pharyngeal pouch (Zenker's diverticulum)

- The patient is usually a middle-aged or elderly person, more commonly a male, who presents with gurgling noises in the neck during meals, dysphagia, swelling in the neck especially during meals, and regurgitation of undigested food after meals.
- There is a lateral neck swelling, usually on the left side at the level of cricoid. The swelling is smooth, soft, cystic, opaque, and nonpulsatile. It enlarges during meals and can be emptied by pressure.

Laryngocele

The patient is usually a middle-aged person who is a glass blower or trumpet player, or has chronic cough. There is a smooth, oval, boggy swelling at the level of cricoid (Fig. 30.14). It increases in size when the patient blows out against closed nose (Valsalva maneuver). It may be resonant on percussion. It may disappear on pressure or by itself with gurgling and discharge of contained mucus into the pharynx.

Carotid body tumor (chemodectoma)

The patient is usually a middle-aged or elderly person who presents with a painless, slow-growing swelling of neck situated at the level of hyoid bone covered by anterior border of sternomastoid muscle. It is smooth or lobulated, vertically oval, and firm to hard in consistency (potato tumor). It is mobile transversely but not vertically, and pressure on it may precipitate a syncopal attack.

Sternomastoid tumor

The patient is an infant who has a firm, smooth, and fusiform swelling in the middle of sternomastoid with its long axis parallel to the long axis of sternocleidomastoid muscle. It is mobile from side to side but not up and down. The medial and lateral borders are distinct but not the upper and lower limits. If it is not treated, it may lead to wry neck or torticollis.

5. LOWER LATERAL NECK SWELLINGS

Enlarged lymph nodes

Like other lymph nodes of the neck, these lymph nodes commonly enlarge due to tuberculosis, metastatic disease, and lymphoma. The metastases in these nodes come from thyroid, upper esophagus, lungs, and breasts. The left supraclavicular lymph nodes may also be enlarged in carcinoma of stomach and testes.

Cystic hygroma

The patient is usually an infant or a child who has a painless and slow-growing swelling in the neck since birth. It is usually situated in the lower part of posterior triangle of neck (Figs 30.15 and 30.16). It can occur in upper neck, axilla, pectoral region, or even groin. It is smooth or lobulated, soft, cystic, and brilliantly transilluminant.

Cervical rib

It is characterized by a bony hard, fixed lump in the lower part of the neck posteriorly.

Cervical rib may be associated with neurovascular pressure symptoms in the upper extremity, that is, pain, numbness, and ulceration. The radial pulse may be weak or absent.

Subclavian artery aneurysm

It presents as a smooth, tense, and pulsatile swelling in the supraclavicular fossa. It has expansile pulsation and bruit. The lesion can be seen by ultrasonography, CT scan, or MRI.

Pancoast's tumor

It is a carcinoma of apex of lung which causes erosion of neck of first rib.

- Clinical features: The patient is usually an elderly male, a chronic smoker who presents with cough maybe with hemoptysis, weight loss, and pain. It may present with tingling, numbness, and paresthesia in the distribution of ulnar nerve (C8T1). There is a lump in lower neck deep to clavicle which is irregular, hard, ill-defined, and fixed.
- It may be associated with Horner's syndrome due to paralysis of cervical sympathetic caused by cancerous infiltration. It is characterized by ipsilateral miosis (small pupil), anhidrosis (absence of sweating in the affected area), ptosis (dropped upper eyelid), and enophthalmos (regression of eyeball).

Lung hernia (pneumatocele)

It is characterized by an intermittent, soft, and resonant swelling at the root of neck. It comes out or becomes more prominent on coughing or blowing with pinched nose, and reduces by itself or on pressing.

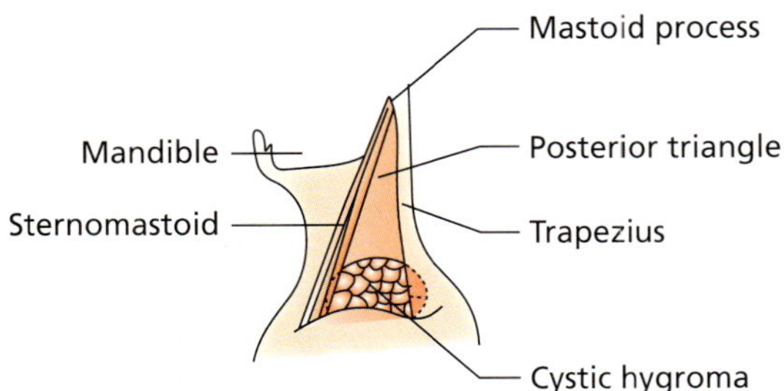

Figure 30.15 Cystic hygroma of lower part of posterior triangle of neck.

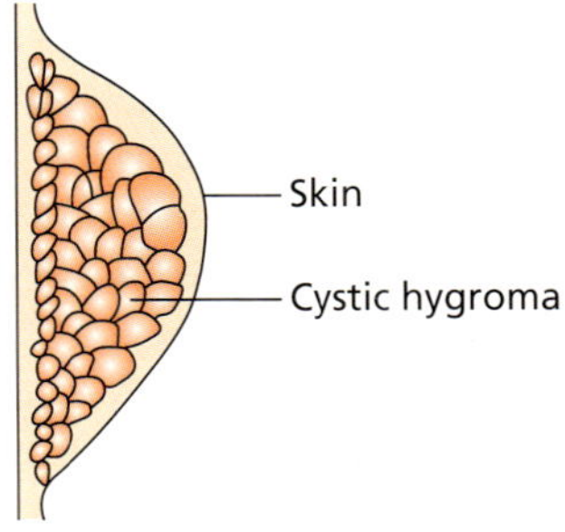

Figure 30.16 Cystic hygroma.

6. SWELLINGS OF NAPE OF NECK

Enlarged suboccipital lymph nodes

Enlarged lymph nodes may be present below the occipital protuberance. They may be enlarged due to scalp infection, secondary syphilis, tuberculosis, and metastatic disease.

Carbuncle

The patient is usually a middle-aged diabetic who presents with a diffuse swelling of the nape of neck of acute onset. It has signs of acute inflammation (red hot tender swelling). It discharges pus from many openings on its surface giving it a sieve-like appearance.

Lipoma

The nape of the neck is a common site of occurrence of a lipoma. It is characterized by a painless, slow-growing swelling of insidious onset which is smooth or lobulated and soft, and has an edge that slips under the finger.

Occipitocervical meningocele

The patient is a child who presents with a swelling in the posterior midline of the neck since birth. It is soft, cystic, globular, and transilluminant (Fig. 30.17). It may be associated with neurological deficit.

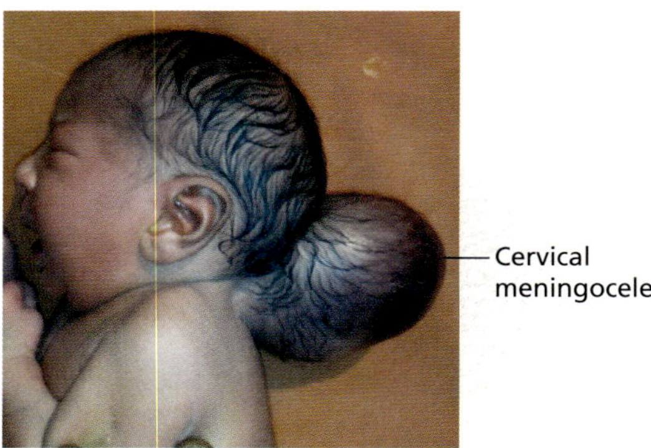

Figure 30.17 Cervical meningocele. (Courtesy: Professor J.D. Rawat)

7. MANAGEMENT OF SWELLINGS OF THE NECK

Investigations

- **Blood studies**: It is examined for hemoglobin, counts, and erythrocyte sedimentation rate (ESR). In acute abscess there is polymorphonuclear leukocytosis and in tuberculous lymphadenitis there is lymphocytosis and elevated ESR. In a thyroid swelling, thyroid hormones and calcitonin are measured. In a toxic goiter and medullary carcinoma, they are elevated, respectively.
- **Radiography of the neck**: It helps in the diagnosis of laryngocele (localized air shadow), erosion of first rib in Pancoast's tumor, and pharyngeal pouch (barium swallow).
- **Ultrasonography**: It helps in the diagnosis of most of the cystic swellings including carotid artery aneurysm.
- **CT scan and MRI**: It may be done to see the further details of various swellings.
- **Others**: In branchial cyst the aspirate has cholesterol crystals. In actinomycosis the discharge is examined which shows ray fungus.

Principles of treatment

The principles of treatment of swellings of neck are described as follows:

- The basic treatment is removal of the cause, but if the cause is not known, most of the swellings are treated with excision.

- Swellings due to infection are treated by appropriate antibiotic therapy. Tuberculous lesions are treated with a full course of antituberculous drugs [rifampicin, INH, pyrazinamide, and ethambutol for 2 months followed by first two drugs for 7 months; total course duration is 9 months]. Faciocervical actinomycosis is treated with prolonged penicillin therapy.
- The puberty goiter is treated with supplemental thyroid hormone.
- The benign tumors and other benign lesions, for example, cysts, are excised completely.
- The malignant tumors are usually treated with wide or radical excision. Chemotherapeutic and/or radiotherapeutic help may be required, for example, lymphoma of neck.

KEY POINTS

- Swellings of the neck are very common. They arise from normal tissues and structures of the neck.
- They may be nonspecific and specific. The nonspecific swellings include lymph node enlargement, sebaceous cyst, boil, acute abscess, cold abscess, and tumors such as papilloma, lipoma, neurofibroma, and hemangioma. They can occur anywhere in the neck.
- The site is the most important point in making the diagnosis of specific swellings. Depending on the site of occurrence, the swelling can be anterior midline, upper lateral neck, middle lateral neck, lower lateral neck, and nape of neck.
- The anterior midline swellings include enlarged anterior midline lymph nodes, Ludwig's angina, sublingual inframylohyoid and suprasternal dermoid, thyroglossal cyst, subhyoid bursa, and solitary nodule of isthmus of thyroid.
- The upper lateral neck swellings include enlarged level I lymph nodes, periauricular dermoid, swellings of cervical part of parotid and submandibular salivary glands, branchial cyst, plunging ranula, and faciocervical actinomycosis.
- The middle lateral neck swellings include enlarged level II lymph nodes, swellings of lateral lobe of thyroid, carotid artery aneurysm, pharyngeal pouch, laryngocele, carotid body tumor, and sternomastoid tumor.
- The lower lateral neck swellings include enlarged level III lymph nodes, cystic hygroma, cervical rib, subclavian artery aneurysm, Pancoast's tumor lung, and hernia (pneumatocele).
- The swellings of nape of neck include enlarged suboccipital lymph nodes, carbuncle, lipoma, and occipitocervical meningocele.
- The neck swellings may be solid or cystic on palpation. Sebaceous cyst and a cold abscess can occur anywhere in the neck. The cystic swellings of anterior midline of neck from above downwards include sublingual inframylohyoid dermoid, thyroglossal cyst, cyst of isthmus of thyroid, and suprasternal dermoid.
- The cystic swellings of the lateral neck include periauricular dermoid, branchial cyst, cervical extension of plunging ranula, laryngocele, pharyngeal pouch, cyst of lateral lobe of thyroid, cystic hygroma, and lung hernia.
- The cystic swellings of the posterior midline of neck include occipitocervical meningocele which is a developmental defect seen in neonates.
- The cystic swellings may be opaque or translucent. The anterior midline translucent swellings include thyroglossal cyst, subhyoid bursal cyst, and cyst isthmus of thyroid.
- The lateral translucent swellings include cervical part of plunging ranula, laryngocele, cyst of lateral lobe of thyroid, and cystic hygroma which is brilliantly transilluminant. The branchial cyst and laryngocele may be opaque.
- The solid swellings are diagnosed by their site, consistency (soft in benign and hard in malignant), and shape (regular in benign and irregular in malignant).
- The main investigations are needle aspiration (including FNAC), biopsy, and imaging.
- The inflammatory swellings are treated with antibiotics and drainage or excision. The cysts and benign tumors are completely excised, and malignant tumors are treated with a combination of wide excision, radiotherapy, and chemotherapy.

SELF-ASSESSMENT

Long answer questions

1. Discuss the differential diagnosis and treatment of anterior midline swellings of neck.
2. Enumerate the cystic swellings of neck. Describe their differential diagnosis and treatment.

Short answer questions

1. Collar-stud abscess
2. Cystic swellings of the neck
3. Plunging ranula
4. Cystic hygroma
5. Branchial cyst
6. Dermoid cyst

Multiple choice questions

1. A middle-aged person has a painless, slow-growing swelling on the side of neck for 5 years. It is hemispherical and smooth, and has a dark spot on the top in the center. What is the diagnosis?
   (a) Lipoma
   (b) Cold abscess
   (c) Cystic hygroma
   (d) Sebaceous cyst
2. Double-chin appearance is a sign of
   (a) Branchial cyst
   (b) Sublingual inframylohyoid dermoid
   (c) Thyroglossal cyst
   (d) Cold abscess
3. A young girl of 14 years presents with a swelling in the neck in upper midline for 6 years. It is cystic and moves up with protrusion of tongue. What is it?
   (a) Sublingual dermoid
   (b) Thyroglossal cyst
   (c) Cyst of isthmus of thyroid
   (d) Cold abscess
4. A 58-year-old female has an intermittent swelling of right submandibular salivary gland which appears during meals. The swelling is smooth, mildly tender, and bimanually palpable. A hard nodule is palpable in floor of mouth of the same side. What is the diagnosis?
   (a) Distended submandibular salivary gland due to stone in the Wharton's duct
   (b) Tuberculosis of submandibular lymph nodes
   (c) Branchial cyst
   (d) Plunging ranula
5. A 55-year-old male complains of noises in the neck during eating and regurgitation of food. A swelling appears nearly in the middle of neck on the left side behind sternomastoid during meals. It empties on pressure with a gurgle. What is the diagnosis?
   (a) Pharyngeal pouch
   (b) Carotid body tumor
   (c) Laryngocele
   (d) Cold abscess
6. A 51-year-old male, a professional flute player, comes with a swelling in the upper neck on one side. It appears when the patient plays the flute and disappears after the playing is stopped with repeated coughing and profuse expectoration. The swelling is soft and compressible and partly dull and partly resonant. What is the diagnosis?
   (a) Laryngocele
   (b) Pharyngeal pouch
   (c) Thyroglossal cyst
   (d) Branchial cyst
7. A neonate is brought with a swelling in the middle of neck on one side of midline. It is firm, smooth, ovoid, and fixed to the sternomastoid muscle. What is the diagnosis?
   (a) Carotid body tumor
   (b) Branchial cyst
   (c) Sternomastoid tumor
   (d) Carotid artery aneurysm
8. A neonate is brought with a lower lateral neck swelling which is smooth, nontender, cystic, and transilluminant. What is the nature of lesion?
   (a) Branchial cyst
   (b) Cyst of lateral lobe of thyroid
   (c) Dermoid cyst
   (d) Cystic hygroma

(CONTD...)

SELF-ASSESSMENT (...CONTD)

9. The patient is a middle-aged woman having radiating pain in the upper arm with signs of ischemia in the index finger. There is a fixed bony mass at the root of neck posteriorly. What is the diagnosis?
   (a) Cervical rib
   (b) Subclavian aneurysm
   (c) Lung hernia
   (d) Cystic hygroma

10. A middle-aged male diabetic presents with a painful swelling of nape of neck. It is red, hot, and tender and discharging pus from many openings. What is the diagnosis?
   (a) Lipoma of neck
   (b) Cellulitis
   (c) Tuberculous sinuses
   (d) Carbuncle

11. A middle-aged person has a painless, slow-growing, soft swelling at the nape of neck of long duration. It has an edge that slips under the finger. What is the nature of the lesion?
   (a) Occipitocervical meningocele
   (b) Carbuncle
   (c) Lipoma
   (d) Lymphangioma

Answers

1. (d) 2. (b) 3. (b) 4. (a) 5. (a) 6. (a) 7. (c) 8. (d) 9. (a) 10. (d) 11. (c)

Anesthesia

31

Introduction

Anesthesia means absence of sensation which is very important for painless performance of any operation. It is of two types: general anesthesia and local anesthesia. Definitions of common terminologies used in anesthesia are given in Box 31.1.

Box 31.1 Definitions of common terminologies in anesthesia

- **Anesthesia**: Loss of feeling or sensation
- **General anesthesia**: A state of unconsciousness associated with absence of pain sensation all over the body, and greater or lesser degree of muscular relaxation
- **Local anesthesia**: Loss of feeling or sensation confined to one part of the body
- **Anxiolysis**: Decrease of anxiety without production of excessive drowsiness
- **Conscious sedation**: Process of calming down, maintaining consciousness
- **Neuroleptanalgesia**: A state of quiescence, altered awareness, and analgesia produced by the use of a combination of a narcotic analgesic and a neuroleptic agent
- **Neuroleptanesthesia**: A state of neuroleptanalgesia and unconsciousness produced by combined use of a narcotic analgesic and a neuroleptic agent, together with the inhalation of nitrous oxide and oxygen

1. GENERAL ANESTHESIA

General anesthesia is characterized by loss of consciousness and all types of sensations and complete muscular relaxation.

Indications of general anesthesia

General anesthesia is indicated in all operations provided the patient is fit for it, but in minor procedures requiring limited invasion local anesthesia is best.

Contraindications of general anesthesia

They include advanced cardiac disease, pulmonary cripples, and uncontrolled hypertension, diabetes mellitus, and hyperthyroidism.

Stages of anesthesia

Arthur Ernest Guedel described four stages of anesthesia when only diethyl ether was used to give anesthesia which is now very much modified. The modern anesthesia has the following stages: **inadequate anesthesia, surgical anesthesia, and deep anesthesia**. The depth of anesthesia is mainly judged by respiration and pupils.

Induction agents

These drugs are used to initiate anesthesia which is subsequently maintained by the use of one or more anesthetic agents. The salient features of common induction agents are described in the subsequent text.

Sodium Thiopental

- It is the oldest drug of this series which causes rapid induction.
- Sodium thiopental is an ultra-short-acting barbiturate which in its usual doses is associated with rapid induction followed by rapid emergence because of redistribution of the agent from brain to peripheral tissues. It reduces the metabolic rate and lowers the intracranial pressure, hence useful in neuro-surgical operations.
- Dose: It is 2–5 mg/kg.
- Disadvantages: It is a poor analgesic and can cause laryngeal spasm. Accidental intra-arterial injection causes vasospasm and gangrene.

Ketamine

- It produces a dissociative state of anesthesia, emergence delirium, and bad dreams.
- Dose: It is 1–2 mg/kg.
- Advantage: It has profound analgesic activity, hence an ideal choice for field anesthesia.
- Disadvantages: It increases blood pressure, heart rate, and intracranial pressure, decreases bronchomotor tone, and is associated with emergence delirium.

Propofol

- It is a widely used short-acting induction agent.
- Dose: It is 1–2 mg/kg.
- Advantages: It is associated with smooth nausea-free emergence. It is an excellent bron-chodilator. It is used for ambulatory surgery, and also for total intravenous anesthesia by continuous infusion. It has good hemody-namic stability and a short duration of action.
- Disadvantage: It causes burning sensation on injection.

Etomidate

- **Dose**: It is 0.3 mg/kg.
- **Advantage**: It is an imidazole compound which produces minimum hemodynamic

changes, hence a good choice in hypovolemia and congestive heart failure.
- **Disadvantages**: Its disadvantages include burning pain on injection, abnormal muscular movements (myoclonus), and adrenocortical suppression when given as a prolonged infusion.

Midazolam

- It is sometimes used for induction.
- Dose: It is 0.15–0.3 mg/kg.
- Advantages: It has a shorter duration of action than diazepam. It causes minimal cardiovascular side effects.
- Disadvantages: Its side effects include light-headedness, lassitude, increased reaction time, motor incoordination, confusion, and anterograde amnesia.

The salient features of common induction agents are described in Table 31.1.

Muscle relaxants

These drugs are used to produce muscular relaxation with the advantage that the operation can be performed under relatively lighter anesthesia (but full pain relief). Also the endotracheal intubation can be done easily. Their main disadvantage is inadequate respiration due to relaxation of muscles of respiration.

Types

There are two types of neuromuscular blockers available: depolarizing (noncompetitive) and nondepolarizing (competitive).

Depolarizing agent—succinylcholine (Scoline)

It is the only depolarizing agent still in clinical use because of rapid onset and short duration of action (5 minutes). It causes muscular fibrillation before paralysis. Its dose is 70–75 mg. The side effects include bradycardia, hyperkalemia, and malignant hyperthermia in susceptible patients. It is not antagonized by neostigmine and it need not be antagonized because of its short duration of action.

Nondepolarizing agents

Pancuronium is used when succinylcholine is contraindicated and when prolonged relaxation is required. Their side effects are often related to vagolysis or release of histamine.

The duration of action and dose of various muscle relaxants are described in Table 31.2.

Table 31.1 Salient features of common induction agents

Agent	Dose (mg/kg)	Comments
Sodium thiopental	2–5	• Commonly used induction agent • No analgesic property • Can cause severe hypotension
Ketamine	1–2	• Potent analgesic • Good bronchodilator • Produces dissociative anesthesia
Propofol	1–2	• Replacing sodium pentothal • Can be used for induction in outpatients • Good bronchodilator • Causes burning sensation on injection
Etomidate	0.1–0.3	• Used for induction in patients in shock • Spontaneous movements during induction • Causes burning sensation on injection
Midazolam	0.15–0.3	• Induction in patients with cardiac contractile dysfunction • Potent amnesia

Table 31.2 Duration of action and dosage of various muscle relaxants

Muscle relaxant	Duration of action (minutes)	Dose (mg/kg)
Depolarizing agent		
Suxamethonium (Scoline)	5–10	1–2
Nondepolarizing agents		
Pancuronium (Pavulon)	20–40	0.08–0.12
Vecuronium	10–20	0.1–0.2
Cisatracurium	20–40	0.15–0.2
Mivacurium	Short	0.15–0.2
Rocuronium	30–60	0.6–1.0

Side Effects of Muscle Relaxants

The side effects of muscle relaxants are described in Table 31.3.

Inhalational anesthetic agents

Diethyl Ether

- **Advantages**: It is a potent and safe anesthetic agent which is very simple to administer. It has very little cardiac toxicity, and has an irritant effect on upper respiratory tract, hence unpleasant to inhale.
- **Disadvantages**: It is highly inflammable and can cause explosion. Hence, it is now less commonly used.

Nitrous Oxide

- **Advantages**: It is a weak anesthetic but good analgesic. It influences respiration and hemodynamics minimally, and has low solubility in blood. It is often combined with one of the potent volatile agents to permit a lower dose of the latter. It reduces the side effects and cost and facilitates rapid induction and emergence.
- **Disadvantage**: It diffuses into closed gas spaces faster than nitrogen; hence, it is contraindicated in pneumothorax and small bowel obstruction.

Halothane (Fluothane)

It is a noninflammable liquid having a pleasant odor.

- **Advantages**: It does not irritate the respiratory tract. It anesthetizes rapidly and smoothly. The recovery is also rapid.
- **Disadvantages**: It causes some fall of blood pressure, hepatotoxicity, and respiratory depression. It is administered with N_2O and oxygen with great care as it sensitizes the myocardium to catecholamines.

Malignant hyperthermia

It is a rapid rise of body temperature and massive increase in the oxygen consumption

Table 31.3 Side effects of muscle relaxants

Muscle relaxant	Side effects
Scoline	Muscle pains, hyperkalemia, arrhythmia, prolonged action in patients with deficiency of pseudocholinesterase
Pancuronium	Tachycardia, hypertension; should be avoided in renal failure
Vecuronium	Bradycardia; should be avoided in renal failure
Cisatracurium	Histamine release
Rocuronium	Rapid onset of block

and production of carbon dioxide following the induction of anesthesia with halothane or any of the halogenated inhalational anesthetic agents. It may result in death unless the anesthetic is discontinued and treatment with dantrolene is begun promptly.

Enflurane

It is pleasant and nonirritating to inhale. Enflurane produces less cardiac sensitization to catecholamines. It is associated with mild renal dysfunction. It is relatively contraindicated in seizure disorder.

Isoflurane

It has replaced halothane and is the most commonly used potent inhalational anesthetic.

- **Advantages**: It reduces the cardiac output but increases the heart rate. It causes less sensitization of myocardium to the arrhythmogenic effects of catecholamines. It enhances coronary perfusion.
- **Disadvantages**: It has a very pungent odor like ether; hence, it is not used for inhalational induction, but used for maintenance of anesthesia.

Desflurane

It is rapidly taken up and eliminated. Desflurane is associated with tachycardia and hypertension if the concentration is increased too rapidly. Desflurane, enflurane, and isoflurane produce more carbon monoxide than halothane or sevoflurane. Hence, one must be careful.

Sevoflurane

It is pleasant to inhale, hence can be used in children for induction. Sevoflurane is good for outpatient surgery. Its relatively low solubility facilitates rapid induction and emergence.

The important features of inhalational anesthetic agents are described in Table 31.4.

Technique/steps of general anesthesia

Preoperative Evaluation and Preparation

A surgical patient may have a concurrent medical illness, for example, hypertension, coronary insufficiency, diabetes mellitus, and pulmonary problems. Hence, the patient should be carefully interrogated, examined, investigated, and the illness controlled and an informed consent is taken before giving anesthesia. Surgery, in general, is performed on empty stomach.

Premedication

It is given half an hour or so before anesthesia to produce sedation, reduce fear and anxiety, and reduce airway secretions. The commonly used drugs include a narcotic (e.g., pethidine), an antihistamine (e.g., promethazine), and an antisecretory agent (e.g., atropine).

Table 31.4 Salient features of inhalational anesthetic agents

Anesthetic agent	Potency	Induction and emergence	Induction suitability
Nitrous oxide	Weak	Fast	Insufficient
Diethyl ether	Potent	Very slow	Suitable
Halothane	Potent	Medium	Suitable
Enflurane	Potent	Medium	Not suitable
Isoflurane	Potent	Medium	Not suitable
Desflurane	Potent	Rapid	Not suitable
Sevoflurane	Potent	Rapid	Suitable

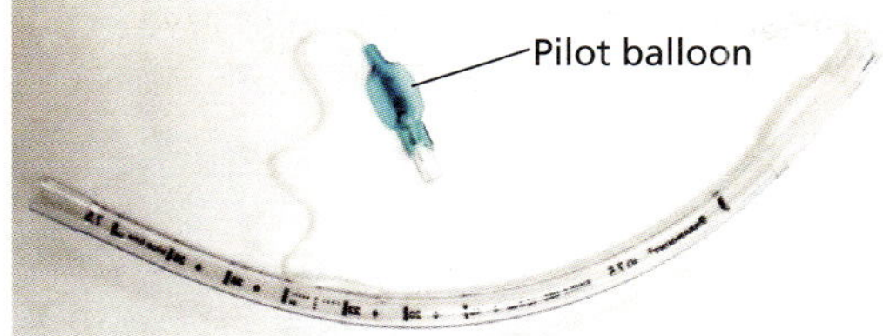

Figure 31.1 Endotracheal tube.

Induction

The patient is made to lie on the operation table and given 100% oxygen for 2–3 minutes and the anesthesia is induced by giving propofol (or thiopentone sodium) intravenously slowly till the patient goes to sleep. It is the usual practice in older children and adults, but inhalation induction is commonly used in younger children.

Endotracheal Intubation

Now a muscle relaxant, for example, succinylcholine (1–2 mg/kg), is given intravenously. As soon as the muscles start relaxing, the breathing is assisted by slowly squeezing the bag of anesthesia machine to give 100% oxygen.

Now a cuffed endotracheal tube is passed into trachea per orally with the help of a laryngoscope (Figs 31.1–31.3) and Magill's forceps (Fig. 31.4) and the cuff is inflated. The nasal route is used less commonly, especially when space in the mouth is required for doing intraoral surgery. Intubation is easy in class I and II Mallampati score and difficult in class III and IV score. The Mallampati score is described in Box 31.2.

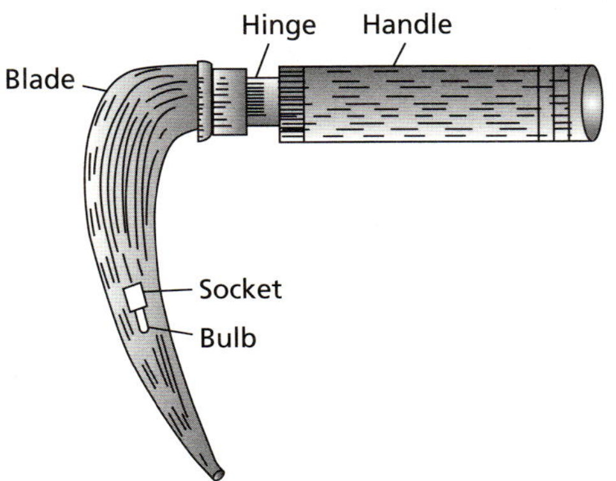

Figure 31.2 Laryngoscope with curved blade used for endotracheal intubation.

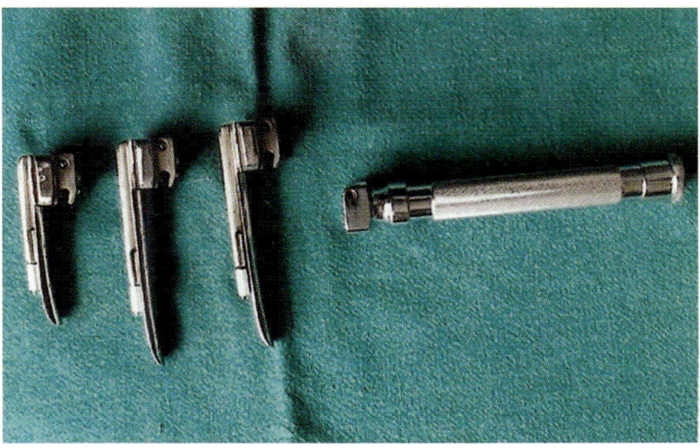

Figure 31.3 Laryngoscope with straight blades.

Box 31.2 Mallampati score to predict ease of endotracheal intubation

Class I: Faucial pillars, soft palate, and uvula are seen **Class II**: Faucial pillars and soft palate seen	Easy intubation
Class III: Only soft palate seen **Class IV**: Up to hard palate seen and not beyond	Difficult intubation

Full Anesthesia and Maintenance

The endotracheal tube is connected to anesthesia machine (Figs 31.5 and 31.6) and manual ventilation is given and continued till the spontaneous respiration returns. Now the patient is fully anesthetized and maintained on ether or isoflurane, N_2O, and O_2 till the operation is completed. The concentration of anesthetic agents is varied depending on the depth of anesthesia required.

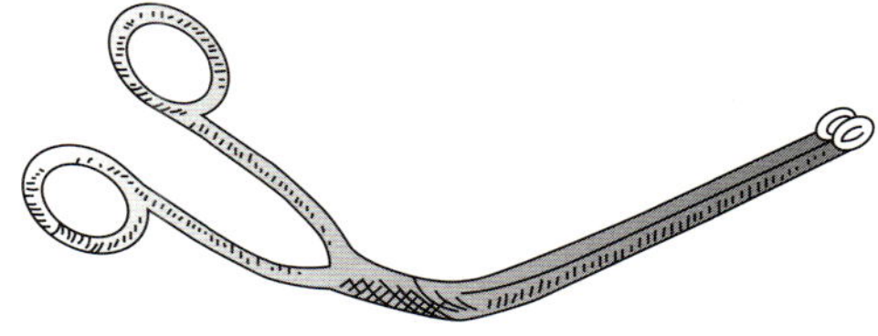

Figure 31.4 Magill's forceps for directing the endotracheal tube into trachea.

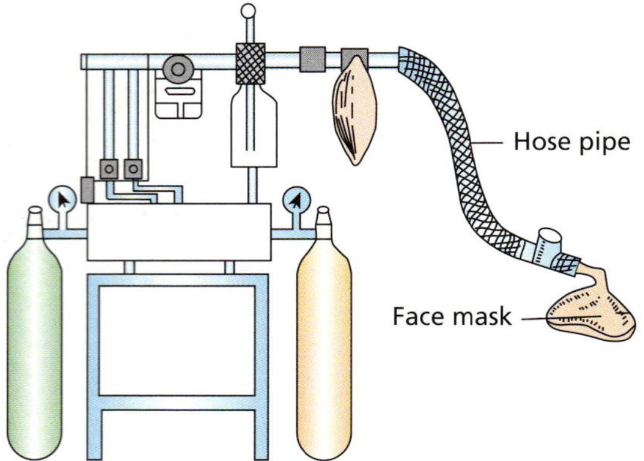

Figure 31.5 Schematic diagram of general anesthesia machine.

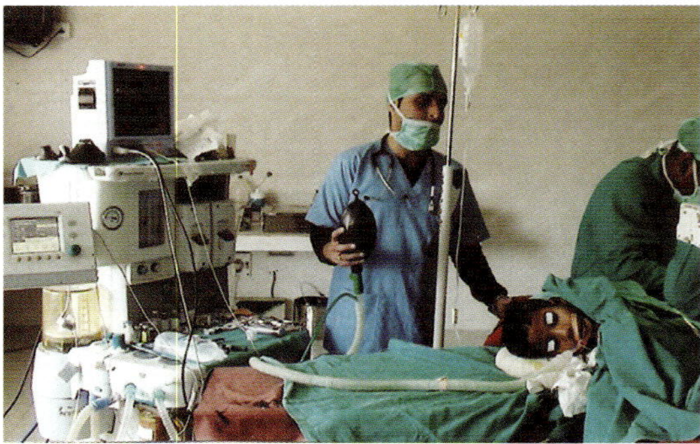

Figure 31.6 General anesthesia in progress.

Termination and Extubation

At the end of operation, the anesthetic agents are stopped, muscle relaxation is reversed, and the patient is ventilated with 100% oxygen so that most of the anesthetic drugs are eliminated. Now the extubation is done, the throat cleared, and the patient sent to recovery room.

Reversal Agents

Neostigmine 2.5 mg has antagonizing effect on depolarizing muscle relaxants. It is commonly used with atropine 1.2 mg (or glycopyrrolate) to neutralize its cholinergic effect. Edrophonium and pyridostigmine are other reversal agents.

Monitoring

Continuous blood pressure, pulse rate, and electrocardiographic monitoring are done during the operation (and even after operation). Pulse oximetry gives information about O_2 saturation at tissue level. Its probe is put on the fingertip or ear lobule.

Complications of general anesthesia

- Airway obstruction
- Endotracheal tube going inadvertently in esophagus
- Cardiovascular complications including arrhythmias, hypotension, hypertension, and cardiac arrest
- Postanesthetic sickness including vomiting and retching
- Postoperative hypoxemia
- Pulmonary atelectasis, pneumonitis
- Mendelson's syndrome
- Malignant hyperthermia

General anesthesia in dental practice

Most of the dental work is done under local anesthesia, but general anesthesia is required to do it in children, and in very anxious patients and for doing major work on the jaws, for example, reduction and fixation of a fracture.

Indications of General Anesthesia in Dental Practice

- Young children 3–8 years of age, especially when multiple extractions in different quadrants of the jaw are required
- Extensive conservative dentistry combined with extraction
- Uncooperative anxious patients
- Acute infective conditions of mouth
- Allergy to local anesthetics but true allergy to local anesthetics is rare (whatever symptoms appear, they may be of vasovagal fainting, or

may be flushing and palpitation due to adrenaline mixed in the local anesthetic)

Problems of General Anesthesia During Orodental Surgery

- Sharing of airway between the dentist and the surgeon, hence the airway problem may crop up during the procedure, for example, aspiration of broken teeth, crowns, and portions of fillings.
- Blood and oropharyngeal secretions may enter the airway. With them, infection may also enter. Hence, packing the airway around the endotracheal tube is very important.
- Most of the work is done in sitting or semisitting position; hence, the anesthesia has to be modified accordingly.
- Pollution of operating room environment may occur with anesthetic gases.
- Endotracheal intubation may be difficult in maxillofacial injuries.
- Nasal intubation is done if full oral cavity is required for surgical work.

Day-Care Surgery

Most of the patients after orodental surgery under general anesthesia can be sent home sometime after operation the same day because of quick and complete recovery and safety of modern anesthesia. The criteria for day-care surgery are described in Box 31.3.

Box 31.3 Criteria for day-care surgery

- The patient must be healthy and fit, and free from cardiorespiratory diseases satisfying ASA categories I and II
- The surgical procedure must not last for more than 1 hour
- There should be no significant risk of complications such as bleeding and vomiting
- The recovery from anesthesia should be rapid and complete
- The patient must be accompanied back home by a responsible adult who will look after the patient for the next 24 hours and will bring back the patient to the hospital if there is a problem

Contribution of dental sciences/dentists in the development of anesthesia

- In 1842, an American medical student, William Clark, administered ether for painless dental extraction.
- Horace Wells, a dentist, used nitrous oxide to extract teeth painlessly in 1844.
- William Mortan, a dentist, administered ether on October 16, 1846, to a young man, when John Collins Warren removed a vascular malformation from the neck at Massachusetts general hospital.

2. LOCAL ANESTHESIA

Introduction

In this anesthesia the part to be operated upon is made numb for painless operation with the use of local anesthetic agents.

Methods of local anesthetic delivery

Surface Anesthesia

In this method, the body surface, for example, oral cavity, is anesthetized by local spray or application of jelly, cream, or ointment of the anesthetic agent, such as cocaine 1%, lignocaine 2–5%, or prilocaine 4%.

Infiltration Anesthesia

It is produced by injecting the anesthetic agent in the proposed line of incision. The point of needle is kept moving as the anesthetic is being injected to minimize the possibility of inadvertent intravenous injection. The drugs used include lignocaine 1–2%, prilocaine 0.25–0.5%, and Marcaine.

Nerve Block

In this method the nerve or nerves supplying sensory twigs to the operating field is/are blocked by local injection of the anesthetic agent. It requires a lot of anatomical accuracy as the nerve concerned must be located exactly. The examples of this anesthesia are brachial plexus block for upper limb operations, and inferior dental and lingual nerve block for operations on mandibular molars.

Field Block

In this method a barrage of local anesthetic is laid across the path of nerves supplying the operating field, for example, field block for doing an inguinal hernia repair.

Indications of local anesthesia

- For taking biopsy from superficial lesions and doing needle biopsy from deep lesions
- For doing all types of dental work except in children and very anxious patients
- For excising small superficial lesions, for example, lipoma and sebaceous cyst

Contraindications of local anesthesia

The main contraindication is hypersensitivity to local anesthetic drugs.

Mechanism of action

The local anesthetics bind to a specific receptor site within the pore of Na^+ channels and prevent the generation and conduction of nerve impulse.

Use of a vasoconstrictor

Sometimes adrenaline is mixed with a local anesthetic. It has two advantages:

1. The drug remains at the local site for a longer period, prolonging the effect of anesthesia.
2. The vasoconstricting effect reduces intraoperative bleeding.

Local anesthetic agents

- **Lidocaine**: It produces faster, more intense, longer-lasting, and more extensive local anesthesia than procaine. Hence, it is widely used.
- **Mepivacaine**: Its action is similar to lidocaine with duration 20% longer than that of lidocaine. It is not effective as a topical anesthetic and toxic to a neonate.
- **Bupivacaine**: It is a potent local anesthetic agent. Its long duration of action and quality to provide more sensory than motor block has made it popular for providing prolonged analgesia. It is cardiotoxic.
- **Ropivacaine**: It is slightly less potent than bupivacaine, but more motor sparing than bupivacaine. Its duration of action is similar to that of bupivacaine.

The salient features of common local anesthetic agents are described in Table 31.5.

Complications of local anesthesia

The complications of local anesthetics depend on the site of injection and the speed of absorption. Inadvertent intravascular injection produces toxicity with much smaller doses. The symptoms

Table 31.5 Salient features of local anesthetic agents

Local anesthetic	Onset of anesthesia (minutes)	Duration of anesthesia (minutes)	Maximal dose (mg/kg)
Lidocaine	10–20	60–180	3
Mepivacaine	10–20	60–180	5
Bupivacaine	15–30	180–360	2
Ropivacaine	15–30	180–360	3

of toxicity involve the central nervous system and the cardiovascular system. The complications of local anesthetic agents are described in Box 31.4.

Fainting on Dental Chair

Sometimes the fear and anxiety combined with orodental work may produce significant autonomic nervous system overactivity leading to sweating and fainting due to reflex vasodilatation, decreased venous return, fall in cardiac output, and severe hypotension. As soon as this happens, the patient is made to lie down and prevented from falling. The head end of the dental chair is lowered to improve cerebral circulation and the patient given supportive treatment including dexamethasone and oxygen.

Box 31.4 Complications of local anesthesia

- Local
  - Infection
  - Hematoma formation
- Systemic usually due to overdose or accidental intravenous injection
  - *Cardiovascular*: Cardiac arrhythmia, cardiac arrest
  - *Neurological*: Depressed consciousness, disorientation, slurring of speech, convulsions
  - *Others*: Metallic taste, tinnitus, visual disturbances

KEY POINTS

- Anesthesia means absence of sensation which is very important for painless performance of any operation. It is of two types: general and local.
- General anesthesia is characterized by loss of consciousness and all types of sensations and complete muscular relaxation. It has following stages: inadequate anesthesia, surgical anesthesia, and deep anesthesia.
- Induction agents are used to initiate anesthesia which is subsequently maintained by one or more anesthetic agents. Examples include sodium thiopental, ketamine, propofol, etomidate, and midazolam.
- Sodium thiopental is an ultra-short-acting barbiturate which in its usual doses is associated with rapid emergence. But it is a poor analgesic and can cause respiratory depression and laryngeal spasm.
- Propofol is a widely used short-acting induction agent associated with smooth nausea-free emergence. It is an excellent bronchodilator and used for ambulatory surgery, and also for total intravenous anesthesia.
- Muscle relaxants are used to produce muscular relaxation with the advantage that the operation can be performed under relatively lighter anesthesia (but with full pain relief) and easy endotracheal intubation. Their main disadvantage is inadequate respiration due to relaxation of muscles of respiration.
- Succinylcholine (Scoline) is the only depolarizing muscle relaxant still in clinical use because of rapid onset and short duration of action (5 minutes). Pancuronium is used when succinylcholine is contraindicated and when prolonged relaxation is required.
- Inhalational anesthetics include diethyl ether, nitrous oxide, halothane, enflurane, isoflurane, desflurane, and sevoflurane.
- Diethyl ether is a potent and safe anesthetic agent with little cardiac toxicity but the main

(CONTD...)

KEY POINTS (...CONTD)

disadvantage is that it is highly inflammable and can cause explosion. Hence, it is now less commonly used.

- Nitrous oxide is a weak anesthetic but a good analgesic. It is often combined with one of the potent volatile agents to permit a lower dose of the latter.
- Halothane is noninflammable, does not irritate the respiratory tract, anesthetizes rapidly and smoothly with rapid recovery. But when it is administered with N_2O and oxygen, it may sensitize the myocardium to catecholamines. Hepatotoxicity is also a salient disadvantage.
- Isoflurane has replaced halothane and is the most commonly used potent inhalational anesthetic. It reduces the cardiac output but increases the heart rate and enhances coronary perfusion. It causes less sensitization of myocardium to the arrhythmogenic effects of catecholamines.
- Premedication is given half an hour or so before anesthesia to produce sedation, reduce fear and anxiety, and reduce airway secretions. The commonly used drugs include a narcotic (e.g., pethidine), an antihistamine (e.g., promethazine), and an antisecretory agent (e.g., atropine).
- In dental practice, general anesthesia is indicated in young patients who need multiple extractions and combined procedures, uncooperative and anxious patients, and patients having allergy to local anesthetics.
- Methods of local anesthetic delivery include surface anesthesia, infiltration anesthesia, nerve blocks, and field blocks.
- The common local anesthetic agents are lidocaine, mepivacaine, bupivacaine, and ropivacaine. Sometimes adrenaline (vasoconstrictor) is mixed with the local anesthetic for prolonging the duration of local anesthesia and reducing the intraoperative bleeding.
- The toxicity of local anesthetics is rare and depends on the site of injection and the speed of absorption.

SELF-ASSESSMENT

Long answer questions

1. What is general anesthesia and what are its indications? Mention briefly about induction agents.
2. Describe the indications, methods of delivery, and complications of local anesthesia.

Short answer questions

3. Propofol
4. Muscle relaxants
5. Ether
6. Nitrous oxide
7. Isoflurane
8. Complications of local anesthesia

Multiple choice questions

1. Anesthesia means
   (a) Absence of touch
   (b) Absence of pain
   (c) Absence of heat and vibration sense
   (d) Absence of all sensations
2. Which of the following is not used as an induction agent?
   (a) Thiopentone sodium
   (b) Ketamine
   (c) Scoline
   (d) Etomidate
3. All of the following statements are true about thiopentone sodium, except
   (a) It is fast acting
   (b) It is associated with rapid emergence
   (c) It is a good analgesic
   (d) It can cause laryngeal spasm
4. All of the following statements are true about ketamine, except
   (a) It produces dissociate state of anesthesia
   (b) It increases blood pressure and heart rate
   (c) It causes emergent delirium
   (d) It has poor analgesic activity

(CONTD...)

SELF-ASSESSMENT *(...CONTD)*

5. All of the following drugs are used as muscle relaxant for endotracheal intubation, except
   (a) Vecuronium
   (b) Diazepam
   (c) Scoline
   (d) Pancuronium (Pavulon)
6. All of the following statements are true about suxamethonium (Scoline), except
   (a) It is a short-acting muscle relaxant
   (b) It is given in the dose of 50–75 mg intravenously
   (c) It causes muscular fibrillation before paralysis
   (d) It is antagonized by neostigmine
7. Which of the following is not a quality of diethyl ether?
   (a) It is a potent and safe inhalation anesthetic agent
   (b) It has a very small cardiotoxicity
   (c) It is not inflammable
   (d) It irritates the upper respiratory tract, hence unpleasant to inhale
8. Which of the following facts is false about halothane?
   (a) It is a noninflammable liquid
   (b) It anesthetizes rapidly and smoothly
   (c) It irritates the respiratory tract
   (d) It is hepatotoxic
9. Which of the following facts is false about isoflurane?
   (a) It is a potent inhalational anesthetic
   (b) It reduces cardiac output but increases heart rate
   (c) It has a very pleasant odor
   (d) It enhances coronary circulation

Answers

1. (d) 2. (c) 3. (c) 4. (d) 5. (b) 6. (d) 7. (c) 8. (c) 9. (c)

Biopsy

32

Definition

Biopsy is the procedure of taking a small portion of tissue from a lesion for microscopic or histological examination. It is the most important investigation for making or confirming the diagnosis of a neoplastic lesion. Most of the biopsies are done under local anesthesia.

Indications of biopsy

Biopsy is indicated to make a diagnosis, if it is not made, or to confirm a clinical diagnosis.

Contraindications of biopsy

Biopsy is not done in bleeding disorders and a pleomorphic adenoma of parotid and testicular tumors.

Types of biopsy

Biopsy is of many types. In the four methods of biopsy described in the subsequent text, a small piece of tissue is taken for microscopic study to provide a tissue diagnosis. Hence, it is the most reliable and accurate method of diagnosis. It takes 3–7 days for the biopsy report to come. The types of biopsy and their indications are described in Table 32.1.

Excisional Biopsy

If the lesion is small, it is totally excised and the whole specimen is sent after putting it in a preserving/fixing solution for histopathological examination, for example, papilloma, solitary neurofibroma, and fibrous epulis (Fig. 32.1a). In a case of suspected lymphoma, one complete lymph node should be removed to study the architecture of the node.

Incisional Biopsy

It is the most common method of biopsy. It is usually done in a large lesion when a small piece is taken out (but sufficient for histopathology) usually from the junction of normal and abnormal tissues (Fig. 32.1b).

Needle Biopsy

In deep-seated lesions and organs (e.g., liver, kidney), a core of tissue can be taken with the help of a large-bore needle under local infiltration

Table 32.1 Types of biopsy and their indications

Types of biopsy	Indication
Excisional biopsy	• Small lesions such as papilloma, solitary neurofibroma, fibrous epulis • In a suspected lymphoma, one complete lymph node is excised to study the architecture
Incisional biopsy	Large lesion when a small piece of tissue is excised usually from the junction of normal and abnormal tissues
Needle biopsy	• Deep-seated lesions and organs such as liver • Performed under ultrasound or CT guidance
Endoscopic biopsy	Lesions situated in hollow organs, tubes, or body cavities, for example, carcinoma of esophagus during esophagoscopy and carcinoma of urinary bladder during cystoscopy
Exfoliative cytology	Examination of exfoliated cells in carcinoma of cervix, lung, and urinary bladder
FNAC	All swellings
Frozen section	Carcinoma of breast

FNAC, fine-needle aspiration cytology.

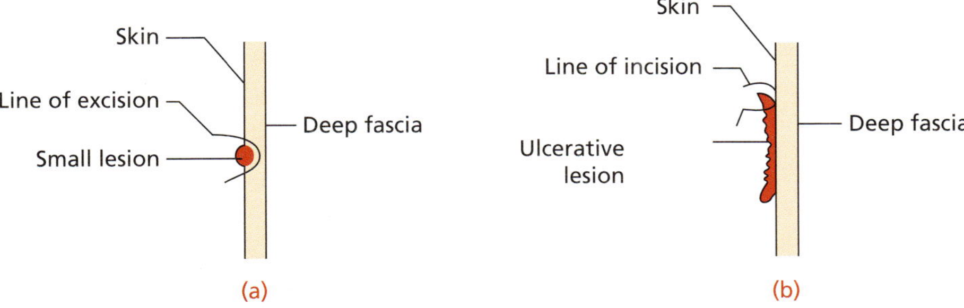

Figure 32.1 Biopsy: (a) excisional and (b) incisional.

anesthesia, for example, Vim-Silverman or Tru-cut needle (Fig. 32.2). For taking the tissue accurately from the lesion, this job is now mostly done under ultrasound or CT guidance (Fig. 32.3). It is a very common modern method of biopsy.

Punch Biopsy

It is a type of biopsy in which the tissue is obtained by punching the lesion with a forceps having sharp cutting tips.

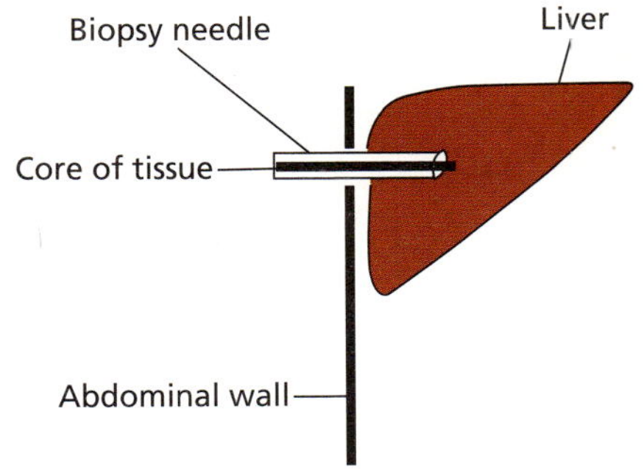

Figure 32.2 Needle biopsy.

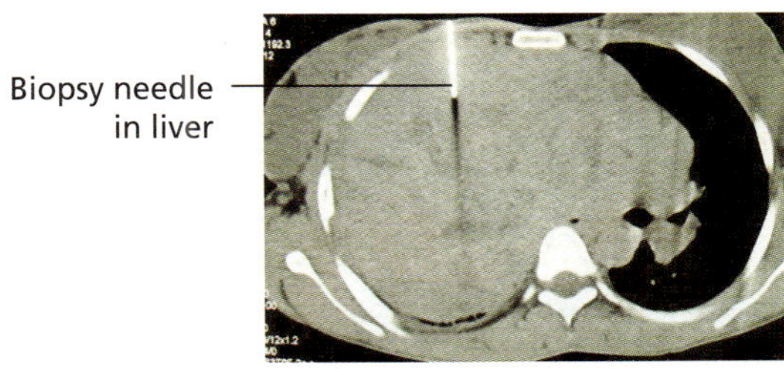

Figure 32.3 Percutaneous axial CT-guided needle biopsy of liver. The lesion in the liver is hepatocellular carcinoma.

Brush Biopsy

It is done by brushing the surface of an ulcerated lesion with a special brush to obtain small particles of tissue for histopathology/cytology. It is done commonly in a bronchogenic carcinoma and carcinoma of stomach.

Endoscopic Biopsy

The biopsy from the lesions situated in hollow organs, tubes, or body cavities can be done when the lesion is being visualized during endoscopy, for example, carcinoma of esophagus during esophagoscopy and carcinoma of urinary bladder during cystoscopy (Fig. 32.4). A special biopsy forceps is available for this purpose.

Rapid methods of diagnosis

To avoid delay in the treatment, rapid methods of diagnosis are being used more and more these days. There are many methods of rapid diagnosis.

Exfoliative Cytology

Principle From all the body surfaces including that of internal organs and body cavities, the surface cells are shed normally into the lumen or cavity from time to time (exfoliation) where they may mix with the contents, for example, in urine of urinary bladder. From the cancer surface too, this phenomenon of exfoliation is going on, probably at a rapid rate. In exfoliative cytology, these shed cells are examined.

Indications This method of diagnosis is employed for the diagnosis of carcinoma of cervix, lung, and urinary bladder.

Method The exfoliated cells may be examined by making a smear from the contents or secretion and stained by Papanicolaou method and examined for malignant cells microscopically. The rate of exfoliation can be increased by putting a proteolytic enzyme, for example, chymotrypsin into the lumen or cavity of that organ to be studied.

Results Depending on the presence or absence of cancer cells, the smear may be "positive" or "negative." A negative smear does not rule out malignancy (may be false-negative). A positive smear is diagnostic of cancer as false-positive is unknown.

Fine-Needle Aspiration Cytology (FNAC)

Indications It is indicated in all the lumps for making a cytological diagnosis except in follicular carcinoma of thyroid.

Method In this method the tissue fluid of the lesion is aspirated into a fine needle (no. 23 needle) attached to a syringe by making a number of passes into the lesion (Fig. 32.5). A smear is made from the aspirate of the needle and examined cytologically.

Advantages This method of rapid diagnosis has become very popular as it is convenient, rapid, and minimally invasive. It has an accuracy rate of 80–96%.

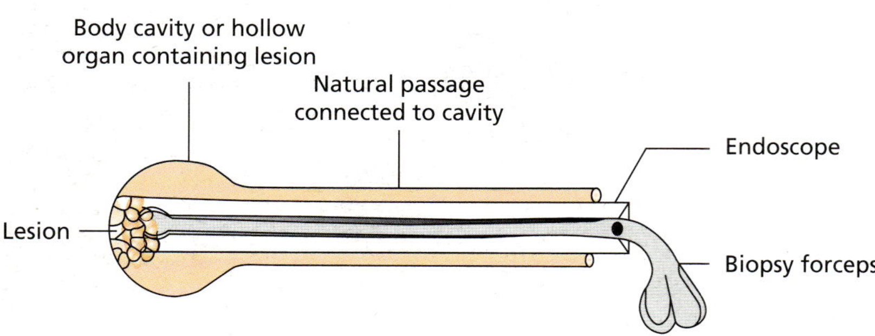

Figure 32.4 Endoscopic biopsy.

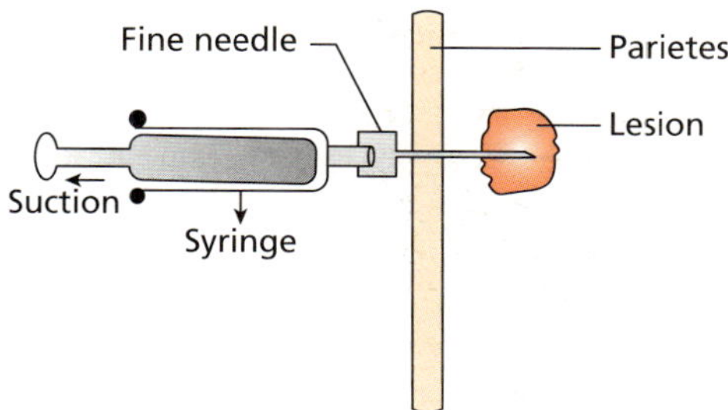

Figure 32.5 Fine needle aspiration cytology.

Frozen Section

Indication It is a common practice employed in the treatment of carcinoma of breast (one-step method).

Method Sometimes in a suspected cancer full preparation is made for the definitive surgical procedure and open biopsy is done first and the biopsy piece is examined then and there in the operating room by frozen section technique. It takes 10–30 minutes to give a diagnosis.

Result If it turns out positive for cancer, definitive surgery is performed at the same time. It has 90–95% accuracy and is convenient to the patient.

Imprint Cytology

Method After making the full arrangement for definitive treatment, the lesion is excised and transected into two pieces. The cut surface of the excised lesion is squeezed on a glass slide to make an imprint smear which is examined cytologically.

Advantages It is a simpler method than frozen section. It gives the diagnosis within 5–10 minutes with 90–95% accuracy.

Complications of biopsy

The complications of biopsy are rare, and include bleeding, infection and risk of dissemination, and local implantation of cancer cells which can be prevented by the following measures:

- Open biopsy must not be done in salivary gland and testicular swellings suspected to be a tumor.
- Instead, a FNAC can be done with the precaution to excise the needle track during excision of tumor.
- During biopsy of a bone tumor, the biopsy site and incision is so planned as to be excised when the tumor is being excised subsequently.

The complications of various types of biopsy are described in Box 32.1.

Box 32.1 Complications of biopsy

- Pain
- Bleeding
- Wound infection
- Risk of dissemination or local implantation of cancer cells

KEY POINTS

- Biopsy is the procedure of taking a small portion of tissue from a lesion for microscopic examination. It is the most important investigation for making a diagnosis of surgical diseases.
- Biopsy can be excisional, incisional, needle, and endoscopic. It is the most reliable and accurate method of diagnosis but it takes 3–7 days for the biopsy report to come.
- Rapid methods of diagnosis include exfoliative cytology, fine-needle aspiration cytology (FNAC), frozen section, and imprint cytology.
- Excisional biopsy is done in small lesions where the entire lesion is excised. In incisional biopsy a small piece is taken out from the junction of normal and abnormal tissues.
- Needle biopsy is performed in deep-seated lesions and organs where a core of tissue can be taken with the help of a large-bore needle such as Vim-Silverman or Tru-cut needle under ultrasound or CT guidance.
- Endoscopic biopsy is performed in the lesions situated in hollow organs, tubes, or body cavities

(CONTD...)

KEY POINTS (...CONTD)

which can be visualized and biopsied with a special biopsy forceps at the same time.

- In exfoliative cytology the exfoliated cells from the surface of lesion mixed with the contents of that organ, for example, urinary bladder, are examined cytologically.
- In FNAC the lesion is aspirated with a fine needle (no. 23) making three to four passes into the lesion and the aspirate is examined cytologically. It has 80–90% accuracy.
- Frozen section is done in a suspected case of carcinoma of breast with full preparation for definitive operation in the operating room. It gives report within 10–30 minutes. If it is positive, a definitive operation is performed.
- Open biopsy must not be done in salivary gland and testicular swellings suspected to be a tumor. Instead, a FNAC can be done with the precaution to excise the needle track during excision of tumor.

SELF-ASSESSMENT

Long answer questions

1. What is biopsy? Describe the indications, types and, complications of biopsy.
2. What are biopsy methods of rapid diagnosis? Describe the indications, technique, and results of exfoliative cytology.

Short answer questions

3. Excision biopsy
4. Needle biopsy
5. Exfoliative cytology
6. FNAC
7. Complications of biopsy

Multiple choice questions

1. For a small lesion anywhere on the body surface or in the oral cavity, which of the following is the biopsy method of choice?
   (a) Incisional biopsy
   (b) Excisional biopsy
   (c) Needle biopsy
   (d) FNAC
2. Smear of exfoliative cytology is usually stained with
   (a) Hematoxylin–eosin
   (b) Giemsa stain
   (c) Papanicolaou method
   (d) None of the above
3. FNAC is done with the help of a
   (a) No. 23 hollow needle
   (b) Tru-cut needle
   (c) Vim-Silverman needle
   (d) No. 18 hollow needle
4. Which of the following is a rapid method of diagnosis?
   (a) Incisional biopsy
   (b) Excisional biopsy
   (c) FNAC
   (d) Endoscopic biopsy

Answers

1. (b) 2. (c) 3. (a) 4. (c)

Radiotherapy (Radiation Treatment)

33

Introduction

Radiation is being used for both diagnostic (radiography, CT scan) and therapeutic purposes. The use of radiation in the treatment of disease is called radiotherapy. It is mainly used in the treatment of a variety of cancers. The use of radiation in the treatment of cancer has become so widespread and its association with surgery is so important that the students of dental surgery should have some knowledge of principles of radiotherapy.

Types of radiation

- **Alpha radiation**: It consists of two protons and two neutrons and has hardly any therapeutic relevance.
- **Beta radiation**: It consists of an electron. It penetrates a few millimeters of tissue.
- **Gamma radiation**: It is identical to X-rays. The penetration of this radiation depends on the energy carried and may be very marked. Hence, it is used in therapy.

Mechanism of action

Radiotherapy acts on different phases of cell cycle to destroy the cancer cells but the cells in "S" phase of cell cycle (when DNA is being synthesized) are radioresistant. After radiation exposure, these cells go into G2 or M phase.

Biological effects of radiotherapy

- **Formation of hydroxyl and peroxide radicals**: The radiation penetrates and collides with the atoms in the tissues to release energy and causes ionization of the water in the cells. The hydroxyl and peroxide radicals thus formed cause breakdown of DNA and chromosomes in the cells.
- **Cell death**: Microscopically vacuoles appear in the cytoplasm of the cells which swell subsequently. The nuclear chromatin forms clumps and the chromosomes break down. The overall effect of these changes is that the cells may die or may not be able to divide again.
- **Effect of oxygen**: The biological effect of radiotherapy is enhanced by oxygen as it increases the chances of forming free radicals which damage the cells. About 10% of cancer cells are hypoxic and the hypoxic tumor cells are radioresistant. Radiotherapy causes reoxygenation of these cells which can be killed by subsequent dose of radiation. Hence, fraction-

ation of radiotherapy makes it more effective (fractionalized radiotherapy). As oxygen is a good radiosensitizer, sometimes hyperbaric oxygenation is used for radiotherapy.

Radiation dose (absorbed dose)

The unit of radiation used for therapy is gray. It is defined as absorption of 1 J of energy by 1 kg of tissue (1 J kg).

- 1 Gy = 100 rad
- 1 rad = 0.01 Gy
- 1 mrad = 10^{-3} cGy

Radioisotopes

They emit beta or gamma radiation or both and are used for both diagnosis (e.g., radioiodine to find the nature of a solitary thyroid nodule and metastasis in follicular carcinoma of thyroid) and treatment (e.g., I^{131} in the treatment of metastatic follicular carcinoma of thyroid). The commonly used radionuclides are:

- $Cesium^{137}$ (Cs^{137})
- $Iridium^{192}$ (Ir^{192})
- $Gold^{198}$ (Au^{198})
- $Iodine^{131}$ (I^{131})

Advantages and disadvantages of radiotherapy

Advantages

- It can cure some early cancers without pain, bloodshed, and other risks of surgery, for example, carcinoma of lip, penis, and larynx and Hodgkin's lymphoma stage IA.
- In advanced cancer, radiotherapy is used for palliation of certain distressing symptoms such as bleeding, fungation, and obstruction.
- Surgically inaccessible lesions, for example, a pituitary tumor, can be treated by this method.

Disadvantages

- The equipment is costly and requires special training to operate it. It is not available freely in our country.
- Radiotherapy damages the normal cells and tissues near the area being treated.
- Second cancer may occur due to exposure of radiation to the surrounding normal tissues.

Overall the advantages of radiotherapy overweigh the disadvantages, and it is a useful and important method of therapy of cancers.

Delivery systems of radiotherapy

Teletherapy

In teletherapy, the source of radiation is kept at a distance from the site of disease to be irradiated (Fig. 33.1). It is also called external beam radiotherapy and is the most commonly used form of radiotherapy.

Types of teletherapy

The types are described in the subsequent text.

Superficial Radiotherapy Here the X-rays are generated at 60–140 kV. They are suitable for treating skin lesions and other lesions up to 4 mm depth.

Deep X-Ray Therapy They are generated (conventional or orthovoltage X-rays) at 200–300 kV. Until 1951, deep X-rays were the only tool

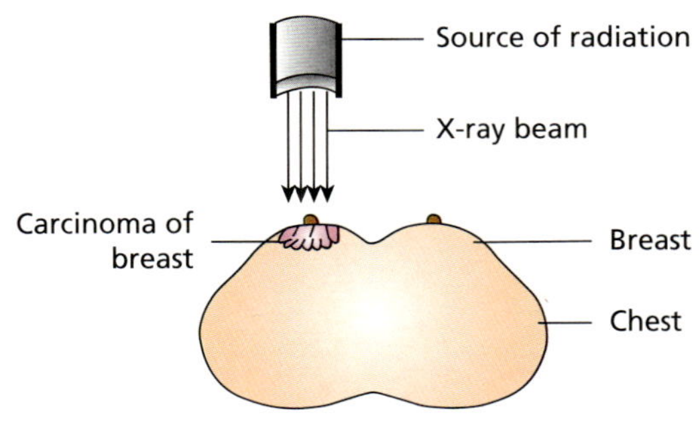

Figure 33.1 Teletherapy of carcinoma of breast.

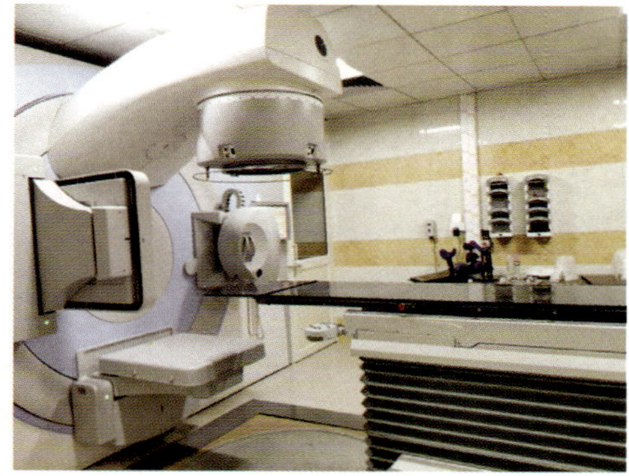

Figure 33.2 Linear accelerator. (Courtesy: Professor M.L.B. Bhatt)

available for treating deep-seated tumors. This therapy has one big disadvantage that a proportion of dose is absorbed by the tissues overlying the tumor causing serious side effects.

Megavoltage Radiation Therapy These X-rays are produced above 1 MV usually by a linear accelerator (Fig. 33.2). The usual working range of these machines is 4–25 MV. They are costly machines, hence are not freely available in our country. The main advantage of megavoltage radiation is greater penetrating power with minimal skin reaction.

Cobalt^{60} It gives a beam of almost monomagnetic radiation which has the penetrating power equal to that produced by an X-ray tube at 3 MV (Fig. 33.3).

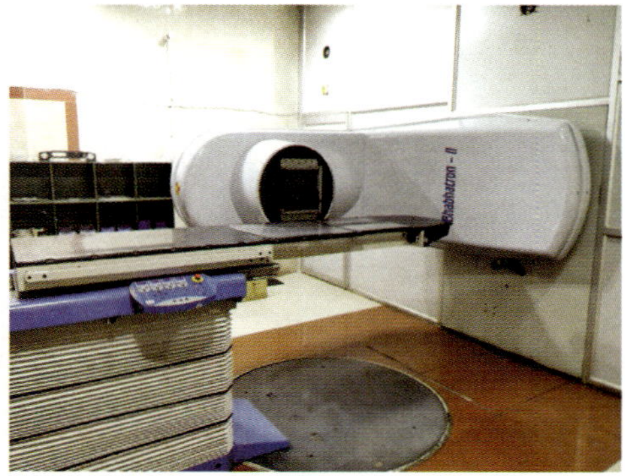

Figure 33.3 Cobalt^{60} radiotherapy machine. (Courtesy: Professor Rajeev Gupta)

Advantages and disadvantages of teletherapy

The advantages of teletherapy include simplicity of administration and no risk of local infection by contact. The disadvantages include risk of scattering of radiation beyond the tumor.

Brachytherapy

In this method of treatment the source of radiation, usually a radioactive isotope, for example, cesium^{137} and iridium^{192}, is kept very near or in the lesion to be treated by localized irradiation. For this an 18-channel high-dose-rate (HDR) brachytherapy unit with iridium^{192} is available. It is one of the oldest forms of radiotherapy which conforms the radiation dose tightly to the target while limiting the side effects. Now image-based brachytherapy is being used for accurate target localization, planning of dosage, and placement of applicators which are MRI and CT compatible.

Types of brachytherapy

It is of three types.

Surface Therapy It includes intracavitary brachytherapy for carcinoma of cervix uteri, intraluminal therapy for esophageal and tracheal cancers, and central vaginal cylinder for postoperative radiotherapy of cancer of cervix and endometrium, and mold brachytherapy for carcinoma of penis (Fig. 33.4).

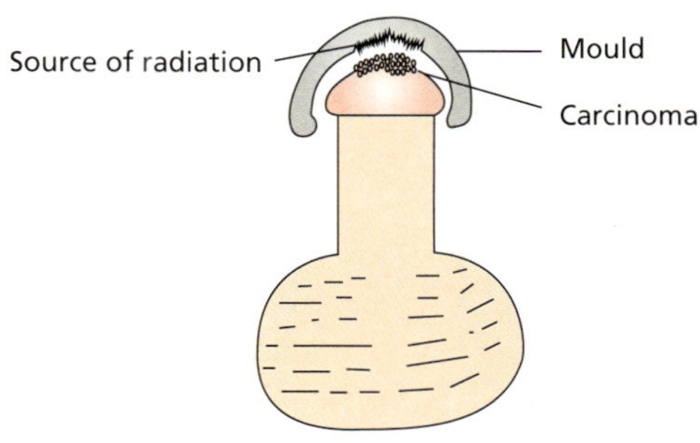

Figure 33.4 Contact or surface irradiation of carcinoma of penis by keeping the source of radiation in the mould.

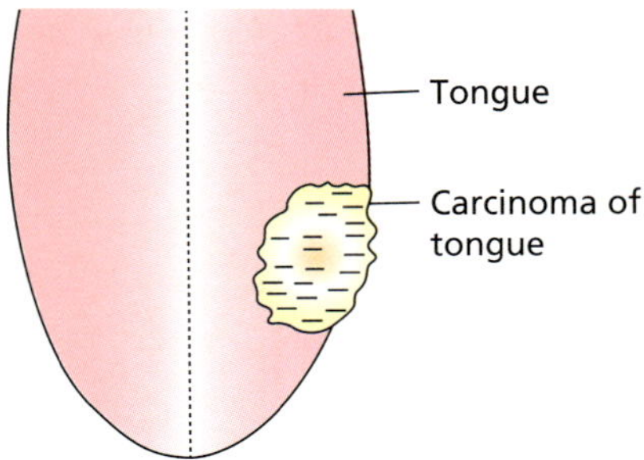

Figure 33.5 Interstitial radiotherapy of carcinoma of tongue by implantation of source of radiation in the tumor.

Interstitial Therapy It is the method of implanting the source of radiation, for example, iridium[192] wire in head and neck cancers (Fig. 33.5), soft-tissue tumors, and carcinoma breast.

Intraoperative Brachytherapy It is given to the operative field during operation, for example, mastectomy for carcinoma of breast.

Advantages of brachytherapy

- Localized radiation can be given in a high continuous dose in a short time.
- Deeper and adjacent normal tissues are spared.
- It is curative in early cancer; hence, surgery can be avoided.
- Now after-loading devices are available which reduce the radiation exposure to treating team.

Disadvantages of brachytherapy

The disadvantages include technical difficulty and requirement of special facilities and complications such as displacement and erosion of the implant.

Recent trends in radiotherapy

Newer developments have occurred in this field which have changed the face of modern radiotherapy completely.

Imaging Methods

CT, MRI, and PET scans help in accurate localization of the lesion as regards its site and size.

Simulators

Now 2D and CT simulators are available which are used in the planning of treatment. Image-controlled simulation allows quick and accurate repositioning of the fields, collimator rotation, and couch position, thereby significantly reducing simulation time and radiation dose (Fig. 33.6). Some new methods of radiotherapy include intensity-modulated radiotherapy, image-guided radiotherapy (IGRT), rapid arc therapy, and stereotaxy.

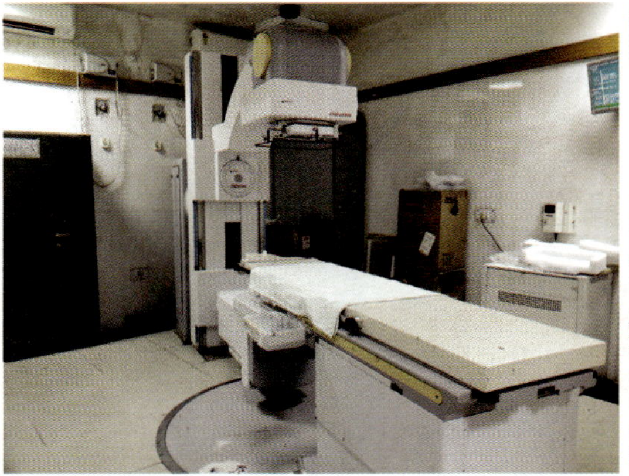

Simulator

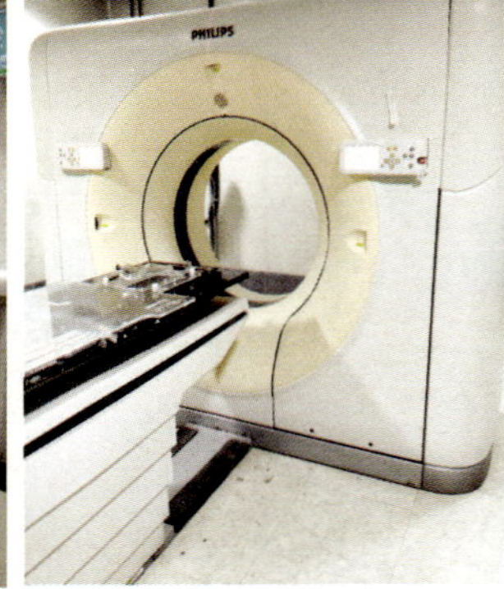

CT simulator

Figure 33.6 CT simulator for treatment planning. (Courtesy: Professor Rajeev Gupta)

Rapid Arc Therapy

- It is a combination of precision and speed with the aim of improving the standards of care and treating more patients in a short time. It is a volumetric arc therapy that delivers a precisely sculpted 3D dose distribution with a single 360° gantry rotation.
- The treatment planning algorithm can change three parameters simultaneously during treatment, that is, rotation speed of gantry, shape of treatment aperture using the movements of multileaf collimator leaves, and delivery dose rate. The availability of high-definition multileaf collimator (HDMLC) consisting of 120 leaves with a leaf thickness of 25 mm each allows improved dose conformity around the target volume, sparing the organs and tissues at risk in the vicinity.

Stereotactic Radiosurgery

- It is done with a gamma knife and the principal area of its use is in neurosurgery.
- It consists of more than 200 separate sources of high-energy radiation arranged in a circular fashion to be focused stereotactically on to a minute area in the brain. The head is held motionless by an external fixation device.
- This therapy is able to destroy finite areas within the brain. Hence, it is used in the treatment of benign and malignant brain tumors including those of pituitary, arteriovenous malformations, and an epileptic focus.

Types of radiotherapy

Radiotherapy is used to treat radiosensitive tumors (Table 33.1). The type of treatment can be curative, palliative, concomitant, and intraoperative radiotherapy (IORT).

Curative Radiotherapy It is given in early cancers which are sensitive to radiotherapy, for example, carcinoma of lip, tongue, and penis.

Palliative Radiotherapy It is given to advanced incurable cancers to relieve certain distressing symptoms, for example, pain in metastatic carcinoma of vertebral column and bleeding in carcinoma of oral cavity are relieved by giving 60 Gy in 30 fractions over 6 weeks. It is also used to give relief in fungation, obstruction, spinal cord compression, and pathological fracture.

Chemoradiation (Concomitant Radiotherapy) It is the use of chemotherapy together with radiotherapy. The commonly used drug is 5-FU. It improves the results of radiotherapy, but adds to the toxicity at the same time. Chemotherapy can also be given before radiotherapy. It is called induction chemotherapy. It reduces the bulk of tumor without altering its vascularity. After radiotherapy usually no chemotherapy is given.

Intraoperative Radiotherapy It is the use of a large single dose of radiation given to the operative field and local potential areas of tumor spread after the excision of tumor before closure of wound. It improves the results of surgery.

Complications of radiotherapy

The radiation is injurious to all organs and tissues of the body. The most sensitive tissues are bone marrow, gonads, eyes, and mucosa

Table 33.1 Radiosensitivity of tumors

Common radiosensitive tumors	Common radioresistant tumors
• Squamous cell carcinoma • Basal cell carcinoma • Carcinoma of urinary bladder • Carcinoma of cervix uteri • Seminoma testis • Hodgkin's lymphoma • Ewing's sarcoma • Carcinoma of prostate	• Gastrointestinal carcinomas • Carcinoma of gallbladder • Malignant melanoma • Chondrosarcoma • Medullary carcinoma of thyroid

of gastrointestinal tract. The adverse effects on various organs and tissues are enumerated in Table 33.2. Although so many side effects are described, the radiotherapy is quite safe and effective if given in correct dosage and by correct technique.

Table 33.2 Complications of radiotherapy

Organ	Effect of radiotherapy
Bone marrow	Myelosuppression
Gonads	Amenorrhea (ovaries), oligospermia (testes)
Eyes	Radiation cataract
Gastrointestinal tract	Mucositis leading to nausea, vomiting, and diarrhea. Later on, stricture and fistulation may occur
Skin	Erythema, desquamation, hair loss, pigmentation, ulceration, fibrosis, telangiectasia
Spinal cord	Myelitis which may present as paraplegia or hemiplegia
Lungs	Radiation pneumonitis presenting as cough and dyspnea. Later on, it may cause pulmonary fibrosis
Oral cavity	Edema, ulceration, xerostomia, loss of taste, oral thrush, dysphagia
Kidneys	Radiation nephritis followed by chronic renal failure
Liver	Hepatic fibrosis
Bones	Avascular necrosis of head of femur or humerus, damage to epiphysis in children
Radiation-induced malignancies	Leukemia, papillary carcinoma of thyroid, lymphoma, carcinoma of breast

KEY POINTS

- The use of radiation in the treatment of disease is called radiotherapy in which gamma radiation is used. It acts on different phases of cell cycle to destroy the cancer cells but the cells in "S" phase of cell cycle (when DNA is being synthesized) are radioresistant.
- The radiation penetrates and collides with the atoms in the tissues to release energy and causes ionization of the water in the cells which leads to breakdown of DNA and chromosomes. The overall effect of these changes is that the cells may die or may not be able to divide again.
- In teletherapy, the source of radiation is kept at a distance from the site of disease to be irradiated. It is also called external beam radiotherapy and is the most commonly used form of radiotherapy.
- Superficial radiotherapy, deep X-ray therapy, and megavoltage radiation therapy are the types of teletherapy.
- Superficial radiotherapy is suitable for treating skin lesions and other lesions up to 4 mm depth. Deep X-ray therapy is used for treating deep-seated tumors. This therapy has one big disadvantage that a proportion of dose is absorbed by the tissues overlying the tumor causing serious side effects.
- In brachytherapy, the source of radiation, usually a radioactive isotope, for example, cesium^{137} and iridium^{192}, is kept very near or in the lesion to be treated by localized irradiation. It conforms the radiation dose tightly to the target while limiting the side effects.
- Types of brachytherapy are surface therapy, interstitial therapy, and intraoperative brachytherapy. The disadvantages include technical difficulty and requirement of special facilities and complications such as displacement and erosion.
- 2D and CT simulators are available which are used in planning of treatment. Some new methods of radiotherapy include intensity-modulated radio-

(CONTD...)

KEY POINTS *(...CONTD)*

therapy, image-guided radiotherapy (IGRT), rapid arc therapy, and stereotaxy.

- Curative radiotherapy is given in early cancers which are sensitive to radiotherapy such as carcinoma of lip, tongue, and penis.
- Palliative radiotherapy is given to advanced incurable cancers to relieve certain distressing symptoms, for example, pain in metastatic carcinoma of vertebral column and bleeding in carcinoma of oral cavity.
- Chemoradiation (concurrent radiotherapy) is the use of chemotherapy with radiotherapy. The commonly used drug is 5-FU. Intraoperative radiotherapy is the use of a large single dose of radiation given to the operative field and local potential areas of tumor spread after the excision of tumor before closure of wound.
- The radiation is injurious to all organs and tissues of the body but the most sensitive tissues are bone marrow, gonads, eyes, and mucosa of gastrointestinal tract.

SELF-ASSESSMENT

Long answer questions

1. What is radiotherapy? What are its types and complications?
2. What is brachytherapy? What are its types, advantages, and disadvantages?

Short answer questions

1. Teletherapy
2. Brachytherapy
3. Stereotactic radiosurgery
4. Chemoradiation
5. Intraoperative radiotherapy

Multiple choice questions

1. Stereotactic radiosurgery is used in the treatment of
   (a) Tumors of pituitary
   (b) Carcinoma of maxilla
   (c) Carcinoma of tongue
   (d) Carcinoma of larynx
2. The drug used in chemoradiation is
   (a) Cyclophosphamide
   (b) Adriamycin
   (c) 5-FU
   (d) Cisplatin
3. Which of the following is the most radiosensitive tumor?
   (a) Chondrosarcoma of maxilla
   (b) Malignant melanoma of face
   (c) Multiple myeloma
   (d) Ewing's tumor
4. The effect of radiotherapy on the bone marrow is
   (a) No effect
   (b) Suppression
   (c) Stimulation
   (d) Initial stimulation followed by suppression

Answers

1. (a) 2. (c) 3. (d) 4. (b)

Diabetes Mellitus in Surgery

34

Introduction

Diabetes mellitus is a very common disease and affects 2–5% of the general population. Its incidence is increasing. Diabetes affects the whole body; thus, every specialty in medical sciences has its own quota of diabetic manifestations. The main feature of this disease is elevated blood sugar level, the normal sugar level being 60–110 mg/dL with panic if it falls below 40 mg/dL or rises above 500 mg/dL. The sugar may also come in urine (glycosuria), the normal urine being sugar-free.

Etiology

The main etiological factor of diabetes is insulin deficiency. The digestion of food occurs at two levels, first in the gastrointestinal tract with the help of digestive enzymes, and then in the tissues at the cell level where the glucose is "digested" with the help of insulin to release energy (and CO_2). Hence, the diabetes is a type of malabsorption syndrome of glucose at the cell level.

Insulin

Insulin was discovered by Dr. Frederick Banting and Charles Best in Canada in 1921. They found that it was effective in decreasing blood glucose levels in diabetic dogs. It is a protein hormone formed by β-cells of islets of Langerhans of pancreas and secreted into the blood to regulate carbohydrate (mainly), lipid, and amino acid metabolism and used therapeutically in diabetes mellitus (insulin-dependent diabetes).

Indications of surgery in a diabetic patient

A diabetic patient comes in surgery for the following reasons:

- **Treatment of complications of diabetes**, for example, diabetic foot and carbuncle (Figs 34.1 and 34.2)

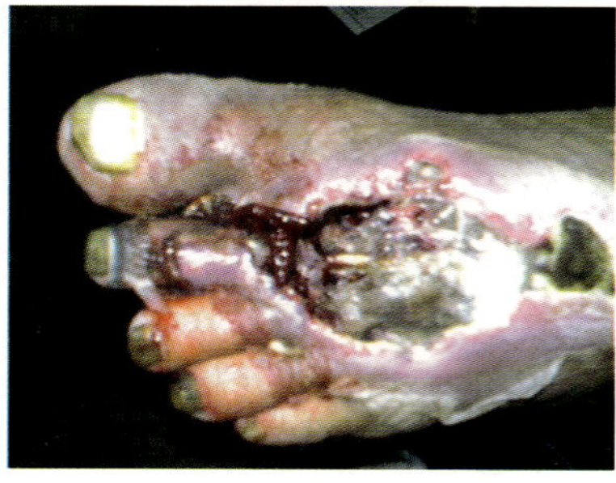

Figure 34.1 Gangrene of foot with gangrene of second toe and part of dorsum with surrounding inflammation in a diabetic patient. (Courtesy: Professor Sandeep Tewari)

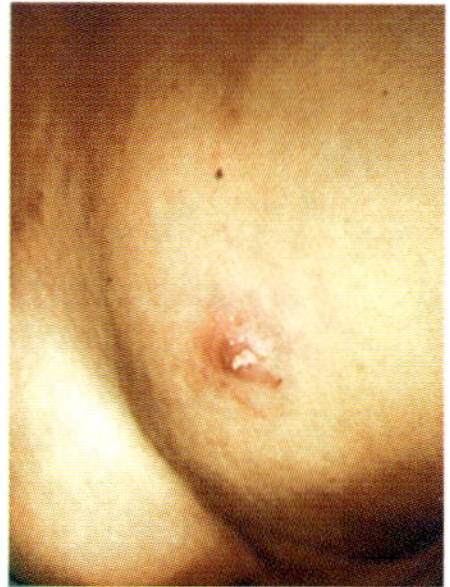

Figure 34.2 A small carbuncle of right scapular region of back.

- **Treatment of surgical diseases**, for example, excision of a jaw tumor, total thyroidectomy for carcinoma of thyroid, and excision of a pharyngeal diverticulum (in these patients the diabetes must be controlled before operation)

Diabetic foot

Diabetic foot has three clinical presentations: diabetic ulcer, diabetic cellulitis, and diabetic gangrene.

- Diabetic ulcer is a nonspecific ulcer occurring in a diabetic person which refuses to heal if the diabetes remains uncontrolled.
- Diabetic cellulitis is a rapidly spreading cellulitis seen in an uncontrolled diabetic. It spreads more under the skin along the tissue planes causing toxemia and septicemia and kills the victim if not urgently treated by broad-spectrum combination antibiotics, quick control of diabetic ketoacidosis, and laying open the infected tissue spaces widely.
- Diabetic gangrene is a stage ahead of diabetic cellulitis which requires urgent amputation.

Problems due to diabetes mellitus in surgery

Infection Diabetic patients are more prone to infections as compared to nondiabetics (due to impaired immune function), and these infections cannot be controlled with antibiotics without controlling the sugar level.

Impaired Wound Healing It is due to changes in soft-tissue matrix, granulation tissue, and microvascular disease. If macrovascular disease (accelerated atherosclerosis) is present, the impaired wound healing is more pronounced.

Mortality The overall mortality of surgery in a diabetic is about 2% mainly due to cardiovascular reasons or sepsis, particularly staphylococcal. The mortality of emergency surgery in diabetes is several times more than that of elective procedures, for example, in emergency cholecystectomy it is 22%, while it is 1% in elective operations. The special problems of diabetes mellitus in a surgical patient are described in Box 34.1.

Box 34.1 Problems due to diabetes mellitus in surgery

- Increased risk of infection due to more sugar in tissues and impaired immune function
- Impaired wound healing due to:
  - Changes in soft-tissue matrix and granulation tissue
  - Microangiopathy and accelerated atherosclerosis
  - Sensory neuropathy

Metabolic response of diabetic patients to surgery

The main factors which may seriously affect the metabolism in these patients include nothing orally for a few hours before operation and secretion of stress hormones, for example, adrenaline and cortisone. They result in an increased risk of diabetic ketoacidosis characterized by hyperglycemia and acetonuria.

Treatment of diabetes mellitus in surgical patients

The treatment depends on severity of diabetes, severity of surgical disease, and the nature and extent of surgery. The basic requirement is that the blood sugar must be normal or near normal before operation by the appropriate use of insulin.

Preoperative Evaluation

It includes blood sugar estimation, careful evaluation of arteries including carotid arteries, and investigations to determine the cardiac status and renal function. The eyes may be seen for retinopathy and the fasting lipids should also be measured.

Glycemic Control

- The patients with mild diabetes controlled by dietary modification require no specific measures other than blood sugar monitoring.
- Oral antidiabetics have hardly any role in the control of surgical diabetes except when a mild diabetic controlled on these drugs needs a minor operation under local anesthesia.

Patients requiring insulin therapy

- In **elective surgery**, enough time is available for full control of blood sugar level.
  - Preoperatively, one-half to two-thirds of daily dose of insulin is usually given and intravenous drip of glucose is started to maintain glucose level and prevent ketoacidosis.
  - Postoperatively, intermittent doses of regular insulin can be titrated to frequently determine blood glucose levels till the patient comes on regular diet and previous stable regimen.
  - Alternatively, an insulin–glucose infusion can be used to maintain normoglycemia.
- In **emergency situation**, the blood sugar levels may be very high due to stress and disease process (infection). These patients require insulin and urgent control of acute disease to control blood sugar level.
  - The blood sugar level is continuously monitored and should be below 250 mg/dL.
  - The diabetic ketoacidosis is corrected by administration of intravenous fluids, insulin, bicarbonate, and potassium.
  - Surgery must not be done until the abnormalities are corrected at least partially.

The essential features of diabetes control in surgery are described in Box 34.2.

Box 34.2 Essential features of diabetes control in surgery

- **Patients controlled on oral hypoglycemics**: Avoiding morning dose
- **Patients controlled on insulin**: Intravenous infusion of dextrose and insulin
- **Monitoring of sugar and potassium levels**: Extra potassium usually required (GKI regime)
- **Gangrenous limb likely to cause instability in diabetes**: Immediate amputation as diabetes control becomes easier after amputation

KEY POINTS

- Diabetes mellitus is due to insulin deficiency, and is a type of malabsorption syndrome of glucose at the cell level.
- A diabetic patient comes in surgery for treatment of complications of diabetes such as diabetic foot, and for treatment of surgical diseases in diabetes.
- Surgical complications of diabetes mellitus include infection, impaired wound healing, and mortality due to cardiovascular reasons or sepsis. The mortality of emergency surgery in diabetes is several times more than that of elective procedures.
- The patients with mild diabetes controlled by dietary modification require no specific measures other than blood sugar monitoring.
- In elective surgery, insulin is used to obtain glycemic control in the perioperative period. In emergency situation the blood sugar levels may be very high due to stress and disease process (infection). These patients require insulin and urgent control of acute disease to control blood sugar level. Surgery must not be done until the abnormalities are corrected at least partially.

SELF-ASSESSMENT

Long answer question

1. What are the surgical complications of diabetes mellitus? Discuss the treatment of diabetes in a surgical patient.

Short answer questions

1. Insulin
2. Problems due to diabetes mellitus in surgery

Multiple choice questions

1. What is normal blood sugar level?
   (a) 60–110 mg%
   (b) 180–220 mg%
   (c) 220–260 mg%
   (d) 260–300 mg%
2. What is normal urinary sugar level?
   (a) 10–20 mg%
   (b) 20–30 mg%
   (c) 30–50 mg%
   (d) Nil
3. Which of the following statements is false?
   (a) Normal urine has no acetone
   (b) Normal urine has significant acetone
   (c) Acetone is present in urine during starvation
   (d) Diabetic ketoacidosis is characterized by hyperglycemia and acetonuria
4. For a major elective operation under general anesthesia, the diabetes should be controlled with
   (a) Diet control
   (b) Oral antidiabetics
   (c) Diet control and oral antidiabetics
   (d) Diet control and insulin

Answers

1. (a) 2. (d) 3. (b) 4. (d)

Surgical Diathermy (Electrocautery) 35

Introduction

Surgical diathermy is one of the commonest and an important equipment of the operating room (Fig. 35.1).

Principle of diathermy

With the help of this machine, a high-frequency alternating current (AC) is passed through the body tissues. The local concentration of the current produces an area of high current density liberating a lot of heat with very high local temperature. The current frequency ranges from 400 kHz to 10 MHz. In this range there is minimal muscular response.

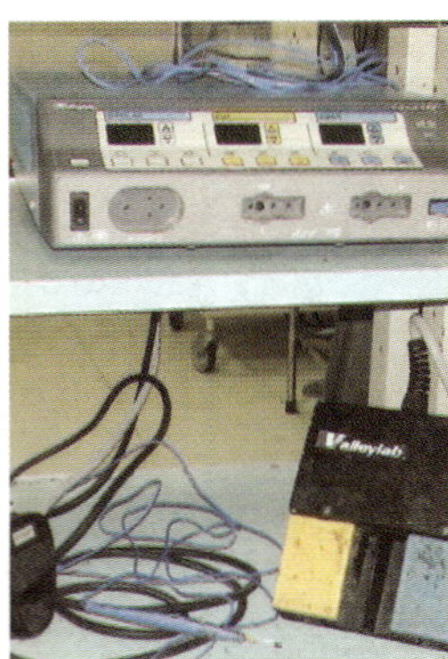

Figure 35.1 Operating diathermy.

Types of diathermy

The diathermy is of two types, that is, unipolar and bipolar.

Unipolar Diathermy

Here the active electrode works at the surgical site from where the current passes through the patient's body to a dispersive electrode or plate to complete the circuit (Fig. 35.2). As the current passes through the body, it may cause harm to a pacemaker.

Mechanism of action

- It consists of a high-frequency AC generator (over 20,000 Hz), regulator to control the intensity of current, foot control, active electrode, and dispersive electrode.

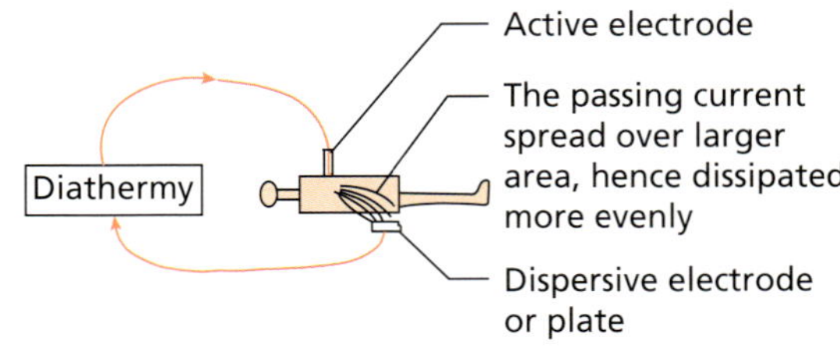

Figure 35.2 Unipolar diathermy.

- When the active electrode tip touches the body tissues directly or indirectly (through a hemostat) and the foot control is pressed, the current passes into the body and goes out through the dispersive electrode which is a flat steel plate that is put in full contact with the patient's back, thigh, or buttocks.
- The contact between the patient's skin and the electrode is increased by either shaving this area or using a conductive jelly. The electrode is usually wrapped in a wet cloth to improve conduction. It acts as earth for current.
- The active electrode is a fine tip; hence, a high current density is available at this point to work on the tissues. By changing the intensity of current, the diathermy can be used for performing various functions.

Functions of unipolar diathermy

The unipolar diathermy can be used to perform coagulation, cutting, and fulguration during operations.

Coagulation

The small bleeders are coagulated to stop bleeding. They are first clamped in a hemostat which is then touched with diathermy point to coagulate the cut end. This function is performed by using blue switch when the temperature of tip reaches 100°C.

Cutting

By increasing the current, the tip of active electrode can be used for cutting the soft tissues (Fig. 35.3). It cuts and coagulates the small vessels; thus, the bleeding stops at the same time. The temperature of tip reaches 1000°C. The color of its controlling switch is yellow.

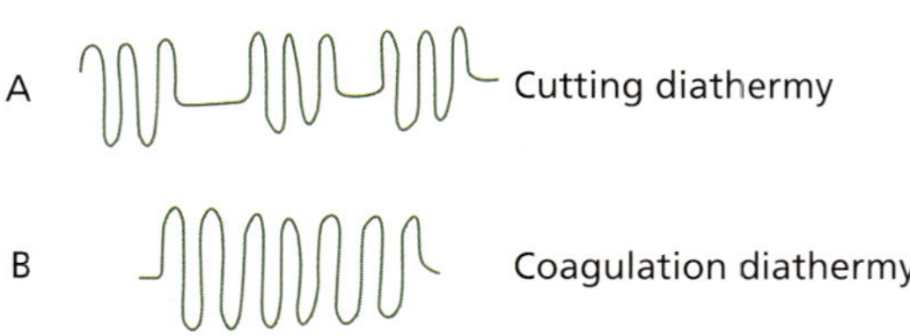

Figure 35.3 Waveform of surgical diathermy.

Fulguration

It is destruction of living tissues by the electric sparks generated by a high-frequency current. It is used to treat small lesions, for example, papilloma and leukoplakia.

Bipolar Diathermy

Mechanism of action

The working electrode consists of two blades of forceps performing the function of both active and dispersive electrodes. The tissue to be treated is grasped in the forceps to complete the circuit (Fig. 35.4).

Functions of bipolar diathermy

As the current generated is smaller, this diathermy can be used only for coagulation and not for other functions. The bipolar diathermy is essential for laparoscopic surgery.

The differences between a unipolar and a bipolar diathermy are described in Table 35.1.

Advantages and disadvantages of bipolar diathermy

The advantages of bipolar diathermy include reduction of risk of burns and interference in the function of ECG unit and pacemaker, and spark ignition of anesthetic gases.

The disadvantage of bipolar diathermy is that it cannot be used for cutting, burning, and fulguration of tissues.

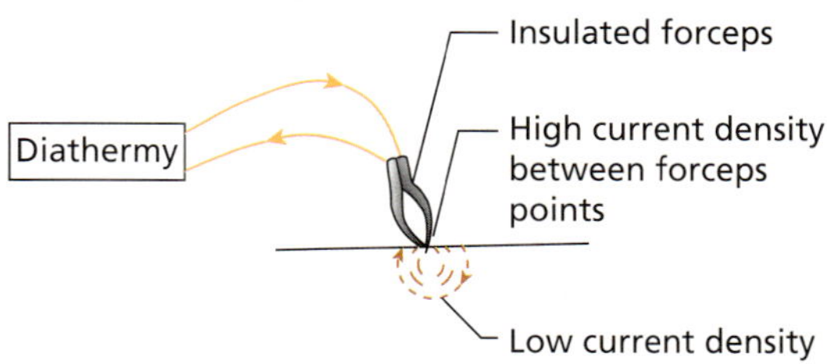

Figure 35.4 Bipolar diathermy.

Table 35.1 Differences between unipolar and bipolar diathermy

Features	Unipolar diathermy	Bipolar diathermy
Uses	Used for coagulation, cutting, and fulguration	Used only for coagulation
Dispersive electrode	Used	Not required
In patients with pacemaker	Should not be used	Can be used
Electrical injury of other tissues	Can occur	Does not occur

Precautions

- The equipment should be checked from time to time, especially the insulation and alarm system.
- The people who are using diathermy should know the rules of the use of diathermy.
- Ensure intimate contact between the patient's body and the indifferent electrode. Avoid point contact, for example, on bony ridges.
- Avoid contact of diathermy point with retractors and other metal instruments when being used.
- The live electrode must be put in a quiver, never on drapes or tray.
- The operator should wear rubber footwear to avoid accidental burn.
- Avoid using ether and cyclopropane for general anesthesia. Alcohol-containing disinfectants should not be used or should be dried before the diathermy is used.

Complications of use of diathermy

- Electrical burns
- Explosion in operating room
- Electrocution
- Pacemaker dysfunction
- Overheating of metallic prostheses (hence, when a monopolar diathermy is used, the dispersive electrode should be sited well away from the prostheses)

KEY POINTS

- Surgical diathermy is one of the commonest and an important equipment of the operating room.
- With the help of this machine, a high-frequency alternating current (AC) is passed through the body tissues. The local concentration of the current produces an area of high current density liberating a lot of heat with very high local temperature which helps in cutting, coagulation, and fulguration of the tissues.
- In unipolar diathermy, active electrode works at the surgical site from where the current passes through the patient's body to a dispersive electrode or plate to complete the circuit. It cannot be used in patients with pacemakers.
- By changing the intensity of current, the unipolar diathermy can be used for performing various functions such as coagulation, cutting, and fulguration.
- For cutting the tissues, the current is increased by controlling the yellow switch and the temperature of the tip of active electrode reaches 1000°C.
- Fulguration is destruction of living tissues by the electric sparks generated by a high-frequency current. It is used to treat small lesions.
- In bipolar diathermy, the working electrode consists of two blades of forceps performing the function of both active and dispersive electrodes. The tissue to be treated is grasped in the forceps to complete the circuit.
- As the current generated is smaller, bipolar diathermy can be used only for coagulation and not for other functions. The bipolar diathermy is essential for laparoscopic surgery.
- When using diathermy for surgery, general anesthetics such as ether and cyclopropane must be avoided. Alcohol-containing disinfectants should not be used or should be dried before the diathermy is used.
- Complications of diathermy in surgery include electrical burns, explosion in operating room, electrocution, pacemaker dysfunction, and overheating of metallic prostheses.

SELF-ASSESSMENT

Long answer questions

1. What are the types of surgical diathermy? Describe their mechanism of action and uses.
2. What are the advantages and disadvantages of surgical diathermy? What are the complications of the use of diathermy and how to prevent them?

Short answer questions

1. Unipolar diathermy
2. Bipolar diathermy
3. Fulguration
4. Dangers of diathermy

Multiple choice questions

1. With diathermy machine, a high-frequency alternating current is passed through the body tissues for all of the following purposes, except
   (a) Fomenting the tissues
   (b) Cutting
   (c) Fulguration
   (d) Dissection
2. What is the current frequency of surgical diathermy?
   (a) 100 kHz to 1 MHz
   (b) 200 kHz to 2 MHz
   (c) 300 kHz to 5 MHz
   (d) 400 kHz to 10 MHz
3. What is the local temperature at the site of use for cutting the tissues by diathermy?
   (a) 100°C
   (b) 500°C
   (c) 800°C
   (d) 1000°C or more

Answers

1. (a) 2. (d) 3. (d)

Part II:

Clinical and Practical

Clinical Cases

36

Introduction

Usually two short cases are allotted to a dental student in the practical clinical examination. A short case is one where the details of history and complete physical examination of the patient are not mandatory for making a clinical diagnosis. Here, the diagnosis is based on symptoms and brief local examination.

Not infrequently the diagnosis is made, just by a "look" at the patient and the lesion. It is called spot diagnosis. It is the usual practice of making a clinical diagnosis in a large number of patients in outpatients department.

In most of the practical examination settings, about 20 minutes per case are given to make a diagnosis and to write in brief about the patient on reply sheet. For following this time schedule, students should do this drill repeatedly during their clinical posting in Surgery Department.

Questioning

Primary Questions

Four primary questions are usually asked from every candidate on an allotted case:

1. What is the diagnosis?
2. What are the reasons for making this diagnosis?
3. What are the investigations to be done in this case? Or how will you investigate this case?
4. How will you treat this patient's disease?

These four are **primary questions**, as they are more or less absolute or fixed questions. Hence, the candidate must organize the answers to these questions while waiting for the viva, so that the correct and "to-the-point" answers are given to these queries. Most of the time, the success in the practical examination is determined by the replies given in response to these questions. Also subsequently in the clinical practice, one has to deal with or solve these four queries throughout one's career.

Secondary Questions

These questions originate from the answers given by the candidate to the primary questions. Hence, they are very variable and not asked from every candidate. If the primary questions are answered well, they may not be asked at all, or lesser number of questions are asked. Some examples of secondary questions are given in the subsequent text.

After Answering the First Primary Question

- How will you differentiate it from .... (name of some other similar diseases you have not diagnosed)?
- Is there any differential diagnosis?
- Can it be ... (name of some other disease resembling the disease you have diagnosed) and not the one you have diagnosed and why?

After Answering the Second Primary Question

- What is the cause of this symptom ... or sign ... this patient has?
- How will you examine the patient for this sign?
- Demonstrate how you elicit this sign.

After Answering the Third Primary Question

- Tell the findings on blood examination.
- What are the normal levels of ... blood sugar, serum calcium, and others?
- What are the radiographic signs of this disease, for example, ameloblastoma and dentigerous cyst?
- What are the indications for doing this investigation?
- What are the causes of this finding ...?

After Answering the Fourth Primary Question The treatment of most of the surgical diseases is an operation. Hence, the candidate usually names the operation in response to this question. The secondary questions of this response are:

- What is done in this operation, for example, complete excision of lining of a sebaceous cyst and excision of a benign tumor with its capsule?
- Under which anesthesia will you do this operation?
- What is the preoperative preparation?
- What are the complications of this operation?
- Is there any medical or nonoperative treatment?

It is not necessary that all the secondary questions described above are asked from every examinee. The number of questions depends on the time available and the prompt response of the candidate. The viva on a short case mostly finishes with the primary questions and some secondary questions.

Tertiary Questions

These questions are asked less frequently, as usually there is no time left for these with most of the candidates. They are usually asked from fast and knowledgeable candidates. They are asked for three reasons:

1. To seek further clarification to the answers given in response to the secondary questions

2. To know the theoretical details about the disease diagnosed

3. To identify the meritorious candidate for giving “distinction or honor”

If the student has attended all the lectures and clinics and adequately studied the subject, there is nothing to worry about as the examination is usually easy and simple. Usually, commonly available cases are kept and common questions are asked. Hence, appear in the examination with hope and confidence—success is awaiting you.

Best of luck for the examination, and for a bright career as a good dental surgeon.

Case sheet writing

Case sheet writing and keeping the records of the patient are important for doing research, for example, analysis of results of treatment, and for medicolegal reasons. The details of case sheet writing are described in Box 36.1.

Box 36.1 Case sheet writing

Name Age Sex Married/single

Profession Residence

Habits: Vegetarian/nonvegeterian/alcohol/tobacco/paan masala

Symptoms in chronological order with duration

- ... days/weeks/months/years
- ...
- ...

History

- **Present illness**
  - Total duration
  - Onset—sudden/gradual or insidious
  - Course—progressive/regressive/stationary/fluctuating
  - Sequence of events
  - Treatment taken
- **Past illness:** Past history of tuberculosis, venereal disease, diabetes mellitus, trauma, or the same types of illness as the present one
- **Family history:** History of any familial disease, tuberculosis, diabetes mellitus, venereal disease

Physical examination

General examination

- Appearance
- Lymph nodes
- BP/pulse
- Respiration
- Edema over feet

Systemic examination

- Nervous system
- Cardiovascular system
- Respiratory system
- Liver/spleen

Local examination

- Inspection (seeing the lesion)
- Palpation (gentle touching and pressing)
- Percussion (striking and hearing the sound)
- Auscultation (hearing as such)

Sample case 1: basal cell carcinoma

Ganesh Prasad, a 68-year-old married male, agricultural laborer, vegetarian, nonalcoholic, non-tobacco user, and resident of Malihabad, presents with ulcer on the face for 3 years and serous discharge for 2 years.

The patient was alright 3 years ago when he noted a small nodule in the left parotid region. Within a few months, it turned into a small ulcer which is not healing and increasing in spite of treatment. It discharges small amount of serous fluid from time to time.

There is no past history suggestive of tuberculosis, venereal disease, and diabetes mellitus. There is no history suggestive of such diseases in family.

Physical Examination

The general and the systemic examinations are within normal limits including pulse 76/minute, blood pressure 130/90 mm Hg, respiration 16/minute, slight anemia, and no edema over feet.

The local examination shows a large shallow ulcer on the left side of face in the parotid region (Fig. 36.1).

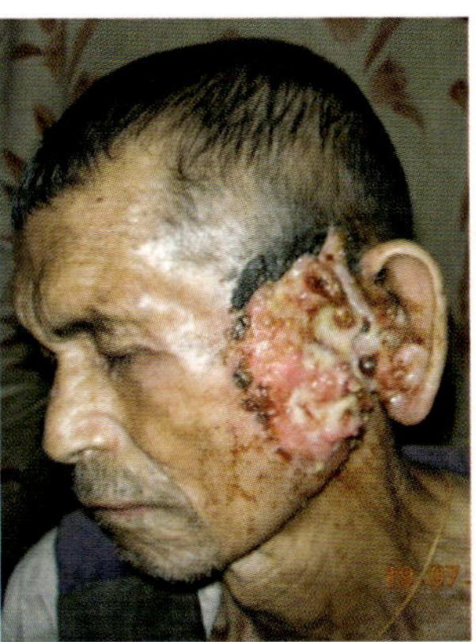

Figure 36.1 A large basal cell carcinoma (rodent ulcer) of left parotid region in an elderly male. (Courtesy: Professor Sandeep Kumar)

- Size: 2 × 2.25 cm
- Color: Blackish red
- Shape: Irregular
- Surface: Irregular, partially ulcerated
- Edge: Raised, beaded, and pigmented
- Firm, nontender, and mobile on underlying tissues on palpation (percussion and auscultation are not required)

Clinical Diagnosis

My clinical diagnosis is basal cell carcinoma of face.

Viva Voce

Q1. What are the reasons for giving this diagnosis?
Answer: The reasons for making this diagnosis are:

- The patient is an elderly male, 68 years of age, and agricultural laborer by profession (works in sun).
- There is a nonhealing ulcer of the left parotid region of 3-year duration.
- It is irregular in shape and has a beaded raised hard edge.
- The regional lymph nodes are not enlarged.

Q2. What is basal cell carcinoma (BCC)?
Answer: It is a malignant tumor of skin that arises from basal cell layer of epidermis.

Q3. You have said in the reasons that the patient is an agricultural laborer. How is this cancer related to agricultural work?
Answer: One of the important risk factors of this cancer is chronic exposure to sunlight and the agricultural laborers are more exposed to it as they work in the fields.

Q4. What is a rodent ulcer?
Answer: It is the ulcerative type of basal cell carcinoma.

Q5. Why is it known as rodent ulcer?
Answer: It is known as rodent ulcer as it gnaws (destroys) the local tissues like a rodent.

Q6. What are the types of BCC?
Answer: It is of four types: nodular, pigmented, cystic, and superficial spreading or "field fire type."

Q7. What is a nodular type of BCC?
Answer: It is characterized by a well-defined elevated lesion with a waxy appearance. It may have a central depression (umbilication) and small blood vessels across the surface of the tumor.

Q8. Describe the pigmented type of BCC.
Answer: Most of the tumors are pink or skin colored but some may have shades of brown or black pigmentation, mimicking a benign mole or melanoma.

Q9. What is the appearance of a cystic BCC?
Answer: It is translucent and may appear blue or gray and may be confused with a blue nevus.

Q10. What is superficial spreading BCC?
Answer: It is a macular lesion that is active at the periphery and appears healing in the center like field fire.

Q11. How does this cancer spread?
Answer: It is a locally malignant tumor that infiltrates the local tissues. It does not spread by lymphatic route and rarely by bloodstream.

Q12. How will you confirm the diagnosis?
Answer: By biopsy.

Q13. What is the microscopic appearance of this cancer?
Answer: It consists of closely packed islands of uniform basophilic epithelial cells disposed in round masses or columns. The peripheral cells are columnar, more deeply staining, and have a palisade arrangement. The central cells are polyhedral. Prickle cells and cell nests are absent.

Q14. How will you treat this case?
Answer: The tumor is excised with a 3- or 4-mm area of histologically tumor-free margin followed by repair.

Q15. How do you treat larger lesions?
Answer: Large cancers, those that invade surrounding structures, and aggressive histological types are treated by surgical excision with 0.5- to 1-cm margin.

Q16. What is Mohs' micrographic excision (MME)?
Answer: It is the technique of excising a tumor close to eyes, nose, or ears to preserve as much tissue as possible with complete removal of tumor.

The procedure is done by a dermatological surgeon along with a histologist. Under local anesthesia, a saucerized excision of the tumor is done and the quadrants of the specimen are mapped with different colors. The excised tissue is studied histologically at the same time. The residual tumor from relevant mapped area is excised and the procedure is repeated until cancer-free margin is achieved all around.

Q17. Is this tumor radiosensitive?
Answer: Yes sir/ma'am.

Q18. Then, why don't you treat this case by radiotherapy?
Answer: This patient can be treated with radiotherapy, but this cancer is not far away from the left eye which may be harmed by radiotherapy.

Q19. What is the role of chemotherapy?
Answer: The chemotherapy has hardly any role in this cancer. However, local 5-FU cream may be tried in small, flat, superficial lesions.

Q20. How does this cancer kill its victim?
Answer: It kills the patient by causing meningitis due to intracranial extension or hemorrhage due to erosion of a large blood vessel.

Q21. What are other methods of treatment of this cancer?
Answer: They include curettage and electrodesiccation, cryosurgery, and laser vaporization.

Q22. What are the results of treatment?
Answer: With adequate treatment, local control rates more than 90% may be obtained.

Sample case 2: ranula of floor of mouth

Kailash, 17-year-old, male, unmarried student, vegetarian, no alcohol, no tobacco, resident of Tanda, Faizabad, presents with swelling in the floor of mouth for 11 months.

The patient was alright 11 months ago when he noted a small swelling in the floor of mouth. Since then it is growing very slowly and painlessly. So far he has not taken any treatment.

There is nothing significant in the past history and family history.

Physical Examination

The general and systemic examinations are within normal limits including pulse 82/minute, blood pressure 118/72 mm Hg, and respiration 18/minute with no anemia and no edema over feet.

The local examination shows a smooth swelling in the floor of the mouth on the right side (Fig. 36.2).

It has a pink bluish color and looks like a frog's belly. It is soft, cystic, sticky, nontender, and brilliantly transilluminant.

Clinical Diagnosis

My clinical diagnosis is ranula of right side of floor of mouth.

Viva Voce

Q1. Why do you say that it is a ranula?
Answer: The reasons for the diagnosis of ranula are:

- The patient is an adolescent person of 17 years of age.
- There is a painless, slow-growing swelling in the floor of mouth, more on one side of midline.
- It is smooth, cystic, nontender, and bluish red in color.
- It is brilliantly transilluminant.

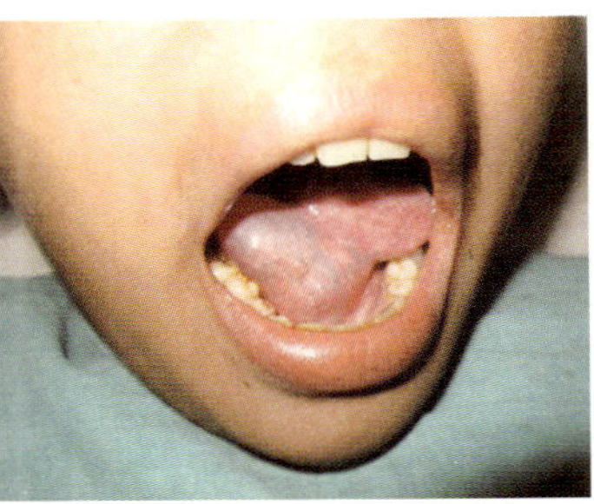

Figure 36.2 Ranula of floor of mouth (R). (Courtesy: Professor Divya Mehrotra)

Q2. What is ranula?

Answer: The term ranula is derived from the Latin word "rana" which means a small frog, as the ranula looks like a frog's belly (soft, bluish, and sticky). Ranula is a cystic swelling of the floor of mouth etiologically related to sublingual salivary gland.

Q3. What is the cause of this cyst?

Answer: It occurs due to slow or chronic extravasation of saliva from the sublingual salivary gland.

Q4. Describe the pathology of ranula.

Answer: It is an ovoid or spherical cyst, 1–5 cm in diameter, and contains viscid or jelly-like fluid. The cyst wall is lined by a layer of macrophages.

Q5. What is a plunging ranula?

Answer: It is a type of ranula having a cervical extension which passes from the floor of mouth to the submandibular region of neck of the same side. It is rare.

Q6. What is the mechanism of formation of a plunging ranula?

Answer: It occurs due to extravasation of saliva from the posterior part of sublingual salivary gland which flows over the posterior border of mylohyoid down in the neck. It may be due to extravasation of saliva from submandibular salivary gland also.

Q7. What are the signs of a plunging ranula?

Answer:

- Apart from the bluish transilluminant swelling of floor of the mouth, there is another swelling in the ipsilateral submandibular region near the angle of mandible.
- The submandibular swelling is smooth, soft, cystic, and nontender.
- Cross-fluctuation is present between oral and cervical swellings.

Q8. What are the investigations that you will do in this case?

Answer: The clinical diagnosis is enough. Hence, apart from routine investigations, no investigation is required.

Q9. Do you know of any specific investigation done in a plunging ranula?

Answer: The full anatomy and the extent of cyst can be visualized by MRI.

Q10. What are the complications of this disease?

Answer: The complications include rupture and reformation, secondary infection, and difficulty in speech, mastication, swallowing, and keeping the mouth closed.

Q11. What is the treatment of this condition?

Answer: The cyst is excised along with the salivary gland from which it is arising.

Q12. What is marsupialization?

Answer: It is another method of treatment in which the top of the cyst is excised and the cut edge of the cyst wall is sutured to the cut edge of the overlying mucosa. Thus, the bottom of the ranula becomes the new floor of the oral cavity.

Q13. What is the treatment of a plunging ranula?

Answer: It is excised completely including the entire sublingual and submandibular salivary glands of that side.

Q14. What are the complications of a plunging ranula excision?

Answer: The complications include injury to hypoglossal nerve and cervical branch of facial nerve, hemorrhage, and recurrence.

Sample case 3: thyroglossal cyst

Kanti, age 21, male, unmarried student, vegetarian, no alcohol, no tobacco, and a resident of Kakori, Lucknow, presents with a swelling in the front of upper neck for 4 years.

The patient was alright 4 years ago when he noted a small swelling in the upper part of front of the neck. It is slowly growing since then without pain. There is no problem with swallowing, speech, and breathing. He has not taken any treatment for it so far.

There is no history of diabetes mellitus, tuberculosis, and venereal disease in the past and in the family.

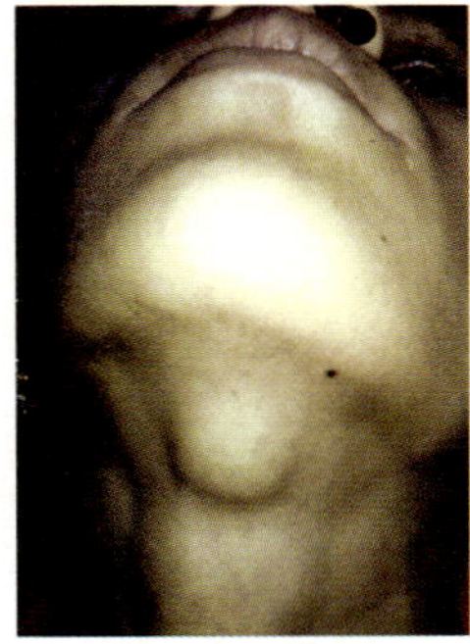

Figure 36.3 Thyroglossal cyst. (Courtesy: Dr. Ravi Mishra)

Physical Examination

- On general examination the patient is not anemic and not jaundiced; there is no cervical lymphadenopathy with normal respiration, pulse, and blood pressure. The systemic examination is within normal limits.
- Local examination
  - *Inspection*
    - Site: A swelling in front of upper neck in midline just above thyroid cartilage a little to the left (Fig. 36.3)
    - Shape: Vertically hemispherical
    - Surface: Smooth
    - Mobility: Moves up with deglutition and protrusion of tongue
  - *Palpation*
- Consistency: Firm but cystic
- Tenderness: Nontender
- Mobility: Mobile from side to side but not vertically up and down
- Translucency: Present
  - *Percussion*: Dull
  - *Auscultation*: Silent

Clinical Diagnosis

My clinical diagnosis is thyroglossal cyst.

Viva Voce

Q1. What are the reasons for making this diagnosis?

Answer: The reasons for making this diagnosis are:

- A young man of 21 years of age is presenting with a painless, slow-growing swelling of 4-year duration.
- It is situated just above the thyroid cartilage in the midline of neck slightly to the left.
- It is vertically ovoid with a smooth surface, nontender, tensely cystic, well defined, and translucent.
- It moves up with deglutition and protrusion of tongue.

Q2. What is a thyroglossal cyst?

Answer: It is a tubulodermoid which arises from the remnants of thyroglossal tract.

Q3. What are the sites of its occurrence?

Answer: It can occur in the midline at the following sites: in front of thyroid cartilage, just below the body of hyoid bone, above the hyoid bone, in the floor of mouth, in front of cricoid cartilage, and in the substance of tongue below the foramen cecum.

Q4. What is the commonest site of occurrence?

Answer: The commonest site of occurrence is just below the hyoid bone a little to the left.

Q5. What is the cause of its movement up with swallowing?

Answer: It is attached to the hyoid bone by fibrous connective tissue and the hyoid bone moves up with deglutition.

Q6. What is the cause of its movement up with protrusion of tongue?

Answer: It moves up with protrusion of tongue as it is attached to the tongue at foramen cecum by obliterated thyroglossal duct.

Q7. What is the cause of this cyst?

Answer: It develops from accumulation of secretion in the unobliterated part of thyroglossal tract.

Q8. Describe the course of thyroglossal tract.

Answer: The thyroglossal tract starts at the foramen cecum of tongue and descends obliquely downwards and forwards through the genioglossi muscles up to the hyoid bone. At the hyoid it may descend in front, through or behind its body and descends up to the upper border of thyroid cartilage and gets attached to isthmus of thyroid gland.

Q9. Describe the gross pathology of the cyst.

Answer: The cyst is ovoid or spherical and variable in size. It contains thick, transparent, jelly-like fluid in which the cholesterol crystals may be present.

Q10. Describe the microscopic appearance.
Answer: It is lined by columnar, cuboidal, or squamous epithelium and surrounded by a layer of lymphoid tissue. It may have small foci of thyroid tissue.

Q11. What are the complications of this cyst?
Answer: The complications include secondary infection leading to abscess formation, rupture with formation of a thyroglossal fistula, and very rarely malignancy.

Q12. What are the investigations that you will do in this case?
Answer: The diagnosis is usually clinical. Hence, apart from routine investigations, no specific investigations are required. However, the diagnosis can be confirmed by:

- Ultrasonography/CT scan of neck
- Radioiodine scintiscan
- Ultrasound-guided needle aspiration

Q13. How do you treat this lesion?
Answer: The cyst is excised completely along with the thyroglossal tract. As the body of hyoid bone may obstruct the complete excision of the tract, it is also excised with the cyst. It is known as Sistrunk's operation.

Q14. What are the complications of this operation?
Answer: The complications of the operation include perforation of larynx, wound infection, infection of cut ends of hyoid bone, and hemorrhage.

Sample case 4: ameloblastoma of mandible

Meraj, 45-year-old, male, married, nonvegetarian, moderate smoker, and resident of Raebareli, presents with swelling of left side of lower jaw near its angle for 3 years.

The patient was alright 3 years ago when he noted gradual painless enlargement of left side of lower jaw (Fig. 36.4). It has never regressed and attained the present size. He has so far not taken any treatment.

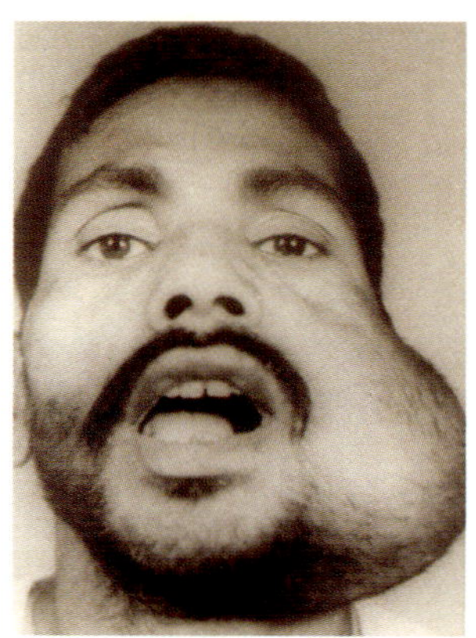

Figure 36.4 Ameloblastoma of mandible near its left angle.

The past history is not suggestive of tuberculosis, diabetes mellitus, and venereal disease.

There is no history of any familial disease or same type of illness in the family.

Physical Examination

The general and systemic examinations are within normal limits including pulse 82/minute regular, blood pressure 122/80 mm Hg, and respiration 16/minute, and no anemia and no edema over feet.

The local examination shows a swelling of lower face of the left side involving the ascending ramus of mandible near its angle.

- Size: 5 × 3 cm
- Shape: Ovoid; bulging only outside, not inside
- Surface: Smooth
- Nontender, firm in consistency with soft areas and disturbed alignment of related teeth on palpation
- Dull on percussion and silent on auscultation

Clinical Diagnosis

My clinical diagnosis is ameloblastoma of ascending ramus of mandible of the left side.

Viva Voce

Q1. What are the reasons for this diagnosis?
Answer: The reasons for making this diagnosis are:

- A 45-year-old patient is presenting with a swelling of mandible of gradual onset.
- The outer table of mandible is expanded, not the inner table.
- The alignment of last molar is disturbed.
- It is firm and nontender with soft areas.
- The regional lymph nodes are not enlarged.

Q2. What is an ameloblastoma?
Answer: It is a tumor of jaw of unknown etiology arising from ameloblasts and characterized by a painless and slow-growing swelling of insidious onset.

Q3. Describe the pathology of this tumor.
Answer: It is a multilocular lesion with loculi lined by tall columnar epithelium. In between the loculi, there are islands of osseous and fibrous tissue.

Q4. What is the nature of this tumor?
Answer: It is a locally malignant tumor.

Q5. What do you mean by a locally malignant tumor?
Answer: A locally malignant tumor infiltrates into the local tissues in the vicinity but does not spread by lymphatic route and bloodstream.

Q6. What investigations will you do in this case?
Answer: The investigations include X-ray of the mandible, orthopantomogram (Fig. 36.5), and biopsy apart from routine investigations.

Q7. What are the radiographic signs of an ameloblastoma?
Answer: The bone is expanded with a radiolucent area which has septa and spaces with smaller spaces or cysts at the periphery (soap-bubble or honeycomb) appearance.

Q8. What are the other causes of soap-bubble appearance on radiography?
Answer: Apart from an ameloblastoma, other causes of soap-bubble appearance are:

- Osteoclastoma (giant cell tumor)
- Brown tumor of hyperparathyroidism
- Giant cell reparative granuloma
- Fibrous dysplasia

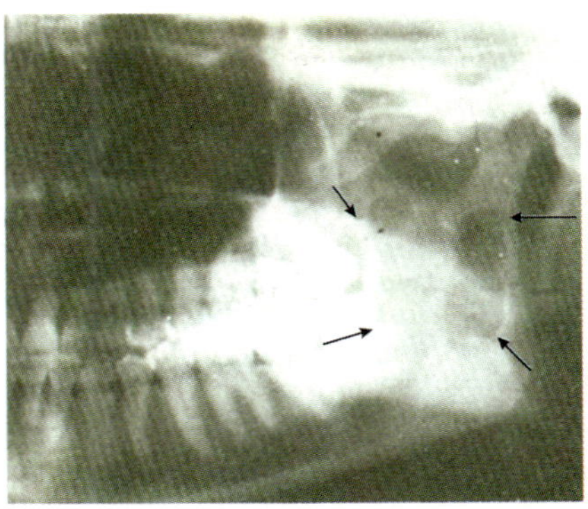

Figure 36.5 Orthopantomogram showing a multiloculated lytic lesion of left ascending ramus of mandible—ameloblastoma. (Courtesy: Professor G.N. Agrawal)

Q9. How will you confirm the diagnosis?
Answer: It is confirmed by biopsy.

Q10. How will you treat this patient?
Answer: The affected segment of the bone will be removed with cancer-free margin of resection along with the soft tissue in the vicinity to extirpate the tumor completely.

Q11. How do you treat an early lesion?
Answer: If the cortical plate is not invaded, subperiosteal excision is done with a margin of up to 1 cm of cancellous bone.

Q12. How will you reconstruct the mandible after resection of horizontal ramus?
Answer: The mandibular defect can be made good by a fibular or iliac crest graft. The help of a plastic and reconstructive surgeon is usually required.

Q13. What is the aim of reconstruction of an alveolar ridge?
Answer: It is reconstructed for the purposes of wearing an artificial denture or doing teeth implantation.

Q14. What is the role of radiotherapy?
Answer: It has no role as this tumor is not sensitive to radiotherapy.

Q15. What is the role of anticancer drugs?
Answer: They do not have any role.

Q16. What is the prognosis?
Answer: The results of treatment are good but the follow-up must be done for a long period of time as recurrence can occur up to 20 years or more.

Sample case 5: oral leukoplakia

Rais Ahmad, 47-year-old, male, married, painter, nonvegetarian, chewing tobacco for 23 years, and resident of Nakkhas, Lucknow, complains of a whitish patch inside left cheek for 6 months and slight burning sensation for 15 days. The patient was alright 6 months ago when he noted a whitish patch in his left cheek which could not be removed by washing or rubbing. It increased in size very slowly and attained the present size. For the past 15 days, there is slight burning sensation which increases at the time of eating. He has not taken any treatment so far.

There is no past history and family history suggestive of tuberculosis, venereal disease, diabetes mellitus and similar illness.

Physical Examination

The **general** and **systemic examinations** are within normal limits including pulse 78/minute, blood pressure 116/74 mm Hg, respiration 18/minute, mild anemia, and no edema over feet.

The local examination shows a white patch in the left cheek near the commissure 3 × 2 cm in size (Fig. 36.6). The right angle of lips also shows early changes (angular stomatitis).

- Irregular in shape
- Slightly elevated from surface
- Feels dry and nontender on palpation, and cannot be rubbed off

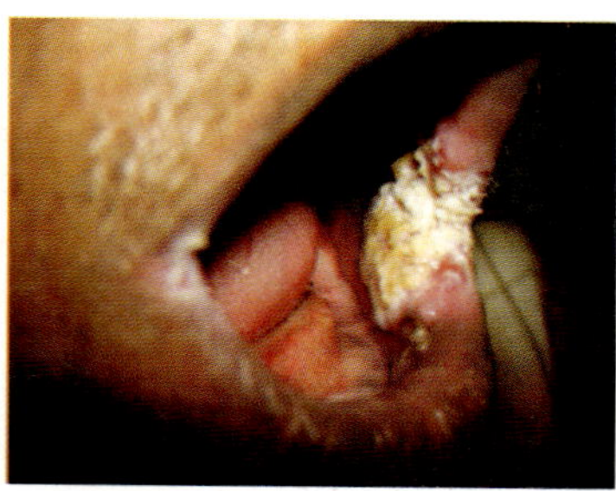

Figure 36.6 Leukoplakia of left cheek undergoing malignant change. The right angle of lips also has some changes. (Courtesy: Professor Surajit Bhattacharya)

Clinical Diagnosis

My clinical diagnosis is leukoplakia of left cheek.

Viva Voce

Q1. What are the reasons for making this diagnosis?

Answer: The reasons are:

- A middle-aged male, tobacco chewer for 23 years, is having a whitish patch in the left cheek.
- It is slightly elevated and feels rough and dry.
- It is irregular and cannot be rubbed off.

Q2. What is leukoplakia?

Answer: It is thickening of mucosa of various surfaces which looks like a patch of old white paint which cannot be rubbed off.

Q3. What is its etiology?

Answer: The risk factors include:

- Tobacco chewing and smoking
- Chronic alcoholism
- Repeated trauma, for example, due to sharp tooth
- Syphilis, chronic sepsis
- Spices

Q4. What are the sites of occurrence in the oral cavity?

Answer: It can occur anywhere in the oral cavity including cheek, lower buccogingival sulcus, tongue, alveolar ridge, palate, and lips.

Q5. Which is the commonest site in the oral cavity?

Answer: The commonest site in the oral cavity is cheek, especially the lower buccogingival sulcus.

Q6. Describe the macropathology of this lesion.

Answer: It has two main features:

1. Cracked white paint appearance due to areas of grayish white plaques of abnormal keratinizing epithelium
2. Raw beef appearance of the areas where the plaques are shed

Q7. What is the microscopic appearance?

Answer: The epithelium is markedly thickened with hyperplasia and all degrees of cellular atypia ranging from mild dysplasia to carcinoma in situ.

Q8. What are the types of leukoplakia?
Answer: The leukoplakia is of following types:

- Homogeneous leukoplakia
- Nonhomogeneous leukoplakia
- Verrucous leukoplakia
- Speckled leukoplakia
- Nodular leukoplakia

Q9. What are the complications of leukoplakia?
Answer: The main complication is malignant transformation.

Q10. What is the nature of malignant transformation?
Answer: Squamous cell carcinoma.

Q11. What are the investigations that you will do in this problem?
Answer: The main investigation is biopsy. The other investigations include serological tests for syphilis and routine investigations.

Q12. How do you treat this problem?
Answer: The principles of treatment include:

- Remove the causative factor—no tobacco and no paan masala chewing, no smoking, no alcohol, and no spices.
- Treat or correct dental problems, for example, rounding off the sharp edges and points of teeth, crowning of decayed teeth, and correction of ill-fitting denture.
- β-Carotene may be taken as it may cause some regression.
- Small lesions may be treated by cryosurgery. Large dysplastic lesions are excised and the raw area may be skin grafted or covered by Prolene mesh (temporary cover till mucosa grows underneath).

Q13. Can you treat this lesion by radiotherapy?
Answer: No. It may promote early malignant change.

Q14. How will you differentiate it from oral candidiasis?
Answer: The differences between these two diseases are described in Table 36.1.

Table 36.1 Differences between leukoplakia and oral candidiasis

Features	Leukoplakia of oral cavity	Oral candidiasis
Wiping off the lesion	Cannot be wiped off	Can be wiped off
Occurrence	• Middle-aged people • Chronic tobacco and paan masala chewers	• Children • Immunocompromised people, for example, AIDS, cancer patients on chemotherapy and/or radiotherapy

KEY POINTS

- The clinical cases, their diagnosis and treatment, are best learnt by attending the clinics in the outpatients and inpatients of the hospital.
- Listen to your patient attentively and inspect the lesion carefully so that you will be able to make a diagnosis in most of the patients.
- Whatever you see in the hospital, read; and whatever you read in your room, see in the hospital (try to find it in the hospital). This is the only method of learning clinical sciences.
- The final result of the examination mainly depends on how you have done your clinical cases. Hence, work and prepare accordingly.

Surgical Instruments

37

Introduction

Every specialty in surgery has its own variety of instruments, and each with its own specific structure and function. Sushruta (600 BC) wrote about the requirements of a surgical instrument:

> समाहितानी यंत्राणि खरश्लक्ष्ण मुखानि च।
> सुदृढाणि सुरूपाणि सुग्रहाणि च कारयेत।। सु.सं., सू.स्था. 7/9

An instrument should be sharp with smooth jaws and should be appropriate for the job it is meant. It should be strong, good looking and should have an easy and comfortable grip.

Although the instruments have changed markedly from the very crude to very fine pieces of art, the requirements of an instrument have not changed very much.

In the practical examination, usually three common instruments are given to be identified and queried. The instrument should be seen carefully and held in the hand as if to be used but one should avoid playing with it. Now the examinee tells about the instrument under the heads described in Box 37.1.

Box 37.1 Description of the instrument

- Name of instrument, for example, hemostat, needle holder, dissecting forceps
- Anatomy or structure—main structural features
- Use or uses
- Method of sterilization

Most of the time, this description satisfies the examiner and he/she may not ask any questions or he/she may probe the candidate deeper for giving "Distinction" or "Honour."

1. COMMON SURGICAL INSTRUMENTS

Cheatle's forceps

Structure It is a long instrument that has two blunt-nosed flat blades. The closed instrument has a beak-like tip. It is bent downwards at the joint. It has no ratchet; one finger grip is like a ring and the other curved like a U (Fig. 37.1).

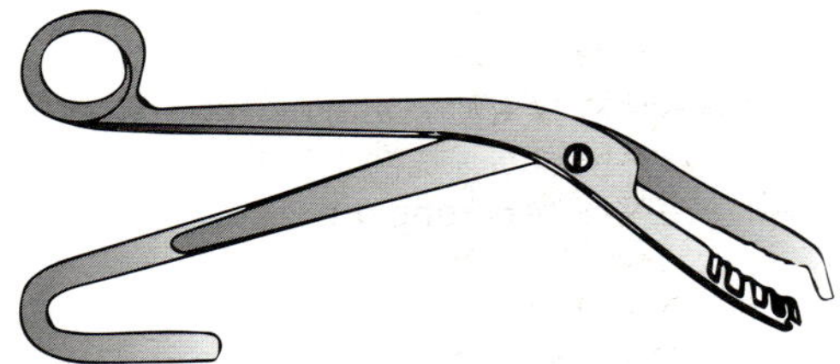

Figure 37.1 Cheatle's forceps.

Uses It is used to pick up sterile instruments and drapes from the drum and to arrange them on the instrument trolley.

Sterilization It is sterilized by autoclaving it from time to time. It is stored vertically in a large bottle with the blades immersed in antiseptic solution ready for use anytime. The antiseptic solution is changed once in 24 hours.

Sponge or swab-holding forceps

Structure It has two blades joined together by a joint nearly in the middle, and a ratchet near the handle. The operating ends are longitudinally oval with fenestration and serrations for a firm grip (Fig. 37.2).

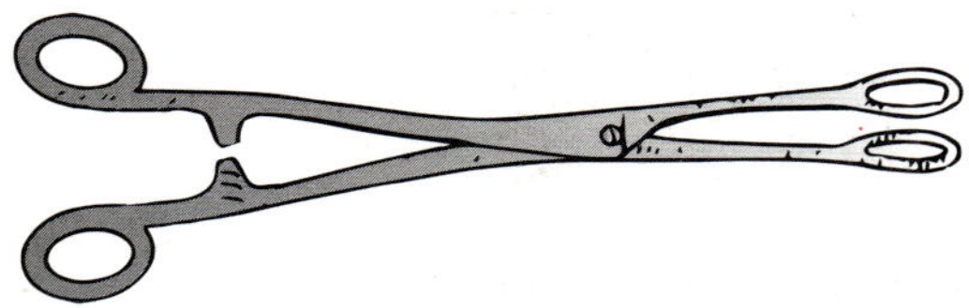

Figure 37.2 Sponge or swab-holding forceps for part preparation.

Uses It is used to hold a swab or gauze to do cleaning and part preparation, hold gallbladder and such structures for dissection, and mop and press a bleeding area in depth.

Sterilization It is sterilized by autoclaving.

Towel clip

Structure Two types of towel clip are available:

1. **Doyen's towel clip**: It has two blades joined together at one end with spring action. The fixing end has two sharp-pointed claws which open when the blades are pressed together and close when the pressure is released (Fig. 37.3).

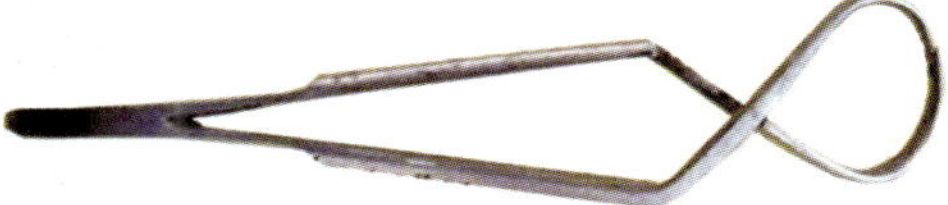

Figure 37.3 Doyen's towel clip.

2. **Mayo's towel clip**: It has two arms joined together at a screw joint. It has claw-like jaws at one end which close when the handles are brought together and has a ratchet arrangement to lock the jaws in closed position (Fig. 37.4).

Uses The towel clips are used:

- To fix sterile drapes in position
- To fix suction tube, diathermy wire, and laparoscopic cables on the operating table
- Commonly to fix ribs in flail chest

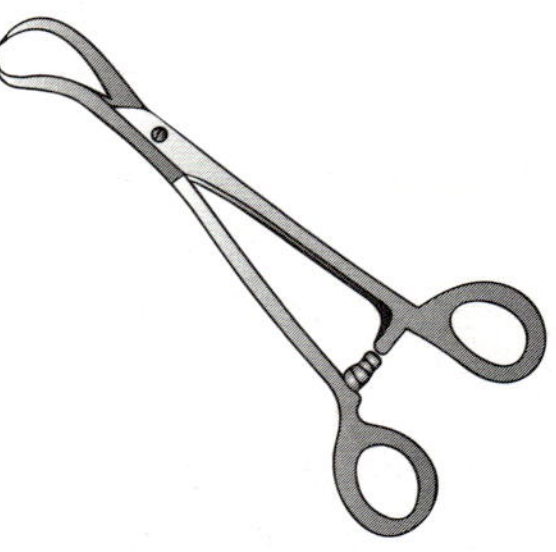

Figure 37.4 Mayo's towel clip.

Sterilization They are sterilized by autoclaving.

Scalpel: Bard-Parker knife with disposable blades

Handle

- **Structure**: It is a flat rod-like structure with serrations in the middle for better grip. Near the tip, it has a narrowed portion with a grove on its edge to hold the blade.
- **Uses**: A smaller handle (3) is used for holding smaller blades, no. 11, 12, and 15; and a larger handle (4) is used for holding larger blades, no. 21, 22, and 23.
- **Sterilization**: It is sterilized by autoclaving (Fig. 37.5).

Blades

- **Uses**: No. 11 blade is used for making stab incisions and no. 15 blade is used for giving incisions in pediatric and plastic surgical procedures.

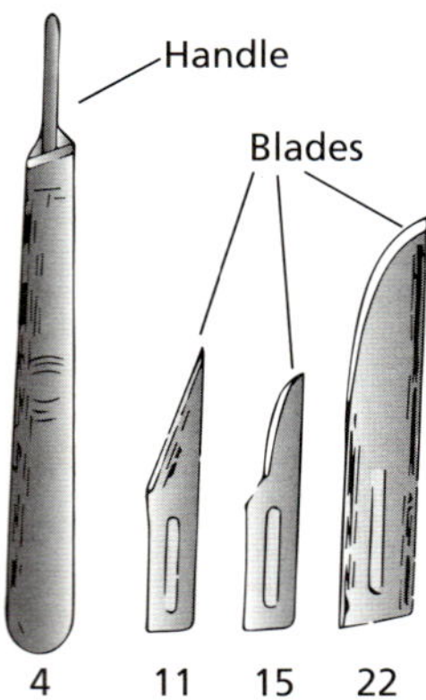

Figure 37.5 Bard-Parker knife—handle and commonly used detachable blades.

- **Sterilization**: They are sterilized by gamma radiation.

Table 37.1 shows types of blades and handles on which they fit.

Hemostat (artery forceps)

Structure It is one of the commonest instruments used during operations. It is of many types depending on its size (small, medium, or large) and shape (straight or curved) (Fig. 37.6). Some common types of hemostats are:

- **Mosquito forceps**: The name is given to this instrument as it is so fine as to be able to catch the proboscis of a mosquito. They are delicate, fine, and short instruments.
- **Kelly's hemostat**: It is the most commonly used artery forceps. It is medium sized and has half serrated jaws.
- **Kocher's clamp**: It has transverse serrations and teeth near the tip. One tooth is present one jaw and two on the other for better grip.

A good hemostat does not allow one to see through the approximated blades on locking the first step of the ratchet, and there is no separation of tips when the ratchet is fully closed.

Uses A hemostat is used for a variety of functions; the most common use is to stop bleeding by catching bleeding vessels; that is why it is called hemostat. The other functions include opening fascial planes, passing a ligature, and holding fascia, peritoneum, stay sutures, and a gauze piece as peanut.

Sterilization It is sterilized by autoclaving.

Table 37.1 Types of blade, handle, and their uses

Blade no.	Handle no.	Uses
10	3/5	Stab incision, pediatric surgery
11	3/5	Stab incision, operations in adults
12	3/5	Tonsillectomy, cardiovascular surgery
15	3/5	Plastic and pediatric surgery
21	4	Skin incisions
23	4	Skin incisions

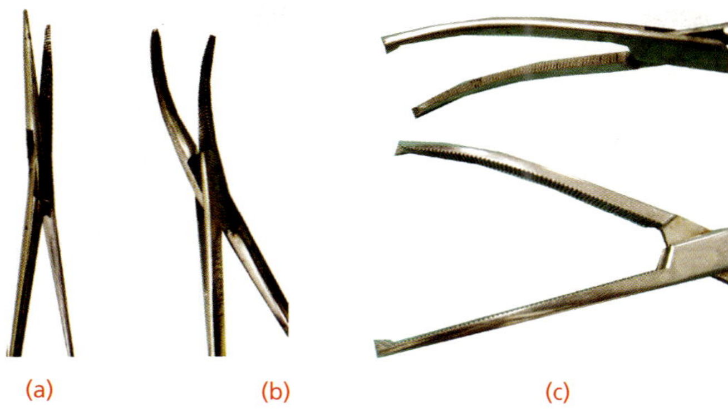

Figure 37.6 Common hemostats. (a) Fine straight hemostat (mosquito artery forceps); (b) fine curved hemostat (mosquito artery forceps); (c) opened jaws of Kocher's artery forceps.

Scissors

Structure The scissors is a sharp cutting instrument which divides the tissues by holding them in between its sharp-edged blades coming together (Fig. 37.7). The blades are joined together by a joint. They are small, medium, or large, straight or curved, narrow-bladed or wide-bladed, sharp pointed or blunt-pointed depending on the operative requirement. Two common types of scissors are:

1. **Metzenbaum scissors**: It is a small, curved-on-flat, blunt-nosed scissors used for fine dissection. Very fine scissors are available for microsurgery, and long and delicate scissors for endoscopic operations.

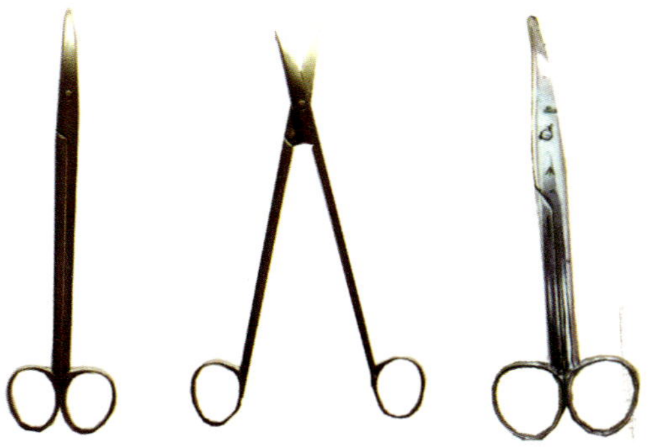

Figure 37.7 Blunt-nosed curved-on-flat scissors for dissection.

2. **Lister's scissors**: It is a stout scissors having two limbs joined together by a screw joint. The lower blade has an olivary tip which prevents damage to the skin when it is inserted under the bandage to cut it (Fig. 37.8). It is used to cut tied bandage during dressing.

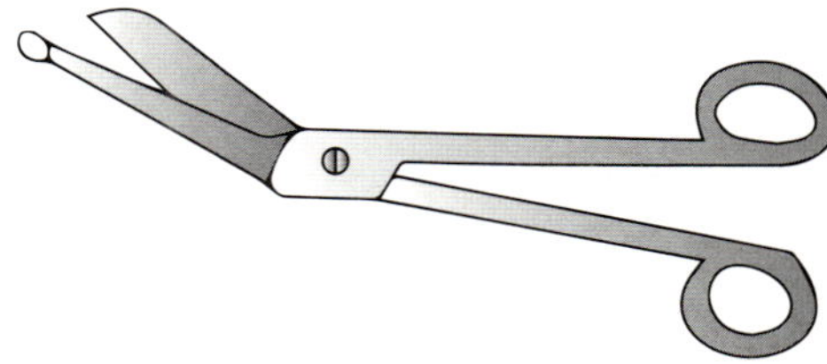

Figure 37.8 Lister's scissors.

Uses Curved-blunt pointed scissors are used for dissection by division of connective tissue and by insertion of closed scissors into tissue planes and then opening the blades.

Sterilization It is sterilized by chemical method (glutaraldehyde, Lysol).

Dissecting forceps

Structure It is one of the commonest instruments which is used nearly in every operation. It has two blades joined together at one end having spring action. On the outer surface of blades nearly in the

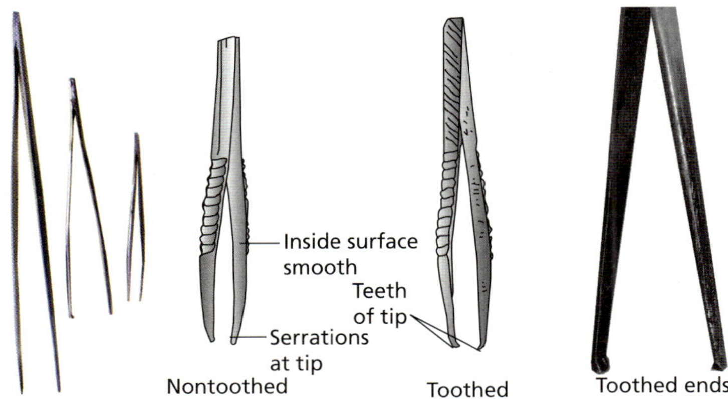

Figure 37.9 Dissecting forceps of various types.

middle, there are serrations for slipless grip. It is of three types:

1. Dissecting forceps without teeth have serrations on the inner aspect of tips for slipless grip.
2. Dissecting forceps with teeth have teeth inside the tips for firm slipless catch (Fig. 37.9).
3. Adson's dissecting forceps are also fine forceps which are used in plastic surgery work (Fig. 37.10).

Uses They are used to hold the tissues for dissection and suturing, and also for suture removal.

Sterilization It is sterilized by autoclaving.

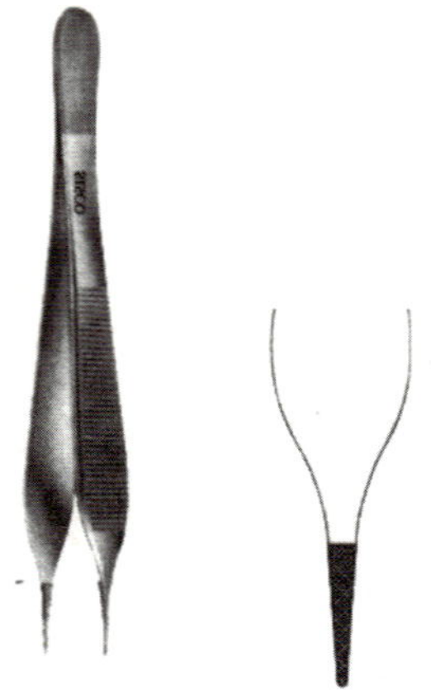

Figure 37.10 Adson's dissecting forceps.

Allis tissue holding forceps

Structure It has two limbs joined together nearly in the middle at a box joint. It has ring-like finger grips for catching, a ratchet for locking and tips which are flattened, curved inwards a little, and fine teeth on distal edge for slipless grip on the structure held (Fig. 37.11).

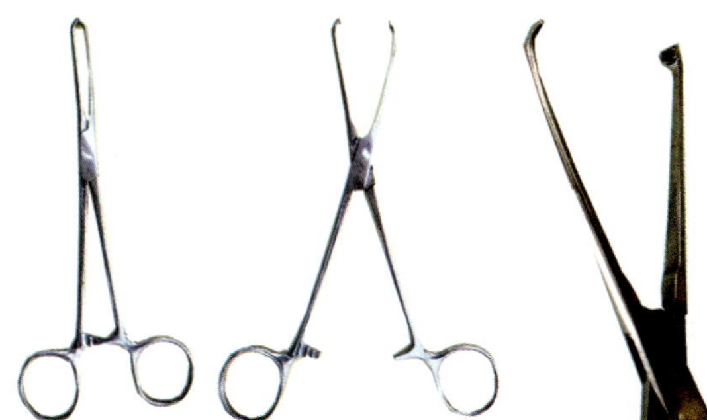

Figure 37.11 Allis tissue forceps with closed/open jaws.

Uses It is used to hold fascia, aponeurosis, capsules of different structures, and many other things.

Sterilization It is sterilized by autoclaving.

Babcock's tissue forceps

Structure It has two thin limbs having two ring-like finger catches at one end, a ratchet

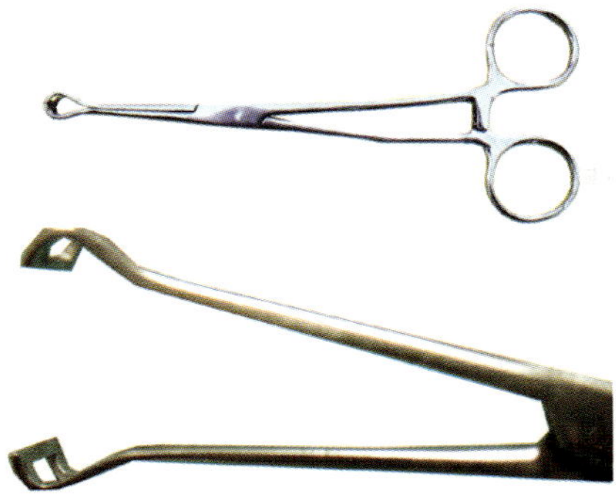

Figure 37.12 Babcock's tissue forceps.

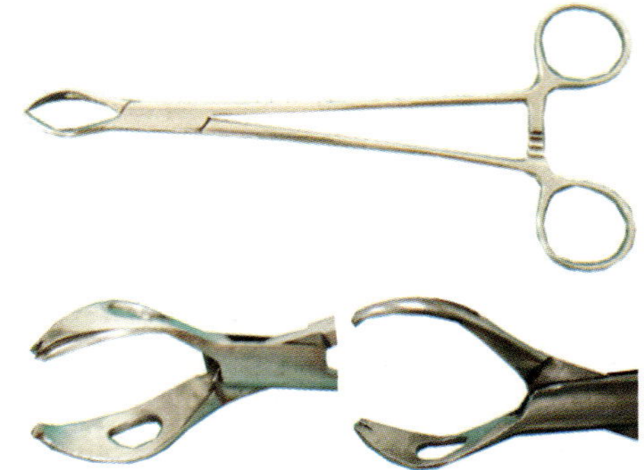

Figure 37.13 Lane's tissue forceps.

at the handles for locking at one end, a joint nearly in the middle, and fenestrated triangular curved blades at the other end. Each blade has a transverse bar at the tip with fine transverse serrations (Fig. 37.12).

Uses It is a nontraumatic tissue holding forceps for holding delicate soft tissues, for example, thyroid and lymph nodes.

Sterilization It is sterilized by autoclaving.

Lane's tissue forceps

Structure It is a strong instrument that has two limbs joined together by a screw joint near its one end. It has two ring-like finger grips at handles, a ratchet, and two curved and fenestrated blades with one-in-two fine teeth at the tip for a secure grip of structures. The hollow between the blades allows the structures to hold without crushing them (Fig. 37.13).

Uses It is a strong instrument to hold and pull the tissues during dissection, for example, fascia and aponeurosis. It may be used as a towel clip.

Sterilization It is sterilized by autoclaving.

A Lane's tissue forceps should be differentiated from a Babcock's tissue forceps. Their differences are described in Table 37.2.

Retractors

Structure These instruments are used to separate and displace the edges and angles of wound and contained structures to the sides to see and work in the depth. Depending on the method of holding, the retractors may be handheld (e.g., single hook retractor, Czerny's retractor, Morris' retractor) or self-retaining (e.g., mastoid retractor, Davis mouth gag). A retractor has to be selected depending on the size and depth of wound and

Table 37.2 Differences between Lane's tissue forceps and Babcock's tissue forceps

Features	Lane's tissue forceps	Babcock's tissue forceps
Overall nature	Heavy, strong, and crude	Light, delicate, and fine
Uses	For holding and pulling crude and strong tissues/structures	For holding and pulling delicate tissues/structures
Jaws	Closed jaws have a long oval space between them	Closed jaws have a near circular space between them
Tip	One tooth on one blade and two teeth on the other to fit into each other	Fine shallow transverse grooves on both blades which fit into each other when the jaws are closed

the nature of operation. The retractors are of many types:

- **Single hook retractor**: It is a simple, flat, rod-like instrument having a handle and a blunt-pointed hook at the using end (Fig. 37.14).

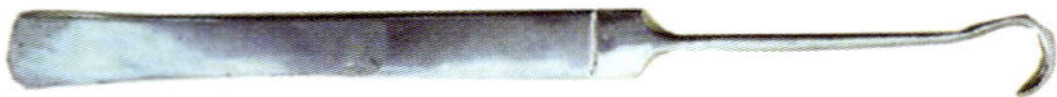

Figure 37.14 Single hook retractor.

- **Double hook retractor**: It has two blunt-pointed hooks at the using end (Fig. 37.15).

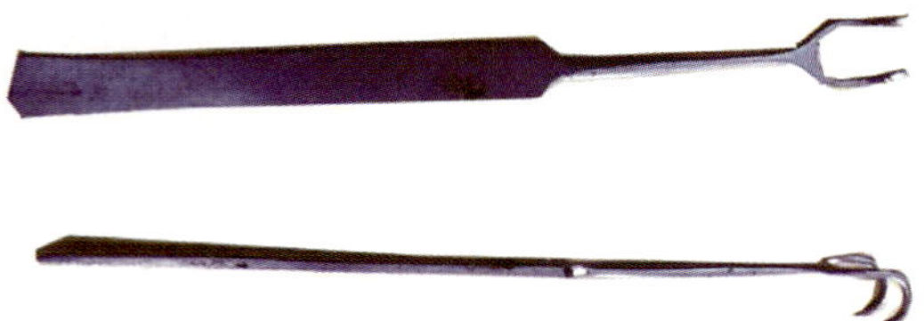

Figure 37.15 Double hook retractor.

- **Cat's paw retractor**: Here the retracting end has many sharp-pointed hooks like a claw or a cat's paw. It is used in scalp operations (Fig. 37.16).

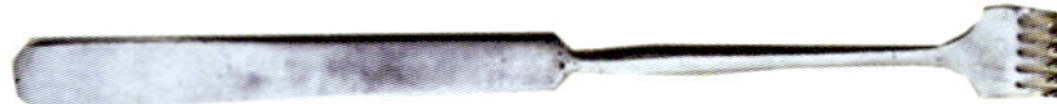

Figure 37.16 Cat's paw retractor.

- **Langenbeck retractor**: It has one narrow and long, flat blade for retraction. It is used in many operations of neck including thyroidectomy (Fig. 37.17).

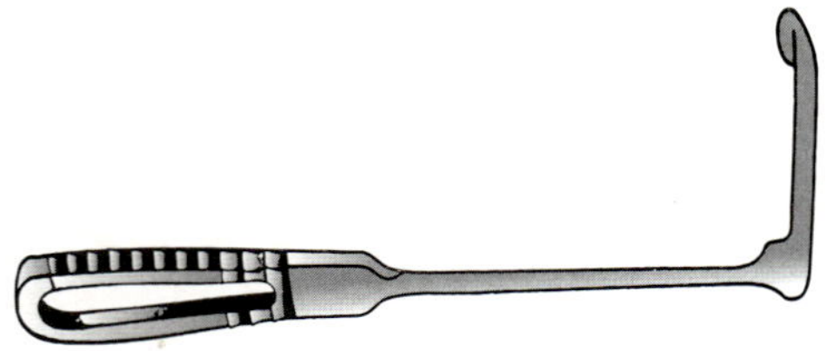

Figure 37.17 Langenbeck retractor.

- **Czerny's retractor**: It is somewhat larger than a Langenbeck retractor. It has a double hooked shape at one end and a single hooked flat blade at the other end with both the ends pointing in opposite directions like "Z" (Fig. 37.18). It is used in many operations of average depth in neck and other places, for example, tracheostomy and inguinal hernioplasty.

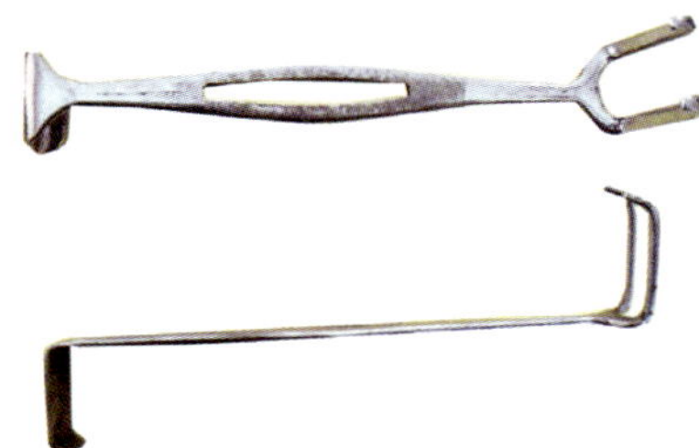

Figure 37.18 Czerny's retractor.

- **Joll's thyroid retractor**: It is a self-retaining retractor consisting of two Doyen's towel clips joined together to make a U-shaped structure. It has got a straight rod-like separator between its two ends near the base of U. It is used to decrease or increase the distance between the towel clips (Fig. 37.19).

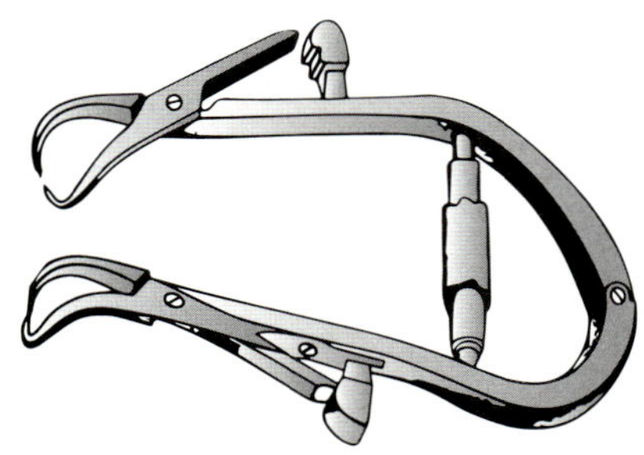

Figure 37.19 Joll's thyroid retractor.

Uses It is used as a self-retaining retractor to retract the skin flaps held in the towel clips during operations on thyroid. Two retractors are used, one on each side.

Sterilization All the retractors are sterilized by autoclaving.

Needle holder

Structure It is a stout and strong instrument having two short blades joined together by a box or screw joint. They have grooves and serrations to firmly grip and hold a stitching needle. The handles have ring-like finger grips and a ratchet (Fig. 37.20).

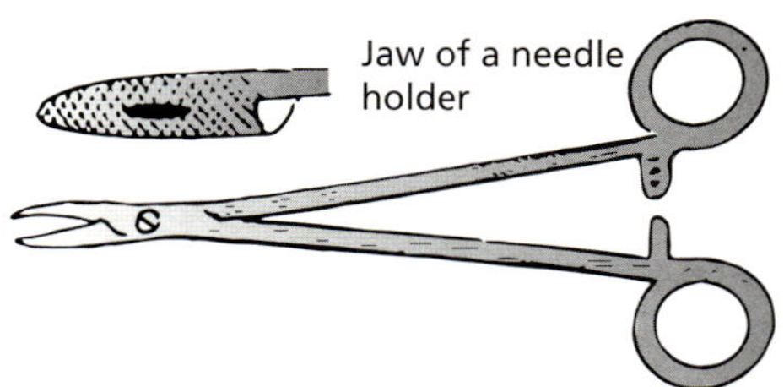

Figure 37.20 Needle holder.

Uses It is used to hold a suturing needle with good grip and control. The needle is usually caught at the junction of proximal two-third and distal one-third of the jaws.

Sterilization It is sterilized by autoclaving.

Sinus forceps

Structure It is a long, slender instrument having two blades joined together nearly in the middle by a screw joint. The name is given to this instrument as it is commonly used for dressing a sinus. There is no ratchet on the handles. It has olivary tips with transverse serrations on inner side (Fig. 37.21).

Uses It is used for dressing and packing a wound or a sinus. It is also used to drain an abscess by Hilton's method to break up the septa.

Sterilization It is sterilized by autoclaving.

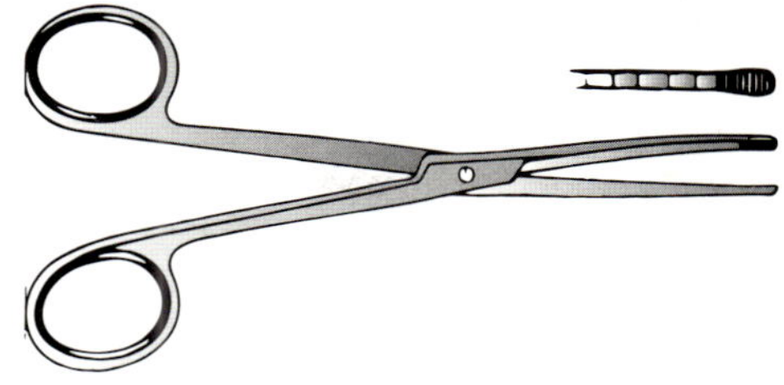

Figure 37.21 Lister's sinus forceps.

Suction tip

Structure It is a long tubular instrument which is suitably curved to one side and has a stout handle in the middle. It has a blunt cap with small holes screwed at one end for sucking in the operative wound. The other end of this tubular structure is connected by a rubber tube to the suction machine (Fig. 37.22).

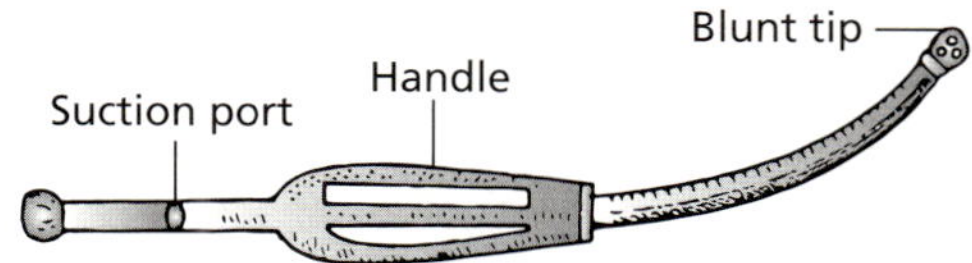

Figure 37.22 Suction tip.

Many other types of suction tips are available depending on the operative requirements.

Uses It is used to suck blood pus, smoke, and other fluids from the operative field to keep the wound clean and field clear.

Sterilization It is sterilized by autoclaving.

2. COMMON BONE INSTRUMENTS

Farabeuf's raspatory (rugine)

Structure It is a strong, and stout instrument with a long, flat, ovoid handle with a flat disc-like finger rest having serrations near its tip. The tip is curved on flat and has a sharp cutting edge (Fig. 37.23).

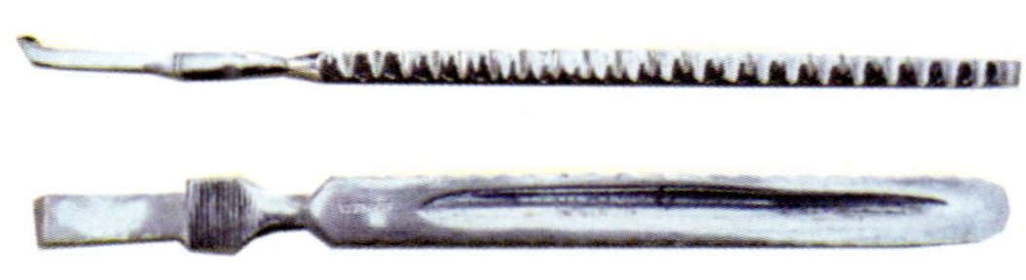

Figure 37.23 Farabeuf's raspatory.

Uses It is used for elevating or stripping the periosteum with its muscular attachments from the bone.

Sterilization It is sterilized by chemical means.

Chisel

Structure It is a strong instrument with a thick polygonal handle with a capped end for striking. The distal half is thin and rectangular in shape and has a cutting edge in the end which is beveled on one side (Fig. 37.24).

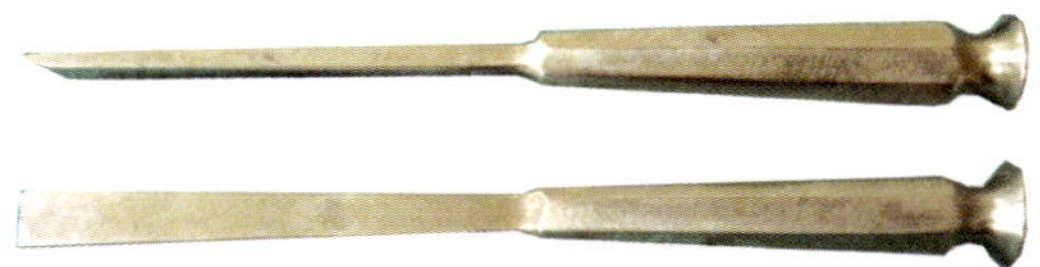

Figure 37.24 Chisel.

Uses It is used for cutting away the bone. The beveled surface should lie on the bone surface and the head is struck with a mallet and the bone is cut away.

Sterilization It is sterilized by chemical means (glutaraldehyde, Lysol).

Osteotome

Structure It is just like a chisel and has a thick polygonal handle with a capped end for striking. The distal half is thin and rectangular in shape. It has a cutting edge in the end which is beveled on both sides and beveling is gradual and not abrupt (Fig. 37.25).

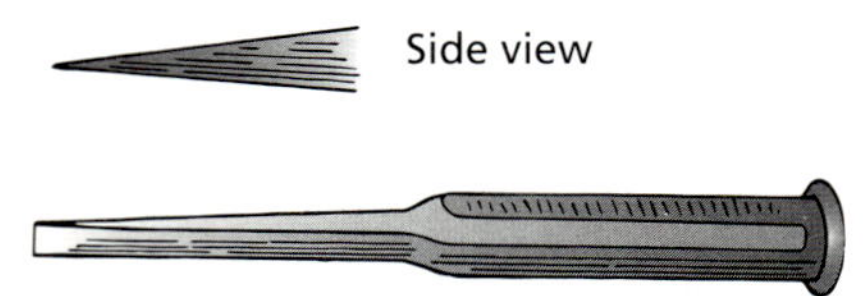

Figure 37.25 Osteotome.

Uses It is used for dividing a bone (osteotomy) in situ.

Sterilization It is sterilized by chemical means.

Bone gouge

Structure Similar to a chisel, it has got a thick, stout, polygonal handle with a capped end. The distal part is thin, flat blade which is concave at one side and has a sharp cutting end (Fig. 37.26).

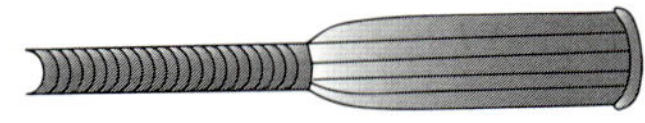

Figure 37.26 Bone gouge.

Uses It is used for making smooth rounded cavities inside a bone (saucerization) and to take bone chips for grafting.

Sterilization It is sterilized by chemical means (glutaraldehyde or Lysol).

Sequestrectomy forceps

Structure It is a strong, stout instrument having two limbs joined together by a screw joint. The jaws are small, strong, and serrated. The handles are large, curved with convexity, and grooves outside. There is no ratchet on the handle (Fig. 37.27).

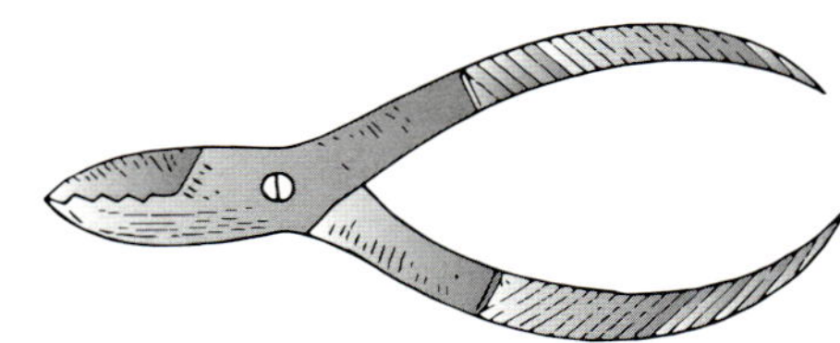

Figure 37.27 Sequestrectomy forceps.

Uses It is used for removing or to pull out a sequestrum from inside a bone.

Sterilization It is sterilized by autoclaving.

Fergusson's lion toothed forceps

Structure It is a very strong, long forceps with jaws having concavity inside. It has two series of teeth near the tip, to give the appearance of a lion's mouth. The handles are curved with outside convexity, have grooves or serrations for a firm grip, and have no ratchet (Fig. 37.28).

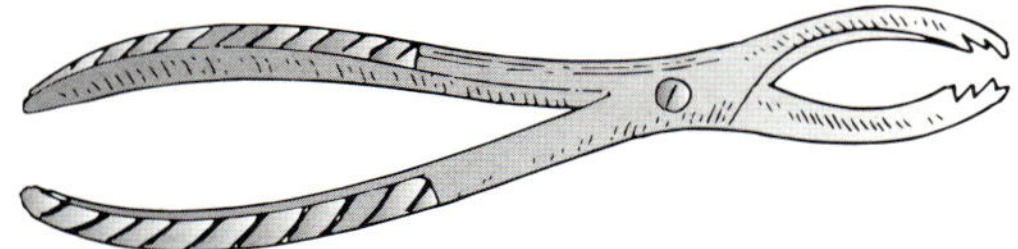

Figure 37.28 Fergusson's lion toothed forceps.

Uses It is used for holding and stabilizing the bone during operations.

Sterilization It is sterilized by autoclaving.

Bone cutting forceps

Structure It is a strong forceps with two limbs joined together by a screw joint. The jaws are short and have cutting edges to cut a bone. The handles are long, curved with convexity outside and have no ratchet (Fig. 37.29).

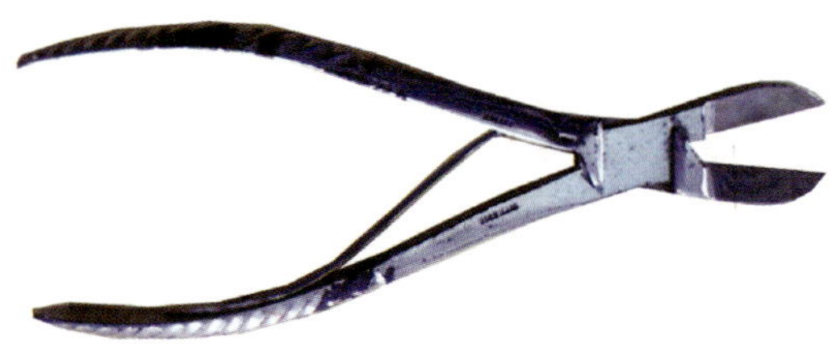

Figure 37.29 Bone cutting forceps.

Use It is used for cutting bones.

Sterilization It is sterilized by chemical means.

Gouge forceps (bone nibbler)

Structure It is a strong forceps having two limbs joined together at a screw joint. The jaws are small and have cupped sharp edge at the tip. The handles are curved and grooved with convexity outside. There is a spring lever in between the handles which opens the forceps when the pressure is released from the handles (Fig. 37.30).

Uses It is used for nibbling the bone for removing the angles and spikes to make the surface smooth and to give shape to the bone.

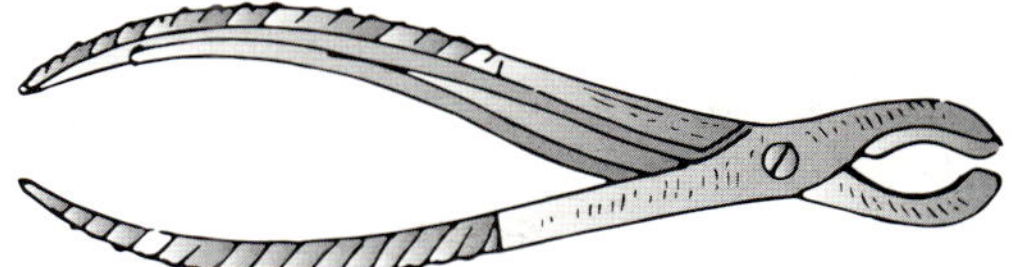

Figure 37.30 Bone gouge forceps.

Sterilization It is sterilized by chemical means.

Gigli wire saw with handles

Structure The wire saw consists of strands of stainless steel twisted together. It is made rough by a series of small bristles on the sides. There are two handles which are small steel rods with a hook in the middle that are connected to the ends of the wire saw. It has a guide to protect the neighboring soft tissues from injury when the wire is being introduced and moved for cutting (Fig. 37.31).

Uses It is used for cutting a bone by rapid side-to-side movements by rubbing during some bone operations, for example, hemimandibulectomy.

Sterilization It is sterilized by chemical means.

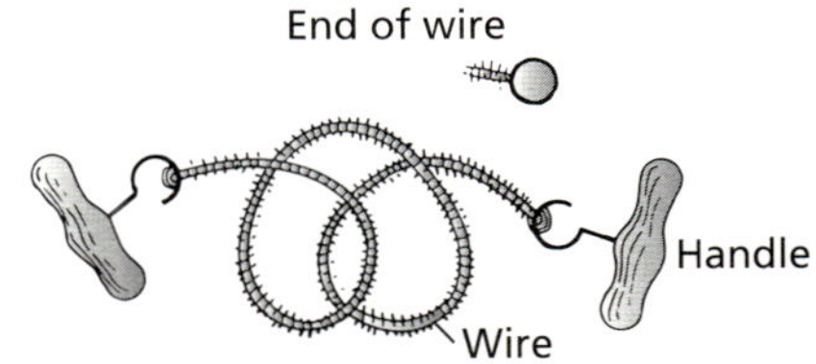

Figure 37.31 Gigli wire saw with handles.

Volkmann's scraping spoon

Structure It is a strong rod-like instrument which is wider in the middle for holding. Both ends are ovoid and small cup-like with a sharp edge (Fig. 37.32).

Use It is used for scraping granulation and necrotic tissue.

Sterilization It is sterilized by chemical means.

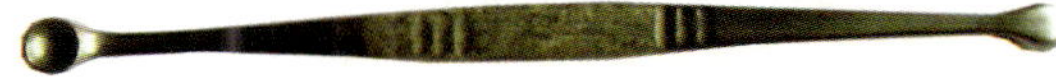

Figure 37.32 Volkmann's scraping spoon.

3. INSTRUMENTS USED IN ORAL SURGERY

Mouth gag (Doyen's)

Structure It has two blades joined together on a joint which is of the type that on approximation of handles the jaws separate out. The handles have finger grips and a long ratchet with many steps. It has broad tooth plates on each blade with serrations to permit a secure grip on the teeth (Fig. 37.33).

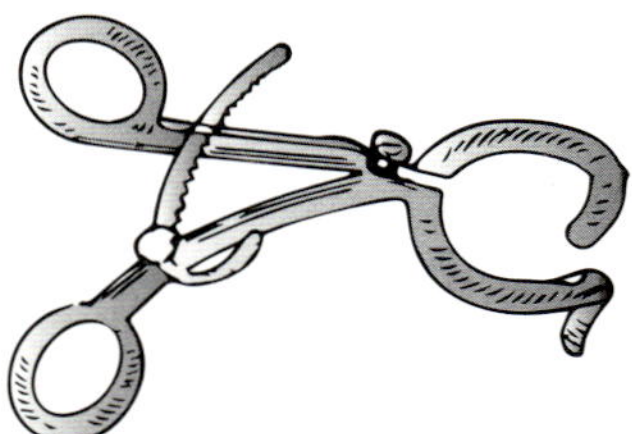

Figure 37.33 Doyen's mouth gag.

Use It is used to open the oral cavity wide by opening the jaws for doing intraoral surgery, for example, tooth extraction under general anesthesia and tonsillectomy.

Sterilization It is sterilized by autoclaving.

Tongue depressor

Structure It is a flat plate of steel which is either short and straight (Fig. 37.34a) or long and right angled in the middle (Fig. 37.34b). The ends are rounded and the edges are blunt and smooth (Fig. 37.34).

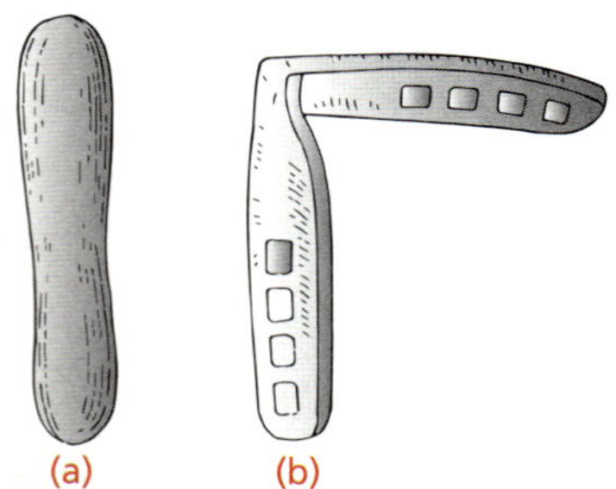

Figure 37.34 Two types of tongue depressor: (a) straight and (b) right angled.

Uses It is used for examination of oral cavity and oropharynx. It is also used in many operative procedures in the oral cavity, for example, drainage of quinsy or retropharyngeal abscess.

Sterilization It is sterilized by autoclaving.

Cheek retractor

Structure It is a small instrument made up of thick metal sheet and has a handle and semicircular curved retracting end whose edges are curled in such a manner that the inner grooved surface takes in the angle of mouth and adjacent portions of lip and cheek. The handle is curved and grooved and has a blunt end (Fig. 37.35).

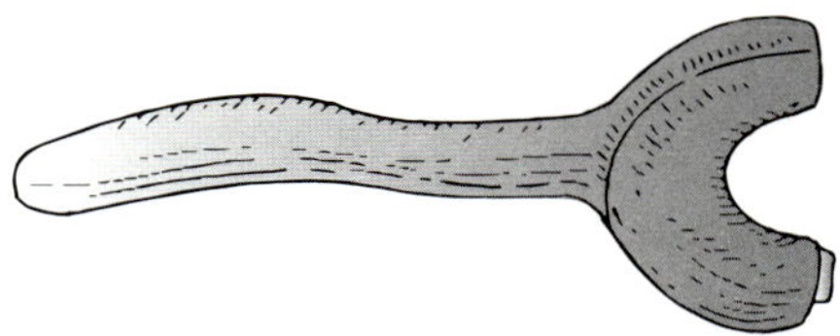

Figure 37.35 Cheek retractor.

Use It is used to open the oral cavity on sides for intraoral operations, for example, interdental wiring, excision of an epulis, and other operations on teeth and alveolus.

Sterilization It is sterilized by autoclaving.

Tongue forceps

Structure It has two limbs joined together by a joint. The jaws have short biconvex blades with fenestrated rounded tips which have oblique serrations on inner surface. A ratchet catch on the handles achieves a secure grip on the tongue (Fig. 37.36).

Uses

- To pull the tongue out in an unconscious patient to relieve airway obstruction

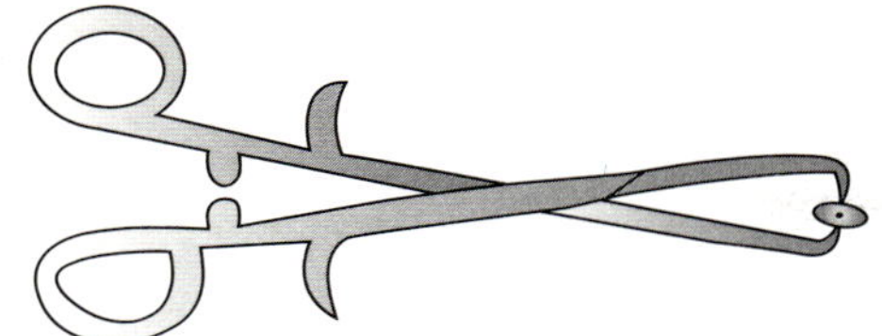

Figure 37.36 Tongue forceps.

- To pull and stabilize the tongue for repair of its lacerations or to do partial glossectomy
- To lift and retract the tongue up for operations on the floor of mouth, for example, excision of ranula and removal of a submandibular stone

Precaution The part of the tongue held by the forceps may undergo pressure necrosis if used for a long time. This may be avoided by releasing the forceps at short intervals and applying it at different places. Other methods of holding the tongue include towel clip and stay sutures.

Sterilization It is sterilized by autoclaving.

Dental extraction forceps

Structure They have suitably curved blades for different teeth. Their handles are stout, slightly convex outside, and serrated to provide a secure grip. There are separate forceps for the upper molars, right and left. All other forceps can be used on either side. The beak of molar forceps is always on the outside where it fits between the two buckle roots (Fig. 37.37).

Uses These forceps are used for extraction of teeth.

Sterilization It is sterilized by autoclaving.

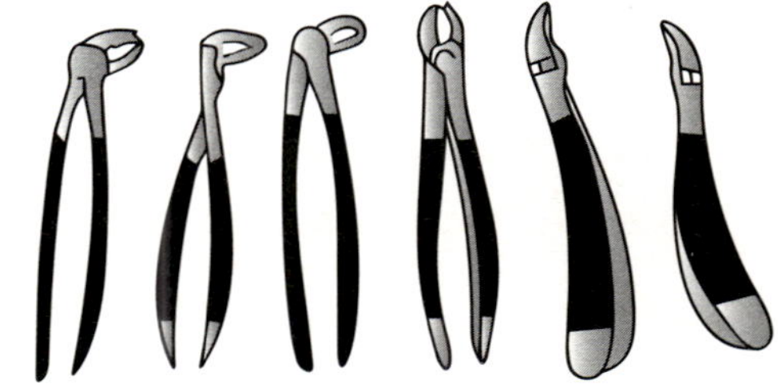

Figure 37.37 Dental extraction forceps of various types.

4. TRACHEOSTOMY INSTRUMENTS

Cricoid hook

Structure It has a broad, flat handle like a single hook retractor with a sharp-pointed hook at the operating end (Fig. 37.38).

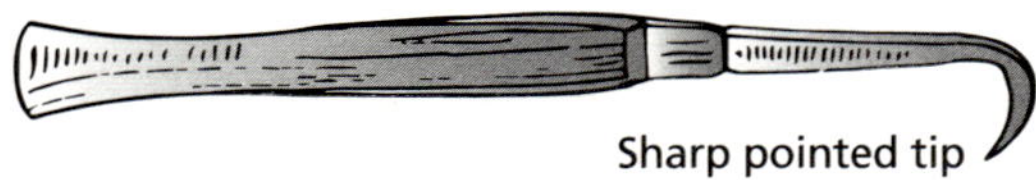

Figure 37.38 Cricoid hook.

Use It is employed to stabilize the trachea by hooking and holding cricoid up during tracheostomy.

Sterilization It is sterilized by autoclaving.

Tracheal dilator

Structure It has two arms joined together at a joint. The jaws are curved down on flat and have olivary ends. The handles have no lock. When the handles are brought together, the jaws open. There is a spring lever between the jaws near the handles which keeps the instrument closed when not in use (Fig. 37.39).

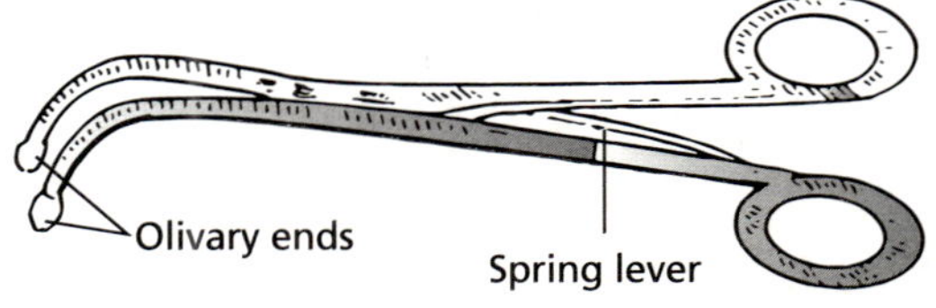

Figure 37.39 Tracheal dilator.

Uses It is used to open the tracheostomy wound for insertion of the tracheostomy tube into the trachea.

Sterilization It is sterilized by autoclaving.

Metal tracheostomy tube

Structure It consists of two tubes telescoped into each other. The inner tube is short and the outer a little long. It is curved on flat. The outer tube is the sheath which retains the inner tube which is breathing tube. The outer end is expanded and has an arrangement for fixing the tube in the neck. When the inner tube is blocked by encrustation of secretions, it is taken out and reinserted after cleaning (Fig. 37.40).

Uses It is used for tracheostomy.

Sterilization It is sterilized by autoclaving.

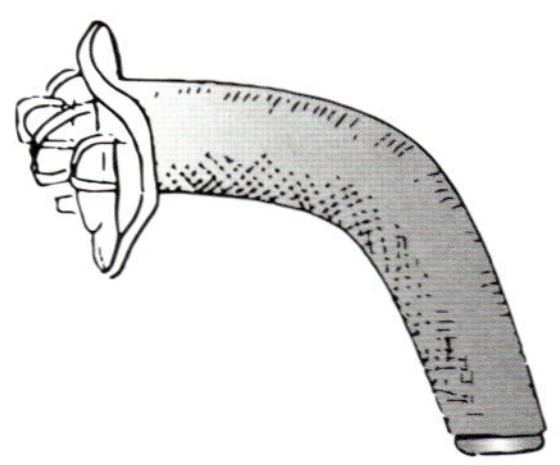

Figure 37.40 Metal tracheostomy tube.

5. ANESTHESIA AND ENDOTRACHEAL EQUIPMENT

Face mask

Structure It is made of rubber (opaque) or plastic (translucent). It has a body which is manipulable or can be molded to fit on the nose and mouth. The rim of the mask (seal) prevents escape of gases between the face and the mask. There is a connector (orifice) at the top of the mask by which it is connected to the breathing system. It may have retaining hooks for fixing the mask on the face (Fig. 37.41).

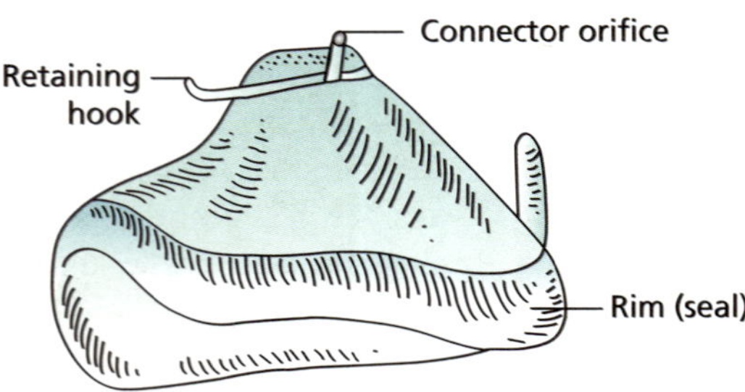

Figure 37.41 Face mask for giving oxygen.

Uses It is used to administer anesthetic gases from the breathing system without introducing a device or tube into the trachea.

Sterilization It is sterilized by chemical means.

Airway

Structure It is made of metal, plastic, or elastomeric material. It is a flat curved tube with a flange at the outer end to prevent the tube slipping lower down into the pharynx. Next to the flange is the bite part of the airway which is straight and fits in between the lips and the teeth. The next is the curved part which is so shaped as to fit on the convexity of tongue.

Uses It is used to maintain the patency of oropharyngeal airway. It also facilitates the suction of oropharynx.

Laryngoscope

Structure It has a handle and a blade joined together at a separable right-angled hinge joint. The handle is a cylindrical tube that contains batteries. The blade may be curved or straight and is available in many different sizes. It has a base, tongue, flange, web, tip, and socket for bearing a small bulb. The tongue is the main

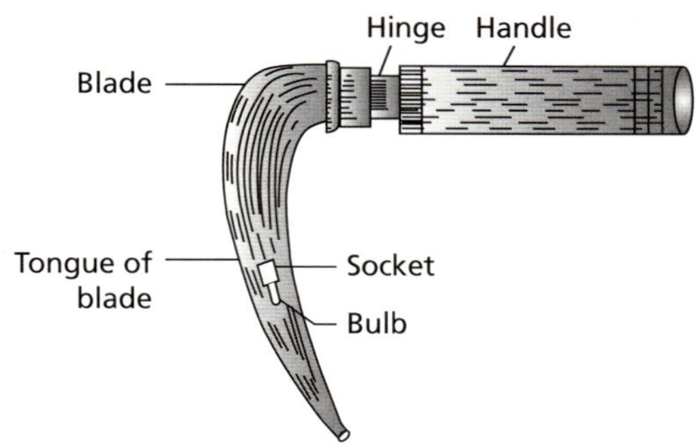

Figure 37.42 Laryngoscope with curved blade used for endotracheal intubation.

component of blade which is used to depress and manipulate the tongue to see the opening of larynx (Fig. 37.42).

Uses It is used to examine oropharyngeal airway and to pass an endotracheal tube.

Sterilization The blade is sterilized by autoclaving.

Magill's forceps

Structure It is a long and thin forceps joined together with a joint nearly in the middle. The handles have finger rings but no ratchet. This forceps has a peculiar bend nearly in its middle so that when the held object in its jaws is taken down, the handles do not obstruct the field of vision. The tips are ovoid, fenestrated, and serrated (Fig. 37.43).

Uses It is used for introducing the endotracheal tube into the larynx. It may be used for removing foreign bodies from oropharynx.

Sterilization It is sterilized by autoclaving.

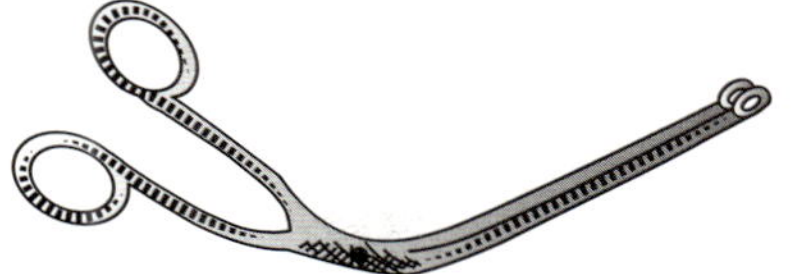

Figure 37.43 Magill's forceps for directing the endotracheal tube into trachea.

Endotracheal tubes

Structure Many types and sizes of endotracheal tubes are available. They are made of rubber, polythene, silicon rubber, or Teflon. They are curved to fit into the anatomy of upper airway. The lower end of the tube is beveled to make it pass easily through the vocal cord slit and to reduce the chances of its obstruction. The tube may be plain or cuffed.

- A cuffed tube has a cuff of 3–4 mL just above its distal end. It communicates with a very thin inflating tube that runs in or with the wall of the tube to communicate with a small pilot balloon. The outer end of the tube has a lid to occlude its opening after the cuff and the pilot balloon are inflated. It is done to occlude the space between the tube and the trachea (Fig. 37.44).
- A plain tube does not have a cuff.

Uses It is used for passing into the trachea to help in breathing and to give endotracheal anesthesia.

Sterilization They are sterilized by gamma irradiation.

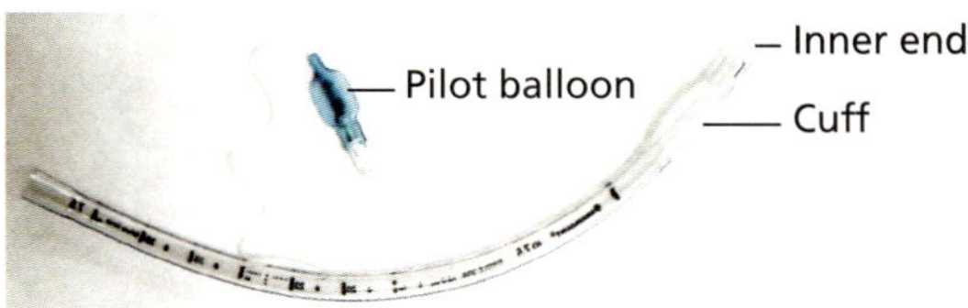

Figure 37.44 Endotracheal tube.

6. OTHER INSTRUMENTS

Kocher's gland holding forceps

Structure It is a long, relatively light instrument having two limbs joined together by a joint. The handles have ring-like catches with a ratchet just above them. The other end of the blades is ring-like, having two hooks each which are directed inwards (Fig. 37.45).

Uses This forceps is used for holding thyroid and lymph nodes during excision.

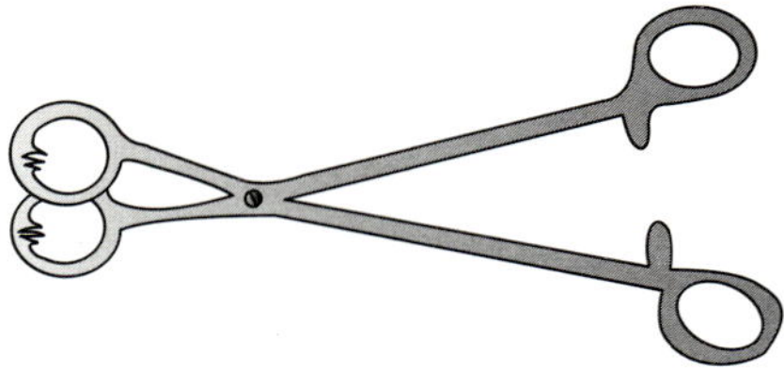

Figure 37.45 Kocher's gland holding forceps.

Sterilization It is sterilized by autoclaving.

Kocher's thyroid dissector

Structure It is a flat instrument that has a long and stout handle roughened by serration. The distal half or operating part is long, narrow, grooved, and somewhat curved. It is blunt tipped and has an eye in the end (Fig. 37.46).

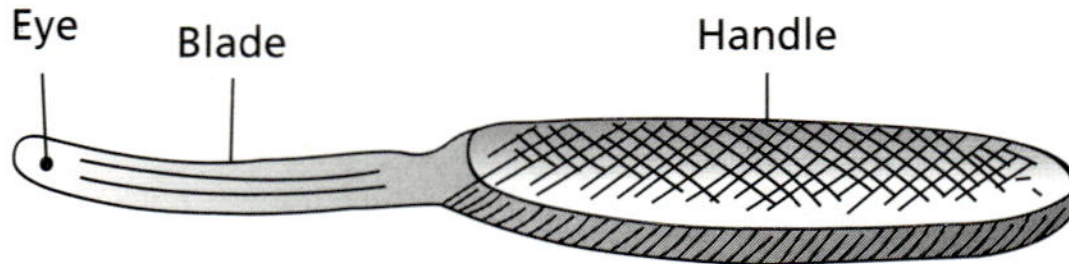

Figure 37.46 Kocher's thyroid dissector.

Uses It helps in dissection of upper pole of thyroid and in separating the isthmus from trachea. It is used for ligation of superior thyroid pedicle.

Sterilization It is sterilized by autoclaving.

Humby's knife with blade

Structure It has a strong handle with a sheath at the other end to hold a long, flat, disposable blade with one sharp edge. It has a screw each at either end of blade holding part which helps in taking the desired thickness of the graft (Fig. 37.47).

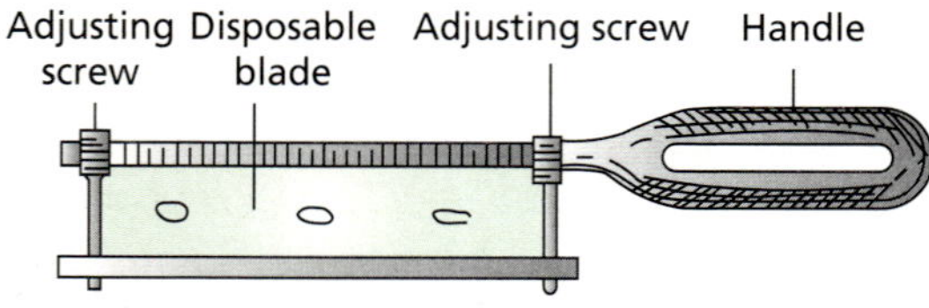

Figure 37.47 Humby's skin grafting knife.

Uses It is the commonest instrument which is used for taking split-thickness or partial-thickness skin grafts.

Sterilization The handle is sterilized by autoclaving and the blade by gamma radiation (and for second use by storing the blade in Lysol).

Aneurysm needle

Structure It is a long instrument with a flat handle. The other end is thin, solid, tubular structure which is curved with a blunt tip and an eye (Fig. 37.48).

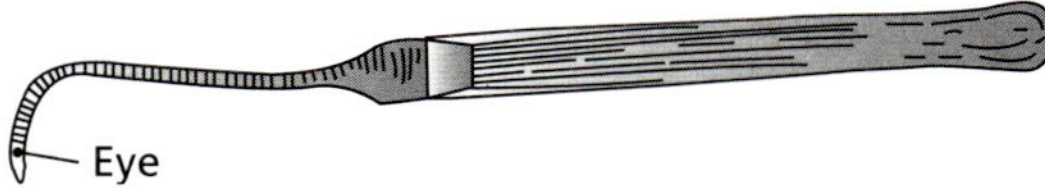

Figure 37.48 Aneurysm needle.

Uses It is used for ligation of a vessel before division by helping in passing a ligature around the vessel.

Sterilization It is sterilized by autoclaving.

Trocar and cannula

Structure It has two parts assembled together; the outer sheath is hollow and known as cannula and used for draining pathological fluids and the inner is a longer, solid tube called trocar. It has a sharp pyramidal point at one end for puncture. The other end is expanded and has a round end for holding (Fig. 37.49).

Uses It is used for draining fluid from closed cystic collections.

Sterilization Cannula is sterilized by autoclaving and trocar by storing in Lysol.

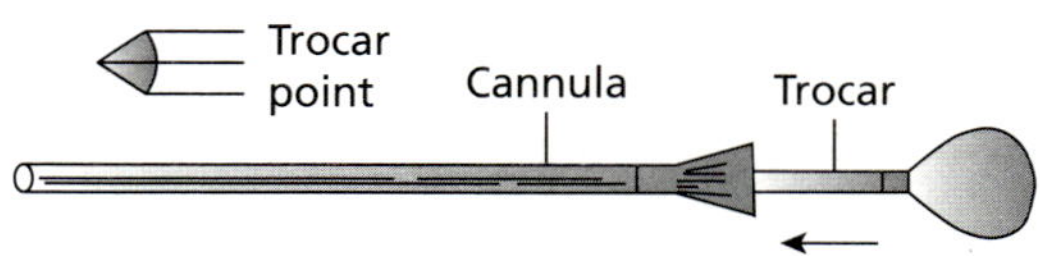

Figure 37.49 Trocar and cannula.

7. RUBBER/POLYTHENE INSTRUMENTS

Plain urethral catheter

Structure It is a straight, long tube of different thicknesses which is open at both ends. It may be made of latex, polythene, or silicon. The inner end is oval or rounded and the outer end is expanded to be fitted to a reservoir bag (Fig. 37.50).

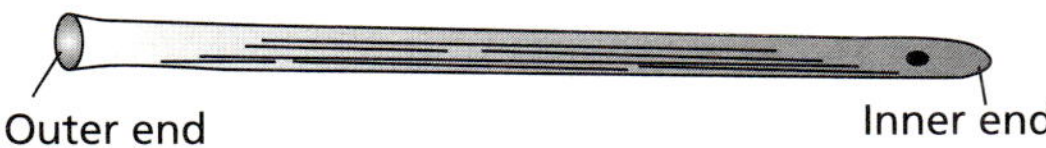

Figure 37.50 Plain urethral catheter.

Uses It is used for many purposes but the commonest use is for evacuating urine from distended bladder. Other uses include giving oxygen and doing suction.

Sterilization It is sterilized by gamma radiation.

Foley's self-retaining catheter

Structure It is a small tube made of latex with silicon coating available in many sizes. Its tip is oval with two subterminal side holes. It has two channels—one large central channel for draining urine and one small side channel embedded in the catheter wall connected to a small balloon around the catheter near its internal end. The outer end is Y-shaped showing both the channels separately (Fig. 37.51).

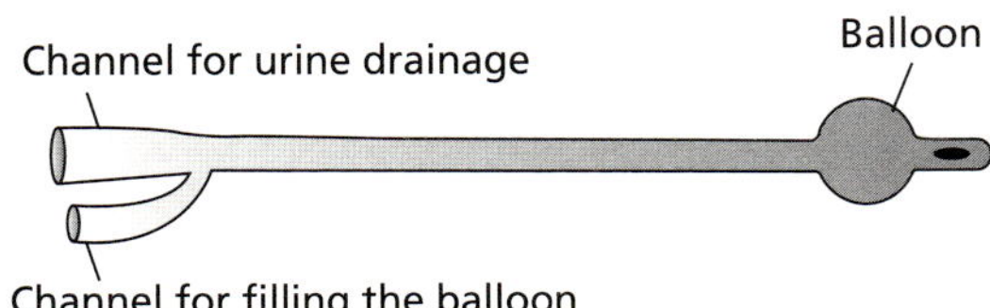

Figure 37.51 Foley's catheter.

Use It is used for long-term drainage of urinary bladder. After passing it in the bladder, the balloon is inflated with distilled water so that the catheter becomes self-retaining and cannot be pulled out.

Precaution Ordinary water or saline should not be used to distend the balloon as the crystals of the salts contained in water and saline may obstruct the fine tube connected to the balloon.

Sterilization It is sterilized by gamma radiation.

Ryle's tube

Structure It is a long, thin tube made of polythene or Portex. It is available in 5–24 FG sizes. Its tip is oval and contains a lead shot to make the tip a little heavy and radio-opaque. There are many subterminal openings on the sides of tube. It has three markings on its surface at 40, 50, and 57 cm; the first indicates the position of tip at cardia, the second in the body of stomach, and the third at pylorus, after tube is inserted in the stomach (Fig. 37.52).

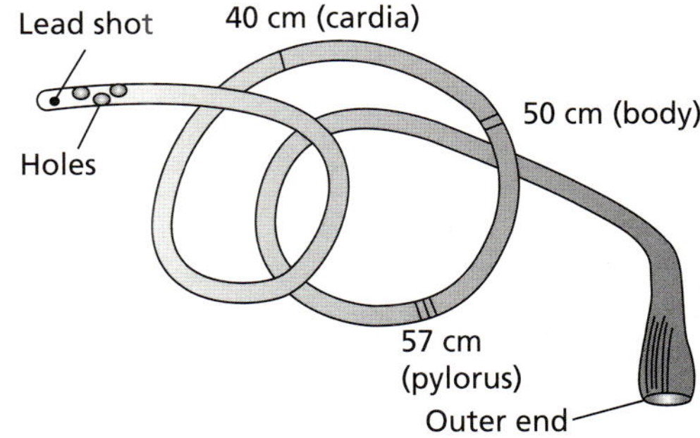

Figure 37.52 Ryle's tube for nasogastric intubation.

Uses It is the commonest tube to be passed in the stomach for diagnostic and therapeutic purposes, for example, gastric aspiration and tube feeding.

Corrugated drain

Structure It is like a sheet made of rubber or polythene that has corrugations on both sides for drainage (Fig. 37.53).

Figure 37.53 Corrugated sheet drain.

Uses It is used for drainage of an operative wound, for example, a thyroidectomy and a parotidectomy wound. Now it is less commonly used as closed system of drainage is being employed more and more.

Sterilization It is sterilized by gamma radiation.

Example of viva voce on a surgical instrument: hemostat

Examiner: See this instrument and tell me its name.

Candidate: It is a straight hemostat.

Viva Voce

Q1. Why do you say it is a hemostat?
Answer: The reasons are:

- It has two limbs joined together by a joint where the limbs cross each other.
- The part proximal to the joint, that is, ringed handles, has a ratchet for locking.
- The part distal to the joint has two jaws or blades having transverse serrations for slipless grip.

Q2. What are the uses of this instrument?
Answer: This instrument is used:

- For catching bleeding points and vessels
- For catching a vessel before it is divided and ligated
- For holding cut edges of fascia and sheaths for dissection, stay sutures, and small rounded swabs (pea nuts) for dissection
- As a substitute for other instruments when they are not available, for example, a needle holder and dressing forceps

Q3. How do you differentiate it from a needle holder?
Answer: A needle holder is a heavier and stronger instrument with smaller jaws having serrations and groove for a firm grip on the stitching needle.

Q4. How do you differentiate it from a sinus forceps?
Answer: A sinus forceps has olivary tipped jaws with a few serrations and no ratchet at the handles.

Q5. Why is it called hemostat?
Answer: It is called hemostat as it is used for stopping bleeding, that is, hemostasis, by catching bleeding points or vessels before division and ligation.

Q6. What is an artery forceps?
Answer: A hemostat was previously called artery forceps, but as it is used to catch both arterial and venous bleeding points, hemostat is a more appropriate name.

Q7. How does a hemostat achieve hemostasis?
Answer: A hemostat achieves hemostasis by the following mechanisms:

- Compression of bleeding point or vessel in the jaws of the instrument
- Crushing of vessel wall with curling in of intima to plug the lumen
- Helping in electrocoagulation of small bleeding points and ligation of large vessels

Q8. What is the purpose of serrations inside the jaws?
Answer: They are present for slipless grip of the bleeding point.

Q9. What are the disadvantages of serrations?
Answer: They may retain tissue debris and clots inside and make the cleaning process of instrument difficult.

Q10. How do you sterilize it?
Answer: It is done by autoclaving.

Q11. How do you autoclave the instruments?
Answer: They are put in autoclave in a drum and treated by steam under 20 lb pressure at 120°C for half an hour.

Q12. Why don't you sterilize it by boiling?
Answer: The boiling does not kill the spores of bacteria and repeated boiling leads to deposition of salts dissolved in water on the instrument.

(There can be many more questions but all the questions are not asked because of time limitation.)

KEY POINTS

- Surgical instruments are the essential basic requirement for doing operative work.
- They are classified into many types, for example, sharp cutting or pointed instruments such as knives, scissors, suturing needles; holding and catching instruments such as hemostat, needle holder, dissecting forceps; retracting instruments such as single hook retractor, Czerney's retractor; bone instruments such as chisel, osteotome, bone cutting forceps; and rubber or plastic goods such as catheter, endotracheal tube.
- Sterilized instruments are used in all operations. The cutting and sharp pointed instruments are sterilized by storing them in Lysol or glutaraldehyde. The blunt instruments are sterilized by autoclaving.
- The basic instruments required for an operation include a knife, scissors, hemostats, retractors, suturing needles, suture material, needle holder, and dissecting forceps.
- The instruments must be counted before and after an operation.

SELF-ASSESSMENT

Long answer questions

1. What is a hemostat? Describe its common types including their structure and function.
2. Give some examples of cutting and puncturing instruments. How do you sterilize them? Describe a Bard-Parker knife, its handle and commonly used detachable blades.

Short answer questions

1. Kocher's artery forceps
2. Mouth gag
3. Bone gouge
4. Needle holder
5. Sinus forceps
6. Towel clip

Multiple choice questions

1. How do you sterilize a hemostat?
   (a) By boiling
   (b) By autoclaving
   (c) By storing in Lysol
   (d) By gamma irradiation
2. An artery forceps is used for, except
   (a) Stopping bleeding by catching bleeders
   (b) Holding stay sutures
   (c) Elevating periosteum
   (d) Dissection of tissue planes by opening its jaws
3. A towel clip is sterilized by
   (a) By autoclaving
   (b) By boiling
   (c) By storing in Lysol
   (d) By gamma irradiation
4. What is false amongst the following with respect to Bard-Parker knife with disposable blades?
   (a) Handle sterilized by autoclaving
   (b) Handle sterilized by boiling
   (c) Blade sterilized by gamma irradiation
   (d) It is used for making incisions

Answers:
1. (b) 2. (c) 3. (a) 4. (b)

Suture Materials and Suturing Techniques

38

Introduction

Suturing of a wound/wounds is an important final step of all operations and also in the management of traumatic wounds. Hence, suturing materials and suturing technique are being described in this chapter.

Armamentarium

Four things are required for suturing a wound—stitching needles, needle holder, dissecting forceps, and suturing material. The needle holder and dissecting forceps have been described in Chapter 37, *Surgical Instruments*. This chapter describes the stitching needles, suturing materials, and suturing technique.

Suturing needles

A large variety of suturing needles are available, the selection of which depends on the type of tissue to be stitched. A needle of appropriate shape and size needs to be selected for least traumatic passage through the tissues. Some of the needle types (Fig. 38.1) are described in the subsequent text.

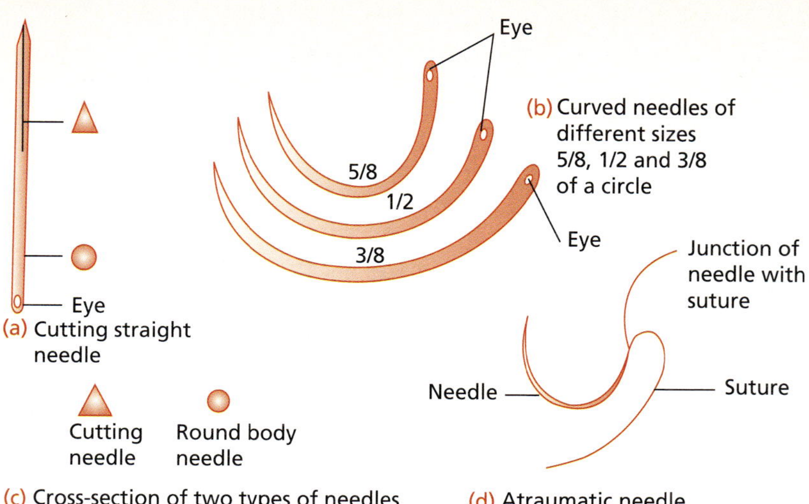

Figure 38.1 Stitching needles.

Straight and Curved Needles The straight needles are used for stitching the skin (plain body surface), while the curved needles are used for stitching in the depth or in a cavity, for example, oral cavity.

Round Body and Cutting Needles The round body needles are used for stitching softer tissues, for example, mucosa, muscles, nerves, and blood vessels. The cutting needles have two or three sharp cutting edges on the sides of needle near the needle point. Hence, they are used for stitching tough tissues such as skin, ligaments, and tendons.

Eyed and Eyeless Needles An ordinary needle has an eye at the blunt end for holding the suture. It is wider than the rest of needle; hence, it traumatizes the tissues more than an eyeless needle where the suture is joined to the end of needle by a special technique (Fig. 38.2.).

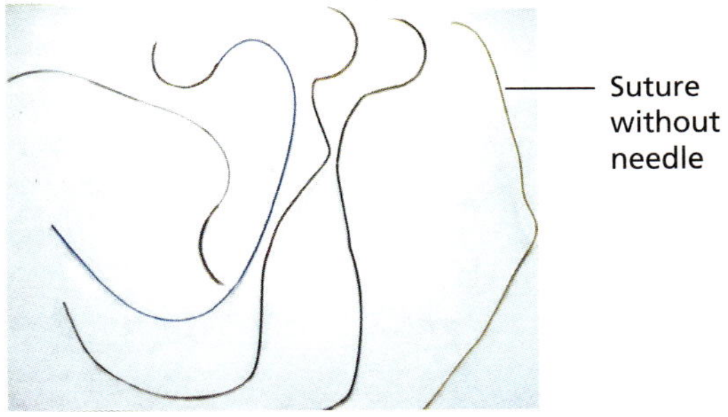

Figure 38.2 Common eyeless needled sutures.

Large and Small Needles Larger needles are used for working on the body surface and for stitching larger and thicker tissues, for example, large muscles and subcutaneous tissue, especially in obese patients. Smaller needles are used for fine work and for stitching in small cavities or spaces. For microvascular work, very fine needles (microneedles) are used.

Suturing materials

They are the materials used for closing surgical or accidental wounds with stitches, for example, cotton thread, silk, catgut, nylon, Prolene, and Vicryl.

Requirements of an Ideal Suture

So far an ideal suture is not known. The qualities of an ideal suture are described in Box 38.1.

Box 38.1 Requirements of an ideal suture

- It should have adequate strength and length
- It should cause no or minimal tissue reaction
- It can be handled easily
- It should have good knotting quality
- It should have no or minimal memory

Classification

Absorbable and Nonabsorbable Sutures Sutures are classified as absorbable and nonabsorbable sutures. They are further classified as natural and synthetic sutures (Box 38.2). All the natural sutures

Box 38.2 Classification of sutures

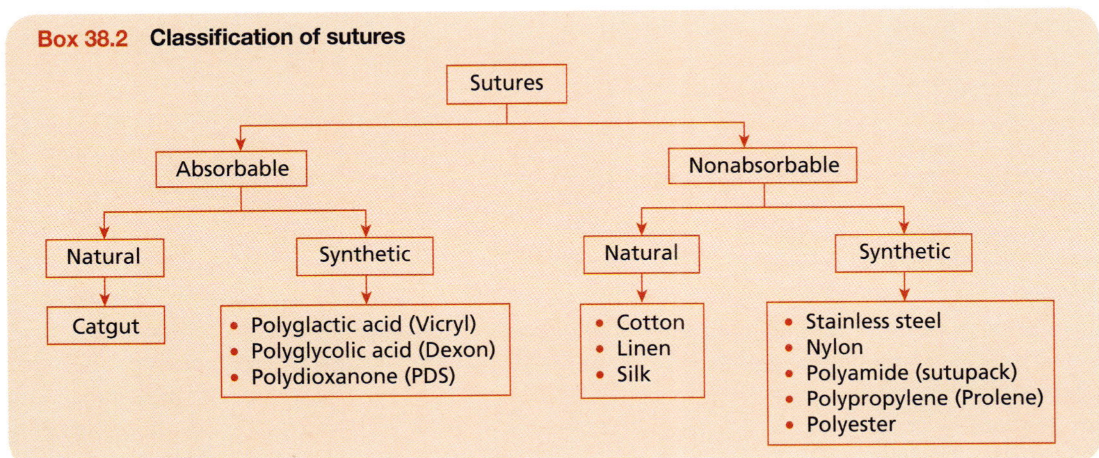

are now being replaced by polymeric synthetic sutures that cause minimal tissue reaction, are of predictable strength, and get absorbed at an appropriate rate.

- **Absorbable sutures**: These sutures get absorbed in the tissues after some time by either the activity of proteolytic enzymes (catgut) or hydrolysis (polyglactic acid).
- **Nonabsorbable sutures**: They are not absorbed in the tissues and may remain throughout life, for example, stainless steel sutures.

Monofilament and Multifilament Sutures Depending on the number of fibers, the sutures can be:

- **Monofilament**: Some nonabsorbable sutures are available as monofilaments which eliminate interstices in the suture and make knots less likely to be a nidus for infection. But they require extra care in tying a secure knot. Examples are polypropylene, PDS, catgut, and steel.
- **Multifilament**: Examples include polyester, polyamide, Vicryl, Dexon, silk, and cotton.

Depending on the Organization and Arrangement of Fibers

- **Braided**: Examples are polyester, polyamide, Vicryl, Dexon, and silk
- **Twisted**: Examples are cotton and linen

Depending on the Treatment of Surface of Sutures

- **Coated**: Coating is done with wax, silicon, or polybutyrate to allow the sutures to run smoothly through tissues and knot securely. Examples are polyamide and polypropylene.
- **Uncoated**: Example includes cotton.

Numbering of Suturing Material

The numbering of suturing material is done from no. 2 to 9/0 which means thickest and thinnest, respectively. A no. 2 suture is used for ligation of pedicles of various organs and large blood vessels, 2/0 for bowel anastomosis, 5/0 for nerve suture or vascular anastomosis, and 9/0 for microvascular work done under operating microscope.

Salient Features of Suture Materials

Catgut It is made from the submucosa of sheep's small intestine. It is of two types:

1. **Plain catgut**: It is yellowish white in color and dissolves in tissues within a week. It is used to stitch subcutaneous tissue and ligate small bleeders.

2. **Chromic catgut**: It is dark brown in color and hardened by chromic salt treatment. It dissolves in tissues in about 21 days by enzymatic digestion. It is used for suturing oral mucosa, lips, and tongue.

The disadvantages of catgut include early loss of strength in tissues and significant tissue reaction. Hence, it is less commonly used now.

Polyglactic Acid (Vicryl) It is a synthetic absorbable suture material that gets absorbed in 90 days by hydrolysis. Polyglactic acid is multifilament, braided, and violet in color. It is twice as strong as catgut. It is used for bowel anastomosis and suturing muscles and oral mucosa. To prevent site infection, especially after prosthetic implantation, it may be impregnated with an antiseptic, for example, Vicryl plus triclosan.

Polyglycolic Acid (Dexon) It is a synthetic absorbable suture which is creamy yellow in color. Silk is inert with good knotting quality.

Polydioxanone It is absorbable suture material which is creamy in color. It has properties like Vicryl but is a little better and costlier.

Cotton and Linen They are twisted, multifilament, natural, nonabsorbable suture materials. They are very cheap and easily available and are usually used for suturing skin. The linen is derived from bark of cotton plant.

Silk It is a natural, multifilament, nonabsorbable suture derived from cocoon of silkworm larvae. Silk is coated with wax to reduce its permeability (capillary action). It is stronger than thread and used for bowel anastomosis and for suturing mucoperiosteal flaps in the oral cavity.

Stainless Steel It is a nonabsorbable suture made up of stainless steel. It is commonly used to suture sternum after median sternotomy and cranial bones after craniotomy.

Nylon It is a synthetic monofilament suture which can be used in the presence of infection. Its knots are slippery.

Polyamide It is a nonabsorbable suture material with good tensile strength, but with poor knotting quality.

Polypropylene (Prolene) It is synthetic, non-absorbable, monofilament suture which is blue in color. It is inert and strong, and has a high memory. (Memory is recoiling tendency of suture after removal from the packet for use. Ideally a suture should have low memory.)

Polyester It is a synthetic polymer. Its fibers are closely braided into a multifilament strand. The advantages of a polyester suture include high tensile strength, low tissue reactivity, and good knot security.

Newer Suture Materials

Metal Sutures, Clips, and Staples Now a variety of stapling devices are available to close wounds in body cavities and many difficult areas. Most of the stapling devices are entirely disposable, relatively expensive, and now also available for minimally invasive surgery.

Tissue Glues The cyanoacrylates have been used for skin closure but they require near-perfect hemostasis. Similarly fibrin tissue glues have been used to cause hemostasis in the liver and spleen, to seal dural tears, and to attach skin grafts without the risk of haemoserous collection under the flaps.

Use of Surgical Sutures

The sutures are used for two purposes, that is, ligating or ligaturing, and suturing or stitching.

Ligating or Ligaturing It means tying tissues or structures with suture material, for example, divided or to be divided blood vessels. Ligating is also required during suturing when the ends of the sutures are tied together to produce a knot.

Suturing or Stitching It is sewing or stitching two structures or divided tissues together by means of a suturing needle threaded with or attached to some type of suture material.

Suturing techniques

The suturing can be interrupted or continuous. Simple and mattress suturing are examples of interrupted sutures while subcuticular and blanket suturing are the examples of continuous sutures. The details of suturing techniques are described in Table 38.1.

Table 38.1 Common methods of suturing

Figure	Suture	Uses
	Interrupted (simple) sutures	For closing a skin or mucosal wound
	Continuous suture	• Used for closing fascia and subcutaneous tissue • Subcuticular stitch is used for closure of skin with least skin puncture and minimal scarring
	Vertical mattress sutures	Used for skin closure with four point vertical distribution of tension on suture line
	Horizontal mattress sutures	Used for skin closure with four-point horizontal distribution of tension on suture line

Knot Tying

Knot tying should be learnt in the initial years of surgical training by repeated practice. The common types of surgical knots are described in Box 38.3.

Box 38.3 Types of surgical knots

Reef knot

- Well-known, reliable knot and universally advocated that has two throws in correct directions
- Must be left "square" by tightening it in correct directions

Triple knot

- A modification of reef knot having three "throws" giving additional security
- Allows ends ("ears") to be cut very short

Surgeon's knot

- Has an extra turn in the first throw
- Best suited for ligation of large vessels and pedicles when thicker ligature is used

Principles of knot tying

- It can be done by using a needle holder with care not to crush or damage the suture material incorporated into the knot.
- Tying knots with fingertips of both the hands is useful when ligating in the depth. All knots should be square.
- The two-throw reef knot (surgeon's knot) does not slip (Fig. 38.3).
- When the knots are cut short, the free ends or "ears" should be left at least 1–2 mm long but not too long.

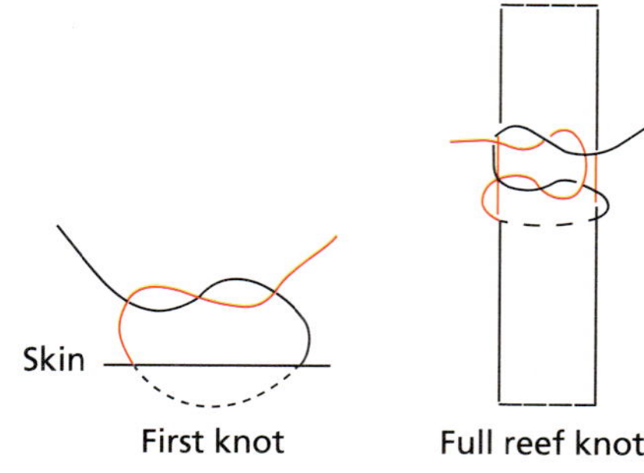

Figure 38.3 Reef knot.

KEY POINTS

- Four things are required for suturing a wound, that is, stitching needles, needle holder, dissecting forceps, and sutures.
- A suturing needle of appropriate shape and size needs to be selected for least traumatic passage through the tissues.
- The straight needles are used for stitching the skin (plain body surface), while the curved needles are used for stitching in the depth or in a cavity, for example, oral cavity.
- The round body needles are used for stitching softer tissues and the cutting needles are used for stitching tough tissues such as skin, ligaments, and tendons.
- An eyed needle traumatizes the tissues more than an eyeless needle where the suture is joined to the end of needle by a special technique.
- Larger needles are used for working on the body surface and for stitching larger and thicker tissues. Smaller needles are used for fine work and for stitching in small cavities or spaces. For microvascular work, very fine needles (microneedles) are used.
- An ideal suture material should have adequate strength and length, cause no or minimal tissue reaction, be easy to handle, have a good knotting quality, and should have no or minimal memory. Sutures are used for ligation of blood vessels and suturing divided tissues.
- Sutures can be absorbable or nonabsorbable. Absorbable sutures get absorbed in the tissues after some time by either the activity of proteolytic enzymes (catgut) or hydrolysis (polyglactic acid).
- Catgut is a natural absorbable suture. Polyglactic acid (Vicryl), polyglycolic acid (Dexon), and polydioxanone (PDS) are synthetic absorbable sutures.
- Cotton, linen, and silk are natural nonabsorbable sutures. Stainless steel, polyamide, nylon,

(CONTD...)

KEY POINTS (...CONTD)

polypropylene (Prolene), and polyester are synthetic nonabsorbable sutures.

- Depending on the number of fibers, sutures can be monofilament (e.g., polypropylene, PDS, catgut, steel) or multifilament (e.g., polyester, polyamide, Vicryl, Dexon, silk, cotton).
- Depending on the organization and arrangement of the fibers, sutures can be braided (e.g., polyester, polyamide, Vicryl, Dexon, silk) or twisted (e.g., cotton, linen).
- Depending on the treatment of the surface of sutures, they can be coated (e.g., polyamide, polypropylene) or uncoated (e.g., cotton). Coating is done with wax, silicon, or polybutyrate to allow them to run smoothly through tissues and knot securely.
- The numbering of suturing material is done from no. 2 to 9/0 which means thickest and thinnest, respectively.
- Plain catgut is yellowish white in color and dissolves in tissues within a week. Chromic catgut is dark brown in color and hardened by chromic salt treatment. It dissolves in tissues in about 21 days by enzymatic digestion.
- Polyglactic acid (Vicryl) is absorbed in 90 days by hydrolysis. It is used for suturing muscles and oral mucosa. To help in prevention of site infection, especially after prosthetic implantation, it may be impregnated with an antiseptic, for example, triclosan.
- Silk is natural, multifilament, nonabsorbable suture and is coated with wax to reduce its permeability. It is used for suturing mucoperiosteal flaps in the oral cavity.
- Nylon is a synthetic monofilament suture which can be used in the presence of infection but its knots are slippery.
- Polypropylene (Prolene) is a synthetic, nonabsorbable, monofilament suture which is blue in color. It is inert and strong, and has a high memory.
- Now a variety of stapling devices, metal sutures, and clips are available to close wounds in body cavities and many difficult areas. Tissue glues such as cyanoacrylates and fibrin glue have been used for skin closure but require near-perfect hemostasis.
- The suturing can be interrupted or continuous. Simple and mattress suturing are examples of interrupted sutures while subcuticular and blanket suturing are the examples of continuous sutures.

SELF-ASSESSMENT

Long answers questions

1. What are the things required for suturing a wound? Describe the types of suturing needles including their structure and function.
2. What are the requirements of an ideal suture? Describe the classification of suture materials.

Short answer questions

1. Requirements of an ideal suture
2. Numbering of suturing material
3. Catgut
4. Polyglactic acid (Vicryl)
5. Tissue glues
6. Use of surgical sutures
7. Surgical knots

Multiple choice questions

1. Catgut is made from the submucous coat of
   (a) Cat's intestine
   (b) Sheep's intestine
   (c) Calf's intestine
   (d) Pig's intestine
2. Which of the following is an absorbable suture material?
   (a) Cotton
   (b) Silk
   (c) Polypropylene
   (d) Polyglactic acid

(CONTD...)

SELF-ASSESSMENT *(...CONTD)*

3. Which of the following is a synthetic suture?
   (a) Cotton
   (b) Polyglactic acid
   (c) Silk
   (d) Linen

4. Which of the following is a natural suture?
   (a) Polydioxanone (PDS)
   (b) Polypropylene
   (c) Polyamide
   (d) Silk

Answers

1. (b) 2. (d) 3. (b) 4. (d)

Clinical Pathology 39

Introduction

The diagnostic signs of many surgical diseases depend on the gross appearance of the lesions. For example, benign lesions are characterized by smooth surface and uniformly soft consistency, and the malignant lesions are recognized by nodular surface and hard or variable consistency. Furthermore, a surgeon has to recognize various diseases during operation by their gross appearances. Hence, a candidate is examined on the specimens of excised lesions. Usually two to three specimens are given in the nonclinical practical examination. The steps in questioning the knowledge of the candidate are given in the subsequent text.

First Step The candidate should examine the specimen carefully from all sides and angles so as not to miss any finding.

Second Step The specimen is described under the following headings:

- Organ or part
- Findings
- Diagnosis

Questioning Three questions are usually asked after the candidate describes and recognizes the disease:

1. What are the reasons for giving this diagnosis?
2. What is this disease?
3. How will you treat it?

Further questioning depends on the candidate's response and the time available. The candidate must remember that your examiner is a surgeon and not a pathologist. Hence, he/she is unlikely to ask you the minor details of pathology. He/she usually limits to the pathology of clinical importance (clinical pathology). Hence, the questioning starts in pathology and ends in surgery.

Pathology specimen 1: Hodgkin's lymphoma

- **Examiner**: See this specimen, describe it, and tell the diagnosis.
- **Candidate**
  - *Organ*: It is one cut opened (bivalved) complete enlarged lymph node.
  - *Findings*: Lymph node is enlarged, smooth, and regular in outline. The cut surface is homogeneous and pale gray in color. There is no evidence of necrosis and liquefaction (Fig. 39.1).
  - *Diagnosis*: It is **Hodgkin's lymphoma**.

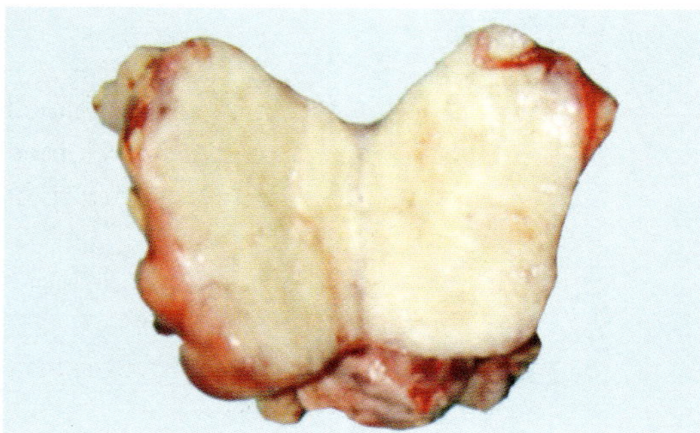

Figure 39.1 Gross appearance of a Hodgkin's lymphomatous lymph node.

Viva Voce

Q1. Why do you say it is Hodgkin's lymphoma?
Answer: It is Hodgkin's lymphoma as the lymph node is enlarged, regular, and discrete. The cut surface is homogeneous and pale gray in color. There is no evidence of necrosis or liquefaction.

Q2. What are the salient features of microscopic picture of Hodgkin's lymphoma?
Answer: Reed–Sternberg cells are the characteristic feature of this disease (Fig. 39.2). They are surrounded by an inflammatory infiltrate consisting of lymphocytes, plasma cells, eosinophils, and histiocytes, the pattern of which determines the pathological type.

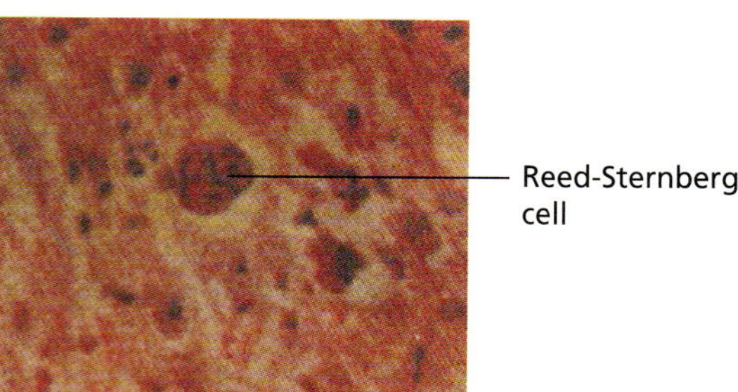

Figure 39.2 Microscopic appearance of Hodgkin's lymphoma showing a large Reed–Sternberg cell in the center. (Courtesy: Professor P.K. Agarwal)

Q3. What are the Reed–Sternberg cells?
Answer: They are the malignant cells of this disease. They are relatively large cells with abundant basophilic or amphophilic cytoplasm, and two or more vesicular nuclei. Each nucleus has a thick nuclear membrane and a single prominent acidophilic or amphophilic nucleolus surrounded by a clear halo (owl eye cells).

Q4. What are the histological types of this disease?
Answer: It is of four histological types: lymphocyte predominance, nodular sclerosis, mixed cellularity, and lymphocyte depletion.

Q5. What is the cause of this disease?
Answer: The cause of this disease is not known. It may be related to certain human leukocyte antigens, immune deficiency, autoimmunity, and an oncogenic virus.

Q6. What is the cell of origin of this disease?
Answer: It originates from B lymphocytes of germinal center origin.

Q7. What are the clinical stages of this disease?
Answer: Clinically it is divided into four stages (Ann Arbor). All of these stages are divided into two stages (A and B) depending on the absence or presence of constitutional symptoms. They are described in Box 39.1.

Box 39.1 Ann Arbor clinical staging of Hodgkin's lymphoma

- **Stage I**: Single lymphatic site involvement
- **Stage II**: Two or more lymphatic sites involved on one side of diaphragm
- **Stag III**: Disease on both sides of diaphragm
- **Stage IV**: Dissemination into extralymphatic sites, for example, liver, lung, bone marrow

Constitutional symptoms

- **A**: Constitutional symptoms absent
- **B**: Constitutional symptoms present

Q8. What are the constitutional symptoms?
Answer: The constitutional symptoms include irregular fever, weight loss (10% weight loss over 6 months), pruritus, and drenching night sweats.

Q9. How will you confirm the diagnosis?
Answer: The diagnosis is confirmed by lymph node biopsy for which a complete lymph node is taken out.

Q10. Why do you take out a complete lymph node?
Answer: It is to see its complete architecture.

Q11. What is the next step after the diagnosis is made?
Answer: The next step is to examine and investigate the patient further, for example, whole-body PET/CT scan and bone marrow biopsy, to find the extent and do staging of the disease.

Q12. How do you treat this disease?
Answer: The treatment of this disease is described in Table 39.1.

Q13. What is the toxicity of this treatment?
Answer: Pulmonary toxicity can occur following chemotherapy and radiation which can lead to pulmonary fibrosis.

Q14. How do you treat relapsing lymphoma?
Answer: It is treated with high-dose chemotherapy and autologous hematopoietic stem cell transplantation.

Q15. How will you treat relapse after autologous stem cell transplantation?
Answer: With antibody drug conjugate, that is, brentuximab.

Q16. What are the results of treatment?
Answer:

- **Stages IA and IIA**: 10-year survival rates in excess of 90%
- **Stage III or IV**: 10-year survival rates of 50–60%

Pathology specimen 2: multinodular goiter

- **Examiner**: Look at this specimen and describe it.
- **Candidate**
  - *Organ*: It is thyroid.
  - *Findings*: The specimen is shield-shaped or like a butterfly with the two lobes joined together by a narrow isthmus. The right lobe is a little larger than the left lobe. The surface is irregular due to multiple nodules of variable size (Fig. 39.3).
  - *Diagnosis*: It is **multinodular goiter**.

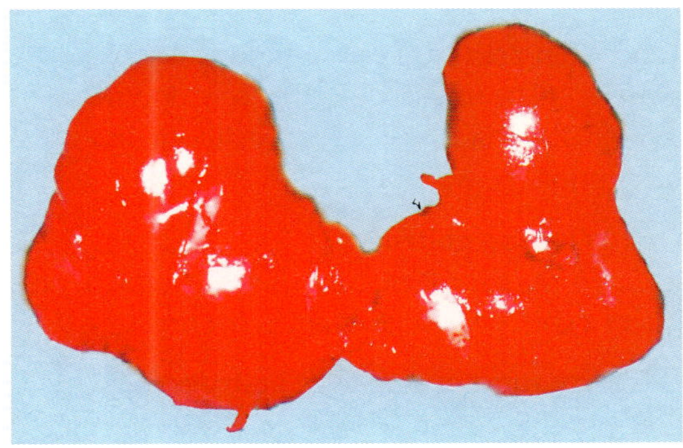

Figure 39.3 Subtotal thyroidectomy specimen of a multinodular goiter. (Courtesy: Dr. Alok)

Viva Voce

Q1. Why do you say it is thyroid?
Answer: It is thyroid because of its butterfly-like shape with two lateral lobes joined together by an isthmus.

Q2. Why do you call it multinodular goiter?
Answer: Because of the presence of many nodules in the thyroid.

Q3. What is a nodular goiter?
Answer: Nodular goiter is a non-neoplastic and noninflammatory swelling of thyroid of varied etiology and characterized by one or more nodules in the thyroid.

Table 39.1 Treatment of Hodgkin's lymphoma

Stage of the disease	Treatment
Stage I and stage II diseases	Combination of short-course chemotherapy (ABVD consisting of doxorubicin, bleomycin, vinblastine, dacarbazine) with involved-field radiotherapy, or a full course of chemotherapy alone
Stage II disease and a large mediastinal or other bulky mass	Full course of ABVD for six cycles with involved-field radiotherapy
Stage III and stage IV diseases	Full course of ABVD

Q4. What is the cause of this disease?
Answer: It is the result of one or more of the following etiological factors:

- Iodine deficiency in food and water (endemic goiter)
- Goitrogens in diet
- Some drugs
- Genetic defects with defects in enzyme system which is necessary for thyroxine synthesis (sporadic goiter)

Q5. What are the causes of iodine deficiency?
Answer: The causes include low iodine content in food and water, and deficient intestinal absorption.

Q6. What is a goitrogen?
Answer: A goitrogen is a chemical which produces a goiter when taken for some time.

Q7. Give some examples of goitrogens.
Answer: The common goitrogens are:

- Vegetables of *Brassica* family, for example, cabbage and rape which contain thiocyanate
- Drugs—PAS, thiocyanates, perchlorate, carbimazole, thiourea compounds, resorcinol

Q8. What is the pathogenesis of this disease?
Answer: Iodine deficiency leads to deficient production of thyroid hormone which results in thyroid-stimulating hormone (TSH) stimulation of thyroid. Persistent stimulation causes diffuse hyperplasia which is initially reversible if TSH stimulation ceases. If the TSH level fluctuates, a mixed-pattern hyperplasia occurs with areas of inactive nodules. Repeated cycles of the above process result in a nodular goiter with most of the nodules that are inactive with active follicles present in the internodular tissue.

Q9. Describe the micropathology of nodules of a nodular goiter.
Answer: The nodules may be colloid or cellular. Cystic degeneration and hemorrhage are common as is subsequent calcification (Fig. 39.4).

Q10. Why do the goiters occur more commonly in females than in males?
Answer: It may be related to estrogen receptors which have been identified in normal thyroid tissue and also in a nodular goiter.

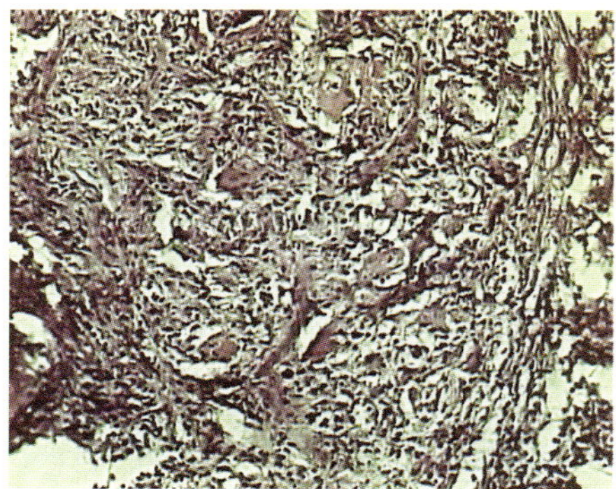

Figure 39.4 Microscopic appearance of a multinodular goiter after subtotal thyroidectomy.

Q11. What are the investigations?
Answer: The investigations include:

- T3, T4, and TSH
- Thyroid antibodies
- X-ray of neck to see the soft-tissue shadow of enlarged thyroid, deviation or distortion of tracheal air shadow, and calcification, if any
- Ultrasonography to see the texture of the goiter and to perform ultrasound guided FNAC from suspicious areas

Q12. What is the functional status of a nodular goiter?
Answer: Usually the patient is euthyroid. Subclinical or mild hypothyroidism may be present.

Q13. What are the complications of a nodular goiter?
Answer: The complications are:

- Tracheal obstruction due to extrinsic pressure
- Secondary thyrotoxicosis
- Carcinoma

Q14. What is the cause of tracheal obstruction?
Answer: The causes of tracheal obstruction include compression or lateral displacement by the goiter and acute compression by hemorrhage into the goiter.

Q15. What is the nature of carcinoma that occurs in a nodular goiter?
Answer: It is usually a follicular carcinoma.

Q16. How do you treat this goiter?
Answer: A small asymptomatic goiter does not need any treatment. A big goiter causing symptoms is treated by doing subtotal thyroidectomy.

Q17. What is done in this operation?
Answer: Most of the thyroid tissue including the nodules is excised and up to 8 g of relatively normal tissue is preserved in each tracheoesophageal groove.

Q18. Can this disease recur after operation?
Answer: Yes, it can recur.

Q19. How do you prevent recurrence?
Answer: The patient is given 0.1–0.2 mg levothyroxine daily postoperatively to do TSH suppression until after the menopause or for an indefinite period.

Q20. Why is it not given after menopause?
Answer: It aggravates osteoporosis, increasing the risk of pathological fractures.

Pathology specimen 3: pleomorphic adenoma of parotid

- **Examiner**: See this specimen and tell me your findings and diagnosis.
- **Candidate**
  - *Part*: It is superficial lobe of parotid salivary gland.
  - *Findings*: An ovoid nodulated swelling (Fig. 39.5) is present with its lower part covered by a thinned-out normal tissue.
  - *Diagnosis*: It is **pleomorphic adenoma of parotid**.

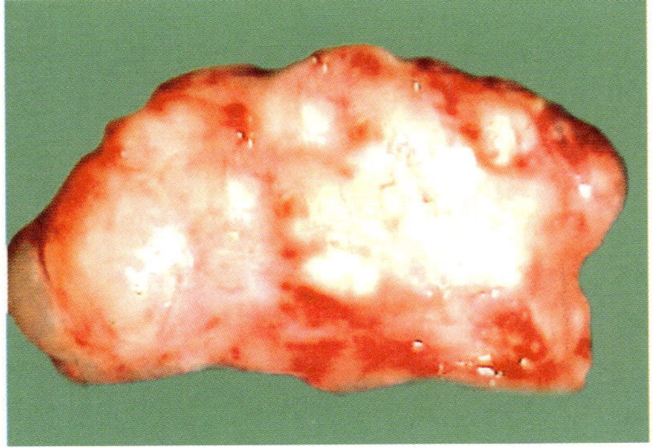

Figure 39.5 Excised specimen of pleomorphic adenoma of parotid with normal tissue around removed. (Courtesy: Professor Sandeep Kumar)

Viva Voce

Q1. Why do you say it is parotid salivary gland?
Answer: It is because of its shape and glandular appearance.

Q2. Why do you say it is pleomorphic adenoma?
Answer: As the swelling is ovoid and lobulated, and it is the commonest swelling of the parotid.

Q3. What are the clinical signs of a pleomorphic adenoma of parotid?
Answer: The clinical signs of a pleomorphic adenoma of parotid are:

- The patient is usually a middle-aged person who presents with a slow-growing swelling in the parotid region.
- It is mostly situated a little in front and above the angle of mandible.
- It is smooth or lobulated, firm, nontender, mobile, and well-defined.
- The ear lobule is lifted up and out.
- The facial nerve and regional lymph nodes are not involved.

Q4. What is micropathology?
Answer: It has a variegated appearance consisting of acini and myxomatous and chondroid tissue.

Q5. What are the sites of occurrence of this tumor?
Answer: It can arise from any salivary gland, but 90% of tumors arise in the parotid gland.

Q6. What is the commonest site of occurrence in the parotid?
Answer: In the tail of parotid.

Q7. Can it occur in minor salivary glands?
Answer: Yes, it can occur in the minor salivary glands of the oral mucosa.

Q8. What is the commonest site of occurrence among the minor salivary glands?
Answer: Minor salivary glands of palate.

Q9. What are the complications of this tumor?
Answer: The main complication is malignant transformation.

Q10. What are the signs of malignant transformation?
Answer: The signs of malignant change are:

- Rapid growth and appearance of pain
- Involvement of facial nerve

- Loss of mobility
- Regional lymph node enlargement
- Ulceration and/or fungation

Q11. How do you confirm the diagnosis?
Answer: The diagnosis is mostly clinical and biopsy should never be done but FNAC can rarely be done.

Q12. Why don't you do incisional biopsy?
Answer: It is not done because of real risk of "spillover" of tumor cells.

Q13. How do you treat this tumor?
Answer: It is treated by superficial parotidectomy.

Q14. What are the complications of this operation?
Answer: The complications of this operation include facial nerve injury, wound infection, salivary fistula, and auriculotemporal syndrome.

Q15. How will you treat a tumor of submandibular salivary gland?
Answer: By complete excision of submandibular salivary gland.

Q16. How do you treat a tumor of palate?
Answer: By wide excision of tumor.

Pathology specimen 4: salivary calculus

- **Examiner**: See this small specimen and tell me what it is.
- **Candidate**
  - *Finding*: It is a small, round structure like pea-seed, gray in color with a slightly uneven surface (Fig. 39.6).
  - *Diagnosis*: It is **salivary calculus**.

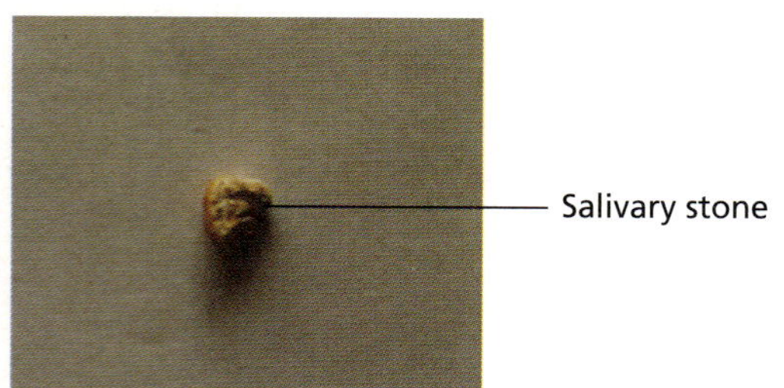

Figure 39.6 Stone removed from the submandibular salivary duct.

Viva Voce

Q1. Why do you say it is a salivary stone?
Answer: Because of its shape and size like a pea-seed and yellowish gray color.

Q2. Which is the salivary gland most commonly affected by calculus disease?
Answer: Submandibular salivary gland and its duct are most commonly affected.

Q3. What is the cause of this disease?
Answer: It is not known. It is nothing to do with serum calcium level. It may be related to the chemical composition of saliva as the chemical structure of the stone resembles that of dental tartar.

Q4. What are the clinical signs of submandibular salivary stone?
Answer: The signs of a submandibular salivary stone are described as follows:

- The patient complains of pain and swelling in the submandibular region which appears or becomes worse during meals.
- The Wharton's duct orifice is inflamed and edematous, and may be pouting. It may exude turbid fluid or purulent saliva which increases on pressing the submandibular swelling.
- The stone may be palpable in the floor of mouth in the submandibular duct as an indurated nodule, or the stone may be visible in the duct orifice and recognized by its grayish yellow color.

Q5. Can this disease occur in the parotid salivary system?
Answer: Yes.

Q6. What are the signs of a stone in the parotid?
Answer: The signs of a stone in the parotid are given as follows:

- The patient presents with attacks of unilateral swelling of whole parotid associated with discomfort of sudden onset at the time of meals.
- It is associated with a sensation of dryness of mouth on the same side.
- The whole of parotid is swollen, smooth, and mildly tender.
- The ipsilateral duct orifice may be edematous, pouting, inflamed and sometimes the projecting tip of the stone may be visible.

- After some time, there is a gush of salty or foul-smelling liquid into the mouth followed by relief.

Q7. What are the complications of a submandibular stone?
Answer: The complications include chronic or recurrent submandibular sialadenitis, secondary salivary calculus, submandibular abscess, and salivary fistula.

Q8. What is a secondary salivary calculus?
Answer: It is a stone that develops in the stagnant ductal system proximal to the primary stone.

Q9. How will you confirm the diagnosis?
Answer: If the stone is visible in the duct orifice, no investigation is required. Otherwise the diagnosis is confirmed by taking a radiograph of the floor of mouth (Fig. 39.7).

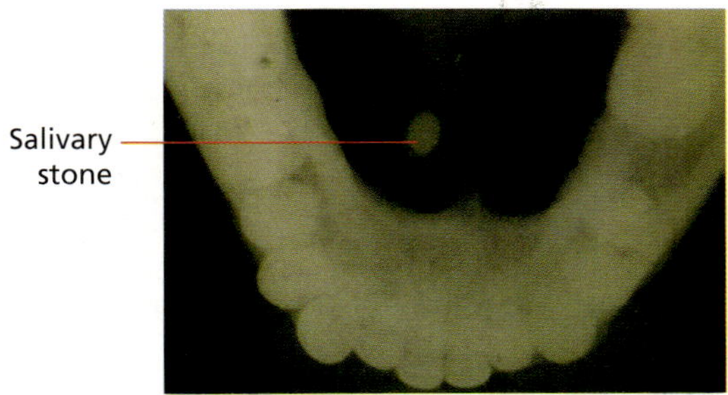

Figure 39.7 Radiograph of floor of mouth showing a small oval radio-opaque shadow on the right side of midline due to a stone in the submandibular salivary duct.

Q10. What are the X-ray signs of submandibular stone?
Answer: It reveals an ovoid or round radio-opacity in the floor of mouth by the side of midline.

Q11. How do you radiograph the stone?
Answer: The patient holds a small plate, for example, a dental film, in the mouth in between the teeth and the X-rays are directed upwards from under the chin.

Q12. How do you treat this disease?
Answer: A stone near the orifice is removed by hooking or meatotomy, while a stone in the duct is removed by making a longitudinal cut on the duct at the site of stone. If the stone is present in the gland, the whole gland is removed.

Q13. What are the precautions during lithotomy?
Answer: A holding stitch is passed around the duct proximal to the stone to prevent it from slipping back into the gland.

Q14. What are the complications of surgical treatment of submandibular stone?
Answer: The complications of lithotomy include injury to the lingual nerve, slipping the stone back into the gland, and stricture of Wharton's duct. The **complications** of submandibular sialadenectomy include injury to cervical branch of facial nerve and hypoglossal nerve, injury to facial artery, and opening of oral mucosa.

Pathological specimen 5: osteosarcoma of mandible

- **Examiner**: Observe this specimen carefully and let me know what it is.
- **Candidate**
  - *Organ/part*: It is a part of excised mandible.
  - *Findings*: Specimen consists of angle of the mandible and a mass of soft tissue attached to its upper part and posterior border. It is irregular in shape and surface and looks fleshy (Fig. 39.8).
  - *Diagnosis*: Its **osteosarcoma of mandible**.

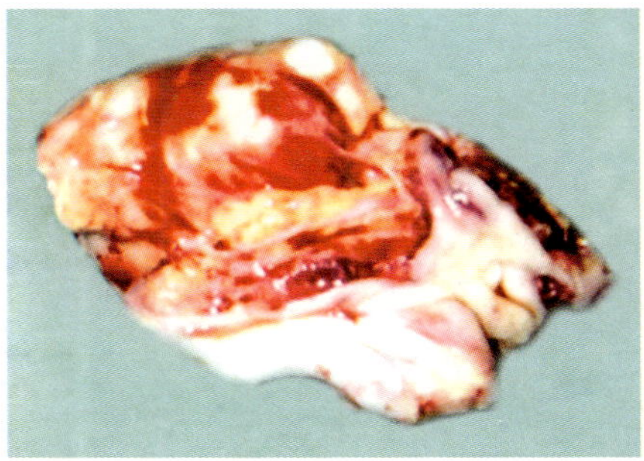

Figure 39.8 Excised specimen of osteosarcoma of mandible. (Courtesy: Dr. Surajit Bhattacharya)

Viva Voce

Q1. Why do you say it is sarcoma of mandible?
Answer: Because it is an irregular fleshy mass involving a part of mandible along the upper

border, retromolar region, and a part of anterior border of ascending ramus.

Q2. What are the clinical signs of osteosarcoma of mandible?

Answer: The patient is usually a young or middle-aged person who presents with a rapidly growing fleshy swelling of the mandible. It is hard or variable in consistency and may be warm and tender.

Q3. How will you confirm the diagnosis?

Answer: The diagnosis is confirmed by radiography and biopsy.

Q4. What are the X-ray signs of osteosarcoma?

Answer: It shows irregular bone destruction and some evidence of new bone formation with soft-tissue shadow of the tumor.

Q5. What will you find on microscopy of biopsy piece?

Answer: It will reveal irregular areas of bone destruction and some evidence of newly formed osteoid tissue. The tumor cells are rounded or oval in shape.

Q6. How will you treat such a case?

Answer: The lesion will be widely excised following a course of preoperative chemotherapy. Local irradiation is usually given postoperatively to look after the inadequacy of surgery.

Q7. How will you make up for the lost mandible?

Answer: The lost part can be made good by using a steel plate or by putting a bone graft obtained from iliac crest or fibula.

KEY POINTS

- Examination on the pathological specimens is important as one has to recognize the nature and extent of the lesion (disease) during operation.
- The specimen must be held correctly in the hands. Make sure that it is not damaged.
- The candidate has to recognize the disease of the specimen by its gross appearance.
- Remember that the examiner is not a pathologist but a surgeon. Hence, he is likely to ask questions on the specimens of clinical importance, not the finer details of pathology.
- During your training period when you are posted in operating room, examine the excised lesions for their gross appearance (and take a photograph if possible) before sending it to the pathology laboratory.

Diagnostic Images

40

Introduction

The internal organs, structures, and tissues of the body can be seen or picturized by radiography (plain and contrast radiography), ultrasonography, computerized axial tomography (CAT scan), magnetic resonance imaging, and radioisotope studies. These methods of imaging have a great value in making/confirming the diagnosis. Hence, a doctor should know when to get them done, how to examine or see them, and how to interpret them. Therefore, an examinee is examined on these pictures in the nonclinical part of practical examination.

The candidate must hold and put the picture correctly on the view box, and see the picture or plate carefully and systemically so as not to miss any finding as the interpretation of the picture depends on the findings. Now the examinee describes the picture under the following headings:

- **Part**: Examples—jaws, neck, skull
- **Nature of picture or imaging**: Radiography, orthopantomography, CT scan/MRI
- **Plain/contrast**
- **View**: AP/lateral
- **Findings**
  - …
  - …
  - …
- **Diagnosis**

Viva Voce If the candidate has correctly read and interpreted the picture, usually two questions are asked:

1. What is this condition or disease?
2. How will you treat it?

The rest of the questioning depends on your response to these questions and the time available. The examiner may ask you any question about the problem you have diagnosed after seeing the picture.

Diagnostic image 1: radiograph of ankylosis of temporomandibular joint

- **Examiner**: See this picture, read it, and describe it.
- **Candidate**
  - *Part*: Both temporomandibular joints (TMJs)
  - *Nature of imaging*: X-ray
  - *View*: Lateral

- *Findings*
  - The joint in the first picture (a) is normal showing articular surfaces and joint space.
  - The joint in the second picture (b) is ossified, that is, the articular surfaces are not seen and the joint cavity is filled with osteoid tissue (Fig. 40.1).
- *Diagnosis*: True (bony) ankylosis of TMJ

Viva Voce

Q1. What is ankylosis of TMJ?
Answer: It is the difficulty or inability to open the mouth due to ankylosis of TMJ.

Q2. What are the types of ankylosis of TMJ?
Answer: It is of two types, that is, extra-articular or false ankylosis and intra-articular or true ankylosis.

Q3. What is extra-articular or false ankylosis?
Answer: It is difficulty or restriction of opening of mouth due to fibrosis around the joint, the joint itself being normal.

Q4. What are the causes of extra-articular ankylosis of TMJ?
Answer: The causes of extra-articular ankylosis of TMJ include submucous fibrosis of cheek, carcinoma of retromolar region, cancrum oris, and postradiation fibrosis of cheek.

Q5. What is intra-articular or true ankylosis?
Answer: It is difficulty or restriction of opening of mouth due to intra-articular fibrosis or deposition of osteoid tissue in the joint.

Q6. What are the causes of intra-articular ankylosis?
Answer: The causes include suppurative arthritis, intra-articular fracture, hemarthrosis, and intra-articular joint surgery.

Q7. How do you clinically differentiate between the two types of ankylosis?
Answer: In extra-articular ankylosis some movement is possible in the joint, that is, the mouth can be opened slightly, while in intra-articular type no movement is possible, that is, the mouth cannot be opened at all.

Q8. What are the X-ray signs of ankylosis TMJ?
Answer: The fibrous ankylosis is characterized by reduced joint space and hazy appearance of the joint but still the normal structure of the joint can be appreciated. Nearly the same findings are seen in extra-articular ankylosis. In bony ankylosis the joint cavity is obliterated by deposition of abnormal bony tissue.

Q9. What are the ill effects of ankylosis of TMJ?
Answer: The ill effects of ankylosis of TMJ are:

- There is early teeth decay as the teeth cannot be cleaned properly and no access is available to the dentist to do dental work.
- If it occurs in the early childhood, especially if it is bilateral, it leads to failure of development of lower jaw leading to receding chin producing a bird-like face or shrew-mouse appearance (Fig. 40.2).

Q10. What are the effects of ankylosis on nutrition?

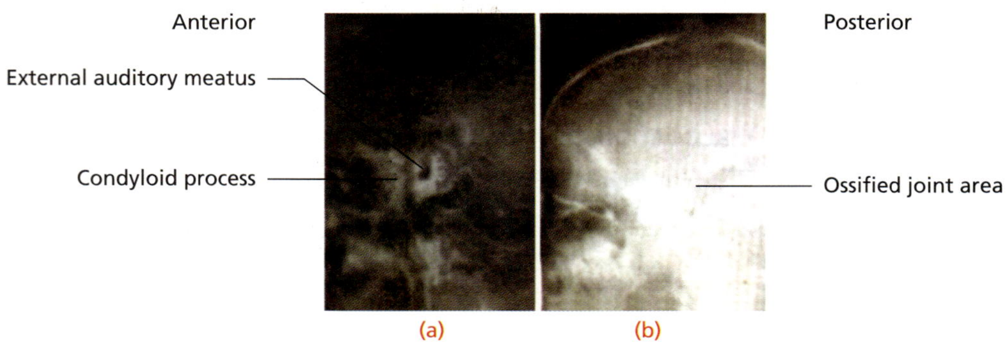

Figure 40.1 Lateral radiograph of central part of face and skull showing (a) normal temporomandibular joint and (b) ankylosed joint.

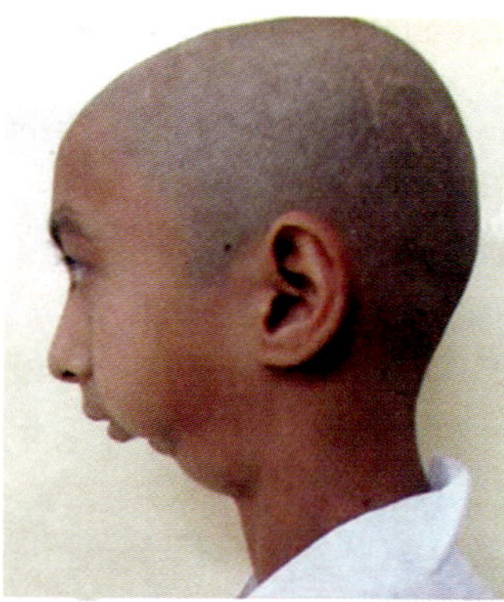

Figure 40.2 Shrew-mouse appearance of face (or bird-like face) due to bilateral ankylosis of temporomandibular joint occurring during early childhood. (Courtesy: Professor Divya Mehrotra)

Answer: The nutrition does not suffer at all as the patient continues to take liquid foods through interdental and retromolar spaces.

Q11. How do you treat extra-articular ankylosis?
Answer: It is treated by passive, repeated, and gradual stretching of fibrous tissue. If it fails, the fibrous tissue is excised followed by skin grafting. If all the measures fail, Esmarch's operation may be done.

Q12. What is Esmarch's operation?
Answer: In this operation a wedge of bone with base down is removed from the mandible near its angle to create a pseudojoint.

Q13. What is the major disadvantage of this operation?
Answer: The grinding or masticatory power of the mandible is markedly reduced as the joint is distal to the attachment of main masticatory muscles which are attached to ascending ramus.

Q14. How do you treat intra-articular ankylosis?
Answer: Three operative procedures are available for treating intra-articular ankylosis—condylectomy, gap arthroplasty, and interpositional arthroplasty.

Q15. What is condylectomy and when do you do this operation?
Answer: It is excision of condyle of mandible and it is done in fibrous ankylosis.

Q16. What are the complications of this procedure?
Answer: Unilateral condylectomy tends to cause deviation of mandible toward the same side on opening the mouth, while the bilateral operation causes anterior open bite due to loss of height of vertical rami of mandible.

Q17. What is gap arthroplasty and what is its indication?
Answer: It is the excision of whole broad, thick area of abnormal bone obliterating the joint, sigmoid notch, and coronoid process by two horizontal osteotomy cuts creating a gap of at least 1 cm to prevent reankylosis. This operation is done in extensive bony ankylosis.

Q18. What is the disadvantage of this operation?
Answer: The main problem of gap arthroplasty is recurrence due to deposition of new bone in the gap.

Q19. What is interpositional arthroplasty?
Answer: It involves creation of a gap and insertion of a barrier between the cut bony surfaces to reduce the risk of recurrence and to maintain the vertical height of the ramus.

Q20. What are the interpositional materials used?
Answer: They include autogenous materials, for example, cartilaginous graft, temporal muscle, and fascia lata; heterogeneous materials, for example, lyophilized bovine cartilage; or alloplastic materials, for example, condylar prosthesis made of steel, Vitallium, or titanium (replacement of joint).

Q21. What are the problems of anesthesia for operation?
Answer: There are two main problems:

1. Endotracheal intubation poses serious problem because the mouth cannot be opened and the mandible is small. Hence, blind nasal intubation is done.
2. Aspiration of blood clot, loose teeth, or foreign bodies can occur during extubation as throat cannot be packed prior to surgery.

Q22. What are the complications of operation?
Answer: The complications of operation include hemorrhage due to injury to superficial temporal

vessels, transverse facial artery, internal maxillary artery, and pterygoid venous plexus; and injury to external auditory meatus, facial nerve, glenoid fossa, auriculotemporal nerve, and parotid gland.

Diagnostic image 2: ultrasonogram showing a thyroid cyst

- **Examiner**: Look at this picture of neck and tell me about it.
- **Candidate**
  - *Part*: Neck
  - *Nature of imaging*: Ultrasonography
  - *Findings*: Presence of a well-defined, homogenous, dark oval area in the thyroid region of neck (Fig. 40.3)
  - *Diagnosis*: Cyst of thyroid

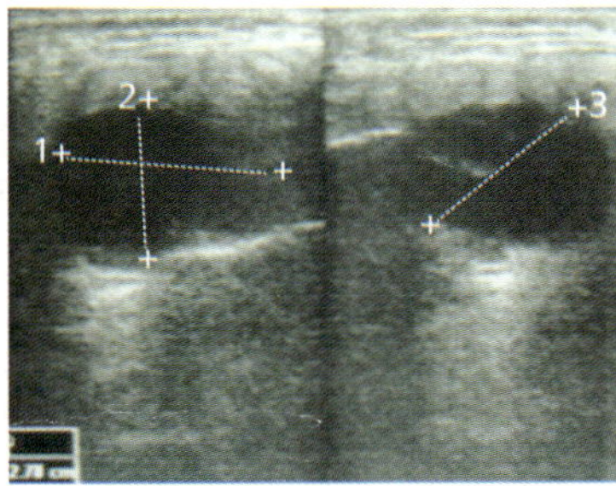

Figure 40.3 Ultrasonography of neck showing a transversely oval, lucent area due to a cyst of thyroid. (Courtesy: Professor Surajit Bhattacharya)

Viva Voce

Q1. Why do you say it is a cyst of thyroid?
Answer: It is a cyst of thyroid as ultrasonography of neck shows a well-defined, ovoid, lucent lesion at the site of thyroid.

Q2. What is a cyst?
Answer: A cyst is a localized swelling of solid organs and tissues that contains clear fluid (other than pus).

Q3. What are the types of cyst?
Answer: Cysts are of two types, that is, true cyst and false cyst.

Q4. What is a true cyst?
Answer: A true cyst is lined by epithelium. Hence, it has a smooth wall.

Q5. What is a false cyst?
Answer: It has a fibrous wall which is not lined by epithelium.

Q6. How does a thyroid cyst present?
Answer: It may be asymptomatic or may present as a solitary thyroid nodule.

Q7. How do you recognize it clinically?
Answer: Usually it is not diagnosed clinically.

Q8. Then, how do you diagnose it?
Answer: It is diagnosed by ultrasound examination of thyroid.

Q9. How do you confirm the diagnosis?
Answer: It is done by ultrasound-guided needle aspiration.

Q10. What are the "dos" to be followed when you do aspiration?
Answer: The "dos" of aspiration of a thyroid cyst are:

- It should be done under ultrasound guidance.
- The cyst should be aspirated completely.
- The aspirate must be sent for cytological examination.

Q11. What are the types of thyroid cyst?
Answer: The types of thyroid cyst are:

- True cysts—they are very rare.
- False cysts are due to colloid degeneration, and necrosis or hemorrhage in benign and malignant tumors.

Q12. Why should a cyst of thyroid be aspirated completely?
Answer: It should be aspirated completely as a benign cyst may be cured by this method.

Q13. Why do you send the aspirate for cytology?
Answer: A thyroid cyst may be neoplastic in origin. Hence, the aspirate is sent for cytology to find if it has tumor in it.

Q14. What are the features of a benign cyst?
Answer: The features of a benign cyst are:

- A well-defined homogeneous lucency in thyroid on ultrasonography
- Clear colorless fluid on aspiration
- Complete disappearance of cyst on aspiration
- Acellular or benign cytology of aspirate

Q15. What is the incidence of neoplastic cysts?
Answer: In one study, 46% of thyroid cysts were neoplastic.

Q16. What is the incidence of cancer in thyroid cysts?
Answer: Fourteen percent of thyroid cysts are cancerous.

Q17. Are all the cancerous cysts diagnosed by cytology?
Answer: No. One-third of malignant thyroid cysts have a false-negative cytology.

Q18. How do you treat a benign cyst?
Answer: If the cyst does not empty completely or refills after aspiration, it is treated by hemithyroidectomy.

Q19. What is the role of local alcohol injection?
Answer: A benign cyst which refills after complete aspiration may be treated by local alcohol (95%) injection.

Q20. How do you treat a malignant cyst?
Answer: It is treated like resectable carcinoma of thyroid by total or near-total thyroidectomy with further treatment depending on the histological nature of the tumor.

Q21. What are the complications of thyroidectomy?
Answer: The complications of thyroidectomy include hemorrhage, compression of trachea, recurrent laryngeal nerve injury, parathyroid tetany, and superior laryngeal nerve injury.

Diagnostic image 3: CT scan of a dentigerous cyst

- **Examiner**: See this picture, read it, and tell me the diagnosis.
- **Candidate**
  - *Part*: Face
  - *Nature of imaging*: CT scan
  - *View*: Coronal
  - *Findings*
    - Obliquely oval, lucent shadow affecting the horizontal ramus of mandible
    - Shadow of unerupted tooth seen inside the lucent area (Fig. 40.4)

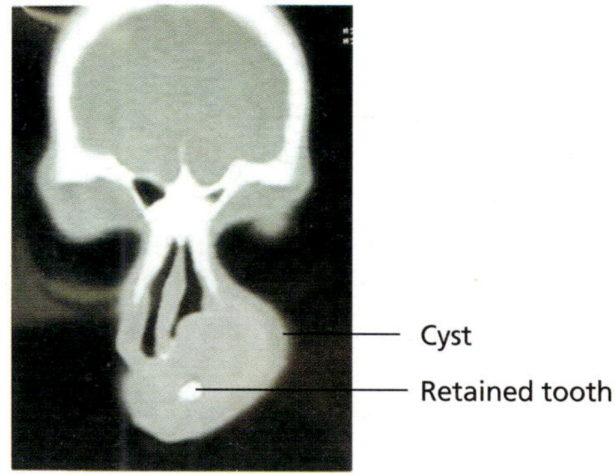

Figure 40.4 Coronal CT scan of face showing a large dentigerous cyst of right horizontal ramus of mandible. The unerupted tooth is seen within the cyst.

  - *Diagnosis*: Dentigerous cyst of horizontal ramus of mandible

Viva Voce

Q1. What is a dentigerous cyst?
Answer: A dentigerous cyst results from enlargement of follicular space of the whole or part of the crown of an impacted or unerupted tooth and is attached to the neck of tooth.

Q2. What is its incidence?
Answer: It is more common than primordial cyst and less common than an apical cyst. It is commonly seen in children and young adults and occurs equally in both sexes.

Q3. What is the site of occurrence?
Answer: It occurs more frequently in the mandible than in the maxilla. Late-erupting teeth are the most frequently involved, being in descending order the lower third molars, upper cuspids (canines), upper third molars, and lower bicuspid (premolar) teeth.

Q4. What are the clinical features?
Answer: The patient presents with a very slow-growing swelling commonly near the angle of jaw causing facial asymmetry. Pain may occur due to secondary infection. There is a smooth, hard, nontender swelling of the jaw with involvement of the outer table. The inner table may be somewhat swollen in large cysts. As the cyst grows

further, it may have egg-shell crackling due to thinning of cyst wall.

Q5. What are the radiographic features?
Answer: A radiograph shows a well-defined unilocular radiolucency containing the crown of unerupted impacted tooth. The pressure of an enlarging cyst may push the unerupted tooth from its direction of eruption, for example, lower third molar may be pushed near the inferior border or into ascending ramus while the upper cuspid may be pushed into maxillary sinus.

Q6. What are the radiographic types?
Answer: Dentigerous cyst is of three radiographic types, that is, circumferential, lateral, and coronal (Fig. 40.5).

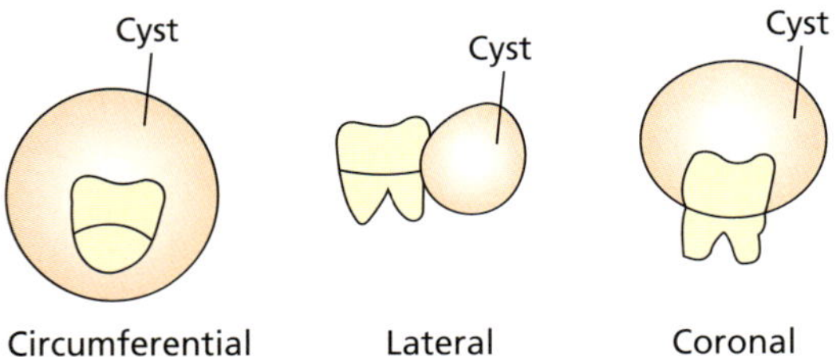

Figure 40.5 Radiographic types of dentigerous cyst.

Q7. What is the nature of cyst fluid?
Answer: The cyst contains clear yellowish fluid which may contain cholesterol crystals. It becomes purulent if secondary infection occurs.

Q8. How will you treat a dentigerous cyst?
Answer: It is treated by any one of two operative procedures—marsupialization and enucleation.

Q9. What is marsupialization?
Answer: It is a surgical procedure in which a part of the wall (outer wall) of the cyst is removed, the contents are removed, and the cut edge of lining of the cyst is sutured to the cut edge of oral mucosa (mucoperiosteum).

Q10. What is the indication of this operation?
Answer: It is indicated in children if the cyst is very large and the intracystic tooth is to be retained.

Q11. What are the results of this operation?
Answer: The tooth may erupt and the defect may heal with normal bone.

Q12. What do you do in enucleation?
Answer: In adults the whole lining of the cyst is excised along with intracystic tooth as the possibility of tooth eruption is low. In children when the root formation of unerupted tooth is complete, the enucleation may be done when the cyst lining is separated from the neck of tooth with a scalpel. As the root formation is complete, the risk of tooth dislodgement is low.

Diagnostic image 4: fibrous dysplasia of mandible

- **Examiner**: See this picture, describe the findings, and tell the diagnosis.
- **Candidate**
  - *Part and type of imaging*: 3D CT reconstruction of face (skull and jaws)
  - *Findings*
    - Multiloculated lesion of the mandible near its angle
    - Similar changes seen in the maxilla just below the lower orbital margin and medial wall of orbit (Fig. 40.6)
  - *Diagnosis*: Fibrous dysplasia of mandible

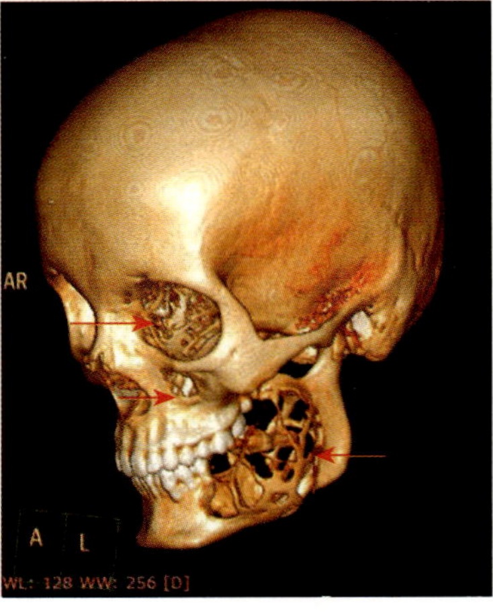

Figure 40.6 Multicystic lytic lesion of mandible near its angle seen in 3D reconstruction CT scan. Similar changes are seen in the orbital wall and in the maxilla just below the lower orbital margin. (Courtesy: Professor Divya Mehrotra)

Viva Voce

Q1. Why do you say it is fibrous dysplasia of mandible?

Answer: The reasons for diagnosing it as fibrous dysplasia are:

- There is multicystic lytic lesion of mandible near its angle causing protuberance of lower border.
- Similar changes are seen in the maxilla just below the lower orbital margin and medial wall of orbit.
- It has an ill-defined border (no capsule).

Q2. What is fibrous dysplasia of bone?

Answer: It is a benign self-limiting disease of bones of unknown etiology in which the normal bony architecture is replaced by abnormal fibrous connective tissue which contains a variable amount of osseous matrix.

Q3. What are the types of this disease?

Answer: This disease is of two types:

1. **Monostotic fibrous dysplasia**: It affects one bone (it can be confirmed by bone scan). It occurs in 80–85% of cases.
2. **Polyostotic fibrous dysplasia**: It affects more than one bone, but the skull and jaws are affected in all patients of this type of dysplasia. Among other bones, the femur is the commonest bone to be affected (shepherd hook deformity). In long bones, it affects metaphysis or shaft, never the epiphysis.

Q4. What are the clinical signs of dysplasia of mandible?

Answer: The clinical signs of fibrous dysplasia of mandible are:

- The patient is usually a child or adolescent person who presents with a painless, slow-growing swelling of lower jaw of insidious onset. The growth of the swelling ceases usually with cessation of skeletal growth.
- Both males and females are affected equally.
- The mandible is less commonly affected than maxilla and the lesion may extend to involve other bones of face.
- Facial asymmetry is usually the patient's chief complaint.
- The swelling is fusiform oval (low plateau), firm, smooth, and nontender with ill-defined borders. It affects the outer table of jaws; the inner table is rarely involved.
- The related teeth are usually firm, but may be displaced by increasing swelling of the jaw.

Q5. How will you confirm the diagnosis?

Answer: The diagnosis is confirmed by radiography of the lesion and biopsy.

Q6. What are the radiographic signs?

Answer: The radiography shows a radiolucent expanding lesion with patchy irregular opacities and a poorly defined border.

Q7. What is the microscopic picture of this disease?

Answer: Microscopy shows proliferating fibroblasts in a compact stroma of interlacing collagen fibers, irregular bony trabeculae scattered haphazardly, or C-shaped trabeculae giving "Chinese character appearance."

Q8. What are the complications of this disease?

Answer: The complications include spontaneous or pathological fracture and sarcoma in polyostotic fibrous dysplasia.

Q9. How do you treat this disease?

Answer: The treatment depends on the extent or size of the lesion.

- **Small lesion disease**: After histological confirmation the patient is put on regular follow-up as the disease stops growing after cessation of skeletal growth.
- **Large lesions with functional or aesthetic problems**: The complete excision of this lesion is not possible and also not required as it is a benign self-limiting disease. Hence, recontouring of the face is undertaken when the disease has stabilized. This procedure entails surgical reduction of the lesion with contouring with a round burr or osteotome, or with a scalpel if it is fibrous tissue. Sometimes it is treated with thorough curetting and cancellous bone grafting.

Q10. What are the results of treatment?

Answer: The overall results are satisfactory, but a variable regrowth of the lesion occurs in 25–50% of patients.

Q11. What is the role of radiotherapy?
Answer: The radiotherapy is contraindicated as it carries the risk of malignant transformation.

Q12. What is the role of bisphosphonates?
Answer: They are used to relieve pain.

Diagnostic image 5: 3D CT reconstruction of face showing a fracture of body of mandible

- **Examiner**: See this picture and tell me the diagnosis.
- **Candidate**
  - *Imaging technique*: 3D CT reconstruction
  - *Part*: Head and face
  - *View*: Anteroposterior with face turned a little to left
  - *Findings*: The body of mandible completely fractured in the right canine region with very little displacement (Fig. 40.7)
  - *Diagnosis*: Fracture of right canine region of body of mandible

Viva Voce

Q1. What is the incidence of this fracture?
Answer: It is the second most common fracture of mandible after the fracture of condylar neck.

Q2. What is the cause of the fracture?
Answer: It is usually due to direct blow.

Q3. What are the clinical signs of this fracture?
Answer: The clinical signs are:

- There is local pain, tenderness, and step deformity of lower border of mandible.
- The dental alignment is disturbed and the saliva is blood-stained.
- Hematoma is present in the floor of mouth.
- The patient may not be able to close the mouth, resulting in drooling of saliva.

Q4. How will you confirm the diagnosis?
Answer: Orthopantomogram (OPG) is the investigation of choice for confirming the diagnosis.

A lateral oblique, lower occlusal, and PA radiograph of the mandible may give valuable information about the degree of displacement in fractures of body and ramus.

Q5. What is orthopantomogram?
Answer: It is plain radiography of mandible by a moving X-ray machine which radiographs the whole mandible straight from condyle to condyle.

Q6. How will you treat this patient?
Answer: The patient should be treated by open reduction and fixation by plating system of stainless steel or titanium.

Q7. Describe the technique in brief.
Answer: The fracture site is opened by extraoral or intraoral approach. To achieve a correct

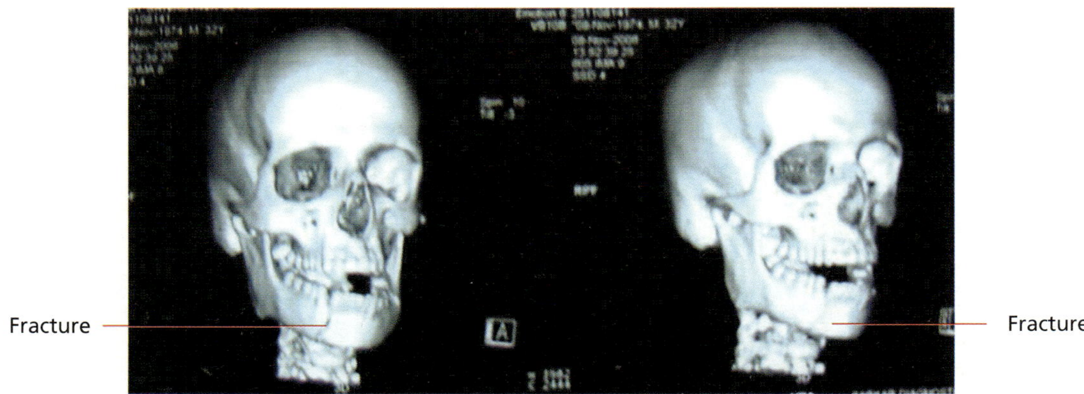

Figure 40.7 3D CT reconstruction of face showing a fracture of right canine region of body of mandible. (Courtesy: Professor Surajit Bhattacharya)

dental occlusion, intraoperative intermaxillary fixation (IMF) utilizing islet wires is done which is removed after the rigid plate fixation is done.

Q8. How will you treat a fracture of edentulous mandible?

Answer: This fracture may be treated by open reduction and miniplating with minimal periosteal mobilization.

Q9. Why is minimal periosteal mobilization done?

Answer: More periosteal mobilization may compromise mandibular blood supply.

Q10. Because of this risk, is there any alternative method of treatment?

Answer: The fracture may be immobilized by putting Gunning splints.

Q11. What is the technique of treatment using Gunning splints?

Answer: The Gunning splints consist of arc-like upper and lower dentures having hooks in place of teeth. These splints are wired to both the jaws—the lower one to the mandible by circummandibular wires and the upper to the maxilla to a stable point in the middle third. The fracture is reduced and the splints are fixed by wires. Finally the intermaxillary fixation is done on the hooks.

Q12. What are the results of treatment?

Answer: The overall results are good, both functional and cosmetic.

KEY POINTS

- The examiner is not a radiologist but a surgeon. Hence, only questions of clinical interest are asked.
- The plate or picture must be held and put on the view box in correct position.
- Note the abnormalities carefully and describe them systematically and conclude with a radiological diagnosis.
- Be ready to answer a few questions about the disease diagnosed after seeing the image.

Appendix

Blood—some important constituents

Constituent	Specimen	Conventional units	SI units
Albumin	Serum or plasma	3.4–4.7 g/dL	34–47 g/L
Bilirubin	Serum or plasma	• Total 0.1–1.2 mg/dL • Conjugated 0.1–0.5 mg/dL • Unconjugated 0.1–0.7 mg/dL	• 2–21 μmol/L • <8 μmol/L • <12 μmol/L
Blood urea nitrogen (BUN)	Serum or plasma	8–20 mg/dL	2.9–7.1 mmol/L
C-reactive protein	Serum or plasma	<0.8 mg/L	–
Calcitonin	Plasma or serum	• Male 0–11.5 pg/mL • Female 0–4.6 pg/mL	• Male 0–11.5 ng/L • Female 0–4.6 ng/L
Calcium	Serum or plasma	• 8.5–10.5 mg/dL • Panic <6.5 or >13.5 mg/dL	• 2.1–2.6 mmol/L • Panic <1.63 or >3.37 mmol/L
Calcium (ionized)	Serum or whole blood	• 4.6–5.3 mg/dL • Panic <3 or >6.2 mg/dL	• 1.15–1.32 mmol/L • Panic <0.75 or >1.55 mmol/L
Carbon dioxide, partial pressure (PCO_2)	Whole blood	32–48 mm Hg	4.26–6.38 kPa
Carbon dioxide total (bicarbonate)	Serum or plasma	• 22–32 mEq/L • Panic <15 or >40 mEq/L	• 22–32 mmol/L • Panic <15 or >40 mmol/L
Carboxyhemoglobin (HbCO)	Whole blood	<9% of total hemoglobin	<0.09 fraction of total hemoglobin
Chloride (Cl^-)	Serum or plasma	101–112 mEq/L	101–112 mmol/L
Cholesterol	Serum or plasma	• Desirable <200 mg/dL • Borderline 200–240 mg/dL • High risk >240 mg/dL	• Desirable <6.0 mmol/L • Borderline 6.0–7.2 mmol/L • High risk >7.2 mmol/L
Cortisol	Serum or plasma	8 AM: 5–20 μg/dL	140–550 nmol/L

(CONTD...)

(...CONTD)

Constituent	Specimen	Conventional units	SI units
Cortisol (urinary free)	Urine	10–110 μg/24 hours	27.6–303.6 nmol/24 hours
Creatinine	Serum or plasma	0.6–1.2 mg/dL	50–100 μmol/L
Eosinophil count	Whole blood	0.04–0.5 × 10^3 μL	0.04–0.5 × 10^9/L
Erythrocyte (RBC) count	Whole blood	4.7–6.1 × 10^6 μL	4.7–6.1 × 10^{12}/L
Erythrocyte sedimentation rate	Whole blood	• Male <10 mm/hour • Female <15 mm/hour	Same
Glucose	Serum or plasma	• 60–110 mg/dL • Panic <40 or >500 mg/dL	• 3.33– 6.11 mmol/L • Panic <2.22 or >27.75 mmol/L
Glycated (glycosylated) hemoglobin (HBA)	Whole blood	3.9–5.6%	–
Hemoglobin, total	Whole blood	• Male 13.6–17.5 g/dL • Female 12.0–15.5 g/dL • Panic ≤7 g/dL	• Male 136–175 g/L • Female 120–155 g/L • Panic ≤70 g/L
Iron	Serum or plasma	50–175 μg/dL	9–31 μmol/L
Lymphocyte count	Whole blood	0.8–3.5 × 10^3/μL	0.8–3.5 × 10^9/L
Magnesium	Serum or plasma	• 1.8–3.0 mg/L • Panic <0.5 or >4.5 mg/dL	• 0.75–1.25 mmol/L • Panic <0.2 or >1.85 mmol/L
Neutrophil count	Whole blood	2.2–8.6 × 10^3 μL	2.2–8.6 × 10^9/L
Osmolality	Serum or plasma	• 275–293 mOsm/kg H_2O • Panic <320 mOsm/kg H_2O	–
Oxygen, partial pressure (PO_2)	Whole blood	83–108 mm Hg	11.04–14.36 kPa
Parathyroid hormone (PTH)	Serum or plasma	Intact PTH 11–54 pg/mL	Intact PTH 1.2–5.7 pmol/L
pH	Whole blood	• Arterial 7.35–7.45 • Venous 7.31–7.41	–
Phosphorus	Serum or plasma	• 2.5–4.5 mg/dL • Panic <1.0 mg/dL	• 0.8–1.45 mmol/L • Panic <0.32 mmol/L
Platelet count	Whole blood	• 150–450 × 10^3/μL • Panic <25 × 10^3/μL	• 150–450 × 10^9/L • Panic <25 × 10^9/L
Potassium (K^+)	Serum or plasma	• 3.5–5.0 mEq/L • Panic <3.0 or >6.0 mEq/L	• 3.5–5.0 mmol/L • Panic <3.0 or >6.0 mmol/L
Protein total	Serum or plasma	6.0–8.0 g/dL	60–80 g/L
Prothrombin time (PT)	Plasma	• 11–15 seconds • Panic ≥30 seconds	–
Red blood cell count	Whole blood	• 4.7–6.1 × 10^6/μL (male) • 3.5–5.5 × 10^6/μL (female)	• 4.7– 6.1 × 10^{12}/L • 3.5–5.5 × 10^{12}/L
Sodium	Serum or plasma	• 135–145 mEq/L • Panic <125 or >155 mEq/L	• 135–145 mmol/L • Panic <125 or >155 mmol/L
Thyroglobulin	Serum or plasma	3–42 ng/mL	3–42 μg/L
Thyroid-stimulating hormone	Serum or plasma	0.4–4 microunits/mL	0.4–4 milliunits/L
Thyroxine, free (FT4)	Serum or plasma	0.7–1.86 ng/dL	9–24 pmol/L

(CONTD...)

(...CONTD)

Constituent	Specimen	Conventional units	SI units
Thyroxine (T4), total	Serum or plasma	5–11 μg/dL	64–142 nmol/L
Triiodothyronine (T3) total	Serum	95–190 ng/dL	1.5–2.9 nmol/L
Uric acid	Serum or plasma	• Male 2.4–7.4 mg/dL • Female 1.4–5.8 mg/dL	• Male 140–440 μmol/L • Female 80–350 μmol/L
White blood cell count	Whole blood	• 4.8–10.8 × 10^3/μL • Panic <1.5 × 10^3/μL	• 4.8–10.8 × 10^9/L • Panic <1.5 × 10^9/L

Normal urine

Features/constituents	Normal values
Color	Clear and amber or straw-colored
Specific gravity	1.010–1.025 (variable)
Reaction	Acidic, pH 6.0 (variable)
Acetone	Nil
Protein	<150 mg/day
Creatinine	1.0–1.6 g/day
17-Hydroxycorticosteroids	2–10 mg/day
Glucose or sugar	Nil
Calcium	<7.8 mmol/day
Potassium	25–100 mmol/day
Sodium	100–250 mEq/day
Bilirubin	Nil
Urobilinogen	1–3.5 mg/day

Normal stool

Features/constituents	Normal values
Color	Brown
Bulk	100–200 g
Water	75%
pH	7.0–7.5
Fat	<7 g/day
Blood, parasite, pus	Nil
Stercobilinogen	<7 g/day

Further reading

1. Bhat SM. SRB's Clinical Methods in Surgery, 1st ed. New Delhi: Jaypee Brothers Medical Publishers (P) Ltd; 2011 (reprinted).

2. Bhat SM. SRB's Manual of Surgery, 4th ed. New Delhi: Jaypee Brothers Medical Publishers (P) Ltd; 2013.
3. Brunicardi FC. Schwartz's Principles of Surgery, 9th ed. New York: McGraw Hill Medical; 2010.
4. Burnand KG, Young AE. The New Aird's Companion in Surgical Studies, 1st ed. Edinburgh: Churchill Livingstone; 1992.
5. Das S. A Manual on Clinical Surgery, 10th ed. Kolkata; 2013 (published by the author).
6. Doherty GM. Current Diagnosis & Treatment: Surgery, 13th ed. New York: McGraw Hill Medical; 2010.
7. Goel TC, Agarwal M, Goel A. Essential Clinical Surgery. New Delhi: Modern Publishers; 2004.
8. Goel TC, Goel A. Clinical Signs of Disease, 2nd ed. Lucknow: Aditya Medical Books Distributors; 1998.
9. Goel TC, Goel A. Practical Surgery—Short Clinical Cases, 3rd ed. New Delhi: Jaypee Brothers Medical Publishers; 2015.
10. Goel TC, Goel A. KGMU Aadhunik Shalya Chikitsa Vigyan. New Delhi: Jaypee Brothers Medical Publishers; 2015.
11. Goel TC, Goel A. KGMU A Method of Clinical Surgery, New Delhi: Ahuja Publishing House; 2016.
12. Henry MM, Thompson JN. Clinical Surgery, 2nd ed. Edinburgh: Elsevier Saunders; 2005.
13. Laskin DM. Oral & Maxillofacial Surgery, 1st ed. St. Louis: Mosby; 2003.
14. Maheshwari J. Essential Orthopaedics, 4th ed. New Delhi; 2013 (published by the author).
15. Maheshwari S, Kumar S. Textbook of ENT, 1st ed. Kala Amb, Himachal Pradesh: Arya Publications; 2003.
16. Malik NA. Textbook of Oral and Maxillofacial Surgery, 2nd ed. New Delhi: Jaypee Brothers Medical Publishers; 2008.
17. Papadakis MA, McPhee SJ. Current Medical Diagnosis and Treatment, 55th ed. New York: McGraw Hill Medical; 2016.
18. Shenoy KR. Manipal Manual of Surgery for Dental Students, 1st ed. New Delhi: CBS Publishers & Distributors; 2003.
19. Townsend CM, Beauchamp RD, Evers BM, Mattox KL. Sabiston Textbook of Surgery, 19th ed. Philadelphia: Elsevier Saunders; 2012.
20. Williams NS, Bulstrode CJK, O'Connell PR. Bailey & Love's Short Practice of Surgery, 26th ed. London: CRC Press; 2013.

Index

B

D

E

F

G

J

K

L

M

N

O

P

Q

R

S

T

U

V

W

X

Z